HOSPITAL FINANCIAL ACCOUNTING
Theory and Practice

Second Edition

L. Vann Seawell, DBA, CPA

Professor of Accounting
Indiana University

1987
Healthcare Financial Management Association
Chicago

KENDALL/HUNT PUBLISHING COMPANY
2460 Kerper Boulevard P.O. Box 539 Dubuque, Iowa 52004-0539

Acknowledgments

The editors are grateful to the following for permission to cite their works as noted in the footnotes.

American Institute of Certified Public Accountants
The Institute of Internal Auditors
Financial Accounting Standards Board
American Hospital Association
Financial Executives Institute
Healthcare Financial Management Association

Dedication

To JOY . . .

She lights up my life.

Contents

Preface to the Second Edition

Strong winds of change have swept across the healthcare industry over the last two decades. Today, the winds of change are increasing in force, with no indication of abatement in the near future. Major adjustments have been made in the organization, operation, and management of the healthcare system, and even more drastic changes are yet to come. Charge-based, cost-based, and per diem payment mechanisms are being discarded. It is likely that the prospective payment system based on diagnosis related groups (DRGs) soon will give way to an arrangement providing for payment on a capitation basis. Hospitals, facing increasing competition for patients, will find themselves in a price war. Much greater emphasis will be given to marketing and public relations. The number of hospital acquisitions and mergers will increase rapidly. Hospitals that are not cost efficient will be forced to close.

Now, more than ever before, there is a need for continued improvement in hospital accounting and financial management. Every effort should be made to upgrade the accounting process so that it produces relevant and reliable information for managerial decision-making purposes. Only through the intelligent utilization of accounting information can hospital managers hope to deal successfully with the new problems and issues that are certain to emerge in the next decade and beyond.

This book is yet another installment in the Healthcare Financial Management Association's long history of educational programs. It is designed primarily for use by students of hospital accounting and finance in courses of an intermediate character, but it also should be useful for general reference purposes to anyone interested in the accounting and financial practices of hospitals. Although major emphasis is given to accounting theory and procedure, an attempt has been made throughout this book to deal also with related financial management considerations.

I sincerely appreciate the favorable response to the first edition of this book. Many readers have offered suggestions for improvements, and I have incorporated many of those recommendations in this edition, while retaining most of the basic features of the previous edition. All questions, exercises, and problems have been updated and revised where necessary. A substantial number of new exercises and problems have been added. Major sections of text of each chapter have been revised in an attempt to improve clarity and to cover recent developments. Two new chapters appear in this edition: (1) Chapter 18, which deals with leases and pension plans, and (2) Chapter 21, which provides a detailed discussion of the statement of changes in financial position. The Glossary has been expanded to include many additional terms. As was the case with the first edition, an Instructor's Manual is available to those teachers who adopt this textbook for their courses.

I could not have written this book without the help of a large number of people. While I wish to acknowledge their valuable and generous assistance, I dare not try to list all of them by name here. I fear that I might inadvertently overlook some who should be recognized in this way. Yet, I must single out several individuals to whom I owe a special debt of gratitude for whatever there may be of value and importance in this writing. None of the people or organizations referred to here, however, have the slightest responsibility for any errors of commission or omission which may appear within these pages. Such responsibility is entirely mine.

I wish to list the names of Louis Block, Ray Everett, Sister Mary Gerald, Harold Hinderer, Henry Hottum, Herman Kohlman, Charlie Mehler, Ralph Miller, Bill Mueller, Bob Penn, Stan Pressler, Bob Schultze, Bob Shelton, John Stagl, and Jeff Steinert who shared their great knowledge of the hospital business with me over many years. They also gave me their friendship, encouragement, and fond memories which I shall always treasure.

A special note of appreciation is extended to Mike Doody, Ron Keener, and Ron Kovener whose kindness, patience, and understanding meant so much to me when I was traveling through troubled waters.

Finally, I particularly want to thank the people of the hospital industry to whom I feel an obligation that is beyond my ability to repay.

L. Vann Seawell
Professor of Accounting
Indiana University

Bloomington, Indiana
August, 1986

PART 1
Basic Concepts, Principles, and Procedures

1
Hospital Management and Accounting

The United States spends more of its gross national product (around 11 percent) on healthcare than any other nation in the world. Healthcare is easily the nation's second largest industry, after construction, with expenditures running at more than $400 billion per year and growing by almost 13 percent annually. Although the healthcare system in the United States has numerous strengths and is far superior to that of any other country, it is argued by some that many Americans do not receive the healthcare services they need while many others receive more healthcare services than necessary. Consequently, the healthcare business continues to be the target of greatly increased public attention, criticism, and controversy concerning its efficiency in managing the huge investment the American people are making in it.

This paradox, often headlined as the "healthcare crisis," is not a single problem, nor is it solvable simply through the expenditure of more money and manpower. Some of the factors involved include financial barriers, weaknesses in the organization of existing healthcare delivery systems, competitive pressures arising from changes in the demand for a variety of healthcare services, unsound financing methods, reimbursement limitations by third-party payers, and changes in medical technology requiring expensive equipment and highly skilled personnel. A satisfactory solution to the many problems involved in the provision of healthcare services has a number of elements, but one can be certain that major emphasis must be given to continued improvement in the efficiency with which healthcare resources are managed. It is to this requirement of more effective accounting and financial management that this book is addressed.

In this book, attention is focused on hospitals, the major component of the healthcare industry. Hospital services currently account for about 40 percent of the healthcare dollar. Today, the nation's 7,000 hospitals have an overall occupancy rate averaging around 67 percent for 1.4 million beds. Annual volume of service at present exceeds 9 million inpatient admissions with a 6.5 day average length of hospital stay and 64 million outpatient visits. Annual spending for patient care is more than $150 billion, compared to only $2 billion in 1946. Hospitals now employ some 4 million persons, compared to 830,000 in 1946, at a payroll cost of some $62 billion per year, which represents about 50 cents of each dollar of operating expenses. Assets per bed vary according to the type of hospital, but the figure averages to about $60,000, compared to $15,000 in 1960. Current per bed construction costs for a new community hospital are in excess of $70,000.

In this era of rapidly rising costs and changes in the socioeconomic environment in which hospitals must function, the financial problems of hospitals have become numerous, severe, and indescribably complex. Indeed, of the many types of modern enterprises, it is difficult to find one whose management offers a greater challenge than does today's hospital. The provision of hospital healthcare services at reasonable costs is an enormously difficult business that requires the fullest application possible of advanced accounting and financial management principles and techniques. Hospital administrators, financial officers, and other members of the hospital management team, in striving for maximum efficiency in the utilization of increasingly expensive and scarce resources, have long since discovered that a high order of accounting is an essential prerequisite to effective financial management. It is this necessary marriage of management with accounting that provides the theme of this book.

THE HOSPITAL CORPORATION

In the United States today, there are more than 7,000 hospitals. Some 5,900 of these are short-term, general hospitals widely referred to as community hospitals. Of these, about 1,700 are government-owned and 800 are proprietary (investor-owned) hospitals. The remaining 3,400 hospitals, 58 percent of the short-term, general hospitals and 48 percent of all hospitals, are voluntary, not-for-profit enterprises which account for more than 70 percent of patient admissions and nearly 80 percent of the total assets of community hospitals. Although long-term and specialized care institutions, government-controlled hospitals, and investor-owned hospitals make up a very important segment of the hospital population, emphasis in this book is on the voluntary, not-for-profit, community hospital. Yet, it should be understood that most of the discussion is relevant to all hospitals because, regardless of type of ownership, hospitals have many common problems with largely the same accounting and financial management solutions.

Definition and Formation

The legal concept of a corporation is that of an artificial person or legal entity created by or under the authority of an act of the legislature to accomplish some purpose which is authorized by the charter or governing statute. A corporation has identity as a legal person with many attributes of an individual; it can buy and sell, it can own real estate, and it can sue and be sued. Because the corporation is a legal entity separate and distinct from its governing board and employees, liability for acts of the corporation rests with the corporate entity and generally does not become the personal obligation of its governing board or management. The widening scope of liability that is being visited upon hospitals by the courts, however, should be recognized by those who are charged with responsibility for wise and prudent direction and control over hospital corporate affairs.

The hospital corporation comes into existence in several ways depending on the laws of the particular state of incorporation. In most states, corporations are formed by act of the legislative body or by administrative action in the office of the secretary of state. A corporate charter is obtained in which the powers to act and conduct business as a corporation are given to the hospital as set forth in its articles of incorporation. These powers are not to be confused with the hospital corporation's bylaws. Bylaws are the rules and regulations adopted by the incorporators or directors to regulate the hospital's internal affairs. The bylaws define the rights, powers, and duties of the hospital's governing board and its administrative officers within the general framework of the corporate charter.

Purpose and Objective

The hospital corporation is somewhat unique in that the purpose of its corporate existence may be described as that of rendering service to persons who are in need of medical attention and hospital care. This is the primary objective of all hospitals, including investor-owned hospital enterprises. The operations of hospitals of all types are directed to the saving of lives, the healing of the sick, and the alleviation of suffering. The investor-owned hospital corporation issues capital stock, seeks a satisfactory return on the stockholders' investment, and distributes profits to the investors. The voluntary not-for-profit hospital corporation, however, does not issue capital stock because, in the absence of profit sharing, there would be no severable value represented by capital stock certificates. Nevertheless, it should not be assumed that "not-for-profit" means that voluntary community hospitals cannot or should not earn a profit. It simply means that no part of the profits earned by such hospitals can inure to the benefit of any private individual. As explained at a later point, there are good reasons why voluntary not-for-profit hospitals should and must have a reasonable profit objective if they are to survive and meet their social objectives.

Tax Status

While the voluntary not-for-profit hospital generally is subject to payroll and certain other taxes, it is an "exempt" organization for purposes of the federal income tax on corporations. The exemption is provided in Section 501(c)3 of the Internal Revenue Code as follows:

> Corporations, and any community chest, fund, or foundation, organized and operated exclusively for religious, charitable, scientific, testing for public safety, literary, or educational purposes, or for the prevention of cruelty to children or animals, no part of the net earnings of which inures to the benefit of any private shareholder or individual, no substantial part of the activities of which is carrying on propaganda, or otherwise attempting to influence legislation, and which does not participate in, or intervene in (including the publishing or distributing of statements), any political campaign on behalf of any candidate for public office.

To qualify for this exemption, the hospital must be organized as a charitable, not-for-profit corporation whose purpose is caring for the sick. It must operate for the benefit of the indigent to the extent of its financial ability. It must not restrict the use of its facilities to any particular group of physicians or surgeons.

In order to maintain its tax exemption, the hospital must not engage in any of the prohibited transactions described in Section 503 of the Internal Revenue Code:

1. Lending money without adequate security or interest.
2. Paying compensation in excess of reasonable levels.
3. Making investments for more than adequate consideration.
4. Selling assets for less than adequate consideration.
5. Subverting in any manner substantial portions of its income or assets.

Thus, the hospital cannot engage in so-called self-dealing with disqualified persons such as board members, officers, employees, donors, and owners. Should a hospital enter into any of these transactions with such individuals, it may lose its tax exempt status. There also is an excise tax imposed on prohibited transactions.

Although the hospital may have an exemption letter from the Internal Revenue Service, it still may incur an income tax liability with respect to unrelated business income. Such income may be derived from an activity regularly carried on by the hospital but which is not substantially related to the exercise or performance of its charitable or other function constituting the basis for its exemption. Income from such activities is taxable at regular corporate income tax rates. Excluded from the definition of unrelated business income are income from hospital research activities, passive investment income in the form of interest, dividends, and rent, and gains on sales of assets.

The application of the above provisions of the federal income tax laws to a particular hospital situation is not always entirely clear. In addition, most states have registration and other requirements that must be met by not-for-profit organizations. It therefore is important that hospitals seek the advice of professional tax advisors on these matters.

Organization

The contemporary hospital utilizes different kinds of specialized resources and makes available on a virtually continuous basis an ever-expanding spectrum of services. These services are provided by personnel employed in a diversity of occupations ranging from housekeepers to medical research scientists. While providing these services, there must be a constant concern for economy. The only way that a hospital will achieve its service and financial objectives is by effectively organizing its physical and human resources. Only by dividing the work of the hospital into manageable units where authority is centralized and responsibility is fixed can efficiency be assured. Duties must be clearly defined and interrelationships among organizational units must be carefully structured so that all individuals and groups work in a coordinated and cooperative manner toward common goals.

A sound organizational structure is an essential requirement for effective management. While certain basic principles of organization are generally applicable to all enterprises, there is no single organization plan that can be regarded as the proper plan for all hospitals. No two hospitals are alike in all respects. What may be a suitable organizational structure for one may not be applicable to another because of differences in size, range of services, type of personnel, management philosophy, and other characteristics. A typical general pattern of organization, however, is indicated in Figure 1-1. More detailed organization charts are examined in Chapters 4 and 9.

Governing Board

Ultimate authority and responsibility for the proper and prudent management of the hospital's affairs rests with its governing board. The governing board of the voluntary not-for-profit hospital has a fiduciary obligation to the community at large to preserve the assets of the hospital and to direct the hospital business in a manner that ensures the continuity of hospital services. Membership on a hospital board involves a serious

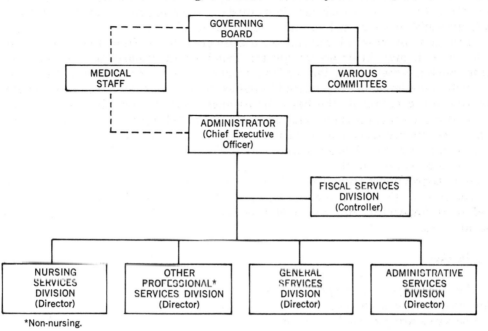

Figure 1-1.
General Organization of the Hospital

*Non-nursing.

moral and legal responsibility, and members should be chosen with great care and circumspection. In many cases the board has a broad membership drawn from various sections of the community, including different ethnic, religious, economic, and cultural groups.

The corporate laws of each state establish qualifications for membership on governing boards. The number of members usually is set within certain limits by statute. The bylaws of the hospital corporation define the duties of the board to include, through the chief executive officer or administrator, the control and use of the physical and financial resources of the hospital. The board must be active; it must direct the hospital's business in good faith and with reasonable care. Failure of the board to function has been held to constitute mismanagement, even though the board is not expected to personally manage the day-to-day operations of the hospital. This authority can and should be delegated to the chief executive officer who is held accountable to the board for compliance with the broad operating policies it establishes. The board, however, cannot rid itself of responsibility in this way.

Medical Staff

The importance of the medical staff in the hospital organization is obvious. Doctors who practice within the hospital usually are organized according to service and specialties. While the staff does not have direct authority in the management of the hospital, it does have a very significant influence on the hospital's operations, policies, and financial success. Therefore, it is essential that a cooperative working relationship be maintained between the medical staff and the hospital's financial managers.

Board Committees

To better fulfill its duties, the hospital governing board generally forms a number of standing committees from its membership. It may, for example, establish committees for finance, budgets, investments, buildings and grounds, professional affairs, and public relations. The chairman of the finance committee often serves as the hospital treasurer, having authority to negotiate bank loans and other financial arrangements. In many cases, the treasurer also has major responsibility for the safeguarding of cash and other hospital assets.

Chief Executive Officer (Administrator)

The chief executive officer (hospital administrator) is responsible to the governing board for implementing its policies relative to the control and effective utilization of the physical and financial resources of the hospital. Within the scope of authority delegated by the governing board, the chief executive officer is responsible for all aspects of providing facilities and personnel for the care and treatment of the hospital's patients. It is not possible, however, for the chief executive officer to exercise continuous and direct personal supervision over all hospital activities. The chief executive can and should delegate much of his (her) authority to a second level of management which is accountable for the effective planning and control of the various organizational units within the hospital.

As shown in Figure 1-1, the hospital is often organized into several broad divisions, each having a director responsible for its operations. For a more detailed organization chart, see Figure 4-11. Emphasis in this book is on the role of the director of fiscal services (sometimes referred to as the hospital controller). The authority for financial management of the hospital comes from the chief executive officer to whom the fiscal services executive is directly responsible. While the director of fiscal services has authority for the day-to-day management of financial operations, the chief executive officer (using various reports and control systems) must constantly ascertain that financial management responsibilities are being carried out in an effective manner.

Director of Fiscal Services (Controller)

In years past, the hospital controller was sometimes little more than a glorified bookkeeper and officer manager. Today, however, the controller, or director of fiscal services, is or should be the most critically important person in the financial management structure. If properly qualified, this manager should be the hospital's chief financial officer and should function at the policy-making level. Governing boards and chief executive officers should clearly recognize the imperative need for, and the value of, top quality financial management that can be developed and maintained through the employment of a first-rate financial manager.

The precise title and role of the fiscal services manager varies somewhat from one hospital to another, but the functions of a well-qualified and experienced hospital financial executive may be generally defined to include the following:[1]

A. **Planning**

Establishment, coordination, and administration, as an integral part of management, of an adequate plan for the control of operations. Such a plan, to the extent required in the hospital, would provide:

1. Long- and short-range financial planning.
2. Budgeting for capital expenditures and operations.
3. Revenue forecasting.
4. Performance evaluation.
5. Pricing policies.
6. Economic appraisal (continuous appraisal of economic and social forces and government influences and interpretation of their effects upon the hospital).
7. Analysis of acquisitions and divestments of operating segments.

B. **Provision of Capital**

Establishment and execution of programs for the provision of capital required by the hospital, including negotiating the procurement of capital and maintaining the required financial arrangements.

C. **Administration of Funds**

1. Management of cash, investments and pension funds.
2. Maintenance of banking arrangements.
3. Receipt, custody, and disbursement of the hospital's monies and securities.
4. Credit and collection management.
5. Custodial responsibilities.

D. **Accounting and Control**

1. Establishment of accounting policies.
2. Development and reporting of accounting data.
3. Cost finding and analysis. Cost standards.
4. Internal auditing.
5. Accounting systems and procedures.
6. Reporting to government agencies.
7. Reporting and interpretation of results of operations to management.
8. Comparison of performance with operating plans and standards.

E. **Protection of Assets**

1. Provision of insurance coverage as required.
2. Assure protection of hospital assets and loss prevention through internal control and internal auditing.
3. Real estate management.

F. **Tax Administration**

1. Establishment and administration of tax policies and procedures.
2. Relations with taxing agencies.
3. Preparation of tax reports.
4. Tax planning.

G. **Relations with External Groups**

Establishment and maintenance of communications with investors, creditors, third-party payers, government agencies, hospital associations, and the general public.

H. **Evaluation and Consulting**

Consultation with and advice to other hospital executives on hospital policies, operations and objectives, and the effectiveness thereof.

I.   Management Information Systems
Development and use of electronic data processing facilities, management information systems, and other systems and procedures.

The functions described constitute the total financial management task in hospitals. Depending upon the size of the hospital, its organizational structure, the capabilities of its management personnel, and other factors, these functions usually are divided among the chief executive officer, the director of fiscal services, and the treasurer in some logical and workable manner. A major share of financial responsibilities naturally is assigned to the director of fiscal services who, because of education and experience in accounting and finance, ordinarily is best equipped to deal with a majority of the functions described.

A simpler, more functionally oriented listing of the responsibilities of the financial executive is provided by Berman and Weeks as follows:[2]

1. Planning (budgeting) operations, for both the short and long run, in order to produce a comprehensive, coordinated approach to the achievement of the hospital's objective(s).
2. Recording and summarizing all of the financial transactions of the hospital in order to provide an accurate statement of financial condition and operating results.
3. Measuring and evaluating actual performance against meaningful standards in order to assist functional managers in controlling operations and accomplishing the operational plan.
4. Reporting the results of operations to various levels of management in order to link the planning, recording and measuring functions into an effective control process.
5. Advising the chief executive officer as to the total operational performance and the impact of external factors in order to both evaluate the current status of operations and establish policies for the future.

Thus, the hospital financial manager's role extends far beyond mere record-keeping; this executive also plans, measures and evaluates, reports, and advises. When these functions are performed well, the hospital financial manager makes an essential contribution to the achievement of hospital operational objectives.

The director of fiscal services generally requires a sizable staff in order to carry out the many important tasks and duties assigned to the fiscal services function. Figure 1-2 provides an organization chart that illustrates the manner in which the fiscal services division or controllership function may be organized in a hospital of medium size.

FINANCIAL MANAGEMENT

As noted, the basic purpose of the hospital enterprise is that of providing healthcare services of the quality and quantity required by the community it serves. The objective of hospital financial management is to plan and control the activities and

Figure 1-2.
Organization Chart
Fiscal Services Division

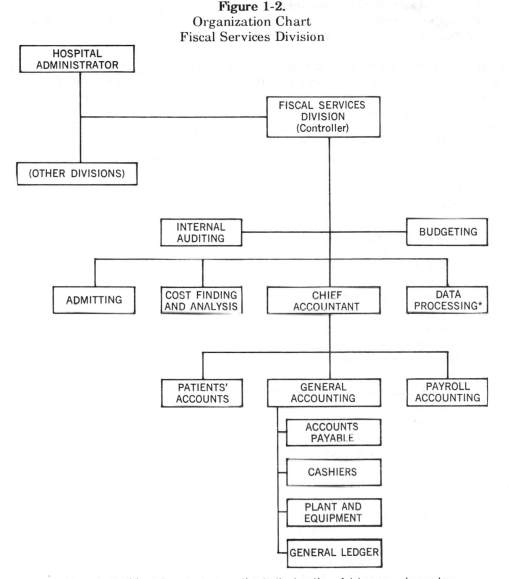

*Some authorities take extreme exception to the location of data processing under the controller and argue, with good reasons, that the function should be organized directly under the hospital administrator or one of his assistants.

affairs of the hospital so that its purpose is achieved at reasonable costs to the community. At the very least, this objective includes the long-run realization of revenues equal to costs, i.e., operating results no worse than the break-even level. This minimum financial performance must be attained because it is necessary to the continued existence of the hospital and, therefore, its continued ability to provide needed healthcare services. Due to current economic and social pressures, however, the management of operations on a break-even basis generally is not sufficient to ensure the perpetuation of the hospital as a viable enterprise. Unless these pressures are relieved, it is incumbent upon hospital managements to pursue financial objectives which result in the control and containment of costs at levels that will provide an excess of revenues over costs.

Whatever the hospital's financial objective may be, it is not realized by chance. Every hospital must develop with great care specific short-run financial programs consistent with sound long-range goals. Once these programs and goals are established, the management task becomes that of procuring the resources necessary to carry out such programs and directing the utilization of available resources so as to produce maximum returns at least costs to the community. The efficient and effective provision of healthcare services requires hospitals that are financially strong and viable, and this can be accomplished only through competent financial management. The quality of financial management planning and control decisions, however, is largely determined by the relevance and reliability of the information generated by the accounting process. In short, the realization of hospital objectives requires competent financial management which, in turn, requires a high order of accounting.

Financial Planning

Financial planning is the process of establishing programs for the achievement of fiscal objectives. It requires decisions as to what amounts of resources will be needed and how such resources can best be secured. It involves the establishment of specific financial objectives and policies through which the overall operating plan becomes an actual achievement. It requires the coordination of all functional units or departments within the organizational structure of the hospital. A hospital building, disarranged equipment, an unorganized complement of personnel, an uncontrolled fund of money, and an unattended pile of supplies will not provide hospital services. Decisions must be made as to what kinds of services will be provided, what functions will be performed by various hospital personnel, and how these services and functions will be financed. These and other operating plans and decisions must be made if the resources of the hospital are to be employed most effectively in the provision of quality care at acceptable costs.

A knowledge and understanding of historical and projected accounting data is the basis upon which sound financial management planning should be established. Without accounting and statistical information and the ability to evaluate and utilize it properly, management plans would be little more than the results of mere hunches, personal whims, and pure guesswork. The critical social role of the hospital obviously deserves a more scientific approach. This does not imply that accounting and statistical information can replace sound management judgment, but that management's judgment can be improved and its administration made more effective by employing the information derived from adequate accounting records. Many decisions are, and should be, influenced by considerations other than those of a purely monetary character.

Financial Control

Financial control is the process by which hospital management secures conformity of the operating results of organizational units with plans and policies so that the hospital's objectives are achieved. Effective control of financial activity and resources requires realistic planning, communication of plans to members of the hospital organization responsible for operating results of their divisions, and the employment of techniques which periodically indicate to management whether or not its plans are being carried out and its objectives are being achieved within the framework of established financial policies. A major feature of financial control is the determination of optimum operating results and financial position (resource allocation and sources of financing) and the direction of activities to the attainment of those goals.

Periodic accounting and statistical reports can reflect how closely the organizational units of the hospital adhere to financial plans and objectives. Accounting techniques such as budgeting, internal control, cost accounting or cost finding, and financial analysis are available as a means of evaluating the performance of the organization and providing assurance that operations conform to established plans and policies. Accounting and statistics do not in themselves control anything; control is achieved only through the actions of people. Accounting and statistical data, however, are essential to managerial control in that such data, when properly reported and evaluated, will point out whether or not and in what areas the organization has departed from established objectives. Such data also serve as the basis for control decisions and for evaluations of the results of those decisions.

HOSPITALS AND COMMERCIAL ENTERPRISES

The basic principles of accounting and financial management are much the same for hospitals as for profit-seeking commercial businesses. In fact, one rather noticeable development over the last 25 years has been the increasing rate at which hospitals have adopted and applied the business methods, accounting procedures, and management techniques of their commercial cousins. This desirable and even necessary trend continues unabated, and the quality of accounting and management practices in many hospitals today is superior to that found in many business ventures. There are, however, certain constraints upon the extent to which "business" methods can be applied to hospital accounting and management. Hospitals are somewhat different from ordinary commercial businesses. Certain unique characteristics of hospitals give rise to problems and responsibilities not found in other types of enterprises. Of course, hospitals and commercial firms have many similar problems, but solutions to some of these common problems often differ in significant ways because certain options open to the private businessman are not available to the hospital executive.

Commercial businesses are formed and operated to produce a profit. They are owned by individuals, either as sole proprietors, partners, or a group of corporate stockholders. For each type of ownership, emphasis is placed on profitable operations, i.e., a satisfactory return on the owners' investments. The primary standard of success is the amount of net income in relation to the capital invested in the enterprise.

Profit-seeking in itself should not be considered wrong or obscene. On the contrary, it is the profit motive and the efforts of business firms to optimize profits that have made possible the unsurpassed standard of living enjoyed by a large majority of the American people; it is no higher anywhere else in the world. While there are short-run inconsistencies, the business which serves the consumer best reaps the largest profits in the long run. Such profits are just rewards for risk-taking and for providing, in an efficient manner, the products and services desired by the public.

On the other hand, hospitals are usually operated as not-for-profit organizations. They exist to care for the sick. They provide care, insofar as they are financially able to do so, for those unable to pay. They do not restrict the use of facilities to some doctors to the exclusion of all other qualified doctors, nor do they permit any of their earnings to inure to the benefit of private shareholders or individuals. Hospitals usually are exempt from many of the taxes assessed on commercial businesses. In this context, the not-for-profit philosophy has a rightful place. The standard of success is the extent to which the hospital can serve the needs of the community and nation while maintaining the quality of its services within certain parameters of cost.

Hospital managements recognize that there is no excuse for careless accounting and management simply because the hospital is operated on a not-for-profit basis and is not a business in the full commercial sense of the word. While the dollar cannot be placed above human life and health, it nevertheless must be considered even by the not-for-profit hospital. The hospital of today must be aware not only of its public service goal but also of its financial responsibilities to the community. A financially distressed hospital cannot provide efficient health care services; a bankrupt hospital renders none.

A hospital is a "business" in that many principles of sound business management are just as applicable to it as they are to a large manufacturing corporation. As a matter of fact, it can be argued that efficient operation is more important to a hospital than to a commercial enterprise. The hospital should periodically ascertain whether it is using to the fullest extent the methods of personnel management, public relations, expenditure control, and other managerial techniques which commercial business firms have found to be useful.

While the equity investment in a commercial business usually comes from a single source, hospitals have been financed through public subscription, governmental assistance, third-party reimbursement, and other sources. Funds received from certain sources are often earmarked for specific purposes by donors. As a result, hospital managements have a responsibility to account to such donors and to the general public for the disposition of those funds. The maintenance of adequate accounting procedures is essential to the discharge of this responsibility to external groups and also for internal administrative purposes. For this reason, the American Hospital Association and other authorities have long recommended that hospitals follow the principles of **fund accounting**, a practice not normally found in commercial ventures. Thus, there is a greater emphasis upon accountability in hospitals than in other types of enterprises.

Commercial organizations formed to produce a profit must adopt policies and employ tactics designed to achieve that objective. Salespeople sell to customers who are selected on the basis of their ability to pay the established prices for products and services. Price negotiations, if any, are conducted with customers on an individual basis. Hospitals, however, do not deny care to those who need it, regardless of their ability to pay. The prices hospitals receive for their services generally are established by a relatively few third-party payers who represent large groups of patients and possess great economic power.

Hospitals operate the workshop in which doctors care for their patients. The hospitals must provide the facilities and services which permit patients to receive the best care at a reasonable cost. The quality and variety of facilities and services offered by the hospital will determine to an extent the quality of care that can be provided by its medical staff. This factor in turn affects the number and type of patients which the hospital is able to accommodate.

Hospitals, in contrast to commercial businesses, have made a practice of rendering a certain amount of services without charge, or at nominal prices. Indigent patients are charged only what they can afford to pay. Reimbursement for the care of indigent patients may be received from social and governmental agencies, but the reimbursements typically are less than the real economic cost of providing such care. While a majority of hospital patients have some form of hospital insurance, reimbursement arrangements with the third-party sponsors of these patients usually fail to generate revenues equal to full economic costs. No single financial matter is more important to the survival of the healthcare industry than the relationship between hospital costs and the revenues generated from third-party reimbursement contracts.

The increase in the purchase of hospital services by government and other contracting agencies, however, has been a significant catalyst for the development of better accounting and management practices in hospitals. Every hospital must be able to determine and control its costs, and to justify the prices charged for its services. This is essential because only those hospitals which are the most efficiently managed will survive.

The accounting systems of many commercial businesses are relatively simple because they deal in relatively few products and services. The hospital, however, provides hundreds of different healthcare services. While primarily service institutions, hospitals also are engaged in manufacturing, processing, and merchandising activities involving products such as pharmaceuticals, medical and surgical supplies, and foodstuffs. The revenues and expenditures related to these products and services generally are more difficult to account for and control than in the commercial business. All in all, the complexity of hospital operations usually is not found in any other type of enterprise.

PROFESSIONAL ORGANIZATIONS

Any established field of worthwhile endeavor eventually will organize itself and develop national professional associations or societies. The hospital accounting and financial management field is particularly fortunate in having several such organizations which have made, and continue to make, significant contributions in the areas of education, research, public relations, professional development, and practical management assistance. These associations include such organizations as the Healthcare Financial Management Association (HFMA) and the American Hospital Association (AHA). There are many other organizations, of course, that have made important contributions to the improvement of hospital accounting and financial management. It is impossible, however, to list all of them. Some of the leading professional accounting organizations are identified in the next chapter.

CHAPTER 1 FOOTNOTES

1. Adapted from "Responsibilities of Financial Executive," **FEI Bulletin** (January, 1970), p. 6.
2. Howard J. Berman and Lewis E. Weeks, **The Financial Management of Hospitals** (Ann Arbor, Michigan: Health Administration Press, School of Public Health, The University of Michigan, 1974), pp. 36-37.

QUESTIONS

1. It has been said that healthcare is big business. What statistics can you provide in support of this contention?
2. Describe the structure and composition of the hospital industry in terms of types and numbers of hospitals.
3. What is the legal concept of the hospital corporation? How do hospital corporations come into existence, i.e., how are they formed?
4. Discuss the purpose and objective of the hospital corporation. Should all hospitals have a profit objective?
5. Certain hospitals are exempt from the federal income tax on corporations. What is the basis for this exemption in the Internal Revenue Code? What are the prohibited transactions in which a hospital must not engage in order to maintain its tax exemption?
6. Why is a sound organizational structure an essential requirement for effective hospital management? What basic principles of organization should be observed in establishing an organization plan for a hospital?
7. Describe the function of the hospital governing board. What is the legal liability of the governing board for appropriate management of resources?
8. What is the function and responsibility of the administrator of a hospital? What is the administrator's relationship to the governing board, medical staff, and controller or chief fiscal officer?
9. List the major functions of the hospital controller or chief financial executive.
10. Define **hospital financial management.** Why is a high order of financial management required in today's hospitals?
11. What is your understanding of the terms **financial planning** and **financial control**?
12. Compare and contrast hospital enterprises with commercial business corporations. What are the major differences in objectives, organization, revenue and capital sources, and customer relations?
13. Name some of the leading professional organizations in the areas of hospital accounting and finance. Briefly describe some of the activities of these organizations.
14. Freitag and Hirsch, writing in an issue of **World** (a publication of Peat, Marwick, Mitchell & Co.), state: "Basic principles of sound business and fiscal management apply to hospitals as they do to any other institution." Do you agree? Explain.
15. Define the responsibilities of the hospital controller. Draw an organizational chart for a medium-sized hospital including some of the major departments within each division of the hospital.
16. A department head would usually be operating in a line capacity but at other times he or she may be operating in a staff capacity. Explain the concepts of **line** and **staff** relationships, and give an example of each in a hospital organization. Is the hospital controller in a line and/or staff relationship? Why?
17. Hospitals vary greatly in their functions and scope of operations. However, there are certain basic functions toward which the efforts of the hospital accountant must be directed. Name these functions.
18. What should be the qualifications for the chief accounting and financial officer of a hospital?

19.   Complete the following five statements:
   1. In the field of management, authorities differ as to the number of the functions of management. If one were to select two functions which could be regarded as encompassing all the functions, these two functions would be _____ and _____.
   2. The management concept which recognizes that there is a definite limit to the number of persons that one person can supervise effectively is known as _____.
   3. The process of assigning supervisory duties to others and thus creating areas of responsibility is known as _____.
   4. The management philosophy which dictates that management's attention should be directed only to those areas where problems exist is known as **management by** _____.
   5. A written statement which sets forth the broad outline or scope within which an activity is conducted is known as _____.

20.   "The most important purpose of financial and statistical data is for the use of managements in planning and controlling the affairs of their hospitals." Do you agree? Discuss.

21.   "The stewardship responsibility of the hospital's governing board does not require it to protect and preserve all capital entrusted to its care." Do you agree? Discuss.

22.   "The not-for-profit hospital has a responsibility to disclose to the public evidence that all its funds are being effectively retained, expanded, or utilized for the sole benefit of its patients." Do you agree? Explain.

23.   You have been employed as the controller for ABC Hospital, and the administrator has told you that you are to be the ambassador of good public relations for the hospital. How would you go about fulfilling this responsibility?

24.   It has been suggested that, due to high hospital costs, a governmental public service commission should regulate hospital charges. List at least four factors that distinguish hospitals from other industries regulated by public service commissions.

25.   The American Hospital Association's "Statement on the Financial Requirements of Health Care Institutions and Services" sets forth guidelines for a program to overcome the financial shortcomings that have plagued healthcare institutions. This statement has several major aims. List some of them.

26.   List the major advantages and disadvantages of having each of the following departments under the direction of the hospital's chief fiscal officer:
   1. Admitting
   2. Purchasing
   3. Data processing

2
Generally Accepted Accounting Principles

Accounting may be described as the accumulation and communication, in conformity with generally accepted principles, of historical and projected economic data relating to the financial position and operating results of an enterprise. It is a service activity whose major function is the provision of quantitative information for use in economic decision-making by groups internal and external to the enterprise. Without this information, intelligent decisions could not be made by managers, by providers of funds, or by creditors, and chaotic conditions would prevail in all sectors of our socioeconomic environment.

It is therefore imperative that there be some reasonably uniform and generally accepted body of concepts and principles underlying the accumulation and communication processes of accounting. Only through the application of commonly observed rules and standards can the myriad and complex affairs of economic entities be recorded and reported in a meaningful and useful manner. Otherwise, the adequacy and reliability of the information generated by the accounting process would be open to question. There must be a consensus among accountants as to generally accepted accounting principles if the end product of accounting is to be understandable and useful to decision-makers.

These observations apply to accounting in all types of organizations, whether profit-seeking or not, that are engaged in economic activity. They seem particularly relevant to hospitals and other organizations in the healthcare industry. In the last two decades, with the tremendous socioeconomic revolution in healthcare and its effects on the future of the industry, the need for continued improvements in hospital accounting and thereby in the quality of the financial information it produces has been greatly magnified.

Today's hospitals are beset with numerous problems, some of which are directly or indirectly attributable to inadequate accounting for financial management and the unfortunate decisions that are based on it. Hospital accountants and financial managers have been occupied with an inferno of governmental regulations, reimbursement contract requirements, rate review and planning agency constraints, and rising costs. Problems are also traceable to the inability or unwillingness of decision-makers to understand and intelligently utilize financial accounting information. Resources have been heavily and necessarily invested in putting out symptomatic fires of the moment while giving insufficient attention to certain of the root causes of these conflagrations.

It is essential that continuing improvements be made in hospital accounting and in the use of the financial information it provides. Better accounting — understandable and reliable accounting in which users have confidence as a sound basis for planning and control — begins with the general acceptance of a body of basic concepts and principles as a theoretical foundation from which more specific and detailed accounting procedures and practices can be derived. Only in this way will the financial information generated by the accounting process become more understandable, useful, and defensible, thereby leading to a more intensive and extensive utilization of such information in the successful management of healthcare organizations.

The purpose of this chapter is to provide a summary of some of the more important basic concepts and principles upon which the accumulation and communication of financial accounting information should be based, given the current stage of development in accounting theory and practice. Subsequent chapters present the more numerous but less permanent specific and detailed principles that appear to be generally accepted at present.

From 1959 to 1973, the Accounting Principles Board (APB) had the responsibility for development of generally accepted accounting principles. While considerable progress was made, the APB was disbanded in 1973 when the Financial Accounting Standards Board (FASB) was created to assume the accounting rule-making function in the United States. Much of the discussion in this chapter is adapted from certain pronouncements of the APB and FASB. In particular, the chapter materials are drawn from APB Statement No. 4 and the Statements of Financial Accounting Concepts (SFACs) which arose from the FASB's conceptual framework project:

SFAC No. 1 – Objectives of Financial Reporting by Business Enterprises (1978)
SFAC No. 2 – Qualitative Characteristics of Accounting Information (1980)
SFAC No. 3 – Elements of Financial Statement of Business Enterprises (1980)
SFAC No. 4 – Objectives of Financial Reporting by Nonbusiness Organizations (1980)

The reader who is concerned with the details of these documents is urged to read them in their official form. They set forth the most authoritative and complete delineation of basic accounting concepts and principles that is currently available.

NATURE OF ACCOUNTING PRINCIPLES

Unlike the natural laws of the physical sciences, the basic concepts and principles of accounting – sometimes called rules, postulates, conventions, or standards – result from a continuing evolutionary process. They are subject to periodic reevaluation and possible change in one degree or another. Some of them are modified or even discarded in response to changes in economic and social conditions, technology, methods of conducting economic activity, and demands of users for more serviceable information. This absence of absolute permanency, however, should not be regarded as entirely undesirable. Accounting is not a science but an art. As such, it must change as its environment and the informational needs of its users change.

The basic concepts and principles of accounting have never been, and probably never will be, fully formulated and completely codified. Enough has been accomplished, however, to provide a substantial framework of fundamental concepts and broad principles within which it has been possible to obtain a consensus on many of the more elusive and detailed principles. It is with this basic framework that this chapter is primarily concerned.

The importance of narrowing or eliminating areas of divergent accounting practices as a means of improving the usefulness of financial information is widely recognized. Major efforts have been made by various organizations and individuals to identify the basic concepts of accounting and to promulgate generally accepted accounting principles.

It is not feasible to attempt here to list the many contributors in this area. The development of generally accepted accounting principles is an unfinished task, and it is likely to remain so, although there are many rather vocal critics who are dissatisfied with the rate of progress to date.

Prior to 1973, the most vigorous and authoritative efforts to establish generally accepted accounting principles were those of the American Institute of Certified Public Accountants through its Committee on Accounting Procedure and its Accounting Principles Board. The Committee (1938-59) issued a series of **Accounting Research Bulletins,** and the APB (1959-73) produced 31 **Opinions** and several other documents. Many of these pronouncements are still in effect, while others have been amended or replaced by **Statements of Financial Accounting Standards (SFAS)** and **Statements of Financial Accounting Concepts (SFAC)** issued since 1973 by the Financial Accounting Standards Board.

Although all of these rule-making bodies have directed their pronouncements largely to profit-seeking business enterprises, the applicability of the financial accounting and reporting standards contained in them generally have been extended to not-for-profit organizations, including hospitals, except where the standards are clearly inapplicable. The **Hospital Audit Guide,** for example, states the following:[1]

> Since financial statements of hospital present financial position, changes in financial position, and results of operations, and are increasingly being used by credit grantors, government agencies, and the community, the Committee on Healthcare Institutions unanimously concludes that they should be prepared in accordance with generally accepted accounting principles.

Accordingly, the general-purpose financial statements of hospitals should be prepared in conformity with the accounting and reporting principles formulated by the AICPA and FASB. The American Hospital Association (AHA) and the Healthcare Financial Management Association (HFMA), through its Principles and Practices Board (P&PB), have in most instances supported the applicability of GAAPs to hospital financial reporting.

At any rate, the position taken in this book is that the basic concepts and broad principles of accounting for enterprises in the profit sector of the economy are, with only slight modification, equally applicable to enterprises in the not-for-profit area. The remainder of this chapter, with the materials drawn from APB Statement No. 4 and the FASB Statements of Financial Accounting Concepts, should demonstrate the universality of the concepts and principles enumerated in those documents, although it is recognized that certain specific and detailed principles may be required for hospital enterprises due to the peculiar characteristics of the industry.

The reader is cautioned, however, that no one textbook (including this book) is to be regarded as authoritative in itself. The consensus of a number of writers, in fact, is only indicative of what may or may not be generally accepted accounting principles.

BASIC FINANCIAL STATEMENTS

Any discussion of basic accounting concepts and principles should begin with a consideration of the end product of accounting, i.e., financial statements. They are the means by which the information accumulated in the accounting process is periodically communicated to those who use it in making economic decisions. These statements are of two major types: (1) statements of financial position and (2) statements of changes in financial position. For purposes of discussion, the latter type is divided into (1) income statements and (2) other statements of changes in financial position.

Statement of Financial Position

Statements of financial position, commonly known as balance sheets, present an indication in conformity with generally accepted accounting principles of the financial status of an enterprise in terms of its resources, obligations, and residual ownership equity at given points in time. A balance sheet may be regarded as a snapshot (photograph) of a resource-and-obligation situation existing at a particular moment in the economic life of an enterprise.

Figure 2-1 presents a balance sheet in a greatly condensed and simplified form. As can be seen, the basic elements of financial position are assets (resources), liabilities (obligations), and owners' equity.

Figure 2-1.
A Hospital Enterprise
Balance Sheet
December 31, 1987

Assets	$\underline{\underline{\$500}}$
Liabilities	$100
Owners' Equity	$\underline{\ \ 400}$
Total Liabilities and Owners' Equity	$\underline{\underline{\$500}}$

Assets. The FASB has defined assets as "probable future economic benefits obtained or controlled by a particular entity as a result of past transactions."[2]   More simply stated assets are the economic resources of an enterprise that are recognized and measured in conformity with generally accepted accounting principles. Were the assets in Figure 2-1 specified in detail, one would find individual categories of assets such as cash, receivables, inventories, land, buildings, and equipment. As discussed later, the assets of not-for-profit hospitals usually are also segregated and classified in groups in accordance with the principles of fund accounting.

It should be noted, however, that a balance sheet does not ordinarily present as assets all of the resources of an enterprise. Good public relations and employee morale, for example, are valuable resources, but they are not formally recognized and measured as assets for balance sheet purposes. On the other hand, balance sheets occasionally may include relatively insignificant items (certain deferred charges, for instance) as assets that technically may not be economic resources.

Generally accepted accounting principles provide criteria which govern the selection of certain resources, and not others, to be recognized and measured as assets in balance sheets. The essential characteristic of all assets is the capacity to provide services or benefits that eventually result in net cash inflows to the enterprise. These probable future benefits are owned or controlled by the enterprise, and they must arise from transactions or events that have already occurred. Another criterion is objective quantification. Accounting does not deal directly at present with subjective psychological and social concepts or attitudes. Resources are not formally recognized unless they can be objectively measured in terms of money and with a reasonable degree of certainty.

Liabilities. The FASB has defined liabilities as "probable future sacrifices of economic benefits arising from present obligations of a particular entity to transfer assets or provide services to other entities in the future as a result of past transactions or events."[3] More simply stated, liabilities are the economic obligations of an enterprise that are recognized and measured in conformity with generally accepted accounting principles. Were the liabilities in Figure 2-1 specified in detail, one would find individual categories of liabilities such as accounts payable, notes payable, salaries and wages payable, mortgages payable, and bonds payable. As is true of assets, liabilities also may be classified by funds.

Under the criteria provided by current generally accepted accounting principles, certain social and nonlegal obligations of the enterprise are excluded from its balance sheet. On the other hand, certain items may be included among the liabilities although such items technically are not economic obligations in the sense that their liquidation will require the release of assets or services in the future. As the socioeconomic environment changes and the informational needs of users change, the principles that govern the selection and measurement of enterprise obligations, and resources, also may change.

Owners' Equity. In a profit-seeking business enterprise, the owners' equity is the residual interest in the assets of the enterprise that remains after deducting its liabilities. The owners' equity is the sum of the owners' investment and enterprise profits minus the amount of investment and profits withdrawn from the enterprise.

The nature of the owners' equity in a not-for-profit hospital enterprise is less easily defined. It is the residual ownership interest in hospital assets; it is the excess of hospital assets over hospital liabilities. But who are the owners of the hospital? The residual ownership interest in a not-for-profit hospital enterprise theoretically resides with the community it serves and with sponsoring organizations, if any, such as a church or university. Legally, however, the rights and duties incident to ownership usually are invested in the governing body, i.e., the board of directors or trustees.

The concept of owners' equity in a not-for-profit hospital is complicated by another factor. Such hospitals typically receive resources whose use and disposition is subject to legal restrictions and against which the general creditors of the hospital may have no claim. In effect, the owners' equity consists of several different residual interests in several different groups of assets, depending upon restrictions imposed by resource donors and other external parties. Hospitals deal with this problem through the vehicle of **fund accounting.** Thus, the owners' equity in not-for-profit hospital enterprises generally is fragmented into a number of **fund balances.** Each fund balance is the difference between the assets and liabilities related to each particular fund. There is an owners' equity element in each fund maintained by the hospital.

Relationship Among Elements. The relationship among the three elements of financial position may be expressed as follows:

$$\text{ASSETS} = \text{LIABILITIES} + \text{OWNERS' EQUITY}$$

This immutable mathematical expression is usually referred to as the accounting equation or model. It is a statement of the equality between the total assets and the total of claims against assets. This equality is maintained throughout the accounting process and it is the basic formula for the balance sheet. A useful variation of the equation is:

$$\text{ASSETS} - \text{LIABILITIES} = \text{OWNERS' EQUITY}$$

In other words, the total of enterprise assets minus the claims of creditors against such assets equals the residual ownership interest in the enterprise.

Income Statements

Income statements present an indication, in conformity with generally accepted accounting principles and in terms of revenues and expenses, of the results of an enterprise's financial operations and activities during a given period of time. These statements are also known as statements of revenues and expenses, or operating statements. Unlike the snapshot picture provided by the balance sheet, the income statement is analogous to a moving picture in that it presents certain changes in financial position that have occurred over a period of time. The basic elements of operating results as shown in an income statement are: (1) revenues, (2) expenses, and (3) net income (or net loss). Figure 2-2 is an illustration of an income statement in a highly condensed and simplified form.

Figure 2-2.
A Hospital Enterprise
Income Statement
Year Ended December 31, 1987

Revenues	$950
Less Expenses	930
Net Income	$ 20

Revenues. The FASB has defined revenues as "inflows or other enhancements of assets of an entity or settlements of its liabilities (or a combination of both) during a period from delivering or producing goods, rendering services, or other activities that constitute the entity's ongoing major or central operations."[4] More simply stated, revenues are gross increases in assets or gross decreases in liabilities, recognized and measured in conformity with generally accepted accounting principles, that result from economic activities of an enterprise that can change the owners' equity. Were the revenues in Figure 2-2 presented in detail, one would find various classifications of revenues. A number of items would be designated as patient service or operating revenues, e.g., revenue derived from room and meal services, laboratory, x-ray, pharmacy, and the like. Another category of revenues would include such items as unrestricted gifts, certain investment income, and other nonoperating revenues.

It should be noted that while many increases in assets and decreases in liabilities are recognized in accounting, not all such changes represent or result in revenue. An increase in cash resulting from a bank loan, for example, is not revenue. Nor is a decrease in a liability resulting from the repayment of such loans to be treated as revenue. It may be helpful to think of revenue as resulting from increases in assets not accompanied by equal increases in liabilities or by equal decreases in other assets.

The term **revenue**, as normally used in accounting, is a **gross** concept while the terms **income** and **gain** usually are used in a **net** sense. The FASB has defined gains as "increases in equity (net assets) from peripheral or incidental transactions of an entity and from all other transactions and other events and circumstances affecting the entity during a period except those that result from revenues or investments by owners."[5]

Use of the term **revenue** is centered largely on the rendering of services to patients or to other activities in the mainstream of a hospital's primary purpose. Values derived from other sources generally are termed **income** or **gains**, and by their nature often require separate classification in income statements. These and other complications involved in accounting for revenues are discussed later.

Expenses. The FASB has defined expenses as "outflows or other using up of assets or incurrences of liabilities (or a combination of both) during a period from delivering or producing goods, rendering services, or carrying out other activities that constitute the entity's ongoing major or central operations."[6] More simply stated, expenses are gross decreases in assets or gross increases in liabilities, recognized and measured in conformity with generally accepted accounting principles, that result from the economic activities of an enterprise that can change owners' equity. Were the expenses in Figure 2-2 detailed, one would find classifications such as salaries and wages, supplies, utilities, and depreciation. Expenses, like revenues, are also classified by hospital department or function, e.g., dietary expense or laboratory expense. Still other expense classifications may be used. In an analysis of expenses, it is customary to classify them as fixed or variable, direct or indirect, and so on.

It should be noted that while many decreases in assets and increases in liabilities are recognized in accounting, not all of them result in expenses. The decrease in cash involved in the repayment of a bank loan, for instance, is not an expense. Nor is the incurrence of a liability for the purchase of an item of equipment to be treated as an expense. In general, an expense may be regarded as a decrease in assets not accompanied by an equal decrease in liabilities or by an equal increase in other assets.

The term **expense**, as normally used in accounting, is a **gross** concept whereas the term **loss** is used in a **net** sense. Like "gains," particular "losses" arising from certain individual transactions often are isolated and reported separately in income statements. The FASB has defined losses as "decreases in equity (net assets) from peripheral or incidental transaction of an entity and from all other transactions and other events and circumstances affecting the entity during a period except those that result from expenses or distributions to owners."[7]

Net Income (Net Loss). Net income is the excess of revenues over expenses, as those elements are recognized and measured in conformity with generally accepted accounting principles, during a given period of time. Net loss is the operating result in periods when expenses exceed revenues. The FASB has not defined the term **earnings**, but has provided a definition of **comprehensive income**, as follows:[8]

Comprehensive income is the change in equity (net assets) of an entity during a period from transactions and other events and circumstances from nonowner sources. It includes all changes in equity during a period except those resulting from investments by owners and distributions to owners.

The relationship among the elements of the income statement is expressed in the following equation:

$$\text{REVENUES} - \text{EXPENSES} = \text{NET INCOME (NET LOSS)}$$

Revenues increase and expenses decrease owners' equity. Net income, then, is the **net** increase in owners' equity resulting from the economic activities of the enterprise during a given period of time.

The determination of net income also includes gains and losses (not to be confused with net loss) from the occasional disposition of assets in transactions more or less incidental to the mainstream of economic activity. These gains and losses result from the matching of revenues and expenses directly identifiable with individual transactions. (No attempt is made in financial accounting, however, to match the mainstream of revenues and expenses on an individual transaction basis.)

Other Statements of Changes in Financial Position

The income statement is but one of the several statements which depict changes in financial position. It presents the changes in assets and in liabilities that represent revenues and expenses during a given time period. The resultant net income (net loss) increases (decreases) the owners' equity, but this does not necessarily account for the total change in the amount of owners' equity during a given time period.

Due to the fact that not all changes in assets, liabilities, and owners' equity are recognized in the income statement, other financial statements are needed to fully disclose all changes in financial position in a given period of time. Two of these statements are described below.

Statement of Changes in Owners' Equity. Income statements, as just noted, present only the changes in owners' equity that result from the revenues, expenses, gains, and losses of a given period. Factors other than these, however, may cause the amount of owners' equity to change. Increases may occur in owners' equity other than from revenues, and decreases may occur other than from expenses. Stockholders of a business corporation, for example, may invest in new issues of capital stock or they may be paid cash dividends. Such events, however, are not encountered in not-for-profit hospital enterprises.

In hospitals, where fund accounting is employed, the owners' equity is termed **fund balance.** Hospital resources and related obligations are segregated into self-balancing groups of accounts called **funds,** and in each fund the excess of assets over liabilities is the fund balance. The **total** owners' equity in a hospital is the total of the individual fund balances, and this total generally is changed in only two ways: (1) by net income or net losses and (2) by the receipt of resources restricted by **donors** to specific operating purposes, the acquisition of plant and equipment, or endowments. Certain interfund transfers of resources may be made, however, that properly increase the equity balance of one fund and decrease that of another fund. But the total of fund balances is not affected by such transfers.

The statement of changes in owners' equity (fund balances) nevertheless is an essential financial statement in the appraisal of a hospital's economic activities. To be most useful, a **single** statement of this kind should present all changes in the balances of **all funds**. The statement also may be presented in combination with the income statement. Further treatment of these matters is deferred to Chapters 19 and 20.

Statement of Changes in Financial Position. A comprehensive statement of changes in financial position provides a summary of all changes in financial position during a given time period. This statement, sometimes called a **statement of sources and applications of funds,** details the more significant changes in individual assets and liabilities occurring in a specified period. It is particularly useful in its disclosure of hospital financing and investing activities. For this reason, it is regarded as one of the primary financial statements. An extended discussion of this statement appears in Chapter 21 of this book.

OBJECTIVES AND CHARACTERISTICS OF ACCOUNTING INFORMATION

The general objectives of financial statements are to present fairly and in accordance with generally accepted accounting principles (1) the financial position of an enterprise in terms of its economic resources and obligations at given points in time, (2) the results of enterprise operations in terms of revenues, expenses, and net income for given periods of time, and (3) other changes in financial position over time. Such information is needed by investors, creditors, and other resource providers, constituents, governing and oversight bodies, managers, and other users in making rational decisions and intelligent assessments of management stewardship and performance. A detailed analysis of the users of hospital financial reports and those users' informational needs appears in Statement 3 of the HFMA's Principles and Practices Board.[9] The objectives of financial reporting by business enterprises and nonbusiness organizations also are discussed at length by the FASB in SFAC No. 1 and SFAC No. 4.[10]

Complementary to these general objectives is a set of qualitative characteristics which greatly influence the content and usefulness of financial statements. In describing the qualitative characteristics of accounting information, the FASB emphasized relevance, reliability, neutrality, comparability, materiality, and cost/benefits, among other matters.[11] Some of these requisite qualities are discussed below. It should be noted that some of these characteristics and objectives may at times be interacting or even conflicting. In addition, the costs of attaining these qualitative objectives must be consistent with the benefits derived by users of the resulting information.

Relevance

Financial statements should present information that bears on the economic decisions made by the users of the statements. Relevance is the most important qualitative objective because information that is not relevant is useless, no matter what other desirable qualities it may possess. The principal problem is to determine users' needs and the kinds of information relevant to them.

Understandability

If accounting information is to be useful, it must be understandable to the user. Much can be done by accountants in choice of format and terminology to enhance the intelligibility of financial statements. There is, however, a presumption that users have an appreciation of the complex economic activities of the enterprise and its industry and some basic familiarity with accounting terminology and processes.

Reliability and Verifiability

If accounting information is to be useful, it must be reliable as well as relevant. Reliability depends upon the extent to which the information is faithfully represented, neutral (free from bias), and verifiable. It is sometimes said that accounting information is based on verifiable, objective evidence. While this is largely true, recognition should be given to the fact that measurements in accounting are not totally free of subjectivity. The measurers (accountants) are human. Yet, a high degree of verifiability is essential as it enhances the credibility and usefulness of financial information. Such information is verifiable if it would be substantially duplicated by other independent accountants using identical measurement methods and principles.

The qualitative objective of verifiability produces the accountant's well-known penchant for the development and use of underlying documents as evidence of transactions and their amounts. Documentary evidence of this type includes purchase orders and invoices, charge tickets, cash receipt slips, and similar forms in common use in hospitals.

Timeliness

The provision of accounting information should be timely, i.e., it should be communicated to users in time to be used as the basis for their economic decisions. If such information is not timely, it loses much of its value and causes delays in the making of critical decisions. Timeliness is an important ancillary aspect of the quality of relevance.

Comparability and Consistency

Financial information is most useful when it possesses the quality of comparability so that points of likeness or difference are readily discerned. Comparisons may be made of financial information at different dates or of different time periods for the same enterprise. Or, such comparisons may be made between enterprises within the same industry although comparability between enterprises is more difficult to achieve. This raises the question of uniform accounting among hospitals, a matter discussed in Chapter 4.

Comparability of financial information rests upon consistency. The format in which comparative data is presented should be consistent, the content of the financial statements must be consistent, and the accounting principles by which the data are measured must be consistent. It is also important that the underlying circumstances of enterprise operation be similar and that reporting periods of equivalent length be involved in comparisons.

The convention of consistency, however, does not preclude a desirable change in any of the above matters. But if such changes are made, they must be disclosed along with an indication of their approximate effect.

Completeness and Disclosure

Completeness is another quality that is essential in financial information. Financial statements should report complete information concerning all important aspects of the financial position and operating results of an enterprise. Adequate disclosure should be made of all significant matters in a manner that promotes understandability and reduces the possibility of erroneous impressions. Significant matters include all information necessary to make the statements not misleading.

To meet the requirements of completeness and full disclosure, the financial statements usually are supplemented with explanatory notes. Such notes should describe accounting policies, provide detailed information concerning specific assets or liabilities, and otherwise inform the user of matters not directly reflected in the financial statements. All significant information of this kind should be clearly reported and not be buried in a mass of trivia.

UNDERLYING CONCEPTS

Underlying the information presented in the financial statements of hospitals are a number of basic concepts. These concepts are derived from the characteristics of the environment within which the hospital accounting function is performed. As this environment changes in the future, certain of these concepts may be modified, or even discarded, and more useful concepts will be developed. Some of the more important basic concepts underlying present-day financial statements are examined in the following section.

Accounting Entity

The individual hospital enterprise is the entity upon which primary attention is focused in hospital accounting. The hospital itself is personified as a being in its own right capable of purchasing and owning resources, providing services, and incurring economic obligations. It is an independent entity whose economic activities are to be accounted for in a manner separate and distinct from the personal affairs of its employees, management, medical staff, and governing board. Hence the expression: "The hospital purchased $50,000 of new equipment."

In the fund accounting system employed by many hospitals, the economic resources and obligations are segregated into funds. These funds are maintained for accounting purposes as separate and independent **subordinate** entities. Even within certain funds, departmentalization of revenues and expenses into responsibility centers results in still another level of sub-entities. (Responsibility accounting is treated in Part 2 of this book.)

The total hospital enterprise nevertheless is the primary entity whose activity is measured, recorded, and reported in the accounting process. This is true even where the hospital is but one facet of a larger organization such as a church, university, or governmental unit. Accounting procedures should be designed, insofar as feasible, so that the financial position and operating results of the hospital alone may be separately determined and not be comingled with that of its parent body.

Going Concern

The accounting entity is assumed to be a "going concern" in the absence of contradictory evidence. That is, the hospital is viewed as having a continuity of existence where the expectation is for the enterprise to continue indefinitely as a viable economic concern. A number of accounting principles are formulated in part on the basis of this basic assumption of relative permanence of economic life. If cessation of all activity and liquidation appeared imminent, the application of those principles based on the going concern concept would not be appropriate. The allocation of certain costs into future periods, for example, clearly would be greatly modified or discontinued altogether.

Periodicity

The operating results (net income or net loss) of an enterprise cannot be determined precisely and finally until the enterprise ceases to exist. Because the users of financial statements frequently require information for decision-making purposes in an enterprise, the continuous activities of a hospital are segmented into relatively short periods of time called **accounting periods**. Information is provided as to operating results and financial position for each such period so as to increase the utility of the data in financial reports.

The accounting period basically is one year in duration, with shorter reporting periods, monthly, for example, being established as required by users' informational needs. Those statements developed for a full-year accounting period together comprise the **annual financial statements**. Those prepared more often are referred to as **interim financial statements**. The time period embraced by a financial statement or report should always be clearly indicated.

Hospitals may have an accounting period that coincides with the calendar year. A "natural business year" that usually ends sometime between April and October, however, is often favored. Many hospitals, for example, have chosen a fiscal year accounting period ending June 30 or September 30. A variation employed by some hospitals is the 13-month accounting period in which the year is divided into 13 "months" of exactly four calendar weeks each. Since each "month" has the same number of days and weekends, interim financial comparisons may be facilitated.

Measurement of Economic Resources and Obligations

Accounting is primarily concerned with the measurement and reporting of economic resources and obligations, and changes in them, in terms of money. An emphasis is given in accounting to economic resources, obligations, and activity that can be quantified. Such measurements are based largely upon objective exchange prices; subjective sociological or psychological value concepts are not yet directly involved in the accounting process.

Accounting is directly concerned, however, with certain nonmonetary measurements. Volume-of-service statistics such as number of meals served, number of laboratory examinations, and number of patient days of care, for example, are particularly useful in the analysis and evaluation of hospital financial data. A discussion of hospital statistics appears in Chapter 4.

Segregation of Resources and Obligations (Fund Accounting)

Many hospitals have a substantial amount of resources whose use is subject to legal and other restrictions. As recommended by the American Hospital Association's **Chart of Accounts for Hospitals**, these hospitals generally have adopted a concept known as **fund accounting**. Basically, fund accounting involves the segregation in the accounting records of hospital resources, and related obligations, into independent subordinate entities called **funds** in accordance with legal and other limitations on the purposes for which they may be employed. A hospital typically will have four or more types of funds, each of which is self-balancing in terms of the accounting equation mentioned earlier in this chapter. Special attention is given to fund accounting in Chapter 4.

Accrual Basis

One of the primary functions of accounting is to measure the changes in economic resources and obligations as they occur over time. This is necessary to the determination of an enterprise's periodic net income (or net loss) and its financial position at various points in time. Such measurements take into account changes in resources and obligations whether or not there is an immediately related cash receipt or disbursement. While most economic transactions eventually lead to a cash receipt or require a cash disbursement, noncash resources and obligations do change significantly in time periods other than those in which the related money, if any, is received or expended. The measurement of these changes, as well as those resulting from current cash flows, is the essence of the accrual basis of accounting.

Under the accrual basis, then, revenue is recognized, measured, and recorded in the time period in which it is **earned**, regardless of when, if ever, the related cash inflow occurs. Revenue, in general, is recognized at the point of sale or when a service is rendered and a claim against the purchaser of the goods or services arises.

Under the accrual basis, expense is recognized, measured, and recorded in the time period when **incurred**, or when economic resources are used up or consumed in the production of revenue, or resources otherwise suffer an expiration of utility to the purposes of the enterprise, regardless of when, if ever, the related cash outflow occurs. Further discussion of the recognition of expense and revenue appears in the treatment of pervasive principles at a later point in this chapter.

The distinction between the **accrual basis** and the **cash basis** of accounting should be made. Under the cash basis, revenue is recorded only when received in cash, and expense is recorded only when paid. The cash basis fails to recognize and measure **all** revenue and expense; it is concerned only with changes in cash resources. Obviously, the information it produces is at best incomplete and is therefore clearly inappropriate as a basis of accounting for enterprises as complex as hospitals.

Matching

The matching of related revenues and expenses is an objective closely associated with the accrual concept. The idea is that the determination of net income requires that the revenue recognized and measured for a given time period in accordance with accrual accounting be matched in the same time period with the expense that was incurred in the production of such revenue. No useful net income figure would be obtained, for example, if a 1987 income statement reported 1987 revenues matched against 1986 expenses! Accomplishment (revenue) and the related effort (expense) must be properly matched in the same time period. This is one of the key problems in accounting.

Approximation, Judgment, and Materiality

The complexities of economic activity often preclude precise measurements in accounting for such activity. For this reason alone, estimates and the attendant exercise of informed judgment are necessary. It is neither possible nor desirable to reduce all accounting to a set of rigid and inflexible rules. The dollar-and-cents balancing feature of balance sheets, unfortunately, often gives rise to misunderstanding among users as to the degree of accuracy actually involved in accounting. Users also may sometimes fail to recognize that matters of opinion and judgment do have a significant influence on financial reporting.

Another concept which also may affect the measurement of economic activity is materiality. Accounting generally is concerned only with a fair statement of information that is of sufficient significance to affect decisions typically made by users of accounting information. Materiality is, of course, a particularly elusive concept. It requires the application of sound judgment to the circumstances peculiar to each individual situation.

General-Purpose, Fundamentally Related Statements

It is presumed that users of financial statements have common needs that are best served by general-purpose financial statements. Such statements are the primary product of accounting, although the same process can provide special-purpose information for management and others when required. All financial statements are fundamentally related in that the information they contain is derived largely from one process governed by a single body of generally accepted accounting principles.

GENERALLY ACCEPTED ACCOUNTING PRINCIPLES

Financial statements are the end product of the accounting process by which quantitative data relating to the economic activities of an enterprise are accumulated and communicated in accordance with generally accepted principles. These principles determine the selection of resources and obligations to enter the accounting process, the method of measuring economic resources and obligations as well as changes in them, the choice of information to be disclosed, and other features of the process. In other words, the utility of the end product of accounting depends mainly upon the accounting principles by which it is produced.

Generally accepted accounting principles embrace all concepts, standards, and rules necessary to define what is or is not accepted accounting practice at a particular time. Such principles are based on the ideas of general acceptance and substantial authoritative support. They become generally accepted by agreement, which is often tacit, and are developed from experience, reason, and custom. The necessary authoritative support is to be found primarily in the pronouncements of organizations such as the Financial Accounting Standards Board, the American Institute of Certified Public Accountants, the HFMA's Principles and Practices Board, and the American Hospital Association. Individual textbooks and writings, no matter who the author may be, do not necessarily in themselves constitute a source of generally accepted accounting principles.

Pervasive Principles

Pervasive principles relate to accounting generally and provide a basis for the other types of principles and for much of the accounting process. They are few in number, and being fundamental in nature are not so prone to change as other types of principles. The pervasive principles are of two kinds: (1) measurement principles and (2) modifying conventions. Pervasive principles indicate the general approach accountants follow in recognizing and measuring the events that enter into the accounting process and provide the elements of financial position and operating results as defined in previous sections of this chapter.

Measurement Principles. The pervasive measurement principles are described briefly:

1. **Initial recording.** The initial recording principle specifies that assets and liabilities are to be recorded on the basis of events in which the enterprise acquires resources from other entities or incurs obligations to other entities and are measured by the exchange prices at which the transfers are effected.

2. **Revenue realization.** Revenue is realized, and is to be recognized, when the earning process is complete, or virtually complete, and an exchange has taken place. The earning process typically is completed when goods are sold, services are performed and are billable, or as time passes, in the case of interest and rent from the use of enterprise resources by others. Revenue should not be recorded before it is earned.

3. **Expense recognition.** Expenses are costs that are directly or indirectly associated with the revenue of a given time period. Three principles govern the recognition of expenses to be deducted from revenue in the determination of the net income or net loss of a period.

   a. **Association of cause and effect.** Certain costs are recognized as expenses because of a presumed direct relationship with specific revenue. The realization of the revenue is accompanied by a recognition of the associated expense. An example is the recognition of inventory costs as expenses when revenue arises from sales of such inventory.

   b. **Systematic and rational allocation.** Where costs cannot be directly associated with specific revenue on a cause and effect basis, costs may be associated instead with specific time periods through a systematic and rational allocation to the time periods to which benefits are provided by such costs. An example of this type of expense recognition is the depreciation of hospital plant and equipment.

    c.   **Immediate recognition.** Certain other costs are given immediate recognition as expense because they provide no discernible benefits that can be associated either with future revenues or with future time periods. In the application of this principle, some costs are charged to expense in the time period in which they are incurred and/or paid.

The **costs** referred to above are historical acquisition costs. In accounting today, assets are initially recorded at acquisition cost and are generally maintained at such historical costs until they are recognized as expense. This convention sometimes is referred to as the **historical cost principle** and reflects a preference for permanent and objective measurements rather than the subjective measurements that would be required in periodic revaluations of assets to replacement cost or to market value.

4. **Unit of measure.** The U.S. dollar, as the medium of exchange, provides the unit of measure for financial accounting. It is the common denominator requisite to the mathematical operations involved in the measurement of operating results and financial position. While the impact of inflation on measurements made in terms of the monetary unit is admitted, the effects have not previously been considered sufficiently important in the United States to require formal recognition in the accounting process. Many large profit-seeking corporations, however, do report the effects of inflation as supplementary information in their annual reports.

These pervasive measurement principles guide the determination of what accounting measures, and how and when it is measured.

    Modifying Conventions. Strict adherence to the pervasive measurement principles is not desirable in all circumstances. For this reason, certain modifying conventions have been generally adopted. These conventions modify the application of the pervasive measurement principles and take their effect through the rules found in the broad operating principles or in the detailed principles.

    One such convention is **conservatism.** Both accountants and users of accounting information historically have exhibited a strong preference for the understatement of net income and net assets when such elements are measured under highly uncertain conditions. This convention, therefore, will result in the determination of net income and net assets at amounts lower than would result from a rigid application of pervasive measurement principles. Deliberate and unwarranted misstatements, however, are not justifiable on grounds of conservatism and cannot be condoned.

    Another convention is the tendency to place primary emphasis on the income statement as opposed to the balance sheet. This is not to say that the balance sheet is unimportant. Rather it is an inclination to adopt accounting principles that are believed to increase the usefulness of the income statement although it is achieved at the expense of the balance sheet. Some emphasis on the determination of operating results is found in hospital accounting, but the reduction of the balance sheet's relative importance is not nearly so pronounced as it has been in accounting for profit-seeking enterprises. In hospital accounting, considerably more attention is given to accountability and stewardship concerns.

    The modifying conventions also serve the purpose of substituting the judgment of the accounting profession as a whole for that of the individual. They allow modification of principles where rigid conformity would yield unreasonable or misleading results in terms of the collective judgment of the accounting profession. This often can be seen in modifications of pervasive principles in accounting for enterprises within a particular industry.

Broad Operating Principles

Broad operating principles, derived from the pervasive principles, are general rules that govern the application of detailed principles. The accounting process consists of a cycle of operations that is repeated in each accounting period. These operations are identified at the beginning of the next chapter. They include the selection and measurement of economic events and the recording and reporting of those events. Broad operating principles are those that guide the performance of the basic operations of accounting. These principles are classified as (1) selection and measurement principles and (2) financial statement presentation principles.

Selection and Measurement Principles. These broad principles govern the selection of events from the stream of economic activity and guide the manner in which their effects are measured. They are organized below in terms of two types of economic events, i.e., external and internal events.

External events selected for measurement in the accounting process are primarily those involving transfers, either reciprocal or nonreciprocal, of resources or obligations to or from other entities (enterprises or individuals). Internal events that are selected and whose effects are measured include those involved in the production of goods and services by the enterprise. The effects of casualties also are considered.

Exchanges (reciprocal transfers) arising from external events usually are recorded when the transfer of resources or obligations occurs or services are provided. Their effects on assets, liabilities, revenues, and expenses are measured at the prices established in the exchanges:

1. **Assets.** The resources acquired in exchanges are recorded as enterprise assets, unless immediately charged to expense as provided for by the pervasive principles. These assets are measured at acquisition cost. When assets are acquired in exchanges involving neither money nor promises to pay money, such assets are measured at the fair market value of assets given up or at the fair market value of assets received, if that is more clearly evident. The exchange price of a group of assets acquired in a single exchange is allocated to the various assets on a relative market value basis. Decreases in assets resulting from exchanges are recorded when the disposition occurs and are measured by the previously recorded acquisition costs of such assets. Measurement of partial dispositions of particular assets is governed by detailed principles such as average cost or first-in, first-out.
2. **Liabilities.** Obligations to transfer assets or provide services in the future are recorded when they are incurred in exchanges. They generally are measured at the amounts to be paid as established in the exchanges, or at the present value of the future amounts to be paid. Decreases in liabilities are recorded when they are paid or otherwise discharged and are measured by the recorded amounts of such liabilities.

3. **Revenues.** Revenue from exchanges involving the sale of products, the provision of services, or the use of enterprise resources by others is recorded when those exchanges occur and is measured by the prices established in such exchanges. Revenue reductions, such as for discounts and allowances, should be recorded separately and on the accrual basis. Revenue from exchanges involving the sale of enterprise assets other than products usually is netted against the costs of such assets and is reported as gains or losses in the income statement.

4. **Expenses.** The costs of assets sold or services provided are recorded as expenses when the revenue from such exchanges is recognized. These expenses are measured by the recorded amounts of the assets transferred or by the costs of providing the services as described in connection with internal events.

In the case of nonreciprocal transfers such as gifts and donations, the assets acquired generally are recorded when such transfers occur and are measured at their fair market value on the date received. Services as well as assets may be donated to hospitals, and the detailed principles that have been developed to determine their proper measurement are indicated at a later point. Nonreciprocal transfers arising from lawsuits and thefts may also occur. In such cases, the assets given up or lost are accounted for at their recorded amounts and imposed liabilities are recorded at the amounts to be paid.

External events other than transfers of resources or obligations may or may not be recorded in accounting. Changes may occur, for example, in the market prices of enterprise assets, in the general price level, in interest rates, or in technology. The general rule is that the **favorable** effects, if any, of such external events are **not** recorded when the events occur. Instead, the recorded amounts of assets and liabilities are retained without adjustment. This principle is derived from such concepts as objectivity, conservatism, and materiality, and from the pervasive principle of realization.

On the other hand, the **unfavorable** effects of the external events noted **are** often measured and recorded in accounting. Adjustments for obsolescence and adjustments of inventories to the lower of cost or market are examples. Application of this broad principle varies according to the type of asset or liability affected and is governed by the specific rules provided by detailed principles.

Internal events not directly involving other entities include production and casualties. Production is considered here in the broad sense, i.e., the economic process in which goods and services are combined to produce other goods and services. Revenue is not recorded at the time of production although utility is added to certain assets. Costs of producing goods and services, however, are measured generally in the amounts of acquisition costs. These costs are shifted to various categories of assets and expenses, or between activities and periods, in a systematic and rational manner as goods and services are used in production operations. The purpose of this part of the accounting process is to determine production costs and provide a basis for relating them to revenue when the products are sold and the services are provided in external transfer events. This book, however, is concerned primarily with financial accounting, and the detailed principles governing production accounting will not be discussed here.

Casualties are internal events such as fires and floods that are not caused by other economic entities. The effects of casualties, when they occur, are recorded by writing down assets to recoverable amounts and recognizing a loss. Insurance proceeds, if any, are treated as a reduction of the amount of loss. Further attention is given to this subject in Chapter 16.

The principle of dual effects, sometimes called double-entry accounting, is seen throughout this discussion. All economic events recorded in the accounting process have interrelated effects. Each recorded event has at least two effects in the accounting records. Consider, for example, the receipt of a bank loan. An asset (cash) is increased and a liability (notes payable to bank) also is increased. When the loan is repaid, the same asset and liability elements are decreased. Other events may result in a decrease in one element and an increase in another. The accountant's shorthand in this increase and decrease process is the debit and credit system. Chapter 3 provides the details of that system.

Financial Statement Presentation Principles. These principles provide the necessary guides to the attainment of the standard of a fair presentation in accordance with generally accepted accounting principles of an enterprise's financial position and operating results. The **minimum** presentation required for hospitals under this standard generally includes (1) a balance sheet, (2) an income statement, (3) a statement of changes in fund balances, (4) a statement of changes in financial position, (5) a statistical summary and (6) supplementary disclosures.

The balance sheet should include, adequately classified by funds, all assets, liabilities, and fund balances as defined by generally accepted accounting principles. The income statement also should be complete, including and adequately describing all revenues and expenses similarly defined. The statement of changes in fund balances should disclose all elements of change in the balance of each fund maintained by the hospital. Particular attention should be given to a proper reporting of interfund transfers. If this statement is presented with the income statement in a combined form, as it often is, the format adopted should clearly reflect the net income or loss of the period. Finally, a complete statement of changes in financial position also should be provided. This statement should fully describe all significant changes in resources and obligations so that the important aspects of the hospital's financing and investing activities are presented. All of these statements should be presented in comparison with those of the preceding period.

In addition to the information contained in the financial statements noted above, an adequate presentation of a hospital's financial position and operating results will include a statistical summary and supplementary notes. The statistical summary generally should report the volume-of-service measurements that pertain to the overall level of hospital activity and that relate to the broad categories of monetary data presented in the financial statements. A last requirement is that there be additional disclosures through explanatory notes to the extent appropriate in the circumstances. These supplementary materials should be regarded as an integral part of the financial statements.

Detailed Accounting Principles

The detailed accounting principles are the numerous rules and procedures that specify the way financial data is to be processed and presented in financial statements. APB Statement No. 4 defines detailed accounting principles as the large body of practices and procedures through which the pervasive and broad operating principles are implemented. No attempt is made in the Statement, however, to enumerate the detailed principles. The reasons given for this omission are (1) that many of these principles could already be found in other authoritative documents, (2) that these principles change so frequently that a comprehensive statement of them would quickly become obsolete and (3) that to attempt to list such principles in detail would involve matters the Board could not consider at the time. The Board's failure to specifically identify the detailed principles was a disappointment in some quarters. It should be noted, however, that the Board's statement of basic concepts, pervasive principles, and broad operating principles was in itself a major achievement.

No effort is made here to itemize in a single chapter all the detailed accounting principles. These principles (or what this writer believes these principles to be) are presented at appropriate points throughout this book. The reader should be aware, however, that the discussion within these pages, including the present chapter, does not have the official approval of any organization.

MATTERS PECULIAR TO HOSPITAL ENTERPRISES

The preceding pages have presented the basic concepts and broad principles generally applicable to all enterprises, with slight adaptions to the not-for-profit hospital. Hospitals, however, have somewhat unique characteristics that give rise to special accounting and financial reporting problems. A full discussion of principles applicable to these problems is deferred to subsequent chapters. It seems appropriate at this point, however, to identify a few of the more important of these principles. An understanding of these presumes a knowledge of fund accounting and other procedural matters to which the reader may not have been sufficiently exposed until subsequent chapters are studied. However that may be, the following discussion is expanded in various parts of this book.

Fund Accounting

As observed earlier in this chapter, a substantial amount of hospital resources may be restricted in use to donor-specified purposes. This situation raises problems of accountability and stewardship that experience indicates can best be dealt with through the mechanism of fund accounting. In fund accounting, hospital assets and liabilities are segregated into independent, self-balancing groups of accounts. Each group constitutes a subordinate entity of which the equity (net assets) is called the **fund balance**. Several different funds, restricted and unrestricted, are usually maintained. Funds are restricted if donors have placed restrictions on the use of the resources. The accounting procedures for funds can become rather complex (see Chapter 4).

Accounting for Plant Assets

Plant assets, including land, buildings, and equipment, should be accounted for as a part of the hospital's Unrestricted Fund. To segregate these assets in a separate fund would imply externally imposed restrictions upon their use, which normally is not the case. If such restrictions do not exist, designations by the hospital governing board do not alter that fact. What a board can do, it can undo, and its designations of resources to particular uses should not be equated with the restrictions placed on resources by their donors.

Depreciation of plant assets should be recognized by hospitals. The periodic charge should be based upon a systematic and rational allocation of the previously recorded acquisition costs of such assets. Although the governing board may provide for amounts larger than the depreciation charge in the accumulation of a replacement and expansion fund, such designations are not expenses but appropriations of the unrestricted fund balance.

If a hospital is reimbursed for depreciation, the amount of such reimbursement should be included in revenue even though all or a portion of it is restricted by third parties to the acquisition of plant assets. Amounts received and restricted in this way should also be shown in the statement of changes in fund balances as transfers from unrestricted to restricted funds. When such amounts are expended, they should be shown as transfers back to the unrestricted fund.

Unrestricted Resources

All resources available at the discretion of the governing board should be shown as unrestricted resources in the financial statements. All resources received that are not donor-restricted should be reported as revenue and **not** be credited directly to fund balances. These resources include so-called board-designated funds. While disclosure should be made of board designations, all funds created by the board should be shown separately from donor-restricted funds. The term **restricted** should not be applied to internally created funds of any kind.

Restricted Resources

Hospitals receive resources whose use is restricted by donors. Such resources may be (1) funds for specified operating purposes, (2) funds for the acquisition of plant assets, and (3) endowment funds.

The receipt of funds that are donor-restricted to specific operating purposes should be accounted for in a restricted fund or as deferred revenue in the unrestricted fund. When expenditures are made for the specified operating purposes, the related donor-restricted resources then are reported in the unrestricted fund as revenue of the same period.

Funds restricted by donors for acquisition of plant assets should be treated as contributions to the hospital's permanent capital and should be credited to a restricted fund balance. When plant asset expenditures are made as specified by donors, such resources should be transferred from the restricted fund balance to the unrestricted fund balance. No revenue is recorded. Upon receipt of plant assets donated in kind, the fair market value of such assets is credited to the unrestricted fund balance.

Endowments received, whether pure endowments or term endowments, are accounted for as restricted funds upon receipt. A pure endowment is one whose principal amount may not be expended. On the other hand, the principal amount of term endowment may be expended after a specified period of time or upon the expiration of restrictions. Income from endowment funds similarly may be restricted or unrestricted, depending upon donors' stipulations. When the principal amount of term endowments becomes available for unrestricted purposes, it should be reported as revenue. If the use of such resources is restricted, the resources should be recorded in the appropriate restricted funds and be accounted for as restricted funds. Endowment-type funds held in trust by others, and not controlled by the hospital, generally should not be included in the hospital balance sheet.[12]

Investment Transactions

The income statement of the hospital should include investment income and realized gains (and losses) relating to all unrestricted resources, including board-designated resources. Income and realized gains on investments of restricted funds should be added to the respective restricted fund balances unless available for unrestricted purposes. Gains and losses on investment transactions between unrestricted and restricted funds should be recognized and disclosed in the financial statements.

Pledges

Pledges may be restricted or unrestricted. Unrestricted pledges (net of provision for uncollectibles) are recorded as revenue of the period in which such pledges are made. If pledges are restricted, they should be accounted for as deferred revenue or as additions to restricted fund balances, depending upon the nature of the donors' restrictions.

Donated Services and Commodities

Hospitals sometimes are recipients of donated services and commodities. Donated services properly are recorded at fair market value when there is an employer-employee relationship and an objective basis for determining the amounts that might otherwise have been paid for such services. Services provided by auxiliaries, guilds, and related organizations, however, generally are not recorded by hospitals, but may be disclosed in notes to the financial statements. Donated commodities which ordinarily would be purchased by hospitals should also be recorded at fair market value when received.

Third-Party Reimbursement

Patient service revenues are recorded on the accrual basis and at the hospital's full established rates, regardless of the amounts the hospital expects to collect from patients or third parties. Differences between gross and realizable revenue, called revenue deductions, also are accounted for on the accrual basis. It should be noted, however, that the HFMA's Principles and Practices Board has recently proposed that patient service revenues be reported at the amount which the payer has an obligation to pay.[13] If payment arrangements provide for a discount, for example, the amount reported as revenue is net of the discount. This proposal has merit, and may become an established practice. In this book, however, the traditional method of accounting for patient service revenues is assumed.

In the case of retroactive cost reimbursement, differences typically arise between estimated settlements and final settlements. Adjustments for such differences generally should be included in the income statement and **not** be treated as direct adjustments of fund balance.

There also may be instances in which certain expenses (depreciation, for example) are properly recognized for financial accounting purposes in one period but enter into cost reimbursement in another period. The effect of such timing differences should be deferred and appropriately reflected in the financial statements so as to match related revenues and expenses.

CHAPTER 2 FOOTNOTES

1. Subcommittee on Health Care Matters, **Hospital Audit Guide—Fourth Edition** (New York: American Institute of Certified Public Accountants, 1982), p. 3.
2. SFAC No. 3, **Elements of Financial Statements of Business Enterprises** (Stamford, Connecticut: FASB, 1980), p. 9. Copyright by Financial Accounting Standards Board, High Ridge Park, Stamford, Connecticut, 06905, U.S.A. Reprinted with permission. Copies of the complete document are available from the FASB. This reprint does not include the appendices. These appendices are an integral part of the document.
3. SFAC No. 3, **Elements of Financial Statements of Business Enterprises** (Stamford, Connecticut: FASB, 1980), p. 12.
4. SFAC No. 3, **Elements of Financial Statements of Business Enterprises** (Stamford, Connecticut: FASB, 1980), pp. 31-32.
5. SFAC No. 3, **Elements of Financial Statements of Business Enterprises** (Stamford, Connecticut: FASB, 1980), p. 34.
6. SFAC No. 3, **Elements of Financial Statements of Business Enterprises** (Stamford, Connecticut: FASB, 1980), p. 33.
7. SFAC No. 3, **Elements of Financial Statements of Business Enterprises** (Stamford, Connecticut: FASB, 1980), p. 34.
8. SFAC No. 3, **Elements of Financial Statements of Business Enterprises** (Stamford, Connecticut: FASB, 1980), p. 27.
9. Principles and Practices Board Statement 3, **Supplementary Reporting of Hospital Financial Requirements** (Oak Brook, Illinois: HFMA, 1980).
10. SFAC No. 1, **Objectives of Financial Reporting by Business Enterprises** (Stamford, Connecticut: FASB, 1978). SFAC No. 4, **Objectives of Financial Reporting by Nonbusiness Organizations** (Stamford, Connecticut: FASB, 1980).
11. SFAC No. 2, **Qualitative Characteristics of Accounting Information** (Stamford, Connecticut: FASB, 1980).
12. Subcommittee on Health Care Matters, **Hospital Audit Guide—Fourth Edition** (New York: AICPA, 1982), pp. 86-89.
13. Principles and Practices Board Exposure Draft, **The Presentation of Patient Service Revenue and Related Issues** (Oak Brook, Illinois: HFMA, 1985), pp. 10-11.

QUESTIONS

1. Define the term **accounting.** What is the major function of accounting in the economy?

2. Describe briefly the nature of accounting principles. Are accounting principles subject to change? Explain.

3. Define the following terms:
    1. Balance sheet
    2. Assets
    3. Liabilities
    4. Owners' equity (fund balance)
    5. Accounting equation

4. Define the following terms:
    1. Income statement
    2. Revenues
    3. Expenses
    4. Net income (or net loss)

5. Distinguish between (1) a statement of changes in owners' equity, or fund balances, and (2) a statement of changes in financial position.

6. What are the three general objectives of financial statements? List and describe briefly some of the principal qualitative objectives of accounting information.

7. What is your understanding of each of the following basic concepts underlying hospital financial statements? Write a brief summary for each item.
    1. Accounting entity
    2. Going concern
    3. Periodicity
    4. Unit of measurement
    5. Fund accounting
    6. Accrual basis
    7. Matching
    8. Materiality

8. What is a generally accepted accounting principle? What is the source of such principles?

9. Distinguish among (1) pervasive principles, (2) modifying conventions, (3) broad operating principles, and (4) detailed operating principles.

10. The unique characteristics of the hospital enterprise give rise to special accounting and reporting problems in the following areas, among others. Briefly state the major principle or principles that have been developed in each of these areas:
    1. Fund accounting
    2. Valuation of donated plant assets
    3. Depreciation
    4. Board-designated assets
    5. Restricted resources
    6. Pledges
    7. Donated services and commodities
    8. Third-party reimbursement

11. Define and illustrate (1) the cash basis of accounting and (2) the accrual basis of accounting. Outline the steps to follow in changing from a cash to an accrual basis.

12. What is **fund accounting**? Define and illustrate. State the advantages of fund accounting. Explain the disadvantages of fund accounting.

13. Indicate whether each of the following statements is true or false. If false, explain why the statement is false.

1. The most important purpose of financial and statistical data is for the use of management in planning and controlling the affairs of hospitals.

2. Consistency refers to the practice of continually changing accounting procedures from one period to another.

3. The concept of full disclosure requires that all significant data be clearly and completely reflected in accounting reports.

4. Historical cost is the amount of replacement value for property, goods, or services.

5. Fund accounting was developed in response to a managerial need for a separate accounting for groups of resources whose use must be limited to particular hospital activities or functions.

6. Board-created funds are donor-restricted specific purpose funds.

7. Under the cash basis system of accounting, revenues are recognized when earned and expenses are recognized when incurred.

8. An amount is material if its exclusion from an accounting statement would cause misleading or incorrect conclusions to be drawn by users of the statement.

9. Unexpired costs are those which are applicable to future periods.

10. Expense in its broadest sense includes all expired costs which are deductible from revenues.

11. Legally, resources that are donor-restricted do not have to be used in conformity with donors' intents.

12. The principal amounts of endowment funds may be used at the hospital governing board's discretion.

13. Donor-restricted specific purpose funds must be used as designated by donors.

14. All receipts of unrestricted funds must be recorded as operating fund income regardless of any action taken by the hospital's governing board or its administrative officers to restrict expenditure to specific purposes.

15. The choice of the dollar as the standard of measurement means that information in accounting reports is limited to those facts that can be related to or translated into dollars and cents.

16. Expenses are expired costs that have been used or consumed in carrying on some activity and from which material benefit will extend beyond the present.

14. The administrator of XYZ Hospital has read a great deal about the controversies over accounting principles for hospitals. Yet, the administrator does not understand why the development of generally accepted principles is so important to the hospital industry. Explain why it is essential that such principles be developed and observed.

15. Give the arguments for and against the use of historical costs as a basis for the valuation of plant assets in hospitals.

16. What is your understanding of the concept of **conservatism** as it is applied in accounting?

17. It has been suggested that hospital investments in securities be valued at current fair market values. Give the arguments for and against this proposal.

18. It has been suggested that hospitals include budgets and forecasts in their published annual financial reports. Do you believe that this should be done? Explain.

19. Many financial managers believe that the income statement is the most important single financial statement prepared by the accountant. Do you agree? Explain.

20. Identify the organizations that have been primarily responsible for the development of current accounting principles. Briefly discuss what has been accomplished by each group.

21. What is your understanding of the following: (1) AICPA, (2) APB, (3) Committee on Health Care Institutions, and (4) FASB?

22. What is a **natural business year**? Do hospitals have a natural business year? If so, what is it?

23. Select the best answer for each of the following multiple-choice items:

1. Which of the following accounting concepts states than an accounting transaction should be supported by sufficient evidence to allow two or more qualified individuals to arrive at essentially similar measures and conclusions?

   a. Matching.
   b. Objectivity.
   c. Periodicity.
   d. Stable monetary unit.

2. What is the underlying concept that supports the immediate recognition of a loss?

   a. Conservatism.
   b. Consistency.
   c. Judgment.
   d. Matching.

3. The principle of objectivity includes the concept of

   a. Summarization.
   b. Classification.
   c. Conservatism.
   d. Verifiability.

4. Objectivity is assumed to be achieved when an accounting transaction

   a. Is recorded in a fixed amount of dollars.
   b. Involves the payment or receipt of cash.
   c. Involves an arm's-length transaction between two independent parties.
   d. Allocates revenues or expenses in a rational and systematic manner.

5. The valuation of a promise to receive cash in the future at present value on the financial statements of a hospital is valid because of the accounting concept of

   a. Entry.
   b. Materiality.
   c. Going concern.
   d. Neutrality.

24. Select the best answer to each of the following multiple-choice items:

1. Which of the following is an example of the expense recognition principle of associating cause and effect?

   a. Allocation of insurance cost.
   b. Sales commissions.
   c. Depreciation of plant assets.
   d. Salaries of department supervisors.

2. Which of the following is considered a pervasive constraint by **Statement of Financial Accounting Concepts No. 2**?

   a. Benefits/cost.
   b. Conservatism.
   c. Timeliness.
   d. Verifiability.

3. According to **Statement of Financial Accounting Concepts No. 2**, relevance and reliability are the two primary qualities that make accounting information useful for decision-making. Predictive value is an ingredient of

	Relevance	Reliability
a.	No	No
b.	No	Yes
c.	Yes	Yes
d.	Yes	No

4. Uncertainty and risks inherent in business situations should be adequately considered in financial reporting. This statement is an example of the concept of

   a. Conservatism.
   b. Completeness.
   c. Neutrality.
   d. Representational faithfulness.

5. What accounting concept justifies the usage of accruals and deferrals?

   a. Going concern.
   b. Materiality.
   c. Consistency.
   d. Stable monetary unit.

25.   Select the best answer for each of the following multiple-choice items:

1.   The financial statement which has as its primary function the summarization of the financing and investing aspects of all significant transactions affecting financial position is the

     a.   Income statement.
     b.   Balance sheet.
     c.   Statement of changes in financial position.
     d.   Statement of changes in fund balances.

2.   During the lifetime of an entity, accounts produce financial statements at arbitrary points in time in accordance with which basic accounting concept?

     a.   Objectivity.
     b.   Periodicity.
     c.   Conservatism.
     d.   Matching.

3.   Which of the following is not a basis for the immediate recognition of a cost during a period?

     a.   The cost provides no discernible future benefit.
     b.   The cost recorded in a prior period no longer produces discernible benefits.
     c.   The federal income tax savings using the immediate write-off method exceed the savings obtained by allocating the cost to several periods.
     d.   Allocation of the cost on the basis of association with revenue or among several accounting periods is considered to serve no useful purpose.

4.   One of the basic features of financial accounting is the

     a.   Direct measurement of economic resources and obligations and changes in them in terms of money and sociological and psychological impact.
     b.   Direct measurement of economic resources and obligations and changes in them in terms of money.
     c.   Direct measurement of economic resources and obligations and changes in them in terms of money and sociological impact.
     d.   Direct measurement of economic resources and obligations and changes in them in terms of money and psychological impact.

5.   Continuation of an accounting entity in the absence of evidence to the contrary is an example of the basis concept of

     a.   Accounting entity.
     b.   Consistency.
     c.   Going concern.
     d.   Substance over form.

3
Review of the Accounting Process

The reader's understanding of much of the materials in this book is dependent to a significant extent upon a previously acquired knowledge of the fundamentals of accounting.[1] A brief and simplified review of the accounting process is presented in this chapter.

BASIC OPERATIONS

APB Statement No. 4 describes the accounting process as consisting of eight basic operations, as follows:[2]

1. **Selecting** the events. Events to be accounted for are identified. Not all events that affect the economic resources and obligations of an enterprise are, or can be, accounted for when they occur.
2. **Analyzing** the events. Events are analyzed to determine their effects on the financial position of an enterprise.
3. **Measuring** the effects. Effects of the events on the financial position of the enterprise are measured and represented by money amounts.
4. **Classifying** the measured effects. The effects are classified according to the individual assets, liabilities, owners' equity items, revenue, or expenses affected.
5. **Recording** the measured effects. The effects are recorded according to the assets, liabilities, owners' equity items, revenue, and expenses affected.
6. **Summarizing** the recorded effects. The amounts of changes recorded for each asset, liability, owners' equity item, revenue, and expense are summed and related data are grouped.
7. **Adjusting** the records. Remeasurements, new data, corrections, or other adjustments are often required after the events have been initially recorded, classified, and summarized.
8. **Communicating** the processed information. The information is communicated to users in the form of financial statements.

Although the operations are listed separately, they overlap conceptually and some of them are performed simultaneously. All operations, of course, are governed by the principles discussed in the preceding chapter.

TRANSACTION ANALYSIS

The first five operations listed constitute the **recording phase** of the accounting process. Events selected to enter the process are **analyzed** as to their increase or decrease effects on the individual asset, liability, fund balance, revenue, and expense classifications employed by the hospital enterprise. As a result of this analysis, the measured effects are formally recorded in the accounting records. The measured effects recorded are then summarized and adjusted for communication to users through financial statements.

Transaction analysis, then is a critical procedure. Only when transactions are properly analyzed and recorded can meaningful financial statements be prepared. The debit and credit system of analysis and balancing therefore evolved as a means of assuring accuracy in recording the effects of transactions.

The mechanics of analyzing and recording transactions in debit and credit terms are derived from the accounting equation stated in the previous chapter:

ASSETS = LIABILITIES + FUND BALANCES

Elements on the left-hand side of the equation (assets) are maintained in an equality with elements on the right-hand side (liabilities and fund balances). After the dual effects of each transaction are considered, the equation must remain balanced; the total of one side equal to the total of the other side.

One may think of the left-hand side of the equation as consisting of **debit elements**, i.e., assets are debit elements. The opposing side logically, then is composed of **credit elements**, i.e., liabilities and fund balances. (This designation of debit side and credit side is an arbitrary one.) It therefore follows that increases in, or additions to, the left-hand side are **debits**; increases in, or additions to, the right-hand side are **credits**. In reverse, it may be said that decreases in elements on the left-hand side are credits and decreases in elements on the right-hand side are debits. In summary:

ASSETS		=	LIABILITIES AND FUND BALANCES	
Debit	Credit		Debit	Credit
Increase	Decrease		Decrease	Increase
(+)	(−)		(−)	(+)

Assume, for example, a hospital with $500 of assets, $100 of liabilities, and a $400 fund balance. The equation would be:

$$\$500 = \$100 + \$400$$

Consider, now, the effects on the equation of a transaction in which the hospital receives a $60 loan from a bank. The revised equation is:

$$\$560 \ = \ \$160 \ + \ \$400$$

Like any other transaction, this has dual effects: (1) the hospital assets (cash) were increased by $60 and (2) the hospital liabilities (bank loan payable) were increased by $60. The amount of the fund balance was not affected by this transaction. In accounting terminology, the transaction is recorded by a **debit** to Cash (the asset increased) and a **credit** to Bank Loan Payable (the liability increased).

Suppose that at a later date $30 of the bank loan was repaid along with $4 of interest. The equation ($560 = $160 + $400) would be restated to read:

$$\$526 \ = \ \$130 \ + \ \$396$$

Assets were decreased by the amount of cash disbursed ($30 + $4); liabilities were decreased by the principal amount of the bank loan repaid ($30); the fund balance was decreased by the interest expense ($4). (The reader will recall that expenses decrease fund balances.) In debit and credit terms, there was (1) a **credit** to Cash (asset) of $34, (2) a **debit** to Bank Loan Payable (liability) of $30, and (3) a **debit** to the fund balance for $4 of expense.

It should not be assumed from the above examples that each transaction results in equal increases or equal decreases. What is true is that each transaction is recorded by equal amounts of debits and credits. Some changes that are recorded by debits are increases (increases in assets), but other debits are made to record decreases (decreases in liabilities and fund balance). The same observation applies to credits. A debit, then, is not always an increase, nor is a credit always a decrease. A debit, furthermore, is not necessarily "bad," nor is a credit necessarily "good," as expressed in terms sometimes used by nonaccountants.

The logic of the debit and credit procedure often escapes those who are just beginning a study of accounting. For them, it generally is helpful to reduce the procedure to two short rules:

1. For assets:
   a. Debit to increase.
   b. Credit to decrease.
2. For liabilities and fund balances, the opposite rule applies:
   a. Debit to decrease.
   b. Credit to increase.

These rules can be easily memorized and applied to the analysis of transactions. Eventually, the logic behind the rules becomes clear.

A slight addition to the rules, however, must be made. The reader is aware that revenue increases and expense decreases the owners' equity (fund balances) element of the equation. While revenues and expenses could be recorded as direct increases and decreases in fund balances as they are recognized, such a practice is not feasible. If this were done, difficult analyses would be required of fund balances to determine the net income or net loss of various time periods. So, in performing the operations of the accounting process during each accounting period, accountants expand the accounting equation as follows:

$$\text{ASSETS} + \text{EXPENSES} = \text{LIABILITIES} + \text{FUND BALANCES} + \text{REVENUES}$$

In this way, revenues and expenses initially are separately accumulated in appropriate categories as the accounting period progresses. At the end of the period, the recorded totals of revenue and expense then are eliminated from the equation. Only then is the fund balance adjusted for the difference (net income or loss).

The rules of debit and credit, based upon the expanded statement of the accounting equation, then become:

1. For assets **and expenses:**
   a. Debit to increase.
   b. Credit to decrease.
2. For liabilities, fund balances, **and revenues**, the opposite rule applies:
   a. Debit to decrease.
   b. Credit to increase.

If the first rule is accepted, the second rule follows automatically. It is the opposite of the first so that an equality will be maintained in debit and credit terms between (1) the total of assets and expenses and (2) the total of liabilities, fund balances, and revenues. This is the well-known balancing feature of accounting which provides assurance that, in certain respects, records of transactions are made accurately.

The terms **debit** and **credit** originally had meanings drawn from the Latin words for debtor and creditor. Even today these terms are abbreviated as **dr.** and **cr.**, but they are used as nouns, as verbs, and as adjectives.

ELEMENTS OF THE ACCOUNTING SYSTEM

Certain essential elements are found in all accounting systems. The most basic of these elements are (1) documentary evidences, (2) a chart of accounts, (3) journals, and (4) ledgers. A brief review of each element is presented in the following discussion.

Documentary Evidences

Accountants obviously must be aware of transactions in the steam of economic activity before they can record them. This awareness is achieved largely through the use of documentary evidences, i.e., business documents such as cash receipt slips, charge tickets, and invoices. These documents provide competent evidence that economic transactions and events have, in fact, occurred. They also provide monetary and other data which permit measurement of the effects of the transactions they represent.

Emphasis is placed on the element of documentary evidences because the accuracy and reliability of the information produced by the accounting process rests heavily upon the extent to which it is based upon competent evidential matter. Although wherever possible the accountant chooses to deal with verifiable, objectively determined data, accounting can never become fully objective. The cost of a depreciable asset, for example, may be ascertained by reference to externally created documents, but the portion of that cost recognized as depreciation expense in a given period is not verifiable in the same way. Even the judgments and estimates in accounting, nevertheless, generally are based in part upon documentary evidence of one kind or another.

Documentary evidences also play a vital role in the hospital's internal control system. This matter is discussed at length in Chapter 5.

Chart of Accounts

Having evidence that transactions have actually occurred, the accountant analyzes the transactions and measures their effects upon established categories of assets, liabilities, fund balances, revenues, and expenses. To do this, a data classification scheme is required. The individual categories into which transaction data are to be classified and recorded is established by a **chart of accounts**, sometimes called a **classification of accounts**. It is designed to provide for a systematic and consistent accumulation of financial data in managerially desired groupings. Legal, tax, and other considerations, however, also influence the design of the chart of accounts. A simple chart of accounts for a hypothetical hospital is presented in Figure 3-1.

Figure 3-1.
Anycity Hospital
Chart of Accounts

100 *Assets*
    101 Cash
    102 Accounts Receivable
    103 Inventories
    151 Plant and Equipment
    152 Accumulated Depreciation

200 *Liabilities*
    201 Accounts Payable
    202 Accrued Salaries and Wages Payable
    203 Deferred Revenue
    251 Mortgage Payable

300 *Owners' Equity*
    301 Fund Balance
    302 Revenue and Expense Summary

400 *Revenues*
    401 Daily Service Revenue
    402 Special Service Revenue
    403 Other Revenues

500 *Expenses*
    501 Salaries and Wages
    502 Supplies
    503 Purchased Services
    504 Insurance
    505 Depreciation
    506 Interest
    507 Other Expenses

The illustrative chart of accounts indicates the classifications in which transaction data are to be accumulated and communicated for Anycity Hospital. Each account in the chart is assigned a number in that the use of numbers rather than account titles saves clerical costs and also promotes accuracy. The numbering system, as well as most other features of the chart, is greatly simplified, but this chart will serve present purposes. A detailed illustration is provided in Chapter 4.

Journals

When the effects of transactions are determined, these effects are recorded in **journals**. The record may be handwritten or it may be machine-written where mechanical and electronic accounting equipment is employed. In any event, the record made is primarily a chronological record of the increase and decrease effects of transactions on the account classifications indicated by the chart of accounts. These increases and decreases are **journalized** in accordance with the debit and credit system described earlier.

Journals, in practice, may be of many different types; the most common being multicolumnar forms. In addition to a general journal, special types of journals are devised for efficient recording of particular kinds of transactions that occur repeatedly in great volume. The journal system of a particular hospital, for example, might include (1) revenue journals or registers, (2) cash receipts journals, (3) voucher registers, and (4) cash disbursements journals, or check registers. Payroll journals are also commonly employed. These journals are not illustrated and discussed here (see the author's **Introduction to Hospital Accounting**). Later in this chapter, however, a series of transaction entries in general journal form are illustrated and described.

Ledgers

The information recorded in the journals generally is in chronological sequence of transactions. Increases and decreases in individual accounts during a particular time period are scattered throughout the many different pages of the various journals. At no place in the journals does the end-of-period balance of any account appear; journals do not provide account balances.

For this reason, it becomes necessary to summarize periodically and to bring together in one place the information recorded in the journals. This involves the transfer of that information from the journals to other accounting records called **ledgers**. The transfer itself is called **posting**, and its purpose is to bring together all recorded increases and decreases in individual accounts so that the balance of each may be determined.

There are many types of ledgers. In addition to the primary ledger (the general ledger), special subsidiary ledgers are employed in which the details underlying the general ledger "control accounts" are maintained. The ledger system of a particular hospital, for example, might include subsidiary ledgers for (1) patient's accounts receivable, (2) inventories, (3) plant and equipment, (4) accounts payable, and (5) payrolls. These ledgers are illustrated and discussed in the author's **Introduction to Hospital Accounting**. Posting to the general ledger, however, is illustrated at a later point in this chapter.

ACCOUNTING CYCLE ILLUSTRATION

The term **accounting cycle** is given to the set of procedures performed during each accounting period. The following is a list of these procedures in their usual sequence.

1. Journalizing the transaction entries of the period.
2. Posting transaction entries to ledgers.
3. Adjusting the accounts:
   a. Journalizing adjusting entries.
   b. Posting adjusting entries.
4. Preparing the financial statements.
5. Closing the books:
   a. Journalizing closing entries.
   b. Posting closing entries.

In order to provide a quick review of these procedures, the remainder of this chapter presents a greatly condensed and simplified illustration of the 1987 accounting cycle for a hypothetical hospital.

Figure 3-2 presents the general ledger balances of Anycity Hospital at the beginning of its 1987 calendar-year accounting period. In an actual situation, of course, this trial balance would include a much larger number of accounts, and they would be grouped by funds. This absence of realism, however, need not detract seriously from the following review of fundamental procedures.

Figure 3-2.
Anycity Hospital
Trial Balance
January 1, 1987

Acct. No.		Dr.	Cr.
101	Cash	$ 65	
102	Accounts Receivable	425	
103	Inventories	110	
151	Plant and Equipment	4,400	
152	Accumulated Depreciation		$1,445
201	Accounts Payable		85
251	Mortgage Payable		1,800
301	Fund Balance		1,670
		$5,000	$5,000

The general ledger of Anycity Hospital at January 1, 1987, is reproduced in Figure 3-3. It contains an account for each classification listed in the chart of accounts previously illustrated in Figure 3-1. The account balances in the ledger are those shown in the above trial balance. Each of these opening balances is labeled OB so that they may subsequently be distinguished from later postings of transaction entries.

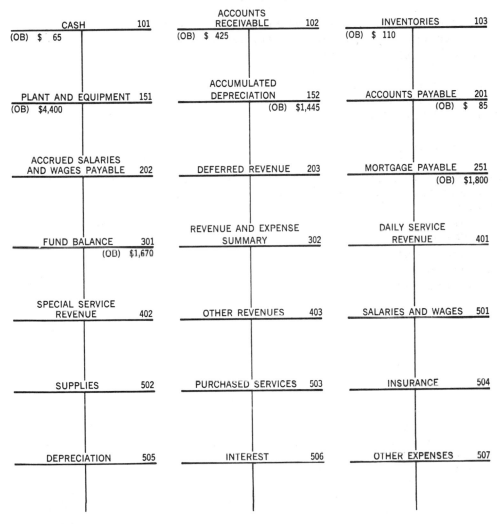

Figure 3-3.
Anycity Hospital
General Ledger
January 1, 1987

Journalizing Transaction Entries

During 1987 Anycity Hospital enters into numerous transactions involving the rendering of services to patients, the purchase and use of supplies, cash receipts, cash disbursements, and other activity. The initial step in the accounting cycle is to analyze these transactions and events, measure their effects on the accounts established in the chart of accounts, and record those effects in the journal. It is assumed that a general journal is used to record all transactions. The assumed transactions, mostly in summary form, are described here, and the required journal entries are illustrated.

Provision of Patient Services. In 1987 Anycity Hospital provided services to patients who were charged at the hospital's established rates:

Daily Services	$1,700
Special Services	1,300
Total	$3,000

Daily services consist of room, meals, and regular nursing care. Special services include laboratory, pharmacy, and radiology. The amounts are totals for the entire year as determined from census reports, charge tickets, and other documents. Adjustments and allowances are not considered here, nor are the usual classifications of revenue by type of patient, revenue center, etc. These and other relevant matters are dealt with in Chapter 7.

The journal entry to record the services described is one charging patients' accounts and crediting revenue accounts as follows:

JE #1

Accounts Receivable	102	$3,000	
Daily Service Revenue	401		$1,700
Special Service Revenue	402		1,300
To record services rendered to patients.			

Transactions of this type are generally recorded in a special journal typically called a revenue register, or revenue journal, and daily postings of charges are made to the patients' subsidiary ledger.

Purchases of Supplies. In 1987 Anycity Hospital purchased $350 of medical and surgical, dietary, and other supplies on account. These transactions are typically recorded in voucher registers, or purchases journals, as follows:

JE #2

Supplies Expense	502	$350	
Accounts Payable	201		$350
To record purchases of supplies.			

It is assumed here that supplies are accounted for under the periodic inventory method. Under the perpetual inventory system, the debit should instead be made to Inventories, the asset account. If the latter system were used, a second entry would be made periodically to debit Supplies Expense and credit Inventories for the cost of supplies requisitioned and used by the various hospital departments. These and related matters are discussed in Chapter 12.

Cash Receipts. The 1987 cash receipts of Anycity Hospital totaled $3,350 as summarized below:

Collections on Patients' Accounts	$2,750
Other Revenues	600
Total	$3,350

For the purposes of this illustration, it is assumed that all patient services are initially charged to Accounts Receivable. This, however, is usually not the case in actual practice where outpatient services are often accounted for on a cash basis.

The appropriate journal entry for the above cash receipts generally is made in a cash receipts journal as follows:

JE #3

Cash	101	$3,350	
Accounts Receivable	102		$2,750
Other Revenues	403		600
To record cash receipts.			

As noted earlier, differences between gross charges and collectible amounts are not considered here. The "other revenues" are assumed to consist of general contributions, grants, and gifts. These and related matters are discussed in detail in Chapters 7, 10 and 11.

Payments on Accounts Payable. Payments made on accounts payable during 1987 amounted to $360. The journal entry generally made in a check register is as follows:

JE #4

Accounts Payable	201	$360	
Cash	101		$360
To record payments on accounts payable.			

It is assumed in this illustration that Accounts Payable consist only of accounts with suppliers. All other expenses are recorded as paid. Details of accounting for current payables are covered in Chapter 13.

Payment on Mortgage. In 1987, Anycity Hospital made payments of $392 on its mortgage liability, of which $92 represented payment of interest. The entry is made as shown below:

JE #5

Mortgage Payable	251	$300	
Interest Expense	506	92	
Cash	101		$392
To record payments on mortgage.			

In addition to mortgages, hospitals may also have long-term debt in the form of bonds. Chapter 17 provides a detailed discussion of this topic.

Payment of Operating Expenses. Cash disbursements in 1987 for various operating expenses were $2,535. Internal control systems usually require that expenses be vouchered prior to payment (see Chapter 5). The entry shown here, however, bypasses this procedure for reasons of simplicity. Instead of debiting expenses and crediting liability accounts in an initial entry and then debiting the liability accounts and crediting cash in a second entry, a single entry is made to record the expense directly as follows:

JE #6

Salaries and Wages Expense	501	$1,900
Purchased Services Expense	503	385
Insurance Expense	504	120
Other Expenses	507	130
Cash	101	$2,535
To record disbursements for expenses.		

Again, the circumstances are greatly simplified, particularly with respect to salaries and wages where payroll taxes are a complicating factor. Payroll accounting is treated at length in Chapter 8; accounting for purchased services and supplies in Chapter 8; accounting for cash disbursements in Chapter 10.

    Summary of Transaction Entries. The six transaction entries for the 1987 economic activity of Anycity Hospital are summarized in Figure 3-4. The entries are numbered, rather than dated, to facilitate their referencing to the general ledger. These summary entries are representative of the thousands of individual transaction entries normally processed in the course of an accounting period.

Figure 3-4.
Anycity Hospital
General Journal
(1987 Transaction Entries)

JE No.	Accounts and Explanations	Acct. No.	Debit	Credit
1	Accounts Receivable	102	$3,000	
	Daily Service Revenue	401		$1,700
	Special Service Revenue	402		1,300
	To record services rendered to patients.			
2	Supplies Expense	502	$ 350	
	Accounts Payable	201		$ 350
	To record purchases of supplies.			
3	Cash	101	$3,350	
	Accounts Receivable	102		$2,750
	Other Revenues	403		600
	To record cash receipts.			
4	Accounts Payable	201	$ 360	
	Cash	101		$ 360
	To record payments on accounts payable.			
5	Mortgage Payable	251	$ 300	
	Interest Expense	506	92	
	Cash	101		$ 392
	To record payments on mortgage.			
6	Salaries and Wages Expense	501	$1,900	
	Purchased Services Expense	503	385	
	Insurance Expense	504	120	
	Other Expenses	507	130	
	Cash	101		$2,535
	To record disbursements for expenses.			

Posting Transaction Entries

In order to obtain the December 31, 1987, balance of each account maintained by Anycity Hospital, the transaction entries must be posted from the journal to the ledger. These debit and credit postings, when combined with the January 1, 1987, balances already in the ledger, produce tentative (before adjustments) balances at year-end as shown in Figure 3-5. Postings of transaction entries are identified by journal entry number.

Figure 3-5.
Anycity Hospital
General Ledger
(With Postings of 1987 Transaction Entries)

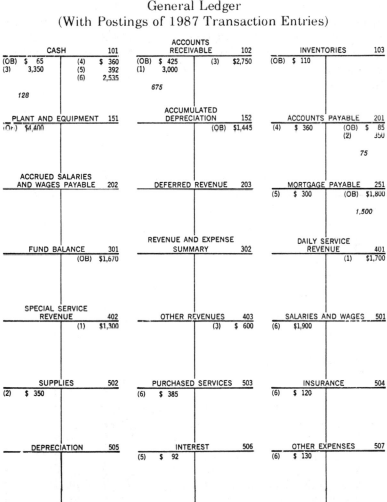

Adjusting the Accounts

The necessary division of the economic life of the hospital into time segments of arbitrary length creates a number of accounting problems. At regular intervals, a summary must be made of the effects of transactions in terms of an enterprise's operating results and financial position. Difficult measurement and reporting problems arise in the preparation of these periodic financial summaries. Particular attention must be given to the inclusion on an accrual basis of all transactions of the period and to the exclusion of all transactions that relate to other periods. Interperiod allocations of revenues and expenses on systematic and rational bases are critical. These allocations have a significant impact on reported financial position as well as a direct effect on the determination of net income or loss for each period.

The **summarizing phase** of the accounting process begins with a trial balance of the ledger accounts after all transaction entries have been posted and updated balances have been determined. Such a trial balance is illustrated for Anycity Hospital in Figure 3-6.

Figure 3-6.
Anycity Hospital
Preadjusting Trial Balance
December 31, 1987

Acct. No.		Dr.	Cr.
101	Cash	$ 128	
102	Accounts Receivable	675	
103	Inventories	110	
151	Plant and Equipment	4,400	
152	Accumulated Depreciation		$1,445
201	Accounts Payable		75
202	Accrued Salaries and Wages Payable		...
203	Deferred Revenue		...
251	Mortgage Payable		1,500
301	Fund Balance		1,670
302	Revenue and Expense Summary		...
401	Daily Service Revenue		1,700
402	Special Service Revenue		1,300
403	Other Revenues		600
501	Salaries and Wages	1,900	
502	Supplies	350	
503	Purchased Services	385	
504	Insurance	120	
505	Depreciation	...	
506	Interest	92	
507	Other Expenses	130	
		$8,290	$8,290

A second step is the examination of the account balances in the trial balance to determine whether or not such balances are properly stated. Many of the accounts usually require adjustments of one kind or another. Typically, adjustments are needed for (1) prepaid and accrued expense, (2) deferred and accrued revenue, (3) depreciation, (4) inventories, (5) uncollectible accounts, and (6) various other matters, including the correction of errors discovered in the transaction entries. Only a sample of these adjustments is illustrated here.

Prepaid and Accrued Expense. A prepaid expense situation arises when, in the current period, payment is made of an expense that relates to a future accounting period. A good example is the prepayment of premiums on fire insurance policies. At the time paid, such premiums may be debited to Prepaid Insurance (an asset account) or to Insurance Expense. In either event, the account that is debited will be overstated at the end of the accounting period, and an adjustment becomes necessary. It is assumed that no adjustment of this kind is needed for Anycity Hospital.

Accrued expense, on the other hand, relates to situations where expense has been incurred in the current period but has not been paid or recorded. Assume, for instance, that Anycity Hospital employees have earned $220 of salaries and wages for which they have not been paid and for which no entry has been made to recognize the hospital expense. The appropriate adjusting entry is:

JE #7

Salaries and Wages Expense	501	$220	
Accrued Salaries and Wages Payable	202		$220
To record accrued payroll.			

This situation arises when the end of a payroll period does not coincide with the end of the reporting period. Accruals of this kind should also take into account the hospital's share of FICA taxes. Matters relating to payroll accounting are discussed fully in Chapters 8 and 13.

Deferred and Accrued Revenue. At the end of an accounting period, certain revenue accounts may be overstated in that amounts received and recorded as revenue in the routine recording procedure may properly relate to future accounting periods. Assume, for example, that the $600 of other revenues recorded earlier includes a $90 grant restricted by the donor to a particular operating purpose that will not be carried out until 1988. Clearly, the $90 grant is not 1987 revenue, even though it has been received in cash. The following adjusting entry therefore must be made:

JE #8

Other Revenues	403	$90	
Deferred Revenue	203		$90
To reclassify grant as deferred revenue.			

If at the date of receipt it was known that the grant was properly deferrable to 1988, the transaction entry might have credited the Deferred Revenue account so that no adjustment would be necessary. Accounting for grants and other donor-restricted resources is treated in Chapter 7.

Depreciation. Depreciation adjustments, like all adjustments noted here, should be made monthly for interim reporting purposes. The illustration in this chapter, however, is framed in terms of annual adjustments. Assuming, then, that the 1987 depreciation expense for Anycity Hospital is $310, the required adjustment at December 31, 1987, is:

JE #9

Depreciation Expense	505	$310	
Accumulated Depreciation	152		$310
To record depreciation for 1987.			

The amount recorded as depreciation expense may be determined by any of several systematic and rational methods. These methods and other matters relating to plant assets and depreciation are discussed in Chapter 16.

Other Adjustments. Assuming that the December 31, 1987, supplies inventory is determined to be $125, the appropriate adjustment would be:

JE #10

Inventories	103	$15	
Supplies Expense	502		$15
To record increase in supplies inventory ($125 - $110).			

The assumption, as noted before, is that Anycity Hospital employs the periodic inventory method in accounting for all supplies. The $125 valuation was obtained on the basis of a physical count and the use of an appropriate costing procedure (see Chapter 12). As a result, the ledger balance for Inventories required an upward adjustment of $15.

Summary of Adjusting Entries. Ordinarily, many other types of adjustments are required. Bank reconciliations give rise to adjustments for returned checks, service charges, and previously undetected errors. Accruals often must be made for interest income earned but not yet received on investments and for interest expense on notes, mortgages, and bond obligations. Reconciliation of subsidiary ledgers of receivables and payables may also indicate needed adjustments. While none of these are illustrated here, they do appear in subsequent chapters of this book.

The December 31, 1987, adjusting entries of Anycity Hospital are summarized in Figure 3-7. Before these entries are journalized in this way, they might have been determined and informally recorded in so-called working papers, or worksheets. Such worksheets are supplementary records developed to facilitate the adjustment and summarization process. A **general worksheet**, for example, may be prepared on which all the adjustments are brought together and an adjusted trial balance is prepared. In such cases, the financial statements often can be prepared directly from the worksheet. (Illustrations of worksheets can be found in the author's **Introduction to Hospital Accounting**.)

After the adjusting entries are recorded in the journal, they are posted to the general ledger. These postings are included in Figure 3-8. At this point, the adjusted balance of each ledger account is determined. If desired, an adjusted or preclosing trial balance may be prepared to ascertain that the ledger balances. No illustration is provided here; it is assumed that the financial statement data are drawn directly from the general ledger accounts.

Figure 3-7.
Anycity Hospital
General Journal
(1987 Adjusting Entries)

JE No.	Accounts and Explanations	Acct. No.	Debit	Credit
7	Salaries and Wages Expense Accrued Salaries and Wages Payable To record accrued payroll.	501 202	$ 220	 $ 220
8	Other Revenues Deferred Revenue To reclassify grant as deferred revenue.	403 203	$ 90	 $ 90
9	Depreciation Expense Accumulated Depreciation To record depreciation for 1975.	505 152	$ 310	 $ 310
10	Inventories Supplies Expense To record increase in supplies inventory	103 502	$ 15	 $ 15

Preparation of Financial Statements

When all the foregoing operations are completed, financial statements can be prepared from the information generated by the process. Two financial statements are illustrated for Anycity Hospital. Figure 3-9 is an income statement and a statement of changes in fund balances in combined form. Figure 3-10 is the December 31, 1987, balance sheet. The usefulness of these illustrations is somewhat limited by the simplifications made in the preceding discussion, but realistic and detailed examples of financial statements are presented in Chapters 19, 20, and 21.

Closing the Books

The final set of procedures in the accounting cycle are those by which the books are **closed** and made ready for the next accounting period when the cycle will begin anew. In closing the books, the objective is to remove all balances from the ledger except those to be carried over into the next accounting period. The accounts carried over, and not eliminated from the ledger, are referred to as **real** or **permanent** accounts; they are the accounts that appear in the balance sheet, i.e., assets, liabilities, and fund balances. All other accounts are called **nominal** or **temporary** accounts, and their balances are removed from the ledger by **closing entries.** If this were not done, there would be some danger of confusing the nominal account balances of one year with those of another, and the determination of operating results in future periods might be impaired. The closing process is also a means of recording the net income or loss for the year in the general ledger fund balance account.

Figure 3-8.
Anycity Hospital
General Ledger
(With Postings of 1987 Adjusting Entries)

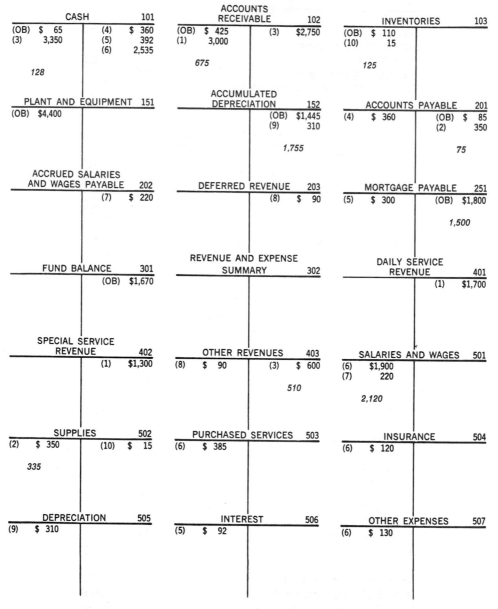

Figure 3-9.
Anycity Hospital
Statement of Income and Changes in Fund Balance
Year Ended December 31, 1987

Assets

Cash		$ 128
Accounts Receivable		675
Inventories		125
Plant and Equipment	$4,400	
Less Accumulated Depreciation	1,755	2,645
Total Assets		$3,573

Liabilities and Fund Balance

Accounts Payable		$ 75
Accrued Salaries and Wages Payable		220
Deferred Revenue		90
Mortgage Payable		1,500
Total Liabilities		1,885
Fund Balance		1,688
Total Liabilities and Fund Balance		$3,573

Figure 3-10.
Anycity Hospital
Balance Sheet
December 31, 1987

Revenues:		
Daily Patient Services	$1,700	
Special Patient Services	1,300	
Other Revenues	510	
Total Revenues		$3,510
Less Expenses:		
Salaries and Wages	$2,120	
Supplies	335	
Purchased Services	385	
Insurance	120	
Depreciation	310	
Interest	92	
Other Expenses	130	
Total Expenses		3,492
Net Income for the Year		18
Fund Balance, January 1		1,670
Fund Balance, December 31		$1,688

Closing entries for Anycity Hospital appear in Figure 3-11. In the closing process, a summary account is used to accumulate the totals of revenues and expenses as those accounts are eliminated from the ledger. A final entry is made to close the summary account and transfer the net income to the fund balance.

Figure 3-11.
Anycity Hospital
General Journal
(1987 Closing Entries)

JE No.	Accounts and Explanations	Acct. No.	Debit	Credit
11	Daily Service Revenue	401	$1,700	
	Special Service Revenue	402	1,300	
	Other Revenues	403	510	
	Revenue and Expense Summary	302		$3,510
	To close revenue accounts.			
12	Revenue and Expense Summary	302	$3,492	
	Salaries and Wages	501		$2,120
	Supplies	502		335
	Purchased Services	503		385
	Insurance	504		120
	Depreciation	505		310
	Interest	506		92
	Other Expenses	507		130
	To close expense accounts.			
13	Revenue and Expense Summary	302	$ 18	
	Fund Balance	301		$ 18
	To close revenue and expense summary to fund balance.			

Once journalized, the closing entries are posted to the ledger. Figure 3-12 presents the general ledger accounts after these postings have been completed. At this point, the only accounts remaining with balances in the general ledger are the balance sheet accounts. These are the account balances to be carried over into the next accounting period. A postclosing trial balance (not shown here) may now be prepared to ascertain that the ledger remains in balance.

ACCOUNTING PROCEDURE SUMMARY

Figure 3-13 provides a summary of the successive steps involved in the accounting cycle, starting with transaction entries and concluding with the closing of the nominal accounts. The numbers are indicative of the general sequence in which the various procedures are performed.

Figure 3-12.
Anycity Hospital
General Ledger
(With Postings of 1987 Closing Entries)

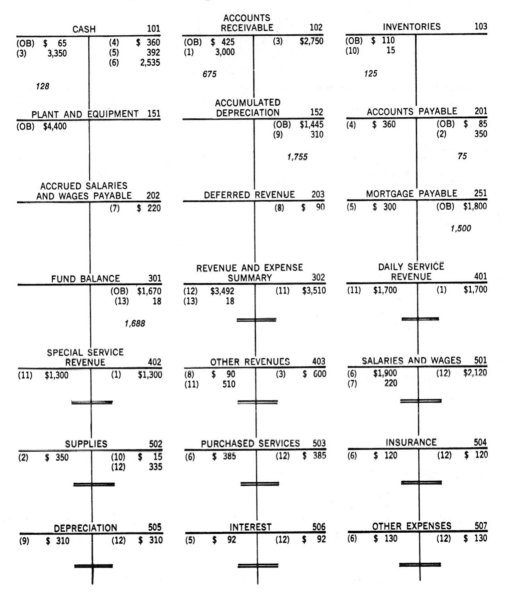

Figure 3-13.
Accounting Procedure Summary

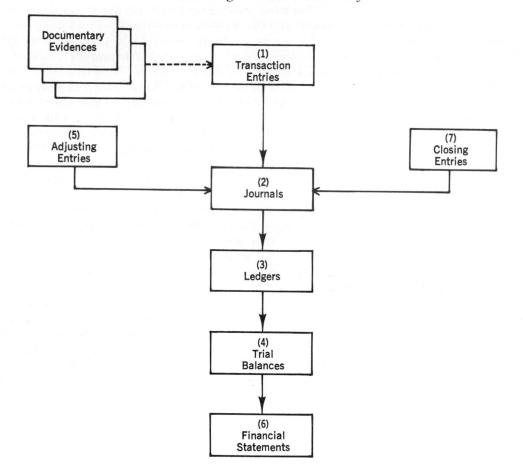

INTERIM FINANCIAL STATEMENTS

The illustration of the accounting cycle was presented in annual terms, assuming that the accounts were adjusted only at the end of the year and that only one set of financial statements was prepared for the entire period. In actual practice, of course, income statements and balance sheets are developed monthly and on a year-to-date basis as the accounting period unfolds. Other financial reports are often prepared weekly or even daily. These statements and reports are referred to as **interim statements and reports**. They relate to reporting periods of less than one year.

All the basic operations described in this chapter are performed on a monthly basis **except** for closing entries. Every month, transactions are journalized and posted, the accounts are adjusted, and financial statements are prepared. Closing entries, however, are journalized and posted only once each year at the end of each accounting period.

MECHANIZED AND ELECTRONIC DATA PROCESSING

The smaller hospital may find that an accounting system involving primarily manual operations is adequate for its needs. As the hospital grows in size and complexity, however, the increased volume of economic activity generally cannot be processed efficiently by manual means alone. Machines, such as posting and billing devices, may be added to the system to replace and supplement manual operations. These machines, using specially designed forms, often are able to prepare original documents and journal and ledger records in a single operation, as well as perform various arithmetic operations.

Larger hospitals find that their requirements for speed, accuracy, and a great amount of detailed information demand some form of electronic system involving magnetic tapes or disks. The computer utilized in these systems has the capability of processing, storing, and recalling vast quantities of data and of performing mathematical functions. Other machines in the system read the stored data and can print out selected information as required.

Despite the capabilities of mechanized and electronic equipment systems, highly skilled accountants are required. The computer cannot think for itself. It must be given explicit instructions for the performance of every operation. Although the accuracy of the computer's arithmetical functions can be assumed, the validity of its output data is totally dependent upon the instructions it receives. Special techniques must be employed to check and verify electronically produced data.

The discussion in this book is framed largely in terms of manual operations in that explanations and illustrations of procedures are more easily presented and comprehended when developed in that way. References are made at appropriate points, however, to machine applications, but the exact manner in which accounting procedures are carried out depends upon the degree of mechanization, the type of equipment, and other considerations. The underlying objectives, principles, and procedures of accounting are the same whether manual, mechanized, or computerized systems are used.

CHAPTER 3 FOOTNOTES

1. For a detailed treatment of basic accounting procedures, see the author's **Introduction to Hospital Accounting** (Chicago: Healthcare Financial Management Association, 1977).
2. Accounting Principles Board, **Statement No. 4** (New York: American Institute of Certified Public Accountants, 1970), pp. 68-69.

QUESTIONS

1. What are the eight basic operations involved in the accounting process?
2. State the rules of debit and credit for each of the following types of accounts:
    1. Expenses
    2. Liabilities
    3. Revenue deductions
    4. Fund balances
    5. Assets
    6. Revenues
3. List the four basic elements of an accounting system.
4. Why does the accountant place great emphasis on documentary evidences?
5. What is a **chart of accounts**? Why are numerical codes assigned to each account listed in the chart? Who decides the design and content of a hospital's chart of accounts?
6. Define the terms **journal** and **ledger**. Name four different types of journals. Name four different types of ledgers.
7. List, in their usual sequence, the procedural steps involved in an accounting cycle.
8. What is the purpose of adjusting entries? Name five different situations for which adjustments usually are required.
9. What is meant by closing the books? Why are the books of a hospital "closed" each year? Briefly describe how a closing of the books is accomplished.
10. Distinguish between **real** and **nominal** accounts.
11. The administrator and governing board of Community Hospital are interested in participating in a central shared computer system rather than installing their own computer. The hospital is a private voluntary general hospital having 400 beds. The hospital has a very limited teaching program but is well diversified in its services. The other hospitals to be included in the system are a university teaching hospital of 700 beds, a city hospital of 800 beds, a 200-bed children's hospital, and another voluntary general hospital of 300 beds. The hospitals are located within a 20-mile radius in an area where seasonal climate presents problems in extreme weather conditions.

    You are asked to evaluate the advantages and disadvantages of entering into the central shared computer system. In addition, it is requested that you estimate the possible cost savings, if any, by joining the shared system as opposed to installing and operating one's own computer.
12. It has been determined that your hospital can no longer process the amount of data required in its business office and service department areas. You have been directed by your administrator to review and report on the feasibility of using data processing techniques to handle this processing workload.
    1. List at least four alternative sources for acquiring data processing service.
    2. What are the most important factors to consider in selecting an optimum approach?
13. Indicate whether the following statements are true or false. If false, explain why.
    1. The human being is the earliest and most integrated data processing system.

    2.   The central processor of a computer is made up of three major components: (1) control unit, (2) memory, and (3) arithmetic unit.

    3.   The term **data processing** encompasses all the operations from the collection of raw data to the final preparation of a meaningful report.

    4.   Memory is the processing device of an electronic data processing system.

14.   The local 350-bed hospital has been using conventional equipment for its accounting requirements. The administrator has requested you to evaluate the feasibility of an integrated data processing system. Outline your approach to this project.

15.   List the principal accounting records that would be used in a general hospital of 90 beds. The hospital participates in the Medicare program.

16.   What are **interim financial statements**?

17.   Distinguish between the general ledger and a subsidiary ledger.

EXERCISES

E1.   Stonecity Hospital completed the following transactions during 1987:

    1.   Services provided to patients who were charged at the hospital's full established rates as follows:

Daily services	$12,400
Special services	9,200
	$21,600

    2.   Purchases of supplies on account, $5,500.

    3.   Cash receipts:

Collections on patients' accounts	$20,300
Other revenues	1,400
	$21,700

    4.   Payments on accounts payable, $5,100.

    5.   Cash disbursements for operating expenses:

Salaries and wages	$13,600
Purchased services	800
Insurance	300
Other expenses	200
	$14,900

    6.   Payment on mortgage:

Principal	$ 5,000
Interest	2,100
	$ 7,100

7.   Purchase of new equipment for $1,500 cash.

Required. Using the classification of accounts provided in Figure 3-3, prepare entries in general journal form to record all the above transactions.

E2.   Refer to the data given in Exercise 1. Assume the following general ledger balances at January 1, 1987:

Cash	$ 14,800	
Accounts receivable	36,000	
Inventories	4,000	
Plant and equipment	245,200	
Accumulated depreciation		$ 94,000
Accounts payable		6,000
Mortgage payable		120,000
Fund balance		80,000
	$300,000	$300,000

Required. (1) Enter the January 1, 1987, balances in general ledger accounts. (2) Post the journal entries of Exercise 1 to the ledger accounts. (3) Prepare a trial balance of the general ledger accounts at December 31, 1987.

E3.   Rockcity Hospital's general ledger reflects the following balances at December 31, 1987:

Mortgage payable	$ 1,600
Accounts receivable	800
Special service revenue	1,400
Purchased services	380
Cash	190
Interest expense	100
Plant and equipment	5,000
Accounts payable	92
Salaries and wages expense	1,950
Other revenues	700
Deferred revenue	65
Insurance expense	110
Accumulated depreciation	1,606
Supplies expense	430
Daily service revenue	1,848
Inventories	120
Depreciation expense	49
Accrued salaries and wages payable	77
Other expenses	88
Fund balance	?

Required. Prepare closing entries in general journal form.

E4. Refer to the information given in Exercise 3.

Required. Prepare (1) a statement of income and changes in fund balance for 1987 and (2) a balance sheet at December 31, 1987.

E5. Newcity Hospital's general ledger at December 31, 1987, reflects the following preadjusted balances, among others:

Accrued interest receivable	$ ...
Allowance for bad debts	400 (dr.)
Prepaid insurance	1,900
Plant and equipment	12,000
Accumulated depreciation	3,500
Inventories	800
Accrued payroll	...
Deferred rental income	600
Accounts receivable	7,500

The hospital, which closes its books annually on December 31 and makes adjusting entries annually at the same date, provides you with the following additional information:

1. Accrued interest receivable at December 31, 1987, is $350.
2. The credit manager estimates that 12 percent of the December 31, 1987, accounts receivable will prove to be uncollectible. 12% × 7,500 = 900.
3. Prepaid insurance at December 31, 1987, is $1,160.
4. Depreciation expense is computed at 10 percent per year. 12,000 × 10%
5. The inventory at December 31, 1987, is $650 by actual count.
6. Unpaid salaries and wages at December 31, 1987, amount to $740.
7. The deferred rental income represents a one-year rental received in advance on September 1, 1987.

Required. Prepare the necessary adjusting entries in general ledger form.

E6. On an answer sheet, write the numbers 1 to 8. Next to each number indicate the letter of your answer choice for each of the following items. Consider each statement separately; they are not related.

86 8788

1. Cade Hospital paid a three-year fire insurance premium in advance on September 1, 1986. The hospital's preadjusted ledger balance of prepaid insurance at December 31, 1987, was $4,640. Cade Hospital adjusts its books annually on December 31 only, i.e., monthly adjustments are not made. The total premium paid on September 1, 1986, must have been

   a. $5,220
   b. $6,960
   c. $9,280
   d. $13,920
   e. Some other amount.

Total was 6960
4640 ÷ 24 = 193 × 3 mo 588
4640 + 579 =

2. Cascade Hospital received two years' rent in advance on May 1, 1986. The hospital's preadjusted ledger balance of deferred rental income at December 31, 1987, was $3,500. Cascade Hospital adjusts its books annually on December 31 only, i.e., monthly adjustments are not made. In its 1987 income statement, Cascade Hospital should report rental income of

    a. $1,750
    b. $2,100
    c. $2,917
    d. $2,625
    e. Some other amount.

    (handwritten: 16÷3500=218.75 x 12 mos.)

3. Curtis Hospital had accounts receivable of $481 at January 1, 1987, and $533 at December 31, 1987. During 1987, $2,735 were collected on account from patients and $39 of uncollectible accounts were written off as bad debts. In its 1976 income statement, Curtis Hospital will show revenues of

    a. $2,722
    b. $2,826
    c. $2,761
    d. $2,865
    e. Some other amount.

    (handwritten: 481 − 533; 52 + 2735 + 39 = 2826)

4. Fall Hospital reported a net income of $500 in 1986 and $600 in 1987. The hospital, however, overlooked and failed to record adjusting entries for accrued interest income as follows:

    | 12/31/86 | $45 |
    | 12/31/87 | 37 |

    The correct net income for 1987 is

    a. $592
    b. $608
    c. $637
    d. $645
    e. Some other amount.

    (handwritten: 600 + 45 + 37 = 592)

5. Fox Hospital reported a net income of $700 in 1986 and $900 in 1987. Adjusting entries for accrued wages payable, however, were overlooked and not recorded as follows:

    | 12/31/86 | $22 |
    | 12/31/87 | 26 |

    The correct 1987 net income is

    a. $904
    b. $864

    (handwritten: 900 + 22 − 26 = 896)

c. $896

d. $922

e. Some other amount.

6. Francis Hospital reported a net income of $300 in 1986 and $400 in 1987. The hospital, however, made errors in recording year-end inventories as follows:

| 12/31/86 | Inventory overstated by $50 |
| 12/31/87 | Inventory understated by $75 |

The correct 1987 net income is

a. $475

b. $525

c. $425

d. $375

e. Some other amount.

7. Kleiser Hospital made cash payments totaling $233 for operating expenses during 1987. Its balance sheets provide the following information:

	12/31/86	12/31/87
Prepaid operating expenses	$ 14	$ 17
Accrued operating expenses payable	11	9

In its 1987 income statement, Kleiser Hospital should report operating expenses of

a. $228

b. $225

c. $234

d. $232

e. Some other amount.

8. Hand Hospital purchased an item of equipment on July 1, 1984. The equipment has a 20 percent salvage value and an estimated useful life of 12 years. At December 31, 1987, accumulated depreciation on this equipment totaled $1,750, after adjustments. This equipment must have been acquired at a cost of

a. $6,000

b. $15,000

c. $7,500

d. $12,000

e. Some other amount.

PROBLEMS

P1.   Bicity Hospital's trial balance at January 1, 1987, is provided below:

	Dr.	Cr.
Cash	$ 102	
Accounts receivable	510	
Inventories	130	
Plant and equipment	5,258	
Accumulated depreciation		$1,260
Accounts payable		72
Mortgage payable		1,500
Fund balance		3,168
	$6,000	$6,000

The hospital completed the following transactions during 1987:

1. Services rendered to patients who were charged at the hospital's full established rates as follows:

Daily services	$1,735
Special services	1,329

2. Supplies purchased on account $346.

3. Cash receipts from patients:

Collections on account	$2,785
Other revenues	677

4. Payments on accounts payable, $356.

5. Payment on mortgage:

Principal	$ 350
Interest	84

6. Payment of other operating expenses:

Salaries and wages	$1,923
Purchased services	391
Insurance	122
Other expenses	106

Adjustment information:

7. Accrued payroll at December 31, 1987, $231.

8. Deferred revenue at December 31, 1987, $82.

9. Depreciation expense for 1987, $325.

10. Inventory at December 31, 1987, $180.

Required. Using the chart of accounts indicated in Figure 3-3, complete all steps in the accounting cycle for 1987.

P2.   Following is a chart of accounts for Tricity Hospital:

101 Cash	301 Fund Balance
102 Accounts Receivable	302 Revenue and Expense Summary
103 Inventory	401 Daily Service Revenue
104 Land	402 Special Service Revenue
105 Buildings and Equipment	501 Salaries and Wages
106 Accumulated Depreciation	502 Supplies and Expense
201 Accounts Payable	503 Depreciation

Tricity decided to build a hospital, and for this purpose an appropriation of $510,000 was made available from city resources as permanent hospital capital. During 1987, the first year of operations, the following summarized transactions were completed:

1. A board of trustees was established, and $510,000 was received from the city. The money was deposited in a bankchecking account opened in the name of Tricity Hospital.

2. Land, suitable for a building site, was acquired at a cost of $10,000.

3. A hospital building was constructed and completely equipped at a total cost of $450,000.

4. Supplies were purchased on account for $45,000.

5. Charges to patients for services rendered:

Daily services	$128,000
Special services	112,000

6. Cash collections on patients' accounts totaled $222,000.

7. Payments of employees' salaries and wages, $170,000.

8. Cash disbursements for other expenses, $44,000.

9. Payments on accounts payable, $37,000.

Adjustment information:

10. Depreciation expense for 1987 is $10,000.

11. The inventory at December 31, 1987, is $5,000.

Required. Complete all steps in the accounting cycle for 1987.

P3.   The following is Tricity Hospital's general ledger trial balance at December 31, 1988, after closing.

	Dr.	Cr.
Cash	$ 21,000	
Accounts receivable	18,000	
Inventory	5,000	
Land	10,000	
Building and Equipment	450,000	
Accumulated depreciation		$ 10,000
Accounts payable		8,000
Fund balance		486,000
	$504,000	$504,000

Transactions completed by Tricity Hospital during 1988 were:

1. Supplies purchased on account, $50,000.

2. Charges to patients for services rendered:

Daily services	$146,000
Special services	140,000

3. Cash collections on patients' accounts, $275,000.

4. Payment of employees' salaries and wages, $190,000.

5. Cash disbursements for other expenses, $41,000.

6. Payments on accounts payable, $52,000.

7. Purchase of new equipment, $4,000.

Adjustment information:

8. Depreciation for 1988, $10,400.

9. The inventory at December 31, 1988, is $12,000.

Required. Complete all steps in the accounting cycle for 1988.

P4.   Community Hospital has kept its books on the cash basis. The following income
statement was prepared for the year ended September 30, 1988:

Cash received from patients		$210,000
Less cash disbursements for expenses:		
Salaries and wages	$104,000	
Supplies	75,000	
Depreciation transferred to plant		
replacement and expansion fund	2,000	
Other expenses	3,000	184,000
Net income for the year		$ 26,000

An analysis of the unrestricted fund accounts and other data revealed the
following information:

1. Balances, 10/1/87:

Cash	$ 20,000
Accounts receivable	75,000
Inventory	15,000
Prepaid expense	2,500
Plant and equipment	200,000
Accumulated depreciation	61,500
Accounts payable	4,000
Accrued salaries and wages	1,500
Due to plant replacement and	
expansion fund	2,000

2. Balances, 9/30/88:

Inventory	$ 25,000
Prepaid expense	1,500
Accounts payable	9,000
Accrued salaries and wages	6,000
Due to plant replacement and	
expansion fund	2,000
Revenue from daily service:	
Inpatients	120,000
Outpatients	10,000
Revenue from special service	70,000
Uncollectible accounts	
receivable	5,000

Required. Prepare financial statements for the year ended September 30, 1988,
on the accrual basis of accounting.

4

Fund Accounting, Chart of Accounts, and Statistics

Widespread employment of fund accounting by not-for-profit, voluntary hospitals is one of the most unique general characteristic of hospital accounting as compared with accounting for profit-seeking industrial enterprises. For this reason, a primary objective of the present chapter is to examine the broad concepts and procedures of fund accounting so as to provide a foundation for the detailed discussions in subsequent chapters. Fund accounting can become rather complex, and it is essential that the reader first obtain a general view of the overall aspects of the system. What is fund accounting? Why is it unique to nonprofit enterprises? What types of funds do hospitals typically maintain? How are interfund transactions recorded? What financial statement presentation problems does fund accounting create?

In addition to presenting the general framework of fund accounting, this chapter also addresses itself to the design and content of an appropriate chart of accounts for hospitals. There has been a continuing effort, spanning more than 60 years, toward the achievement of a reasonable degree of uniformity among hospitals in the manner by which financial and statistical data are accumulated and communicated. If the desired degree of consistency and comparability is to be obtained within the hospital industry, basic agreements must be reached as to the design of charts of accounts and as to definitions of hospital statistical terms. While rigid uniformity is neither desirable nor apparently possible, a higher standard of comparability than exists at present in the reported data of hospital enterprises has been a major goal of the industry.

FUND ACCOUNTING

Besides the resources directly generated from charges made for healthcare and related services provided to patients and others, hospitals also receive gifts, grants, and endowments. A portion of these resources are available, at the discretion of the governing board, for the financing of the general day-to-day operating activities of the hospital. Other hospital resources are donor-restricted to specific uses and purposes such as construction, equipment, research, charity work, and education. Some donors may permit the expenditure and eventual exhaustion of the principal amount of resources contributed by them. Other donors, however, often stipulate that the principal amount of resources given in trust to be kept intact through investment, with only the income therefrom to be expended. Aside from the legal and moral obligation to strictly observe such restrictions, an administrative or managerial need arises to maintain in the accounting records a precise distinction between **unrestricted** and **restricted** resources. A hospital's management, in making financing and investing decisions, must have information as to those resources available for general operating requirements and those which are not so available but whose use is limited to particular donor-restricted purposes. Otherwise, unauthorized and even illegal use might be made of hospital resources. Furthermore, donors often require an accounting from the hospital for its use of resources provided by them as restricted endowments and gifts.

The system of accounting known as **fund accounting** evolved in response to these stewardship and accountability needs. Some may argue that fund accounting unduly complicates the accounting and reporting process and that the same objectives can be accomplished more easily by other means. While there might be some truth in this position, fund accounting is a firmly entrenched, generally accepted accounting practice in the hospital industry and is likely to remain so. It is the common sense answer to an accounting and reporting problem unique to not-for-profit organizations. Accountants, however, must continue in their efforts to make financial statements drawn from records maintained on a fund accounting basis more intelligible to users. Special attention must be given to disclosure of restrictions on resources and to clear presentations of interfund activity.

Nature of Fund Accounting

Fund accounting may be described as a system of accounting in which the economic resources and related obligations of a hospital are segregated in the accounting records into self-balancing sets of accounts regarded as independent fiscal and accounting entities, called **funds**, for the purpose of carrying on specific activities and attaining particular objectives in accordance with legal and other restrictions or limitations. Perhaps the nature of fund accounting can be best explained with a brief illustration.

Assume that Simple Hospital has $900 of assets and $500 of liabilities. The excess of assets over liabilities (owners' equity, capital, or fund balances) therefore is $400. A balance sheet might be prepared for Simple Hospital as shown in Figure 4-1.

Figure 4-1.
Simple Hospital
Balance Sheet
December 31, 1987

Assets	$900
Liabilities	$500
Owners' Equity	400
Total Liabilities and Owners' Equity	$900

Such a balance sheet, however, could be quite misleading as to the financial position of Simple Hospital if (1) there are legal restrictions on the hospital's use of certain assets and (2) creditors' claims therefore may be satisfied only from particular groups of assets. Assuming this to be the case, a revised balance sheet for Simple Hospital is presented in Figure 4-2 as it would appear in accordance with the concept of fund accounting.

Figure 4-2.
Simple Hospital
Balance Sheet
December 31, 1987

	Unrestricted Fund	Restricted Funds		Total All Funds
		Fund A	Fund B	
Assets	$475	$270	$155	$900
Liabilities	$425	$ 55	$ 20	$500
Fund Balances	50	215	135	400
	$475	$270	$155	$900

The revised balance sheet provides a different impression of Simple hospital's financial position! Of the $900 of total assets, only $475 are not restricted and therefore available at the discretion of the governing board for general operating purposes. Creditors' claims against these assets amount to $425, leaving an uncomfortably small excess of assets over liabilities: the fund balance of $50.

Hospital assets that are donor-restricted are presented as **restricted funds**. Fund A, for example, might be an Endowment Fund whose principal amount may not be expended. (Income from Endowment Fund investments may or may not be available to the Unrestricted Fund.) There are only $55 of liabilities to be paid from the assets of this fund, and there is a sizable fund balance ($215).

Fund B includes the remaining $155 of Simple Hospital assets. The use of these assets is also limited by donor's stipulations. This restricted fund could be, for instance, a Plant Replacement and Expansion Fund whose resources may be used only to acquire new property and equipment. The liabilities of this fund are $20, and the fund balance therefore is $135.

The total column in Figure 4-2, then, has no particular significance and might be misinterpreted by the reader. Totaling all hospital assets and liabilities is about as meaningful as adding together the assets and liabilities of General Motors Corporation and the State of Mississippi. Note that such totals are not shown in the more complex balance sheet illustrated in Figure 4-5.

Thus, in fund accounting, assets and related liabilities are segregated into unrestricted and restricted funds depending upon the existence of donor restrictions. Restricted resources, as will be seen, are further categorized according to the major types of restrictions externally imposed. Observe that each fund, unrestricted and restricted, consists of self-balancing accounts. In each fund, debits (assets) equal credits (liabilities and fund balance). This equality is maintained throughout all operations in the accounting process.

A condensed income statement for Simple Hospital is presented in Figure 4-3. It reflects the results of operations for the period with respect to general hospital operating activities financed primarily from unrestricted funds. The statement includes all unrestricted revenues of Simple Hospital and all expenses either directly associated with such revenues or otherwise allocated to the 1987 accounting period as expired general operating costs. (For an explanation of this principle, see Chapter 2.)

Figure 4-3.
Simple Hospital
Income Statement
Year Ended December 31, 1987

Operating Revenues	$800
Less Operating Expenses	796
Operating Income	4
Nonoperating Revenue	21
Net Income for the Year	$ 25

Restricted revenues and related expenses (if any) are recorded in the appropriate restricted fund. If and when these revenues become available for general operating purposes, they are reported as unrestricted fund revenues. Depending upon the circumstances, they may be classified as operating revenues or as nonoperating revenues. Certain revenues of restricted funds, however, may never be recognized as unrestricted fund revenues, although resources frequently are transferred to the unrestricted fund from restricted funds. The proper treatment of interfund resource transfers therefore is extremely important. This matter is governed by rather strict principles; it must not be left to the opinion of the individual accountant nor to the dictates of the governing board.

Because of the importance of interfund transactions, a statement of changes in fund balances is essential to a fair presentation of a hospital's operating results and financial position. The statement of Simple Hospital is presented in condensed form in Figure 4-4. (A more detailed illustration is given in Figure 4-7.)

Figure 4-4.
Simple Hospital
Statement of Changes in Fund Balances
Year Ended December 31, 1987

	Unrestricted Fund	Restricted Funds	
		Fund A	Fund B
Fund Balances, January 1	$ 7	$140	$ 90
Net Income for the Year	25		
Restricted Gifts Received		75	45
Restricted Income from Investments			18
Transfer from Unrestricted Fund to Fund B	(22)		22
Transfer from Fund B to Unrestricted Fund	40		(40)
Fund Balances, December 31	$ 50	$215	$135

The statement begins with the fund balances at the beginning of the year, and it concludes with the fund balances at the end of the year. In between are the changes that occurred during the period:

1. The net income for 1987, as indicated by Figure 4-3, is added to the Unrestricted Fund Balance.

2. Restricted gifts received are added to the appropriate fund balances. As noted earlier, the receipt of restricted resources is not treated as revenue of the Unrestricted Fund.

3. Restricted income from the investments of Fund B is added to the fund balance of that restricted fund. Had that income not been restricted, it would have appeared as revenue in Simple Hospital's income statement in Figure 4-3.

4. The nature of the interfund transfers is not indicated, but it should be. These transfers are shown here to make the point that not all resource transfers from restricted funds to the Unrestricted Fund are treated as Unrestricted Fund revenue, although that is the exception rather than the rule. Similarly, transfers in the other direction may not be treated as expenses of the Unrestricted Fund.

The reader may now have some appreciation of the difficult problems that arise in fund accounting, particularly with respect to recording and reporting interfund activity. Applicable general principles relating to these matters are provided in this chapter; detailed procedures are described in later sections of this book, particularly in Chapters 7, 15, and 16.

Types of Funds

In fund accounting as employed by hospitals, the two major categories of funds (unrestricted and restricted) are each divided into three parts, as follows:

1. Unrestricted Fund.
    a. Current Operating Accounts.
    b. Board-Designated Accounts.
    c. Plant Asset and Related Debt Accounts.
2. Restricted Funds.
    a. Specific Purpose Funds.
    b. Plant Replacement and Expansion Funds.
    c. Endowment Funds.

The use of the singular and plural in the above outline should be noted. There is one, and **only one**, Unrestricted Fund. Although it often is divided into the three parts indicated, its parts are **not** separate funds. They are groups of accounts, sometimes self-balancing by groups, established for accounting purposes. Although for internal hospital management purposes they may be referred to as funds, and even accounted for as such, they must be reported together as a single Unrestricted Fund. On the other hand, there generally are several different funds in the restricted category, and each of them is a distinctive entity to be separately accounted for and reported.

Unrestricted Fund

An Unrestricted Fund is common to the accounting system of all hospitals. This fund includes all hospital resources, with related obligations, not restricted to particular purposes by donors or any other external authority. All resources of this fund are available for general operating activities at the discretion of the hospital's governing board. In addition, the accounts of the Unrestricted Fund include all of the revenues and expenses that are reported in the hospital's income statement.

To repeat, there is but one Unrestricted Fund in terms of external financial reporting by hospitals. This fund, however, may be divided into three parts or groups for internal accounting and reporting purposes. Each account group, in fact, may be self-balancing and accounted for as a separate fund, i.e., current operating fund, board-designated fund, and plant fund. This practice has little or no value for external financial reporting purposes and is generally undesirable due to the mechanical problems it creates. Most of the discussion in this book assumes that the Unrestricted Fund accounts are not maintained by groups on an individually self-balancing or fund basis.

Current Operating Accounts. The current operating accounts of the Unrestricted Fund include unrestricted current resources such as cash, receivables, inventories, and prepaid expenses. Current obligations to be discharged by the use of such resources are also included. The liabilities consist of short-term notes and accounts payable, accrued expenses payable, withheld payroll taxes, and similar accounts. The difference between these current assets and liabilities is the unrestricted working capital of the hospital.

The operating accounts are also comprised of revenue and expense classifications in which the general operating results of the hospital are recorded. The revenue classification includes (1) patient service revenues, (2) other operating revenues, (3) revenue deductions, and (4) nonoperating revenues. The expenses are classified as (1) operating expenses and (2) nonoperating expenses, although the latter category usually is netted against nonoperating revenues. Each of these broad categories of revenue and expense, as subsequently illustrated, is broken down into specific accounts organized principally by responsibility centers within the hospital.

Before continuing with this discussion, the reader will find it helpful to examine Figures 4-5, 4-6 and 4-7, which present a fairly detailed and realistic set of financial statements for a hypothetical hospital. Additional illustrations and discussion of hospital financial statements are in Chapters 19, 20, and 21.

Board-Designated Accounts. Hospital governing boards at times may choose to designate or earmark certain otherwise unrestricted resources for various reasons. As a result, the accountant may establish special board-designated cash and investment accounts in an effort to assist financial managers in using certain resources in accordance with the board's wishes. These accounts may be set up in a board-created "fund" that is self-balancing. Where this is done, such resources are not to be reported as a part of the restricted funds of the hospital.

Properly, the term **restricted** should be applied only to arm's length restrictions established by resource donors and other external authorities. The term should **not** be used in references to resources set aside by action of the governing board for whatever purpose. Such appropriations of otherwise generally available resources must be accounted for and reported as a part of the Unrestricted Fund; they should not be comingled with donor-restricted funds. The point to be made is that so-called board-designated funds carry no legal restrictions as donor-restricted funds do. Board actions can be rescinded whereas donor restrictions can be changed only by approval of the donor or by the court. No special accounting method should be adopted if it would cloud or confuse this important distinction.

Figure 4-5.
Hoosier Hospital
Balance Sheet
December 31, 1987

ASSETS			LIABILITIES AND FUND BALANCES		

UNRESTRICTED FUND

Current Assets:			*Current Liabilities:*		
Cash		$ 11	Notes payable to banks		$ 10
Receivables	$ 55		Accounts payable		29
Less estimated uncollect-			Accrued expenses payable		12
ibles and allowances	13	42	Current portion of long-		
Inventories		18	term debt		6
Prepaid expenses		4	Deferred revenue		3
Total current assets		75	Total current liabilities		60
Board-Designated Assets:			*Long-Term Liabilities:*		
Cash	$ 6		Bonds payable	$ 50	
Investments	59		Mortgage payable	120	
Total board-designated assets		65	Total long-term liabilities		170
Plant Assets:			Total liabilities		230
Land, buildings and			Fund balance		270
equipment	$587				
Less accumulated depre-					
ciation	227				
Net plant assets		360			
Total Unrestricted Fund			Total Unrestricted Fund		
Assets		$500	Liabilities and Fund Balance		$500

RESTRICTED FUNDS

Specific Purpose Fund

Cash	$ 5	Liabilities	$ -
Investments	95	Fund balance	100
Total Specific Purpose Fund		Total Specific Purpose Fund	
Assets	$100	Liabilities and Fund Balance	$100

Plant Replacement and Expansion Fund

Cash	$ 15	Liabilities	$ -
Investments	185	Fund balance	200
		Total Plant Replacement and	
Total Plant Replacement and		Expansion Fund Liabilities and	
Expansion Fund Assets	$200	Fund Balance	$200

Endowment Fund

Cash	$ 21	Liabilities	$ -
Investments	279	Fund balance	300
		Total Endowment Fund	
Total Endowment Fund Assets	$300	Liabilities and Fund Balance	$300

Figure 4-6.
Hoosier Hospital
Income Statement
Year Ended December 31, 1987

Patient service revenues		$415
Less allowances and uncollectibles (after deduction of $12 of related gifts)		102
Net patient service revenues		$313
Other operating revenues (including $14 from Specific Purpose Fund)		25
Total operating revenues		338
Less Operating Expenses:		
Nursing services	$131	
Other professional services	93	
General services	112	
Fiscal services	14	
Administrative services (including interest expense of $4)	19	
Provision for depreciation	13	
Total operating expenses		382
Loss from operations		(44)
Nonoperating Revenues:		
Unrestricted gifts and bequests	$ 40	
Unrestricted income from Endowment Fund	13	
Income and gains from board-designated assets	8	
Total nonoperating revenues		61
Net income for the year		$ 17

If used intelligently, appropriations of resources by hospitals for board-specified purposes may have some merit. Even so, they are fictions, and accountants should not go through the motions of creating new funds for every resolution passed by the governing board, except where the board or situations dictate such accounting as appropriate. The greater the number of such appropriations, the more artificial they become. In no case should board appropriations be treated as expense.

Plant Asset and Related Debt Accounts. The plant accounts of the Unrestricted Fund include asset accounts reflecting the hospital's actual investment in plant assets, i.e., land, buildings, and equipment. These assets should not be reported in the restricted funds as this would imply restrictions upon their use or disposition, and such restrictions do not ordinarily exist. If there are any restrictions, they should be disclosed. Also related to the plant asset accounts within the Unrestricted Fund are mortgages payable and certain other noncurrent liabilities; long-term leases, for example. Previously, plant assets and long-term debt accounts were often combined in a so-called plant fund, but this practice is no longer generally accepted.

Plant assets, on occasion, may be donated in kind to the hospital. Upon receipt of such assets, they should be recorded at fair market value, at date of donation, in the Unrestricted Fund. The offsetting credit should be made directly to the Unrestricted Fund Balance account as a contribution to capital and **not** to revenue. At times, however, a hospital will receive land, buildings, and equipment that are donor-designated for endowment or other restricted purposes. Such donations are not recorded in the Unrestricted Fund but are entered in the appropriate restricted fund at fair market value.

Figure 4-7.
Hoosier Hospital
Statement of Changes in Fund Balances
Year Ended December 31, 1987
UNRESTRICTED FUND

Fund balance, January 1	$247
Net income for the year	17
Transfers from Plant Replacement and Expansion Fund for plant asset acquisitions	16
Transfers to Plant Replacement and Expansion Fund of third-party reimbursement restricted to plant asset acquisitions	(10)
Fund balance, December 31	$270

RESTRICTED FUNDS

Specific Purpose Fund:

Fund balance, January 1		$ 86
Restricted gifts and bequests received		12
Research grants received		11
Restricted income from investments		6
Gain on sale of investments		2
Transfers to Unrestricted Fund for:		
Allowances and uncollectible accounts	$ (3)	
Other operating revenue	(14)	(17)
Fund balance, December 31		$100

Plant Replacement and Expansion Fund:

Fund balance, January 1	$169
Restricted gifts and bequests received	25
Restricted income from investments	12
Transfers to Unrestricted Fund (described above)	(16)
Transfers from Unrestricted Fund (described above)	10
Fund balance, December 31	$200

Endowment Fund:

Fund balance, January 1	$238
Restricted gifts and bequests received	53
Gain on sale of investments	9
Fund balance, December 31	$300

Resources accumulated for plant asset replacement or expansion through a governing board designation are reflected among the board-designated assets in the Unrestricted Fund. Such appropriations by the board are not to be treated as expense even though resources actually are set aside or transferred to a specially created fund. Neither should such resources be transferred to and merged with donor-restricted funds.

In some instances, a portion of the reimbursement received by a hospital may be restricted by third parties to the acquisition of plant assets. While these payments are includable in Unrestricted Fund revenue in order to properly match revenue and expense (depreciation), the amount of such payments should be shown as a transfer from the Unrestricted Fund to restricted funds, i.e., the Plant Replacement and Expansion Fund. When these amounts are expended for new plant assets, they are returned to the Unrestricted Fund and accounted for as direct additions to the Fund Balance account. This procedure is illustrated in Figure 4-7.

Restricted Funds

Hospitals ordinarily receive a substantial amount of resources by way of gifts, contributions, donations, bequests, and grants. If there are no strings attached by donors, such resources are recorded as unrestricted revenues regardless of any action that might be taken by the hospital governing board. It must be presumed that if the donor wished to restrict the use of the resources, it would have been done at the time of contribution. If no such restriction is made by the donors, the governing board cannot do it for them. The board has the power to designate unrestricted resources to whatever use it desires, but its designations are not legally binding on the hospital's general creditors.

A majority of donated resources generally are restricted in some way by the donors. These resources are of three types: (1) resources restricted for specific operating purposes, (2) resources restricted for acquisition of plant assets, and (3) resources restricted as endowments. The types of restricted funds conform to this classification.

Specific Purpose Funds. Resources restricted by donors for purposes other than plant asset acquisitions or endowments are recorded in Specific Purpose Funds. Contributed resources of this kind received from different donors but having substantially identical restrictions generally may be combined into a single Specific Purpose Fund. Otherwise, insofar as feasible, a different Specific purpose Fund must be established for each major donor so that a separate accounting can be made for each.

Once recorded in Specific Purpose Funds, these resources remain restricted until such time as the restrictions lapse, either through the completion of the specified purposes or passage of time. As expenditures are made for specified purposes, periodic transfers of the previously restricted resources may be made to the Unrestricted Fund where the transfers are recorded as revenues or are offset against revenue deductions (see Figure 4-6). On the other hand, if accomplishment of purpose is related to the passage of time, periodic transfers might be made on that basis. However determined, the periodic transfers must meet the requirement of matching revenues and expenses, or must otherwise be systematic and rational, as explained in Chapter 2. Neither the amounts nor the timing of such transfers should be subject to the discretion of the governing board or the accountant.

Restricted income and gains on investments of Specific Purpose Funds normally should be added to the fund balance of such funds. Investment losses and expenses are deducted. Transfers of investment income and net gains are recorded in the same manner as transfers of the principal amounts of such funds.

Eventually, the resources of a Specific Purpose Fund are exhausted, and that particular fund goes out of existence. Specific Purpose Funds thus are not permanent funds. They have sometimes been referred to as **temporary** funds. Endowments, excluding term endowments, are the only permanently restricted funds maintained by hospitals.

Plant Replacement and Expansion Funds. Cash and other assets received by the hospital from donors and third-party payers who restrict the use of those resources to the acquisition of plant assets are included in this fund. Note, however, that plant assets, including those purchased with Plant Replacement and Expansion Fund resources, are not recorded here but in the Unrestricted Fund as discussed above.

Investment income from Endowment Fund investments, if such income is restricted by donors to plant asset acquisitions, should be recorded in the Plant Replacement and Expansion Fund directly. It is not appropriate to record such income initially in the Endowment Fund and later transfer it to this fund. The Plant Replacement and Expansion Fund, as noted before, may also receive transfers from the Unrestricted Fund of third-party reimbursements restricted to plant asset acquisition. Transfers **from** the Plant Replacement and Expansion Fund are **always** made to the Unrestricted Fund as plant asset expenditures are incurred. A transfer of this type is illustrated in Figure 4-7.

Income and gains on investments of the Plant Replacement and Expansion Fund are added to the Fund Balance. Investment expenses and losses are deducted. Transfers of investment income and gains are recorded in the same manner as transfers of the principal amounts of such funds.

Pledges (net of a provision for uncollectibles) restricted to the purchase of plant assets are recorded as additions to the Fund Balance of the Plant Replacement and Expansion Fund. Unrestricted pledges received are recorded as revenue in the Unrestricted Fund of the hospital.

Endowment Funds. Endowments consist of contributed resources which, by donor restriction, are to be held intact for the production of income. These resources, to be endowments, must carry legal restrictions that the governing board cannot normally alter and that prohibit expenditure of their principal amount. **Pure** endowments are permanent (perpetual) in nature whereas **term** endowments may be expended after the donors' requirements have been met and the prohibition upon expenditure of principal is legally released. Both types of endowments are recorded as restricted funds when received. The resources should, of course, be prudently invested within the framework imposed by donors and applicable laws.

Income from investments of endowment funds may be donor-restricted or it may be immediately available for general operating purposes. If donor-restricted to specified operating purposes, this income is recorded as earned in the Specific Purpose Fund(s) and there accounted for as previously described. If donor-restricted to the purchase of plant assets, such income should be recorded as earned in the Plant Replacement and Expansion Fund where it is accounted for as previously discussed. When, on the other hand, investment income on endowment funds is **not** donor-restricted, it is recorded as earned in the Unrestricted Fund.

In each situation noted, investment income on endowment funds is directly recorded in a fund other than the Endowment Fund. It is not correct to record such income in the Endowment Fund initially and later transfer it to another fund. This income is not restricted endowment resources (unless so restricted by donors) and therefore should never be recorded in the Endowment Fund. To do so would open the door to manipulative abuses in the amounts and the timing of the transfers of such resources to other funds.

Thus, income from Endowment Fund investments is not recorded in the Endowment Fund. On the other hand, gains and losses on investment transactions generally are recorded as adjustments of the Endowment Fund Balance unless such items are legally available for other use or are chargeable against other funds. Hospitals should seek the advice of legal counsel on this point.

In reporting Endowment Funds in hospital financial statements, separate disclosure should be made of term endowments. The nature and term of such endowments should be clearly indicated. For both pure and term endowments, full disclosure should be made of the amount of investment income and its disposition to the purpose for which it is restricted or available. Board-created endowments must be reported as unrestricted funds and should not be merged with externally created endowments. Endowment Fund accounting is treated in detail in Chapter 15.

Interfund Transactions

As indicated, particular emphasis is given in fund accounting to the segregation of resources and related obligations into independent sets of accounts called funds. A separate accounting is made of the activity within the individual funds. Interfund activity, however, is unavoidable, and special care must be given to a proper accounting for this activity.

Interfund Transfers. By far the most common interfund transaction is the transfer of previously restricted resources from restricted funds to the Unrestricted Fund. These resources initially are recorded in restricted funds, but, as they become available, they are transferred to the Unrestricted Fund. Upon receipt in the Unrestricted Fund, these resources are credited to (1) revenue, if transferred from Specific Purpose or Endowment Funds or (2) Unrestricted Fund Balance, if transferred from the Plant Replacement and Expansion Fund. This may be regarded as the general principle governing the accounting treatment of interfund resource transfers from restricted to unrestricted funds under ordinary circumstances.

The application of this principle is illustrated by the following entries recording various types of interfund transfers:

1. Transfer of $14 from the Specific Purpose Fund to the Unrestricted Fund.

Specific Purpose Fund

— Transfer to Unrestricted Fund	$14	
Cash		$14
To record transfer of resources available		
for specific operating purposes to		
Unrestricted Fund.		

Unrestricted Fund

Cash	$14	
Other Operating Revenues*		$14
To record receipt of resources available for		
specific operating purposes from the Specific		
Purpose Fund.		

*In certain instances, the credit is made to revenue deductions in the income statement.

2. Transfer of $16 from the Plant Replacement and Expansion Fund to the Unrestricted Fund.

Plant Replacement and Expansion Fund

Transfer to Unrestricted Fund $16
    Cash $16
    To record transfer of resources to the
    Unrestricted Fund for purchases of plant
    assets.

Unrestricted Fund

Cash $16
    Transfer Received from Restricted Funds $16
    To record receipt of resources from Plant
    Replacement and Expansion Fund for purchase
    of plant assets.

In the examples shown, the **transfer** accounts are closed to the respective fund balance accounts at the end of the accounting period. It should also be noted that the transfer accounts should be more precisely and descriptively titled than indicated here.

Much less common are resource transfers from the Unrestricted Fund to one of the restricted funds. Entries for the example provided in Figure 4-7 are given below:

Unrestricted Fund

Transfer to Restricted Funds $10
    Cash $10
    To record transfer to Plant Replacement and
    Expansion Fund of third-party reimbursement
    restricted to plant asset acquisition.

Plant Replacement and Expansion Fund

Cash $10
    Transfer Received from Unrestricted Fund $10
    To record transfer received from Unrestricted
    Fund of third-party reimbursement restricted
    to plant asset acquisitions.

Again, the transfer accounts, which should be more descriptively titled than shown, are closed to the respective fund balances at the end of the accounting period. Note also that this transfer is not treated as an expense of the Unrestricted Fund.

Investment Income, Gains, and Losses. As has earlier been indicated, investment income, gains, and losses relating to restricted funds generally should not require immediate interfund resource transfers. This is true because investment income earned from Endowment Fund investments, for example, is not recorded in the Endowment Fund but directly in the fund of which such income becomes a part of the fund principal. At a later point determined by different criteria, the principal finds its way into the Unrestricted Fund through resource transfers.

Investment gains and losses, however, are recorded directly in the fund in which the related investment assets are carried. Legal interpretations do differ somewhat on this point, but the general rule normally prevails. A contrary legal opinion may suggest another accounting procedure such as the recognition of restricted fund investment gains and losses in Unrestricted Fund revenue and expense accounts.

Unrealized gains and losses on investments in non-equity (debt) securities generally are not recognized in the accounts. The valuation of long-term investments in debt securities at market value, for example, is not a generally accepted practice at present. Yet, if such market values are materially lower than cost and judged to be permanently impaired, write-downs of such investments and recognition of loss are appropriate. Losses of this type on investments of restricted funds are charged against the respective fund balances. In any event, the disclosure of the market values of all hospital security investments in the financial statements is a desirable practice. This may be done parenthetically or by footnotes to the financial statements.

As discussed in Chapter 15, investments in marketable equity securities (corporate stocks, for example) are valued at the lower of aggregate cost or aggregate market value in both unrestricted and restricted funds. Unrealized as well as realized gains and losses on such investments are recognized in the accounts. In addition, extensive disclosure requirements must be met.

Interfund Borrowings. As a general rule, interfund resource transfers should occur only if a failure to transfer resources would be in violation of legal requirements or generally accepted accounting principles. There may be good "business" reasons for deferring or accelerating otherwise valid interfund transfers, but legal and accounting considerations should govern the timing and amount of such transfers. If transfers are in order but resources are not available at the time, the interfund relationships can be reflected in the financial statements through the use of interfund receivable and payable accounts as follows:

Restricted Fund

Fund Balance	$75	
Due to Unrestricted Fund		$75
To record obligation to transfer resources		
to Unrestricted Fund.		

Unrestricted Fund

Due from Restricted Fund	$75	
Revenues		$75
To record resource transfer due from Restricted		
Fund available for general operating purposes.		

Interfund obligations should be discharged as soon as practicable. Large and unrealistic build-ups in the interfund "due to" and "due from" accounts should not be permitted.

The management of an enterprise at times may be somewhat embarrassed by a large surplus in one fund or by a deficit in another. Some tendency may exist to attempt to "window dress" the unwanted situation through otherwise unnecessary interfund resource transfers, ambiguously labeled so as to provide a smoke screen of sorts. Transfers that are essentially bookkeeping devices to suit such objectives are never appropriate.

Interfund borrowings, in particular, can be an abused practice. All interfund borrowing should be documented by debt instruments and be formally approved by the hospital's governing board. In general, no fund should be permitted to borrow from another unless it has **both** a need for the resources and an evident ability to repay them on reasonable terms. This is not to say that no good reason ever exists for resource transfers made solely on the basis of a governing board action. They should never be made, however, when the real purpose is to confuse or mislead the user of financial statements. Even bona fide transfers can do this if not properly and fully presented. Transfers that serve no valid purpose only magnify the problem.

CHART OF ACCOUNTS

As noted in Chapter 3, a basic element of any accounting system is a chart of accounts, sometimes called a classification of accounts. The chart is a listing of the categories into which economic data relating to a hospital's financial position and operating results are to be accumulated in the accounting process. It is a data classification scheme tailored to the informational needs of the individual organization. Yet, enterprises within a particular industry generally have sufficient characteristics in common to produce basic similarities in their charts of accounts. Leaders in the hospital field, for example, have stressed for many years the need for a greater degree of comparability among hospitals in terms of the financial and statistical data reported by them. This has been reflected in a continuing effort toward adoption of an industry-wide uniform chart of accounts, along with uniform definitions of statistical terms.

Until 1922 there was no national pattern of uniform accounting among American hospitals, although the hospitals of certain cities (notably in Cleveland) engaged to some extent in similar accounting practices. It was in 1922 that the American Hospital Association published a recommended chart of accounts that was based in part on the chart that had been developed by the Cleveland hospitals. The 1922 chart was revised by the Association and re-issued in 1935 under the title **Hospital Accounting and Statistics**. A new and amplified edition of this document appeared in 1940, and it was the first attempt to present a more or less complete statement of uniform accounting for hospitals. Ten years later, in 1950, the Association updated that document and published it as **Uniform Hospital Statistics and Classification of Accounts**. This work, in turn, was superseded by the 1959 publication titled **Uniform Chart of Accounts and Definitions for Hospitals**.

The most recent versions of the American Hospital Association's long series of efforts in this area appeared in 1966 and 1976 as **Chart of Accounts for Hospitals**. These manuals made important contributions and even anticipated currently emerging forces. Revisions of the Chart of Accounts manual likely will appear in the future. Although one cannot predict with certainty what changes might be forthcoming, it would appear that a major restructuring of funds and an expansion of the statement of hospital accounting principles would be among them. For this reason, the following discussion departs in several respects from the recommendations of the AHA's 1976 manual. The reader, however, is urged to review that publication, or its successor, in that a reference to uniform hospital accounting is accepted in most quarters to mean the current pronouncements of the American Hospital Association.

Numerical Coding System

Each account in a chart of accounts is usually assigned a numerical code to facilitate the completion of various operations in the accounting process. The numerical coding system described here is drawn from the system presented in the AHA's **Chart of Accounts for Hospitals** (1976). Some modifications have been made here, but it is substantially the same numerical coding system. The system is illustrative only; each hospital tends to develop its own numbering system, particularly with respect to digits subsequent to the fourth digit of account numbers. However that may be, each digit of the numerical code, insofar as feasible, should have a specific and consistent meaning throughout the chart of accounts.

Balance Sheet Accounts. The AHA numerical coding system for balance sheet accounts is shown in Figure 4-8. The first digit designates the financial statement classification of the account, the second digit identifies the fund to which the account is related, the third and fourth digits specify control accounts, and the fifth and sixth digits may be used by hospitals according to their individual needs. A condensed outline of balance sheet accounts is provided in Figure 4-9.

Figure 4-8.
AHA Numerical Coding System
Balance Sheet Accounts

FIRST DIGIT	SECOND DIGIT	THIRD AND FOURTH DIGITS	DECIMAL POINT	FIFTH AND SIXTH DIGITS
0 Not used	0	0	•	0
1 Asset	1	1	•	1
2 Liability and equity	2 General funds	2	•	2
3	3	3	•	3
4	4	4	•	4
5	5 Plant replacement and expansion fund	5 Primary subclassification	•	5 Classification according to individual hospital requirements
6 Income statement	6 Specific-purpose fund	6	•	6
7	7 Endowment fund	7	•	7
8	8 Other funds	8	•	8
9	9	9	•	9

Figure 4-9.
Hypothetical Hospital
Chart of Balance Sheet Accounts

UNRESTRICTED FUND

<u>Assets</u>

1010	Cash in Bank
1014	Petty Cash
1020	Temporary Investments
1030	Accounts Receivable – Inpatients
1044	Accounts Receivable – Outpatients
1060	Allowance for Uncollectible Accounts
1086	Accrued Receivables
1090	Due from Other Funds
1110	Inventories
1120	Prepaid Expenses
1130	Land
1140	Land Improvements
1150	Buildings
1170	Fixed Equipment
1180	Major Movable Equipment
1190	Minor Equipment
1240	Accumulated Depreciation – Land Improvements
1250	Accumulated Depreciation – Buildings
1270	Accumulated Depreciation – Fixed Equipment
1280	Accumulated Depreciation – Major Movable Equipment
1420	Long-Term Investments

<u>Liabilities</u>

2010	Notes Payable
2020	Accounts Payable
2031	Salaries, Wages, and Fees Payable
2035	Payroll Taxes and Deductions Payable
2050	Accrued Expenses Payable
2060	Advances from Third-Party Payers
2080	Due to Other Funds
2111	Deferred Revenues
2119	Current Portion of Long-Term Debt
2150	Mortgages Payable
2190	Bonds Payable

Fund Balance

2210	Unrestricted Fund Balance
2211	Revenue and Expense Summary
2212	Nonrevenue Transfers from Other Funds
2213	Value of Donated Plant Assets
2214	Transfers to Other Funds

SPECIFIC PURPOSE FUNDS

Assets

1610	Cash in Bank
1620	Investments
1681	Pledges Receivable
1682	Allowance for Uncollectible Pledges
1690	Due from Other Funds

Liabilities

2620	Accounts Payable
2680	Due to Other Funds

Fund Balance

2610	Specific Purpose Fund Balance
2611	Restricted Gifts Received
2612	Investment Income
2613	Gains and Losses on Investments
2614	Transfers Received from Other Funds
2615	Transfers to Other Funds

PLANT REPLACEMENT AND EXPANSION FUNDS

Assets

1510	Cash in Bank
1520	Investments
1581	Pledges Receivable
1582	Allowance for Uncollectible Pledges
1590	Due from Other Funds

Liabilities

2520	Accounts Payable
2580	Due to Other Funds

Fund Balance

2510	Plant Replacement and Expansion Fund Balance
2511	Restricted Gifts Received
2512	Investment Income
2513	Gains and Losses on Investments
2514	Transfers Received from Other Funds
2515	Transfers to Other Funds

ENDOWMENT FUNDS

Assets

1710	Cash in Bank
1720	Investments
1790	Due from Other Funds

Liabilities

2720	Accounts Payable
2780	Due to Other Funds

Fund Balance

2710	Endowment Fund Balance
2711	Restricted Gifts Received
2712	Gains and Losses on Investments
2713	Transfers to Other Funds

Income Statement Accounts. The AHA numerical coding system for income statement accounts is indicated in Figures 4-10 and 4-11. The first six digits are used to code transactions for purposes of responsibility accounting and reporting. The seventh, eighth, and ninth digits may be used to provide a standard functional classification of revenues and expenses to meet the requirements of external reporting and allow hospitals to participate in uniform reporting programs. A condensed outline of the income statement accounts is provided in Figure 4-12.

A basic consideration in the design of a chart of accounts for revenues and expenses is the manner in which the particular hospital is organized. No two hospitals are organized in precisely the same way because of differences in size, types of services rendered, and other factors. The individual organization plan employed, whatever its form, must be sound. It must reflect how a particular hospital **actually** gets things done. It should embrace time-proven principles of organization such as unity of command and span of control, i.e., an individual should not be responsible to more than one superior, and no manager should attempt to directly supervise the work of an excessive number of subordinates. Clear lines of authority and definitions of responsibilities must be established.

Figure 4-10.
AHA Numerical Coding System
Revenue Accounts

FIRST DIGIT	SECOND, THIRD, AND FOURTH DIGITS	DECIMAL POINT	FIFTH DIGIT	SIXTH DIGIT	DECIMAL POINT	SEVENTH, EIGHTH, AND NINTH DIGITS
0 Not used		•	Inpatient acute		•	
1		•	Inpatient long-term		•	
Balance sheet accounts						
2		•	Outpatient emergency		•	
3	Classification by organizational units	•	Outpatient referred	Classification according to individual hospital requirements	•	Classification by functional units
Routine and other professional service revenue						
4		•	Outpatient clinic		•	
5 Other operating revenue and deductions from revenue		•	Day care		•	
6		•	Home health care		•	
7 Expense accounts		•			•	
8		•	Other classifications		•	
9 Nonoperating revenue		•			•	

A hypothetical organization chart is presented in Figure 4-13. It is provided for illustrative purposes only and not as a recommended plan of organization for any particular hospital. Note also that it is open-ended and does not list all departments within divisions. Certain departments are organized under different divisions in different hospitals and any one of several placements may be "correct" in given circumstances.

Figure 4-11.
AHA Numerical Coding System
Expense Accounts

FIRST DIGIT	SECOND, THIRD, AND FOURTH DIGITS	DECIMAL POINT	FIFTH AND SIXTH DIGITS	DECIMAL POINT	SEVENTH, EIGHTH, AND NINTH DIGITS
0 Not used		•		•	
1 ⎫		•		•	
⎬ Balance sheet accounts					
2 ⎭		•		•	
3	Classification by organizational units	•	Natural classification of expense	•	Classification by functional units
4 Revenue accounts		•		•	
5		•		•	
6 ⎫		•		•	
⎬ Nursing and other professional services expense					
7 ⎭		•		•	
8 Other services expense		•		•	
9 Nonoperating expense		•		•	

Figure 4-12.
Hypothetical Hospital
Chart of Income Statement Accounts

OPERATING REVENUE ACCOUNTS

Patient Service Revenues

Daily Patient Services

3021 Medical and Surgical Nursing Unit A
3022 Medical and Surgical Nursing Unit B
3080 Obstetric Nursing Unit
3090 Newborn Nursery

Other Nursing Services

3210 Operating Rooms
3211 Delivery Rooms

3250 Central Services and Supply
3260 Intravenous Therapy
3265 Emergency Service

Other Professional Services

4020 Laboratory
4040 Radiology
4070 Pharmacy
4080 Anesthesiology
4091 Physical Therapy

Other Operating Revenues and Revenue Deductions

Other Operating Revenues

5011 Income Transfers from Specific Purpose Funds
5041 Tuition from Educational Programs
5061 Cafeteria Sales
5071 Telephone and Telegraph
5081 Television and Radio Rentals
5085 Medical Record Fees
5171 Purchase Discounts

Deductions From Patient Service Revenues

5510 Provision for Bad Debts
5520 Contractual Adjustments
5540 Charity Service
5555 Administrative and Policy Adjustments

OPERATING EXPENSE ACCOUNTS

Patient Service Expenses

Nursing Services Division

6010 Nursing Services Division – Administrative Office
6021 Medical and Surgical Nursing Unit A
6022 Medical and Surgical Nursing Unit B
6080 Obstetric Nursing Unit
6090 Newborn Nursery
6210 Operating Rooms
6211 Delivery Rooms
6250 Central Services and Supply
6260 Intravenous Therapy
6265 Emergency Service

Other Professional Services Division

7010 Other Professional Services Division—Administrative Office
7020 Laboratory
7040 Radiology
7070 Pharmacy
7080 Anesthesiology
7091 Physical Therapy
7180 Medical Records

General Services Division

8040 General Services Division—Administrative Office
8050 Dietary
8060 Plant Operation and Maintenance
8090 Housekeeping
8110 Laundry and Linen
8113 Personnel Quarters

Fiscal Services Division

8211 Fiscal Services Division—Administrative Office
8212 General Accounting
8213 Patient Accounts
8214 Payroll Accounting
8215 Admitting
8216 Cashiers
8217 Costs and Budgets
8231 Data Processing

Administrative Services Division

8310 Administrative Services Division—Administrative Office
8311 Personnel
8312 Purchasing
8313 Communications

Unassigned Expenses

8510 Depreciation
8610 Insurance
8680 Taxes
8710 Employee Benefits
8720 Interest

NONOPERATING REVENUES AND EXPENSES

9041 General Unrestricted Contributions
9051 Investment Income
9055 Unrestricted Income from Endowment Funds

Figure 4-13.
Hypothetical Hospital
Organization Chart

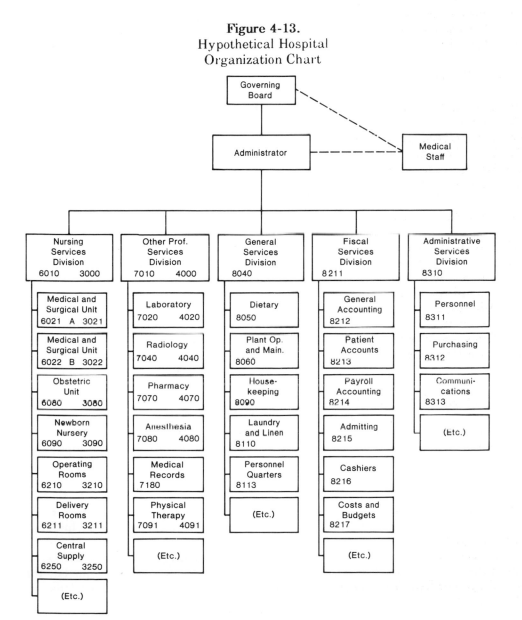

Assuming a sound organizational structure, the design of the chart of accounts for revenues and expenses should conform with that structure. In other words, the hospital organization is comprised of numerous well-defined departments, or **responsibility centers**, each having a manager or department head responsible for its activities. Each center incurs expenses, and many centers also generate revenues from services rendered to patients. The chart of accounts, then, should provide separate expense accounts and, where appropriate, separate revenue accounts for each center to permit the accumulation of (1) controllable expenses incurred by each center and (2) revenues generated by each center. This accumulation in the accounts of revenues and expenses according to decision-making centers is a principal feature of **responsibility accounting** (see Chapter 6).

Note, for example, that Pharmacy is one of the departmental units organized under the Other Professional Services Division in Figure 4-13. The numerical code for this responsibility center is 70. All expenses directly related to the activity of this center and over which the department head (chief pharmacist) exerts substantial control are charged to expense classification 7070. This control account number appears on the left-hand side of the box for Pharmacy in the organization chart (Figure 4-13). As noted earlier, this expense center account is subclassified to provide the details of Pharmacy expense in a natural or object of expenditure classification, i.e., salaries and wages, supplies, purchased service, and other expense items. A similar sub-classification is made, of all expense center control accounts.

Since the Pharmacy is also a revenue-producing center, it has a separate revenue account number — 4070 — as shown in Figure 4-13. All revenues directly generated by Pharmacy activities will be credited to this account. Additional digits may be used, as indicated before, to provide details of this revenue classified by type of patient, category of pharmaceutical, or some other useful information.

Thus, revenues and expenses are accumulated in the accounts in a manner that associates them directly with responsible managers in the hospital. The accounting information that results from such a classification is highly relevant to managerial planning and control decisions involving budgeting and performance appraisal.

HOSPITAL STATISTICS

While accounting is concerned primarily with the accumulation and communication of economic activity in terms of money, it also has a very substantial interest in the compilation and utilization of nonmonetary data. In hospitals, in fact, the amounts of third-party reimbursements are determined in part by statistical data. Inaccurate determinations of patient days, for example, can mean thousands of dollars of lost revenues. It is not surprising that the task of compiling, reporting, and interpreting statistics has fallen largely upon the hospital accountant.

The activities of a hospital are so numerous and diverse that its management requires measurements of service volume in statistical, as well as financial, terms. Consider, for example, the following comparison of the expenses of a dietary department:

	1987	1986
Dietary expense	$277,200	$252,000

From this presentation, it is possible to conclude only that the 1987 dietary expense was $25,200 higher than in 1986. Suppose, however, that it was also known that 210,000 meals were served in 1987 against only 180,000 meals in 1986? With this statistical information, the cost per meal served can be computed as $1.40 for 1986 and $1.32 for 1987. Had there not been any change in cost per meal, the 1987 dietary expense would have been $294,000 (210,000 X $1.40)! The gross dollar data tends to indicate higher, perhaps excessive, costs and decreased efficiency. By relating the dollar data to the number of meals served, it is clear that the unit cost is 8 cents lower per meal, thereby resulting in a cost savings of $16,800 ($294,000 − $277,200). That accounting and statistical data are fundamentally interrelated in this way can be demonstrated in numerous other areas of hospital activity.

The management uses of statistical measurements of hospital activity (both professional and nonprofessional) are generally enumerated as follows:

1. To establish administrative control over functional activities.
2. To serve as a basis for the preparation of operating budgets.
3. To meet reporting requirements of governing boards, outside agencies, and other organizations.
4. To provide a basis for the distribution of expenses when computing cost of operations.
5. To provide a basis for the calculation of average income and costs per unit of service rendered.

To be most useful to these purposes, hospital statistics must be accurately compiled and classified in a manner consistent with the chart of accounts so that statistical and monetary measurements of departmental activity can be related. In addition, statistics should be uniform among hospitals. Otherwise, third-party payers and other health care agencies might be led to erroneous and inequitable interpretations and judgments.

The American Hospital Association has made a considerable effort toward the development of uniform hospital statistics. Its manual titled **Uniform Hospital Definitions** presents recommended definitions of hospital patients by age, by financial status, by type of accommodation, by type of medical care provided, and by other categories. Definitions relating to bed facilities and departmental occasions of service are also included. These definitions are not reproduced here; the reader is urged to read the AHA manual.

It does seem appropriate to include in this discussion the definition and computations of (1) admissions, (2) patient days of service, (3) average daily census, (4) percentage of occupancy and (5) average length of stay.

Admissions

An inpatient admission is the formal acceptance by a hospital of a patient who is to receive physician, dentist, or allied services while lodged in the hospital. An outpatient admission is the formal acceptance by the hospital of a patient who is not to be lodged in the hospital while receiving physician, dentist, or allied services at the hospital.

Patient Days of Services

An illustration of the procedure for computing the number of patient days of service rendered for one day is presented in Figure 4-14. Note that a patient day is counted for any patient who is both admitted and discharged the same day, provided the patient occupied a regular hospital bed and a hospital chart was maintained for the patient. In the computation shown, four patients were both admitted and discharged on May 22. These same four were included in the 37 patients admitted and the 31 patients discharged that day.

Figure 4-14.
Computation of Patient Days of Service

Midnight census, May 21	240
Add patients admitted, May 22	37
Total	277
Less patients discharged (including deaths), May 22	31
Midnight census, May 22	246
Add patients both admitted and discharged (including deaths) after midnight May 21 and before midnight May 22	4
Patient days of service rendered on May 22	250

Average Daily Census

The average daily census is the average number of inpatients maintained in the hospital each day for a given period of time. It is computed for any inpatient classification by dividing the total number of patient days of service rendered during a given period by the number of calendar days in that period. Assume, for example, that a hospital rendered a total of 7,502 patient days of service to adult inpatients during the month of May. This hospital, then, had an average daily census during May of 242 (7,502/31) adult inpatients.

Percentage of Occupancy

Percentage of occupancy is the ratio of actual patient days to maximum patients days, as determined by bed capacity, during any given period of time. It is computed by dividing the actual patient days by the number of patient days of service which would have been provided if every bed had been occupied each day of the period. Assume, for example, that a hospital had an adult inpatient bed capacity of 260 beds from January 1 to June 30 and 300 beds from July 1 to December 31. The maximum adult patient days for the year therefore were 102,250 (260 x 181 + 300 x 184). If the actual patient days for the year were, say, 96,124, the percentage of occupancy was about 94 percent (96,124/102,260).

Average Length of Stay

Average length of stay is the average number of days of service rendered to each inpatient discharged during a given period. It is computed by dividing (1) the total number of days of service rendered to patients discharged during a given time period by (2) the number of inpatients discharged (including deaths) during the same period. If, for example, a hospital has 7,500 patient days of service during a month when 1,120 inpatients were discharged, the average length of stay is about 6.7 days (7,500/1,120).

In addition to the general measurements of utilization and volume of service, specific statistical data must also be compiled on a departmental basis for use in budgeting and cost finding. While general consideration is given to budgeting in Chapter 6 of this book, the topics of cost finding and rate setting are not covered in any detailed manner. The reader with a major interest in these areas may refer to AHA's **Cost Finding and Rate Setting for Hospitals** manual. Adequate departmental statistics are basic elements of the financial accounting system. For this reason, a summary of generally accepted occasions of service for hospital departments is provided in Figure 4-15.

Figure 4-15.
Summary of Occasions of Service

Department	Occasion of Service
Anesthesiology	(1) Number of patients served (2) Time required to administer
Central Services and Supply	Dollar value of processed requisitions
Delivery Rooms	Number of deliveries
Dietary	Number of meals served
Electrocardiology	Number of examinations
Housekeeping	Hours of service
Inhalation Therapy	Time administered
Laboratory	Number of tests
Laundry	Pounds processed
Nursing Service	Hours of service
Operating Rooms	(1) Number of operations (2) Hours of use
Pharmacy	Dollar value of processed requisitions
Physical Therapy	Number of treatments
Plant Maintenance	Employee hours of service
Plant Operation	Pounds of steam produced Tons of ice manufactured Pounds of coal consumed Gallons of oil consumed Cubic feet of gas consumed
Radiology	Number of examinations

QUESTIONS

1. Define **fund accounting**. Why is fund accounting a recommended system of accounting for hospitals?
2. List and briefly describe the two major classifications funds and the four types of funds usually maintained in hospital accounting.
3. What is a board-designated fund? Explain why the resources of such funds are not classified as restricted resources.
4. A hospital receives (1) a donation of an item of medical equipment having a market value of $100,000 and (2) a donation of $100,000 cash restricted by the donor to the purchase of medical equipment. How should each of these donations be accounted for when received? Explain why the treatment differs.
5. A hospital receives a $100,000 cash donation that is restricted by the donor. Should this $100,000 be recorded in the Specific Purpose Fund, the Plant Replacement and Expansion Fund, or the Endowment Fund? Explain how this decision is made by the hospital accountant.
6. When should resources be transferred from the Specific Purpose Fund to the Unrestricted Fund?
7. When should resources be transferred from the Plant Replacement and Expansion Fund to the Unrestricted Fund? From the Unrestricted Fund to the Plant Replacement and Expansion Fund? Give an example of each.
8. If investments held in a restricted fund are sold at a gain, in what fund should the gain be recorded?
9. Distinguish between **pure** and **term** endowments. At the expiration of a term endowment, what disposition is made of the resources of such endowments?
10. In what fund should unrestricted investment income earned on Endowment Fund investments be recorded? Explain.
11. Explain why for many years there has been a considerable interest in the development of a uniform classification of accounts for hospitals. What is the present status of this movement?
12. What is the relationship between a hospital's organizational structure and the proper design of its chart of accounts?
13. List the major management uses of statistical measurements of hospital activity.
14. What is meant by the following terms: (1) patient day, (2) inpatient census, (3) referred outpatient, (4) billed charges, and (5) per diem reimbursable rate?
15. Indicate whether the following statements are true or false and explain why:
    1. The hospital inpatient bed capacity is the number of beds regularly maintained for use by inpatients and outpatients.
    2. The percentage of occupancy is the ratio of actual patient days to the maximum patient days as determined by bed capacity during any given period of time.
    3. The hospital inpatient census is the number of inpatients occupying beds in the hospital at a given time.
    4. An outpatient occasion of service should be recorded each time an outpatient receives an examination, a consultation or a treatment in any of the services or facilities of the hospital.
    5. Each admission to Emergency constitutes an occasion of service.
    6. The occasion of service for Emergency is a visit.

      7. An outpatient admission is the formal acceptance by the hospital of a patient who is not to be lodged in the hospital while receiving physician, dentist, or allied services at the hospital.

      8. Only one outpatient admission should be counted for an outpatient during the period of continued treatment.

16. What is meant by the following terms: (1) full-time equivalents, (2) weighting factors, (3) occasions of service, (4) treatments, and (5) referred outpatient?

17. Indicate whether the following statements are true or false. If a statement is false, alter the wording to make the statement true.

      1. The normal bed complement is the number of hospital beds (including newborn infant bassinets) normally maintained for use by inpatients.

      2. When counting patient days, count the number of days of service rendered including the day of admission and the day of discharge.

      3. The daily census is the sum of the actual patient days for a single day (including the newborn infant days).

      4. The daily census is the sum of the midnight census (beginning of day) plus one patient day for each patient both admitted and discharged this same day.

      5. The percentage of occupancy is the ratio of maximum patient days to actual patient days.

      6. To compute the average daily census, divide the number of inpatient days, including newborn, during a given period of time by the number of calendar days in the period.

      7. The percentage of occupancy is the ratio of average daily census to average bed complement.

      8. The average length of stay is computed by dividing the maximum number of patient days during a period by the number of discharges during the same period.

      9. The normal bed complement includes all beds in patients' rooms, labor rooms, recovery rooms, and emergency rooms.

      10. The days for a newborn remaining in the newborn infant nursery after the discharge of the mother are counted in the computation of actual patient days.

18. There are at least five basic reasons, administratively, for gathering correct and complete statistics. Name four of these reasons.

19. Define the following or provide the formula for the computation of each:

      1. Average daily census

      2. Percentage of occupancy

      3. Average length of stay

      4. Outpatient admission

EXERCISES

E1. Given the following statistical data relating to XYZ Hospital:

Patients admitted, June 1	30
Patient census at midnight, May 31	220
Inpatients discharged, June 1	25
Inpatients admitted and discharged, June 1*	5

*Included in patients admitted and discharged, June 1.

Required. Compute the number of patient days of care rendered on June 1.

E2. Given the following statistical data for the month of June:

Total patient days	8,190
Hospital bed capacity	300
Inpatient admissions	1,050
Inpatient discharges	1,092

Required. Compute (1) the percentage of occupancy, (2) the average length of stay, and (3) the average daily census. Are the data complete?

E3. General Hospital, with 400 beds and 40 bassinets, has accumulated the following statistics during the year:

1.	Patient days (census days)	
	−adults and children	137,700
	−newborn	11,000
2.	Admissions−adults and children	15,500
3.	Births	2,430
4.	Discharges (and deaths)	
	−adults and children	15,300
	−newborn	2,400

Required. Compute the following measurements and show the correct presentation of the statistical report: (1) Average daily census, (2) Average length of stay, and (3) Percentage of occupancy. If any computation cannot be made from the data given, or is made differently than required, give an explanation.

E4. Given the following statistical data for May:

1.	Hospital inpatient bed capacity	200
2.	Inpatient admissions	786
3.	Total patient days	3,930
4.	Inpatient discharges	655
5.	Outpatient admissions	1,965

Required. Compute (1) the average daily census, (2) the percentage of occupancy, and (3) the average length of stay.

E5.   Assume the following at the end of the last day in September:

Patient	Date Admitted	In-house Days
A	9/19	12
B	9/25	6
C	9/27	4

On October 1, the patient activity was as follows:

Patient A discharged
Patient D admitted
Patient E admitted
Patient F admitted

Required. Using the conventional method, compute the daily census for October 1. Reconcile the in-house days and discharge days to the census for October 1.

E6.   Hartful Hospital employs fund accounting in the manner specified in the AICPA's **Hospital Audit Guide.** During 1987, the following interfund transactions were completed:

1.   The Specific Purpose Fund transferred $16 to the Unrestricted Fund to finance charity work.
2.   The Plant Replacement and Expansion Fund transferred $27 to the Unrestricted Fund to finance the purchase of plant assets.
3.   The Unrestricted Fund transferred $19 to the Plant Replacement and Expansion Fund. This $19 represented third-party reimbursement restricted by third parties to plant asset acquisitions.
4.   The Unrestricted Fund borrowed $25 from the Specific Purpose Fund.

Required. Prepare entries in all funds involved to record the above transactions.

E7.   Following are multiple-choice questions relating to the use of fund accounting by hospitals:

1.   Resources set aside by action of the hospital's governing board for use in acquiring new plant assets should be reported as assets of the
    a.   Endowment Fund.
    b.   Unrestricted Fund.
    c.   Plant Replacement and Expansion Fund.
    d.   Specific Purpose Fund.

2. Which of the following accounts would not be included in the Plant Replacement and Expansion Fund?
   a. Cash.
   b. Investments in stocks and bonds.
   c. Property, plant, and equipment.
   d. Pledges receivable.

3. Gilmore Hospital's property, plant, and equipment (net of accumulated depreciation) consists of the following:

Land	$ 500,000
Buildings	10,000,000
Equipment	8,000,000

   What amount should be included in the hospital's restricted funds?
   a. $-0-
   b. $500,000
   c. $10,500,000
   d. $18,500,000

4. Depreciation expense should be recognized in the financial statements of
   a. Investor-owned hospitals only.
   b. Not-for-profit hospitals only.
   c. Both investor-owned and not-for-profit hospitals.
   d. Neither investor-owned nor not-for-profit hospitals.

5. On July 1, 1987, Lilydale Hospital's board of trustees designated $200,000 for expansion of outpatient facilities. The $200,000 is expected to be expended in the fiscal year ending June 30, 1990. In Lilydale's balance sheet at June 30, 1988, the $200,000 should be classified as a (an)
   a. Restricted current asset.
   b. Restricted noncurrent asset.
   c. Unrestricted current asset.
   d. Unrestricted noncurrent asset.

6. The long-term debt of a hospital should be recorded in the
   a. Unrestricted Fund.
   b. Specific Purpose Funds.
   c. Plant Replacement and Expansion Funds.
   d. Endowment Funds.

7. An unrestricted pledge from an annual contributor to a voluntary not-for-profit hospital made in December of 1987 and received in cash in March of 1988 would generally be credited to
   a. Nonoperating revenues in 1987.
   b. Nonoperating revenues in 1988.
   c. Operating revenues in 1987.
   d. Operating revenues in 1988.

8.   The income statement of a hospital is drawn from the accounts of
   a.   All funds maintained by the hospital.
   b.   The Unrestricted Fund only.
   c.   The Unrestricted Fund and the Specific Purpose Funds.
   d.   All funds except the Endowment Funds.

Required. Select the best answer to each of the above multiple-choice items.

PROBLEMS

P1.   Metro Hospital provides you with the following account balances at September 30, 1987:

Notes payable to banks	$ 11
Receivables patients	57
Investments – specific purpose fund	92
Bonds payable	80
Prepaid expenses	5
Investments – unrestricted fund (current)	14
Accrued expenses payable	13
Cash – board-designated	5
Investments – endowment fund	303
Accounts payable	41
Land	8
Allowance for uncollectible accounts	15
Mortgage payable	135
Equipment	260
Cash – plant replacement and expansion fund	17
Cash – unrestricted fund (current)	14
Building	320
Current portion of long-term debt	10
Investments – plant replacement and expansion fund	174
Cash – specific purpose fund	3
Investments – board-designated	47
Accumulated depreciation	242
Deferred revenue (current)	6
Inventories	27
Cash – endowment fund	18

Required. Prepare an all-funds balance sheet for Metro Hospital at September 30, 1987.

P2.   Cosmo Hospital provides you with the following information taken from its
accounting records at June 30, 1987, the end of its fiscal year:

Nursing services expense	$134
Deductions from revenues	99
Income and gains from board-designated investments	7
General services expense	108
Depreciation	12
Unrestricted gifts and bequests	36
Gross patient service revenues	422
Fiscal services expense	29
Unrestricted income from endowment fund	21
Other professional services expense	101
Other operating revenues	31
Administrative services expense	22
Unrestricted fund balance, July 1, 1986	325
Interest expense	11
Transfer received from specific purpose fund for:	
Free service	14
Education	9
Transfer received from plant replacement and	
expansion fund for purchase of plant assets	52

Required. Prepare (1) an income statement and (2) a statement of changes in
unrestricted fund balance for the year ended June 30, 1987.

P3.   Central Hospital is preparing its annual report for the fiscal year ended
September 30, 1987. The following statistical data are available:

1.   Patient days:

Adult	51,000
Pediatric	3,600
Newborn	2,300

2.   The hospital had the following beds available through the year:

10/1/86-11/30/86	175
12/1/86- 3/31/87	180
6/1/87- 7/31/87	180
8/1/87- 9/30/87	170

On April 1, 1987, the administration closed 30 beds for redecorating, which
were reopened on June 1, 1987.
3.   Discharge days (adult and pediatric), 52,325.
4.   Number of admissions (adult and pediatric), 8,900.
5.   Number of discharges (adult and pediatric), 9,100.

Required. Compute (1) average daily census, (2) average length of stay, and (3)
percentage of occupancy.

P4.   On January 1, 1987, your hospital had 50 ward beds, 60 private and 140 semiprivate beds. These beds were staffed throughout the year. You also had 8 recovery beds, 3 beds in the emergency room for patients to use following treatments or minor operations, 7 labor room beds, and 40 bassinets. During the year, you had 75,990 patient days and 12,145 discharges. Of these, there were 10,110 newborn days and 2,010 newborn discharges.

At midnight on July 10, 1987, the census at your hospital was 210 adults and 30 newborn. During the next 24-hour period, the following occurred:

1.   Thirty-two adults were admitted; 28 adults were discharged.
2.   Of the 32 adults admitted, 2 were discharged the same day.
3.   One patient, who had been hospitalized 8 days, expired.
4.   Ten babies were delivered plus 1 stillborn delivered and 1 baby transferred to pediatrics. Eight babies having an accumulated stay of 36 days were discharged.

Required. Answer the following questions: (1) What was your census at midnight on July 11? (2) How many patient days of care were rendered on July 11? (3) What is your bed complement? (4) What is your percentage of occupancy for the year? (5) What is the average length of stay for the year?

P5.   Given the following statistical data (the statistics contained in one statement are not included in any other statement):

1.   Inpatients both admitted and discharged after midnight May 1 and before midnight May 2   3
2.   Inpatient deaths of patients admitted after midnight May 1 and before midnight May 2   2
3.   Inpatients remaining in hospital at midnight May 1   100
4.   Patients in the emergency room just prior to midnight May 2   8
5.   Inpatients admitted after midnight May 1 and before midnight May 2   15
6.   Inpatient deaths occurring after midnight May 1 but before midnight May 2 (inpatient deaths of patients admitted May 2 excluded)   1
7.   Fetal deaths occurring after midnight May 1 and before midnight May 2   2
8.   Inpatient discharges after midnight May 1 and before midnight 2   9
9.   Transfer from newborn nursery to pediatrics   1

Required. Compute the total number of patient days of service rendered to inpatients on May 2.

5
Fundamentals of Internal Control and Auditing

This chapter is directed mainly to a logical development of the broad principles of internal control and auditing for hospitals. These fundamental considerations apply, however, to all types of organizations engaged in economic activity, whether profit-seeking or not. A knowledge of the basic features of internal control and auditing is essential to an understanding of the detailed control procedures and practices employed by a particular hospital to meet its own needs. Thus, while there are universal principles on which all internal control systems are based, the manner of their application will differ to some degree from hospital to hospital. It therefore is impossible to describe, in a single chapter, all these variations. Many of the detailed methods and measures not covered in this chapter are discussed in subsequent chapters. The discussion of the details of internal control systems often is suggestive only; it may or may not have direct application to the circumstances of a specific hospital.

Some readers will wish to pursue the subjects of internal control and internal auditing in greater depth. Particularly useful for this purpose are HFMA's **Safeguarding the Hospital's Assets**, AHA's **Internal Control and Internal Auditing for Hospitals**, and AICPA's **Internal Control**. Much of the material in this chapter is drawn from these sources.

NATURE OF INTERNAL CONTROL

The term **internal control** is sometimes defined so as to limit it to a narrow accounting concept. Properly viewed, however, internal control is a broad concept embracing management operations as well as accounting functions. This broader and more useful concept of internal control is reflected in the following widely quoted definition:[1]

> Internal control comprises the plan of organization and all of the coordinate methods and measures adopted within a business to safeguard its assets, check the accuracy and reliability of its accounting data, promote operational efficiency, and encourage adherence to prescribed managerial policies.

Internal control therefore involves considerably more than the completion of a set of routine accounting procedures such as the reconciliation of bank checking accounts and the periodic balancing of detailed subsidiary ledgers against the general ledger control accounts. The broader concept of internal control includes budgeting, statistical performance standards, employee training programs, internal auditing, responsibility reporting, and all other measures by which a management attempts to improve operating efficiency and assures that activities are carried out in accordance with approved policies and procedures.

Thus, a distinction is often made between administrative controls and accounting controls. **Administrative controls** consist of those methods and measures in the internal control system whose primary purposes are to improve the efficiency with which hospital activities are performed and to secure a high degree of compliance with established managerial policies. These controls relate only in an indirect way to the accounting records. On the other hand, **accounting controls** consist of those methods and measures whose primary purposes are to safeguard assets and to assure a high degree of reliability in the information generated by the accounting process. Both types of controls will be found in any fully satisfactory system of internal control.

The discussion in this book deals with administrative controls as well as with accounting controls. All too often, the narrow accounting concept of internal control is given undue emphasis. An inordinate amount of attention may be given to the safeguarding of assets against error and fraud, and dollars may be spent to catch dimes. The hospital manager and accountant have an obligation to protect hospital assets from such dangers, but internal control dollars can often be invested more productively in administrative controls to eliminate the waste that results from operating inefficiency. This idea is not new, but some healthcare organizations have been somewhat slow to extend their accounting-oriented internal control systems into the administrative controls area. It must be recognized that the development and maintenance of effective administrative controls is perhaps even more important than accounting controls.

REASONS FOR INTERNAL CONTROL

It would be quite incorrect to assume that hospitals, being not-for-profit organizations, do not need internal control systems. To the contrary, hospitals require internal control systems precisely because they **are** organized on a not-for-profit basis. The profit-seeking corporation with poor internal controls may be able, at least for a time, to absorb the resultant waste and losses in its profits and in its stockholders' investments. Hospitals have no profits or other resources to use in this way, and sound internal control systems consequently are needed as much as they are in commercial enterprises.

It also would be most incorrect to maintain that hospitals, being not-for-profit organizations, cannot afford to install and maintain a sophisticated internal control system. The fact of the matter is that hospitals cannot afford **not** to have such systems. While internal control systems can be rather expensive, the lack of a good system is likely to prove even more expensive! Sometimes, a system may be too sophisticated for a particular set of circumstances. Such a system, by involving unnecessary procedures, may even impair operating efficiency to some extent. Yet, it probably can be said that an overly elaborate internal control system is far better than no system at all.

There are several major reasons why strong internal control systems are essential in hospitals. These are (1) the size and complexity of the hospital enterprise, (2) the importance of accurate and reliable accounting data, (3) the obligation to safeguard hospital assets from error and fraud, and (4) the economic impracticability of detailed audits by independent accountants. Each of these reasons is discussed here briefly.

Size and Complexity of Hospitals

Consider the operation of a small retail store in which the sole owner also acts as manager. While there may be three or four employees, the owner-manager generally can exercise continuous personal and direct supervision of all employees as they perform their assigned duties. Should the work of an employee not be efficient or be at variance with prescribed methods and policies, the manager is in a position to observe and correct this immediately on a first-hand basis. The employees are constantly aware of the manager's presence. The manager is almost always in rather close proximity, and much of what the employees do and say is easily seen or overheard.

In spite of this, the owner-manager typically will not need or choose to delegate much authority to the employees. The manager usually performs all of the more important and sensitive duties. In other words, the manager will do all the purchasing, process and pay all bills, hire and discharge employees, prepare and distribute payroll checks, and make bank deposits. The more of this the manager can do, the less the business needs in the way of internal controls.

The hospital manager, however, is hardly in this position. Even the 50-bed hospital facility is "large" compared to most retail businesses, and it is many times more complex. Administrative personnel, even at intermediate levels of management, are physically unable to supervise their subordinates in a continuous and direct manner. Personal observation of the work of individual employees is severely limited. In the absence of other controls, inefficiencies and violations of established policies might go undetected and uncorrected for long periods of time. Nor can the hospital manager "do it all himself (herself)" due to the skills required in a variety of tasks and the large volume of activity.

In hospitals, then, important duties must be assigned to numerous employees working in a variety of occupations at many different locations. These employees are informed of approved methods and procedures for performing their duties, and they will be made aware of hospital policies pertinent to their tasks. How can those charged with administrative responsibilities have any reasonable degree of assurance that approved methods and procedures are followed, that established policies are observed, and that the performance of subordinates is efficient? Where direct and continuous supervision is not feasible, there is but one answer: a system of administrative and accounting controls.

Accurate and Reliable Accounting Data

It seems reasonable to assume that the best management decisions can be made only after all relevant information is carefully considered. The information most relevant to a majority of financial management decisions is the monetary and statistical data provided in accounting reports and analyses. If these data are not accurate and reliable, management decisions based upon them are likely to be unwise. It therefore is imperative that such information not be inaccurate and unreliable, and this should be a major objective of internal control systems. It is accomplished through a system of checks and balances which greatly reduces the possibility of serious errors in the accumulation and communication processes of accounting. An effective internal control system will give managers greater confidence in accounting information and, consequently, in decisions based upon such information.

Obligation to Safeguard Assets

A hospital obtains its assets from a variety of sources. In some cases, certain assets may be donor-restricted in use to specified purposes, and methods must be employed to assure that such restrictions are fully observed. Other assets may be unrestricted and available for general operating purposes at the discretion of the governing board. Whether restricted or not, the assets of the hospital must be protected from loss caused by fraud, by error, or by inefficiency. In return for the use of resources given to it and for its not-for-profit status, the hospital has an obligation to make the most effective possible use of resources in providing healthcare services. Its resources must not be wasted in any manner, and particularly not by fraud and error.

The legal and moral obligation for the proper and effective utilization of assets rests primarily with the governing board. The board, of course, assigns operating authority and responsibility for this obligation to the chief executive officer, or administrator. Since the hospital administrator cannot possibly perform all hospital functions personally, he or she must delegate authority to others who, in turn, delegate it to still others. As a result, there are several levels of management authority and responsibility in the hospital organization. At each level there are department heads, managers, or supervisors with a common factor. They have given to subordinates the authority to carry on specified activities, but they remain fully responsible for their subordinates' performances. Administrative personnel, of necessity, therefore depend heavily upon internal controls for assurance that the activities and performances of their departments are efficient, in accord with prescribed policies and free of fraud or significant error. Without such assurance, the administrative task would be an intolerable responsibility.

While inefficiency and policy or procedural violations are perhaps the major causes of waste in hospitals, the safeguarding of assets from fraud and error also must be emphasized. The author's experience leads to an opinion that hospital people generally are possessed of a somewhat greater dedication and concern than their counterparts in profit-seeking enterprises. However this may be, the possibility of fraud and honest error in the handling of hospital resources should never be discounted.

Unintentional errors will occur; they can never be entirely eliminated so long as human beings are involved. Yet, every effort should be made to minimize errors, particularly those resulting from carelessness and slipshod procedures. The hospital's internal control system, for example, should include procedures that preclude the payment of any invoice whose quantity, unit price, extensions, and totals have not been verified. This point may be obvious, but it is not in the least trivial. Thousands of dollars can be lost annually in the payment of unaudited invoices.

Losses arising from inefficiency and error tend to go almost unnoticed, and this is one reason why they are so deadly. Fraud, on the other hand, generally produces spectacular newspaper headlines: "Trusted Hospital Employee Admitted Embezzler." Such publicity can be as damaging as the loss itself. Hospital governing boards and administrations should recognize that their primary obligation in this area is to **deter** fraud. Internal control systems, insofar as is feasible, should make it as difficult as possible for employees to commit a successful theft or other fraudulent manipulation of hospital assets. Opportunities and temptations to engage in such activity should be eliminated. This should be accepted by hospital management as a basic obligation to its employees. The **detection** of fraud, when it does occur, is an important feature of an internal control system, but it is a secondary consideration. Locking the barn door after the horse has been stolen is a fruitless procedure. A management that leaves the barn doors open in the first place is doing a disservice to employees.

Impracticability of Detailed Audits

Apparently, managements sometime feel that an internal control system is unnecessary because "we have regular annual audits by independent professional accountants." Then, if after such audits a substantial fraud is exposed, the same managements express surprise and outrage that it was not uncovered by the auditors. This reflects a somewhat common misconception about the nature and general purpose of the typical audit.

The ordinary audit by external accountants involves an extensive use of sampling techniques. The auditors will not examine in detail every transaction record of the hospital. Instead, auditors make a thorough examination of a carefully selected sample of activity to the extent necessary to permit them to render an opinion as to the fairness of the hospital's financial statements taken as a whole. Completely detailed audits simply are not economically practicable. Statistical sampling is the only feasible approach.

The size of the auditor's sample is determined largely by an evaluation of the effectiveness of the hospital's internal control system. If the internal control system is discovered to be highly effective, the sample size usually is rather small. If the internal control system is deemed to be weak, a much larger sample of recorded information must be examined in considerable detail. This, of course, results in a higher audit fee. In cases where the hospital's internal control system is grossly inadequate, the auditors may not be in a position to express an opinion on the financial statements. This raises very serious problems for the hospital in its relationships with third-party payers, creditors, and other external parties.

Thus, external audits typically are not completely detailed examinations of the accounts of a hospital. They are not necessarily designed to detect all instances of fraud and error. It is true that audits often will expose frauds, but by then the damage has been done. The emphasis therefore should be upon the determent of fraud and error in the first place, and this is best accomplished through a strong internal control system.

BASIC ELEMENTS OF INTERNAL CONTROL

The basic elements, or characteristics, of a satisfactory system of internal control are (1) a sound plan of organization, (2) a system of authorization and record procedures, (3) sound practices, and (4) qualified personnel. These elements are fundamentally interrelated in that a serious deficiency in any one so impairs the others that the effective operation of the internal control system is precluded. All four elements are required in a satisfactory system.

Plan of Organization

It has been noted that the complexity of hospital enterprises makes direct and continuous personal supervision of all employees impossible. As a result, a sound plan of organization must exist if effective administrative control is to be achieved. While no two organization plans are likely to be identical, they nevertheless should be based upon proven principles of organization that generally apply to any situation. The organizational structure should provide, for example, for unity of command and a reasonable span of control. The plan should establish clear lines of authority and responsibility. These features, of course, are prerequisites to the system of responsibility accounting and reporting that is essential to effective management.

Another characteristic of a plan of organization that is required for internal control purposes is the appropriate segregation of functional responsibilities. While cooperation among departments of a hospital and coordination of their activities are essential objectives, a careful separation of functional responsibilities — operating, custodial, and accounting — should be maintained to the extent feasible. A similar division of powers can be seen in the organization of the federal government into executive, legislative, and judicial branches.

What this means in a hospital is that no operating or custodial department should have absolute control of, or even access to, the accounting records. More simply, the "players" should not be allowed to keep the "score." The hospital pharmacy, for example, should not keep its own revenue and expense records, at least not without adequate provision for independent verification of such records. Otherwise, the integrity of the records might be impaired. The segregation of functional responsibilities also means that individuals who handle cash or have custody of securities, inventories, and other assets should not have access to accounting records that measure their custodial responsibility. By the same token, it follows that the accounting or "scorekeeping" function should be divorced organizationally from operational and custodial functions. The accountant, with no direct personal interest in the outcome of the "game" and with no organizational obligation to any particular "player," therefore can render unbiased "scores" concerning the performance of each participant.

In hospital enterprises, however, it is difficult to avoid a certain amount of overlapping in operating, custodial, and accounting functions. The smaller the hospital, the more difficult it becomes to maintain the ideal degree of organizational independence in these three areas. Cashiers, for example, may handle cash receipts and, at the same time, make accounting records of such receipts involving access to accounts receivable ledgers. It simply may not be economical or feasible to provide for a complete segregation of all functional responsibilities. All such situations, however practical, should be recognized as fundamentally undesirable in that they weaken the effectiveness of the internal control system. Special supplementary and compensating measures therefore must be adopted to assure that such weaknesses do not lead to fraud and error.

System of Authorization

A second characteristic of a satisfactory internal control plan is an adequate system of authorization and record procedures. The system employed by a hospital should be completely described in a formal, written manual of policies and procedures. This manual should set forth the prescribed manner for dealing with all types of events and transactions. It should include a detailed chart of organization with job titles and descriptions of duties. It should present the hospital's chart of accounts with clear indications of the nature and content of each account. The accounting plan also should be set forth in a full discussion of all forms and records used. Clear statements should be made as to the authorizations and approvals required for initiating and completing all types of transactions. The manual should be kept current, being revised often to reflect changes that may occur in established policies and procedures.

Documentary evidences such as purchase orders, charge tickets, and supplies requisition forms are essential requirements of the system of authorization and record procedures. These documents, properly executed, serve as authorizations for initiating transactions and as media for making records of transactions. They also provide a basis for subsequent verification and analysis. Periodically, studies should be made of the forms and documents employed so as to improve their design and to eliminate those which may no longer serve a useful purpose. There must be a constant effort to minimize excessive red tape and yet retain adequate documentation of adherence to prescribed management policies and procedures at each significant stage of transactions from initiation to completion.

Sound Practices

Sound practices consist of the tactical measures taken to provide assurance that transactions are properly authorized and accurately recorded, and that an appropriate accounting is made of the responsibility for asset custody. It is important to recognize that the establishment of an organization plan and a system of authorizations and record procedures is no guarantee that it actually works in the manner intended. Sound practices must be followed to insure that the prescribed plan and system is, in fact, effectively observed. Such practices are centered on a division of duties and responsibilities — within and between departments — so that no one individual will handle a transaction completely from beginning to end. Ideally, the person who authorizes or initiates a transaction should have no part in either recording the transaction or in the stewardship of the asset (if any) arising from the transaction. This tends to provide an automatic check of the accuracy of the work and substantially enhances the probability that errors and fraud will be detected promptly unless there is collusion among individual employees. If circumstances do not permit this division of duties and responsibilities, other protective practices must be instituted.

There is an almost endless number of sound practices, and therefore it is not practical to attempt to list all of them here. Briefly, sound practices generally to be observed for cash receipts and cash disbursements would include:

1. The opening of all incoming mail by persons independent of cashiering and accounting.
2. The making of an immediate record of cash receipts in the form of mail remittance lists, cash receipt slips, cash logs, or cash register tapes.
3. The depositing of all cash receipts intact and on a daily basis.
4. The comparing of authenticated bank deposit slips with cash receipt records of the accounting department.
5. The prenumbering of all documents, and accounting for such documents on the basis of numerical sequence.
6. The bonding of all employees who handle cash receipts or who sign checks or otherwise have access to signed checks.
7. The securing of competitive bids from suppliers.
8. The comparing of the data of purchase orders, receiving reports, and vendor's invoices before payments are authorized.

9. The reconciling of bank statements by persons other than those who approve invoices for payment or prepare, sign, or enter checks in the accounting records.

Sound practices such as those described are needed because the organization plan and the system of authorization and record procedures, no matter how well designed, will not automatically provide effective internal control. The organization plan identifies authority and responsibility as it **should** exist with respect to various types of transactions; the system of authorization and record procedures prescribes the use of particular forms and their orderly flow within and among departments; the development and observance of sound practices provides assurance that actual operations are carried out in conformity with such plans and systems. Practices such as these assure the accuracy and integrity of the recorded information in the chain of events from the initiation to the completion of transactions.

Adequacy of Personnel

Of the four elements of a satisfactory system of internal control, the most important is that the quality of personnel be commensurate with responsibilities. It has been said that accounting controls nothing! This is very true. Control is obtained and achieved by people, not by journals and ledgers or by organization charts and authorization systems. Unless hospitals attract and retain personnel of adequate competence, no internal control system will prove satisfactory. For this reason, plus the fact that employee compensation is the major component of healthcare costs, considerable emphasis must be placed on personnel management, particularly employment practices, employee training programs, and performance appraisals.

Much of the waste that can occur in any enterprise can be attributed to poorly qualified personnel. In the labor-intensive hospital industry, this can be an especially critical factor. It therefore is essential that a hospital give careful attention to the initial selection of employees. Every position in the hospital should be analyzed in terms of the qualifications of the person required to fill it capably. Efforts must then be made to engage the services of such a person on competitive employment terms. This must be accomplished if high rates of turnover and other labor-related wastes are to be avoided.

Formal employee training programs also are quite important in hospitals. Much can be done in training programs to increase employee morale as well as efficiency. Explanations of hospital policies and procedures provide an understanding and appreciation among employees of the contribution each makes to the overall internal control system. With appropriate training, job rotation also becomes possible as a means of providing variety, improving employee performance, and adding versatility. Personnel can also be motivated by the possibility of moving upward into positions of greater responsibility.

In addition to sound employment practices and training programs, it is essential that means be developed to appraise employee performance. One method, already noted, is to arrange duties so that the work of employees is complementary, i.e., the work of one employee provides an automatic check on the work of another. Thus, if prescribed procedures are not being observed, they will be discovered and can be corrected. Other methods include the development, with employee participation, of budgets and standards against which actual performances are measured in a responsibility reporting system.

Internal auditing can also be an important means of evaluating the performance of employees with respect to administrative and accounting controls.

INTERNAL AUDITING

Internal auditing is an independent appraisal activity carried on within a hospital by employees designated as internal auditors. These auditors perform functions similar to those of external auditors, but they also carry out many assignments that are beyond the scope of ordinary audits by independent certified public accountants.

Nature of Internal Auditing

Internal auditing is more than merely a number-checking function; it should be a management tool for the appraisal of all activities to promote the attainment of the objectives of the hospital. The most authoritative discussion of the nature of internal auditing is the **Statement of the Responsibilities of the Internal Auditor** issued by the Institute of Internal Auditors. A major portion of the statement is reproduced here.

Internal auditing is the independent appraisal activity within an organization for the review of the accounting, financial, and other operations as a basis for protective and constructive service to management. It is a type of control which functions by measuring and evaluating the effectiveness of other types of control. It deals primarily with accounting and financial matters, but it may also properly deal with matters of an operating nature.

The overall objective of internal auditing is to assist management in achieving in the most efficient administration of the operations of the organization. This total objective has two major phases, as follows:

1. The protection of the interests of the organization, including the pointing out of existing deficiencies to provide a basis for appropriate corrective action. The attainment of this objective involves such activities of the internal auditor as:
    a. Ascertaining the degree of reliability of the accounting and statistical data developed within the organization.
    b. Ascertaining the extent to which the organization's assets are properly accounted for and safeguarded from losses of all kinds.
    c. Ascertaining the extent of compliances with established policies, plans, and procedures.
2. The furtherance of the interests of the organization, including the recommendation of changes for the improvement of the various phases of the operations. The attainment of this objective involves such activities of the internal auditor as:
    a. Reviewing and appraising the policies and plans of the organization in the light of the related data and other evidence.
    b. Reviewing and appraising the internal records and procedures of the organization in terms of their adequacy and effectiveness.

    c.   Reviewing and appraising performance under the policies, plans, and procedures.

Internal auditing is a staff or advisory function rather than a line or operating function. Therefore the internal auditor does not exercise direct authority over other persons in the organization.

The internal auditor should be free to review and appraise policies, plans, and procedures, but his review and appraisal does not in any way relieve other persons in the organization of the primary responsibilities assigned to them.

Independence is basic to the effectiveness of the internal auditing program. This independence has two major aspects, as follows:

1.   The head of the internal auditing department should be made responsible to an officer of sufficient rank in the organization as will assure adequate consideration and action on the findings or recommendations. The organizational status of the internal auditor and the support accorded to him by management are major determinants of the range and value of the services which management will obtain from the internal auditing function.
2.   Internal auditing should not include responsibilities for procedures which are essentially a part of the regular operations of a complete and adequate accounting system or of a properly organized operating department. In some instances, management may assign current operating responsibilities to the internal auditing department, but in such cases the execution of the current operating responsibilities should be performed by separate personnel and be subjected to the same review and appraisal as is accorded other operations.

Thus, it can be seen that internal auditing extends far beyond the routine detailed verification of financial data. It can be, and often is, a complete periodic survey and analysis of all operations for the purpose of improving the efficiency with which such operations are conducted.

    Among hospitals, internal auditing generally has been associated only with the larger institutions. An increasing number of smaller hospitals, however, have found it desirable and feasible to establish internal auditing functions. While the use of regular employees on a part-time basis has met with moderate success in certain cases, it usually is preferable to employ one or more internal auditors on a full-time arrangement. This permits organizational independence and avoids conflicts of loyalties and fears of reprisals that might otherwise exist. The internal auditor should not have direct authority over, nor be responsible to, those individuals whose work is reviewed and evaluated. Typically, the internal auditor reports directly to the director of fiscal affairs, the hospital controller or, in some cases, to the administrator.

    Although the internal auditor does considerable work of an auditing nature, he does not compete with the external auditor. Instead, the two cooperate and supplement each other's somewhat parallel efforts. The internal auditor, through continuous review of the internal control system, greatly facilitates the work of the external auditor. The existence of an effective internal auditing function puts the external auditor in a much stronger position to render an authoritative opinion as to the fairness of the hospital's financial statements. On the other hand, the external auditor can bring greater objectivity and broad experience to bear on problem areas in which the internal auditor may need assistance.

Evaluation of Internal Control

A significant portion of the internal auditing function is a continuous and constructive evaluation of the hospital's internal control system. The internal auditor, like the external auditor, will often employ internal control check-lists or questionnaires in this effort. Figure 5-1 is an illustration of the types of questions that might be included in a preliminary survey of cash receipts and disbursements in an attempt to appraise the effectiveness of internal controls in that area. Similar questionnaires may be developed for investments, revenues and receivables, inventories, plant assets, accounts and notes payable, payrolls, purchasing, and for any other function or account group with which the internal auditor may become concerned. Most leading textbooks on auditing include many examples of questionnaires that are easily adapted to the hospital enterprise. The hospital's external auditors also would be a good source of additional information on internal control checklists.

Answers to the questionnaire items are obtained by the internal auditor by investigation and by interviews with various hospital personnel. The internal auditor's primary objectives are (1) to become acquainted with the employees and with what they do or do not do, (2) to acquire an understanding of particular hospital activities and operations, (3) to determine existing control methods and procedures, (4) to identify apparent weaknesses and areas which may require closer investigation, and (5) to obtain the information needed to devise appropriate internal audit programs. In this process, valuable impressions may be acquired concerning the efficiency of individual employees and their understanding of particular procedures in relation to the internal control system taken as a whole.

System Flow-Charting

From the information secured by observation and questionnaires, the internal auditor can develop flow charts of internal control procedures. Flow charts are visual or pictorial plans that show the flow of information and the sequence of procedures involved in control systems for various functions and activities. The flow-charting of an actual situation is an effective method for (1) determining how a particular system actually works, (2) evaluating the effectiveness of the existing internal control procedures, (3) developing more effective procedures, and (4) instructing employees of their individual duties in relation to the total system. External auditors also make extensive use of flow charts in obtaining a comprehensive picture of a client's internal control program.

The flow chart illustrated in Figure 5-2 provides a graphic portrayal of the principal procedures in an internal control system for purchasing and cash disbursements. Considerably more sophistication and detail can be built into such presentations by the use of different symbols (squares, circles, triangles, ovals, and diamond shapes) and lines (solid, dotted, wavy, and doubled) as well as with brief commentary within the chart itself. The art of flow-charting, particularly for automated systems, can be rather complex.

Figure 5-1.
Internal Control Questionnaire
Cash Receipts and Cash Disbursements

Genera

1. Are all bank checking accounts properly authorized by the governing board?
2. How many different checking accounts are maintained and what is the purpose of each account?
3. Are there any inactive checking accounts? If so, why are they maintained?
4. Is responsibility for the receipt and deposit of cash centralized?
5. Are all employees who participate in the receiving, paying and handling of cash:
   a. Adequately bonded?
   b. Required to take annual vacations?
6. Are employees in departments such as billing, credit and collection and purchasing, and those who might be in a position to participate in irregularities involving cash also adequately covered by fidelity bonds?
7. Is the hospital safe combination changed frequently and is access to the safe properly limited?
8. Are duties within the cashier's department segregated to provide the maximum practical degree of control within that department?
9. Do the employees of the cashier's department perform any of the following duties:
   a. Prepare charge tickets or other revenue records?
   b. Keep or have access to patients' ledgers?
   c. Assist in balancing the patients' ledgers with general ledger controls?
   d. Participate in the preparation and mailing of patients' statements?
   e. Approve discounts or allowances on patients' accounts?
   f. Approve the write-off of uncollectible accounts?
   g. Have custody of securities?
   h. Prepare or approve disbursement vouchers or sign checks?
   i. Prepare, sign or distribute payroll checks?
   j. Have custody of unclaimed payroll checks?
   k. Keep records of patients' safekeeping deposits?
   l. Keep or have access to petty cash?
10. Are bank statements and canceled checks obtained directly from the mail room or the bank by the person who prepares the bank reconciliation?
11. Are bank reconciliations made in the accounting or internal auditing department, rather than in the treasurer's or cashier's department, by employees who do not participate in the receipt or disbursement of cash?
12. Are bank reconciliations reviewed critically each month by a person not directly involved with the processing of cash receipts and disbursements?

Cash Receipts

1. At how many locations and by whom is cash received?
2. What kinds of cash receipts records are kept and who keeps them?
3. Is the mail opened by a person:
   a. Who does not prepare bank deposits?
   b. Who does not have access to the patients' ledgers?
4. Does the person who opens the mail list the receipts in detail?
5. Is the mail receipts list compared with the accounting records by an independent person?
6. Are cash receipts deposited daily and intact?
7. Does the cashier retain control of cash receipts until they are deposited?
8. Does someone independent of the cashier, and having no other access to cash or patients' ledgers, occasionally make a surprise check of the cash items against the bank deposit slip after the deposit has been prepared but before the deposit is actually made?

Figure 5-1 — *Continued*

9. Is a duplicate deposit ticket, after authentication by the bank, received directly from the bank by an employee independent of the cashier?
10. Are authenticated bank deposit slips compared with cash receipts records?
11. Does the cashier cash checks out of current receipts?
12. Have the banks been instructed in writing to cash no checks made payable to the hospital?
13. Are all persons who handle cash receipts adequately bonded?
14. Does the cashier receive incoming counter receipts directly from patients?
15. If cash register tapes, cash receipt slips and daily cash logs are used in proving the cash receipts, is the proof made by an employee independent of the cashier?
16. If the names of patients are not determinable from remittances,
    a. Does the cashier make deposit of remittances without delay?
    b. If not, does the cashier turn over such remittances to a responsible employee having no access to cash or patients' ledgers?
    c. Are such undeposited remittances controlled by recording them in a temporary account such as "undeposited remittances"?
17. Is independent accounting control established, outside of the cashier's department, over miscellaneous cash receipts such as interest, dividends and sales of supplies to employees?
18. Are patients' deposits and advance payments deposited promptly and properly accounted for?

Cash Disbursements

1. What kinds of cash disbursements records are kept and who is responsible for keeping these records?
2. Are all cash disbursements, except for petty cash items, made by check?
3. Are disbursements made only on the basis of approved vouchers that have supporting documents attached?
4. Are the supporting documents and approvals on the vouchers reviewed by the check signers at the time of signature?
5. Is notation of payment made on supporting documents to prevent duplicate payment? If so, how, when and by whom are such notations made?
6. Who are the check signers? Have all check signers been properly authorized by the governing board?
7. How many signatures are required on checks?
8. Are checks prenumbered and on protected paper?
9. Is a check protector used? If used, are signature machines properly controlled?
10. Are voided checks mutilated to avoid reuse?
11. Are voided checks retained and properly filed?
12. Are unused checks properly controlled?
13. Are all checks made payable to a person or company? Have banks been instructed not to cash checks made payable to the hospital?
14. Are checks signed *only* after they have been prepared in full?
15. Does any person authorized to sign checks have any of the following duties:
    a. Open the mail or list mail receipts?
    b. Act as cashier or have any access to the cash receipts?
    c. Prepare the bank reconciliation?
    d. Prepare or audit the disbursement vouchers?
    e. Have custody of petty cash funds?
16. Who has access to the checks after signature and who mails out the signed checks?
17. Are checks ever drawn payable to:
    a. Employees (other than for compensation)?
    b. Cash or bearer?

Figure 5-1—*Continued*

18. Does the person preparing the bank reconciliation:
    a. Account for all check numbers?
    b. Examine signatures?
    c. Examine endorsements?
    d. Compare canceled checks with entries in the accounting records?
19. With respect to long-outstanding checks:
    a. Are such checks investigated?
    b. Is payment on such checks stopped?
20. Are transfers between bank accounts promptly recorded?

Figure 5-2.
Internal Control Flow Chart
Purchasing and Cash Disbursements

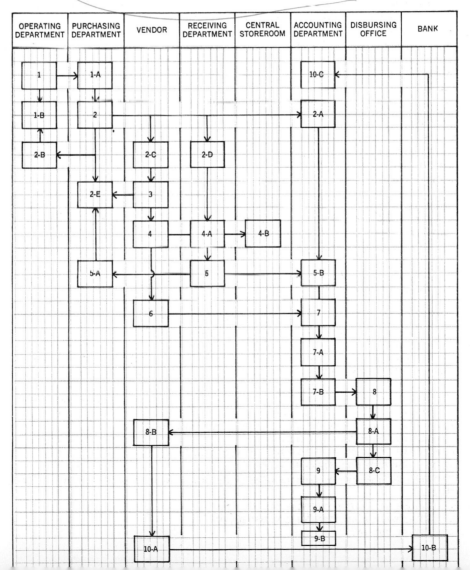

Figure 5-2 assumes that the hypothetical hospital is of sufficient size to have a centralized purchasing department and an otherwise reasonably good division of functions. The chart, however, does not directly reflect the necessary separation of duties within the accounting department. The system described is illustrative only; different circumstances require somewhat different systems. In the interests of clarity, the procedures depicted in the flow chart are briefly outlined rather than explained in the body of the chart.

1. An operating department, dietary or radiology, for example, notes that the inventory of certain supplies it uses has approached the order-point level. The department head consequently prepares a **purchase requisition** to inform the purchasing department of the **need to purchase** these supplies.

   A. One copy of the purchase requisition, properly executed, is sent to the purchasing department.

   B. A second copy is retained in a file by the operating department as evidence that the request was made.

2. The purchasing department, noting that the purchase request is properly authorized, makes appropriate determinations of quantity, price, and vendor and prepares a **purchase order** to acquire the supplies.

   A. One copy of the purchase order is sent to the accounting department for subsequent use in invoice audit and approval.

   B. A second copy is sent to the requisitioning department as notification that the order has been placed. The operating department will match this with its retained copy of the requisition.

   C. Two copies are sent to the vendor company. One of these is for the vendor's own use; the other is signed and returned to the hospital as acknowledgment of the order.

   D. Another copy of the purchase order is routed to the receiving department to assist that department in identifying incoming shipments. This copy, however, often does not provide information as to quantities ordered.

   E. A final copy is retained by the purchasing department in an unfilled orders file.

3. The vendor returns the acknowledgment copy of the purchase order to indicate acceptance of the order. The purchasing department matches this document with the purchase order copy in the unfilled orders file.

4. The supplies are shipped by the vendor to the hospital.

   A. In the receiving department, the supplies are counted, weighed, and otherwise inspected.

   B. The supplies are transferred to the inventory storeroom. (A discussion of inventory procedures appears in Chapter 12.)

5. A **receiving report** is prepared by receiving department personnel as a record of the quantity of supplies actually received. In some cases, a copy of the purchase order, with appropriate notations, is used as the receiving report.

   A. A copy of the receiving report is sent to the purchasing department where it is used to clear the related purchase order from the unfilled orders file.

   B. A second copy is routed to the accounting department to be used in subsequent invoice audit and approval procedures.

6. The vendor bills the hospital for the shipment. The **vendor's invoice**, while it may go through the purchasing department for approval, should be sent directly from the mail room to the accounting department.

7. In the accounting department, the three documents relating to the purchase are matched. These documents are the purchase order, receiving report, and vendor invoice or other billing. In a voucher system, a **voucher** is prepared and attached to the other three documents to form a **voucher package**. (For a description of how the purchase is audited, see Chapter 10.) In many cases, a check is prepared, but not signed, at this time.

   A. The purchase is recorded in the accounting records by an appropriate entry in a voucher register or purchases journal. The voucher package is placed in an unpaid vouchers file which constitutes the **accounts payable subsidiary ledger**. This file is regularly reconciled with the accounts payable control account in the general ledger.

   B. Just prior to its due date, the voucher package is removed from the unpaid vouchers file. The package is approved for payment and is transferred to the office of the hospital's disbursing authority.

8. The approved voucher package, with check included, is received by the disbursing officer. If desired, the documentary evidence in the package may be examined; other verifications also may be made.

   A. The check is signed by the disbursing officer and is mailed directly to the vendor. Signed checks are not returned to accounting department.

   B. The vendor receives the signed check by mail directly from the hospital disbursing office.

   C. All documents in the voucher package are indelibly stamped PAID to prevent their reuse in support of another disbursement. The package then is returned to the accounting department.

9. The paid voucher package is received by the accounting department in a personnel unit independent of the one in which the package was prepared and approved.

   A. An appropriate entry is made in the accounting records, check register, or cash disbursements journal, to record the payment of the purchase liability.

B.   The paid voucher package is placed in a paid vouchers file where it is kept for the period specified by the hospital's record retention policies.

10.   The movement of the hospital's check completes the last stage of the purchasing and cash disbursement cycle.

A.   The vendor company deposits the check in its bank.

B.   The check reaches the hospital's bank where its amount is deducted from the hospital's cash account balance.

C.   An independent unit of the accounting department receives the canceled check in a monthly bank statement. An individual in this unit, in the process of reconciling this bank account, will compare the canceled check with its entry in the accounting records.

These are only the highlights of a commonly employed system of internal control over purchasing and cash disbursements. A detailed discussion of these matters appears in Chapters 9 and 10. The presentation here, however, does give the reader an immediate opportunity to see how the considerations dealt with earlier in this chapter are fundamentally related to a specific system of controls. It also should be noted that many of the basic principles indicated by the questionnaire (Figure 5-1) are embraced in the description accompanying the flow chart.

Internal Audit Programs

The internal auditor's tentative conclusions as to the apparent effectiveness of the internal control system constitute the basis for the formulation of internal audit programs such as the one illustrated in Figure 5-3. This is a typical program for the audit of a bank checking account. As can be seen, an audit program is an orderly listing of auditing procedures to be completed in an examination or investigation of a particular account, group of accounts, or function. Some of the general objectives of such programs are (1) to verify that account balances are fairly stated in accordance with generally accepted accounting principles, (2) to detect fraud and errors, (3) to evaluate the effectiveness of internal control procedures as they **actually** exist, and (4) to determine the degree of compliance by employees with administrative and financial policies as prescribed by management. Programs in areas other than the one shown in Figure 5-3 can be obtained from the hospital's external auditor and from auditing textbooks.

Figure 5-3.
Illustrative Audit Program
Cash In Bank

1. Obtain current bank statement directly from the bank or directly from the mail room, unopened.
2. Prepare a bank reconciliation at the current date.
3. Obtain and review the bank reconciliation for the previous period.
4. Count and list all cash and cash items on hand awaiting deposit.
5. Trace prior period deposits in transit to current bank statement.
6. Trace checks listed as outstanding in prior period reconciliation to the current bank statement, listing and investigating all checks still outstanding.
7. Compare a sample of daily cash receipts entries in the accounting records to authenticated deposit tickets, cash register tapes and cash receipt slips.
8. Compare a sample of canceled checks returned with current bank statement with entries in the accounting records.

Figure 5-3. — *Continued*

9. List and investigate all checks made payable to cash, bearer, payroll, banks, employees (other than payroll checks) and unusual creditors.
10. Vouch cash disbursement journal debits to accounts other than accounts or vouchers payable.
11. Investigate the treatment of patients' checks returned by the bank.
12. Test for lapping.
13. Test for kiting.
14. Determine proper receipts and disbursements cutoff.
15. Investigate all interbank and interfund transfers during the period.
16. Verify footings of cash columns in cash receipt and disbursement records.
17. Obtain a bank statement for an immediately subsequent period directly from the bank and prepare a second (cutoff) bank reconciliation.
18. Prepare a proof of cash for the cutoff period.

Internal Audit Reports

Periodically, the internal auditor will prepare written reports of significant matters that are discovered in the course of routine internal audit activities. Reports will also be made of the results of special projects and investigations assigned to the internal auditor by the director of fiscal affairs, controller, or administrator. The auditor's findings and recommendations ordinarily should be discussed in advance with the persons responsible for inefficiencies and who might be directly affected by the auditor's recommendations. In this way, internal auditing may come to be regarded as a helpful and constructive function rather than as a force to be distrusted and feared. The executive receiving the audit report should consider the auditor's findings and recommendations seriously, being careful to carry all of them to a definite and final conclusion. If recommendations are to be implemented, all persons involved should be formally notified. The fact that the internal audit function has the attention and support of top management personnel should be clearly evident to hospital employees.

GENERAL INTERNAL CONTROL PRINCIPLES

The preceding discussion has indicated the nature of internal control and auditing, set forth the major reasons for adoption of internal control systems, and described the basic elements of a satisfactory system. With these introductory considerations in mind, the reader should examine the following listing of general internal control principles. The listing is by no means complete, but it is representative of the types of principles incorporated into the internal control systems of many hospitals. Specific applications of these principles, which vary from hospital to hospital because of differences in the prevailing circumstances, are described in detail in subsequent chapters of this book.

Cash

Internal control over cash is accorded special attention because of the large number of cash transactions and because cash is particularly susceptible to fraud. The control of cash is a topic treated in detail in Chapter 10, but some of the cardinal principles are provided here.

1. Employees who handle cash should be adequately bonded and should have no access to the accounting records. Similarly, persons who keep the accounting records should not have access to cash.

2. Incoming mail should be opened by someone independent of the cashier's office and the accounting department.

3. An immediate record should be made of cash receipts, and all such receipts should be deposited intact on a daily basis. No disbursements should be made directly from cash receipts.

4. The cash receiving function should be centralized to the extent practicable in the circumstances.

5. If minor disbursements are to be made in cash, petty cash funds should be established on an imprest basis for this purpose.

6. Except for petty cash expenditures, all disbursements should be made by serially prenumbered checks.

7. The person responsible for signing checks should not also have invoice auditing and recording functions.

8. Checks should not be signed unless accompanied by documentation evidencing the validity of the disbursements.

9. Surprise counts of cash should be made at irregular intervals by the internal auditor.

10. Bank statements should be reconciled on a regular basis by a person who does not prepare bank deposits or sign checks.

As will be seen in Chapter 10, the most effective administrative controls over cash are cash budgets and daily cash reports.

Investments

Hospital investments of a temporary nature are discussed in Chapter 10; investments in long-term securities are dealt with in Chapter 15. The principal features of internal control with regard to these investments are:

1. Investments should not be purchased or sold without appropriate authorization of the governing board or finance committee.

2. The person having physical custody of securities should not be the same person who maintains the detailed subsidiary ledger records of hospital investments.

3. Investment securities should be kept in a fireproof safe or bank safe-deposit box with access being denied to one person alone.

4. The internal auditor should periodically compare the actual securities with the detailed ledger records and reconcile them with the general ledger control accounts.

Internal control procedures must also be maintained with respect to income from investments, i.e., interest, dividends, and gains.

Receivables

Some of the major measures generally employed in the control of accounts receivable from patients are briefly identified below:

1. There should be a frequent balancing of patients' subsidiary ledgers against the respective control accounts in the general ledger, and this should be done by persons who do not maintain the subsidiary ledgers. Differences should be thoroughly investigated.

2. Ideally, someone other than the patients' ledger bookkeeper should prepare and mail patients' statements. If the billing function is performed by the receivables bookkeeper, another person should compare the statements with the subsidiary ledger records before mailing them.

3. All complaints received with respect to incorrect billings should be carefully investigated by an employee independent of the receivables bookkeeping, billing, and cashiering functions.

4. Internal auditors should compare admission registers, medical records, charge tickets, and census reports with entries made in the patients' ledger records to obtain assurance that charges were accurately and promptly made for all services rendered.

5. Daily totals of payments received on accounts receivable should be balanced against the individual credit postings to patients' accounts. All noncash credits to patients' accounts should be approved by a responsible employee other than the patients' ledger bookkeeper or the cashier.

6. Patients' accounts receivable should be aged at regular intervals, and the aging should be reviewed by an independent person.

Certain control procedures indicated for revenues and cash receipts also provide a measure of control over receivables.

Inventories

Detailed consideration is given to the matter of supplies inventories in Chapter 12. Control procedures with respect to this important asset include:

1. Prenumbered receiving and requisitioning records should be employed, and these records should be accounted for in numerical sequence.

2. Employees responsible for receiving, storing, and issuing supplies should have no access to the accounting records of inventories.

3. Physical controls should be established over inventories of supplies.

4. Periodic physical inventories should be taken at irregular intervals on a surprise basis under the internal auditor's supervision.

5. Perpetual inventory records should be maintained to the extent practicable in the circumstances and reconciled with physical inventories and general ledger control accounts. Significant discrepancies should be closely investigated.

Inventory reports should also be developed to provide periodic information as to slow-moving, obsolete, damaged, and overstocked (or understocked) supply items.

Plant Assets

The hospital investment in land, buildings and equipment is the subject of Chapter 16. Following is a summary of some of the internal controls discussed in that chapter:

1. Subsidiary records should be maintained and reconciled regularly with the general ledger control accounts. Such reconciliations should be performed by someone other than the plant ledger bookkeeper.

2. A physical inventory of movable equipment should be taken annually under the supervision of the internal auditor to verify the existence of such assets and to determine the accuracy of the detailed subsidiary records.

3. Plant assets should be acquired only by proper requisition and authorization by the governing board in accordance with an approved capital expenditures budget.

4. Retirements and disposals of plant assets should be by appropriate authorization, and measures should be adopted to assure a proper accounting for such events.

5. Plant assets should be adequately insured against fire and other risks.

It is extremely important that careful consideration be given to the development of effective methods for evaluating proposed capital expenditures.

Liabilities

The internal control of liabilities, discussed in Chapters 13 and 17, is concerned principally with assuring the validity of obligations prior to recording and paying them. Some general controls are:

1. Borrowings of funds through notes, mortgages, and bonds should be formally authorized by the governing board.

2. Purchases of all types should be properly supported by requisitions, purchase orders, receiving reports, and other documentation evidencing the validity of the related liabilities.

3. Detailed subsidiary records should be maintained and periodically reconciled with general ledger control accounts. These responsibilities should rest with different persons.

4. Measures should be taken to assure timely payment of liabilities to obtain discounts, to maintain a high credit rating, to comply with tax laws, and to meet debt retirement schedules without default.

Internal control procedures for payrolls, purchases, and cash disbursements are also applicable to liabilities in the sense that they represent opposite sides of the same coin.

Revenues and Expenses

Control procedures for revenues and expenses (see Chapters 6-9) are directly related to the controls indicated above for the balance sheet items of receivables, liabilities, and cash. While control over balance sheet items provides a degree of control over revenues and expenses, special controls are necessary for the effective management of the latter. Some of the major requirements for revenue and expense control are:

1. Assurances must be obtained through prenumbered charge ticket systems, departmental service logs, census reports, and other record procedures that **all** services rendered are recorded at established rates. It must be emphasized that unrecorded revenues are unbilled revenues and, if unbilled, are uncollected.

2. Ideally, the recording of revenue and the collection of cash should be independent functions, one providing a check on the other.

3. The personnel function should be centralized, but the authority and responsibility for hiring employees, keeping and approving time records, recording payrolls, and paying employees should be independently performed functions.

   a. Payrolls should be compared with master files of active employees maintained by the personnel department. Steps must be taken to assure that new employees added to the payroll are authorized in accordance with position control plans and other policies.

   b. Accurate data must be obtained as to hours worked by appropriate use of time clocks, time sheets, and other work records certified by department heads and supervisors.

   c. Promotions and changes in rates of pay should be approved by the administrator and reported promptly to the personnel department.

   d. General ledger payroll records should be reconciled with employee individual earnings records.

   e. Occasionally, paychecks should be distributed by the internal auditor instead of the person routinely authorized to do so. Special attention should be given to unclaimed checks.

4. The purchasing function should be centralized to the extent practicable, but receiving, storing, requisitioning, recording, and paying for purchased supplies should be independent activities, each requiring separate authorizations.

5. Recorded dollar amounts of revenues and expenses should be evaluated on the basis of independently accumulated statistics of volume of services provided to patients.

6. Revenues and expenses should be carefully budgeted, recorded, and reported on the basis of a responsibility accounting system.

7. Special controls should exist for nonoperating revenues such as investment income and contributions, and for unassigned expenses such as interest and depreciation.

That the budgeting of revenues and expenses is an absolutely essential requirement for effective hospital management can hardly be overemphasized. The next chapter is devoted to this very important subject.

CHAPTER 5 FOOTNOTES

1. Committee on Auditing Procedure, **Internal Control** (New York: AICPA, 1949), p. 6.

QUESTIONS

1. Define the term **internal control**. Distinguish between accounting controls and administrative controls.

2. State the reasons why an adequate system of internal control is essential in hospitals.

3. One of the basic elements of internal control is sound practices. Give five examples of sound practices.

4. Define the term **internal auditing**. What are the major objectives of internal auditing?

5. Distinguish between internal and external auditing. How are the two related?

6. Prepare an internal control flow chart for mail receipts in a hospital of medium size. Describe the operation of the system.

7. Prepare an internal control questionnaire for cash disbursements in a hospital of medium size.

8. What are the general objectives of an internal audit program?

9. Is internal auditing a line or staff function? How is the independence of the internal auditor maintained?

10. What are the purposes of good internal control? List the basic elements necessary for a general plan of internal control within a hospital. Why is a segregation of functional responsibilities of advantage in a system of internal control?

11. You have been made controller of a medium-sized hospital. The former controller, an honest man, was replaced because the operating fund bank account was found to be $10,000 short when it was reconciled after the vacation period. The weakness of the system of internal control made it difficult to determine responsibility for the shortage. What ten points would you check to assure an adequate system of internal control?

12. Name five basic elements or characteristics of a satisfactory system of internal control in any organization, and describe briefly the role each element or characteristic plays in the system. Do not describe methods or areas that require internal control.

13. Briefly describe the imprest system for operating a cash fund. State the principal advantages of the imprest system from the standpoint of internal control. Prepare a detailed questionnaire to be used in internal auditing in evaluating the internal control over a petty cash fund.

14. The independent auditors of Community Hospital have suggested that internal control be strengthened by the establishment of an internal auditing function. The Board is uncertain as to what this position would involve and has asked you the following questions:
    1. Why do we need such a position when there is no evidence of dishonesty in our organization?
    2. If the internal audit function is established, should the internal auditor report directly to the controller, to the treasurer, or to the administrator?
    3. If the internal audit function is established, will the hospital have any further need for annual audits by certified public accountants?
    4. If the internal audit function is established, how should we explain the purpose and functions of the internal auditor to the other employees?

Required. Answer each of the questions of the Board. Give your reasoning in each case.

15. Define internal control. Describe in detail the elements that are necessary for good internal control of (1) payroll, (2) cash receipts, and (3) cash disbursements.

16. What are the purposes of good internal control? How can good internal control be established and maintained?

17. List the requirements for a good system of internal control over cash receipts.

18. What are the functions and objectives of internal auditing?

19. List the principal internal controls which should be established for the dietary department.

20. List the principal internal controls which should be established for the plant operation and maintenance department.

21. An expansion is being planned for the hospital of which you are controller. Expansion plans call for an additional building and facilities which will increase the hospital's capacity from 150 beds to 250 beds. Since private gifts are needed to match a Federal grant, a building fund drive is anticipated. Your administrator requests you to set up proper controls for the receipt of the special-drive monies.

Before preparing a list of controls for building fund receipts, you decide to review existing forms and records to determine if any controls are in effect for present gift receipts. (The promotion of miscellaneous gift receipts is less than formerly because of a new cost-recovery philosophy of the hospital). The review indicates the following:

1. No source document is prepared for money received from a donor.
2. Miscellaneous gifts are listed in a book either from memory or from a scratch-paper notation.
3. When about a certain total is collected, the listings are pencil-summarized into subtotals for account distribution purposes.
4. A deposit slip in duplicate with the account distribution on it is prepared; the bank authenticated carbon being given to the bookkeeper in charge of the cash receipts journal.

Required. (1) What control procedures would you revise and adapt to building fund donations? (2) What control procedures for miscellaneous receipts would you change, and how? (3) Prepare a list of business controls from the receipt of each gift to its insertion into records.

22. Sunrise Hospital, a medium-sized hospital in a stage of expansion, consists of two divisions in the same location: the outpatient clinical division and the hospital services division.

The administrator is in charge of both divisions. Certified public accountants, in making their annual audit of the hospital, notice that there is a general need for improvement in the system of internal control; they recommend that an internal auditor be employed. This position is authorized. The administrator, knowing that the current operating budget is somewhat restricted, decides to employ a young man just graduated from college. His school record does not show specific courses in internal auditing, but it does reveal part-time work experience in the auditing department of the college he attended. Although his grades in accounting are not outstanding, his personality is excellent. The administrator feels that the latter quality will overshadow other qualities in the development of a successful internal auditing department.

Preliminary to preparing an audit program for his first year, the new auditor studies the hospital's organization chart. He notices that in the hospital services division of Sunrise Hospital, the functions of personnel employment and payroll preparation are in the same department under the same head. This discovery makes him feel that he should undertake immediately a major audit of this department. He discusses his plan with his superior, the comptroller. The comptroller, not having operated with an internal auditor, but feeling that the ambitious plan of the young auditor is in error, decides to call in a consultant, a retired auditor of a large industrial firm. The consultant, in a conference with the internal auditor and the comptroller, advises them to resort to a "get-acquainted" audit program for the first year through small functional audits such as counting inventories on a test basis and delivering department payroll checks.

Required. Prepare answers to the following questions, explaining briefly the reasoning for each answer.

1. Despite the consultant's advice, do you think the course of action as pointed out by the new internal auditor should be followed?
2. If you think the consultant's advice is to be followed, would you stand by your decision if there was knowledge that some of the "seeds" of fraudulent activity other than a lack of a separation of duties existed in the personnel-payroll department of the hospital services division?
3. Do you think a third and different course of action should be followed, with or without the knowledge that some of the causal factors of fraud were present in the personnel-payroll department?

23. Select the best answer to each of the following multiple-choice items relating to internal control:

1. For good internal control, which of the following functions should not be the responsibility of the treasurer?
   a. Data processing.
   b. Handling of cash.
   c. Custody of securities.
   d. Establishing credit policies.

2. Which of the following would be least likely to be considered an objective of a system of internal control?
   a. Checking the accuracy and reliability of accounting data.
   b. Detecting management fraud.
   c. Encouraging adherence to managerial policies.
   d. Safeguarding assets.

3. Which of the following is an administrative control?
   a. Authorizing credit terms.
   b. Execution of transactions.
   c. Recording original data.
   d. Accountability over source data.

4. For an appropriate segregation of duties, journalizing and posting summary payroll transactions should be assigned to
   a. The treasurer's department.
   b. General accounting.
   c. Payroll accounting.
   d. The timekeeping department.

5. To strengthen internal accounting control over the custody of major movable equipment, a hospital would most likely institute a policy requiring a periodic
   a. Increase in insurance coverage.
   b. Inspection of equipment and reconciliation with accounting records.
   c. Verification of liens, pledges, and collateralizations.
   d. Accounting for purchase orders.

6. Internal accounting controls are not designed to provide reasonable assurance that
   a. Transactions are executed in accordance with managerial authorization.
   b. Irregularities will be eliminated.
   c. Access to assets is permitted only in accordance with managerial authorization.
   d. The recorded accountability for assets is compared with the existing assets at reasonable intervals.

7. An independent auditor might consider the procedures performed by the internal auditors because
   a. They are employees whose work must be reviewed during substantive testing.
   b. They are employees whose work might be relied upon.
   c. Their work impacts upon the cost/benefit tradeoff in evaluating inherent limitations.
   d. Their degree of independence may be inferred by the nature of their work.

8. Which one of the following would the internal auditor consider to be an incompatible operation if the cashier receives remittances from the mailroom?
   a. The cashier prepares the daily deposit.
   b. The cashier makes the daily deposit at a local bank.
   c. The cashier posts the receipts to the accounts receivable subsidiary ledgers.
   d. The cashier endorses the checks.

24.   Ajax Hospital's internal auditor is about to begin a study and evaluation of the hospital's system of internal control.

Required. (1) What are the objectives of a system of internal accounting control? (2) What are the reasonable assurances that are intended to be provided by the system of internal accounting control? (3) When considering the potential effectiveness of any system of internal accounting control, what are the inherent limitations that should be recognized?

6
Budgeting Principles and Procedures

The hospital's basic objective is the provision of health care services of the type and quality required by the public. There is no other good reason for the existence of a hospital, or any other enterprise, except to render socially needed services. In striving to meet this objective, the hospital – as any other economic entity – must live within its means; its operations are subject to fiscal constraints. If the hospital is to continue as a viable enterprise, it must obtain revenues in amounts at least equal to the costs incurred in providing the services demanded of it. Or, stated in reverse fashion, the activities of the hospital must be so managed that incurred costs are less than, or not in excess of, revenues for any extended period. The hospital that fails to establish and attain this fundamental fiscal objective will soon find its ability to achieve its social objective severely impaired.

This does not mean that fiscal objectives are more important than social objectives. They are not. Nor does it necessarily follow that the social objectives will always be totally fulfilled if fiscal objectives are met. But, in the economic environment within which hospitals function, it is true that social objectives cannot be effectively achieved without the aid of appropriate fiscal objectives. The hospital does not succeed in achieving its social objectives by mere chance. It requires careful planning and effective control with respect to the resources required in the provision of healthcare services. There must be fiscal plans for securing the necessary resources and for using them in the most efficient manner. There must be fiscal controls by which the effective realization of such plans is reasonably assured.

In short, the preparation and use of a budget is essential to the successful management of today's hospital. It is an absolutely necessary requirement in the administration of the affairs of all hospitals, regardless of size, type, or other characteristic. Securing adequate financing and keeping expenses below revenues are universal and increasingly complex problems that cannot be solved merely by acting on a day-to-day basis to the many internal and external forces of change currently buffeting hospitals. Long-range planning is required as a logical framework within which consistent and meaningful short-range goals may be established. Plans alone, however, are not sufficient; controls are needed to assure their realization. The best method so far developed for effective management planning and control of hospital activities is a well-conceived budgetary program. Such a program, properly integrated with the accounting system, is the most important tool available to hospital management.

This is not, however, a budgeting textbook. But it is a book directly concerned with the financial management of hospitals, and no treatise of this kind would be complete without considerable attention being given to the critical importance of budgeting. While specific budgeting techniques and procedures are not emphasized here, the basic concepts and general principles of budgeting are described at some length. The purpose of this chapter is to present a broad view of the process of budgeting as it relates to management planning and control in hospital enterprises. More detailed considerations of the applications of budgeting principles to particular areas appear in subsequent chapters. Revenue budgeting and expense budgeting, for example, are discussed in Chapter 9, cash budgeting in Chapter 10, and capital expenditure budgeting in Chapter 16.

TYPES OF BUDGETS

A budget, defined in its broadest sense, is a formal plan of future operations expressed in quantitative terms and serving as a basis for subsequent control of such operations. It is a written document in which the objectives of the hospital are reflected in dollars and in various nonmonetary statistical units. The dietary department budget, for example, may be expressed as $800,000 and as 200,000 meals. Budgeting is the process by which budgets are prepared and used not only as a device for planning but also for control. Thus, one often hears the expression "budgetary planning and control."

Comprehensive vs. Partial Budgets

The term **comprehensive budget** refers to the total management plan for the hospital as a whole and for each of its subdivisions and major activities. Thus, it is an overall budget comprised of subbudgets for revenues, expenses, and capital expenditures. These subbudgets, in turn, are broken down further by source of revenue and objective of expenditure in a manner consistent with the hospital organizational structure and chart of accounts. The comprehensive budget brings together the subbudgets, consolidating them into a coordinated master plan of projected operating results and financial position. This includes cash flow, levels of receivables and inventories, purchasing and personnel requirements, plant asset additions, and debt retirement schedules. Such a plan becomes a detailed blueprint for the conduct of operations to achieve established objectives.

The word **budget** is also used to refer to the various components (subbudgets) of the overall plan. Reference may be made, for example, to the revenue budget, the cash budget, the dietary department budget, and so on. Some hospitals, in fact, do not develop comprehensive budgets but practice **partial budgeting**. They may prepare a budget of revenues and a budget of salaries and wages only, and perhaps also a capital expenditures budget. They may employ budgeting for planning but not for control purposes. This is unfortunate in that the full potential of budgeting is realized only through a comprehensive plan embracing all operations and used for both planning and control. Only by comprehensive budgeting is it possible to fully evaluate the adequacy and desirability of the courses of action reflected in the segmental budgets as coordinated and nonconflicting components of a cohesive overall program.

Nevertheless, partial budgeting is far better than no budgeting at all. It should be regarded as a step in the right direction with every effort being made to move toward comprehensive budgeting as rapidly as feasible. It must be recognized that comprehensive budgeting is a formidable task involving the development of budgets for **all** phases of hospital operations and the consolidation of the individual budgets into pro forma financial statements. This is a tall order for hospitals with little or no previous experience with budgeting, and it often is unwise to attempt to install a comprehensive budgeting system in a single year. Instead, such hospitals should begin with partial budgeting, bringing additional areas of operations into the program gradually until the goal of comprehensive budgeting is finally attained. The management of the hospital must not hurry the process unduly or attempt to install a total budgetary system all at once by edict. It will not work, and it can be most harmful in creating undesirable attitudes toward budgets on the part of hospital personnel. The need for comprehensive budgeting in hospitals is urgent, but it cannot as a practical matter be accomplished overnight.

Flexible vs. Fixed Budgets

The preparation of a budget requires that an assumption be made concerning the level of activity at which operations will be conducted. If a budget of dietary department expense, for example, is to be prepared, the probable number of patient meals to be served must be determined at the outset. This is the basis for estimating what the dollar budget should be. Should a dietary department activity level of, say, 200,000 patient meals be anticipated, a budget of perhaps $800,000 might be established. But if a greater or lesser workload is forecasted, a higher or lower number of dollars for this function would be budgeted. Expenses, in this way, tend to increase or decrease in total with increases and decreases in the departmental level of activity.

A **fixed budget** is a budget prepared under a single assumption as to anticipated activity level, e.g., 200,000 meals. Subsequently, this budget could be compared with actual performance as follows:

	Actual	Budget
Dietary Department Expense	$900,000	$800,000
Number of Meals Served	240,000	200,000

Such a comparison is virtually useless, although this is precisely what some hospitals may be doing. It is meaningless, and even misleading, to compare the actual cost of serving 240,000 meals with the budgeted cost of serving only 200,000 meals! The two dollar amounts are simply not comparable. While fixed budgets admittedly offer some benefits from the standpoint of planning, they are almost worthless for the purposes of control when the actual level of activity differs significantly from the anticipated level. And that quite often is exactly what happens.

To secure the fullest benefits from budgeting as a tool of planning and control, hospitals develop **flexible budgets**, sometimes called **variable budgets**. In effect, flexible budgets are a series of fixed budgets prepared under various assumptions as to the possible levels of activity that may be actually experienced. This procedure is facilitated by the identification of expenses as either fixed or variable. Given a relevant range determined by the highest and lowest levels of activity that reasonably can be anticipated, **fixed expenses** are those that do not change in total within that range. **Variable expenses**, on the other hand, vary directly with and are proportionate to changes in the level of activity. Raw food cost, for instance, is a completely variable expense whereas the dietitian's salary is a purely fixed expense. Other specific costs, called semivariable or semifixed costs, may exhibit both variable and fixed characteristics within the relevant range. Various techniques are available for isolating the variable and fixed components of such costs, but this matter is not considered at this point.

In budgeting departmental expenses, it generally is possible to develop a number of different budgets for planning purposes somewhat as shown:

	Estimated Level of Activity		
	Lowest Probable	Most Likely	Highest Probable
Dietary Department:			
Number of Patient Meals	150,000	200,000	250,000
Fixed Expenses	$200,000	$200,000	$200,000
Variable Expenses	450,000	60,000	750,000
Total Expenses	$650,000	$800,000	$950,000

Fixed expenses, as indicated, remain unchanged at any level of activity between 150,000 and 250,000 patient meals whereas variable expenses respond directly to changes in service volume at the rate of $3.00 per meal ($450,000/150,000, $600,000/200,000, or $750,000/250,000 = $3.00). Presentations of this kind can be extremely useful in helping department heads to understand the manner in which costs behave and respond to changes in service volume. This unquestionably leads to better planning for the utilization of resources.

From a control standpoint, the flexible budgeting approach permits the development of budget figures for any level of activity within the relevant range that is actually experienced. If, for example, the actual number of meals served turns out to be 240,000, the actual expenses at that level of activity can be compared with budgeted expenses **at the same level**, as follows:

	Actual	Budget
Dietary Department Expense	$900,000	$920,000
Number of Meals Served	240,000	240,000

The budgeted expense can be determined by interpolation, i.e., since 240,000 meals is 80 percent of the difference between 200,000 and 250,000 meals, the budgeted cost of 240,000 meals therefore is $600,000 + 80% of $150,000 ($950,000 $800,000), or a total of $920,000. If, on the other hand, dietary expenses have been resolved into fixed and variable classifications as shown, the budgeted cost of 240,000 meals is simply the total of fixed costs ($200,000) and variable costs at that level of activity (240,000 x $3.00), or $920,000. The latter procedure usually is necessary when a significant amount of semivariable (semifixed) expense is involved in departmental budgets.

The comparison of $900,000 of actual expense with $920,000 of budgeted expense is a valid and meaningful comparison because the actual and budgeted levels of activity are identical. It is basically a matter of comparing the actual cost of doing something with the budgeted cost of doing the same thing. This naturally permits a more intelligent evaluation of actual performance and a considerably more effective use of the budget as an instrument of control. To be most worthwhile for these purposes, actual and budgeted expenses must both relate to the **same** level of activity. Without this common denominator, such comparisons are invalid.

Long-Range vs. Annual Budgets

One of the major developments in the hospital field in recent years has been the increasing recognition of the importance of long-range planning. It is no longer sufficient, if it ever was, to plan ahead or budget only for a year at a time. In this era of socioeconomic and technological change, the contemporary hospital must engage continuously in long-range planning that reaches five or more years into the future. Should hospitals show an inability or an unwillingness to plan beyond one year, the long-range planning function may be vested entirely in areawide planning agencies or other authorities. Long-range planning is a job that obviously must be done in one way or another. If hospitals fail to accept full responsibility for developing appropriate long-range plans, it will be done for them through some external mechanism. Progressive management of hospitals will be marked by its ability to shape its own future to a substantial extent whereas the less successful managements will concentrate mainly on reacting month-by-month to changes forced upon them.

It may be argued incorrectly that long-range planning is too difficult, or even impossible, because of the great uncertainty that clouds the future of the hospital industry. The very fact that the future **is** highly uncertain, however, is itself indicative of the imperative need for long-range planning. The greater the degree of uncertainty characterizing the future, the greater the need for long-range planning and for annual budgets that are related to long-term objectives and goals. Decisions concerning the preparation of annual budgets cannot be made intelligently unless long-range plans for growth and change have been formulated with all possible precision. Many plans require more than one year for their execution; many plans that can be executed immediately involve investments in resources committed for an extended period of years; and many of today's policies have long-run implications. The annual budget therefore should be viewed as but a single segment of a larger and long-term strategic plan. It should not include planned actions of a tactical nature that are inconsistent with the desired long-term posture of the hospital.

In developing long-range plans, the individual hospital should begin with a detailed analysis of the demographic characteristics of the community it serves. This study includes an investigation of trends in population size, age groups, occupations, economic status, industrialization, and other factors. Consideration must also be given to emerging national and regional changes in medical and other relevant technology, to patterns of financing health care services, and to the characteristics of other health care facilities. Particular attention should be given to directions being taken by other hospitals serving the same community. Such forecast data of a factual nature constitutes **planning premises** for the purpose of establishing patient-service objectives and policies relating both to the primary and secondary care services to be offered. Alternative courses of action must be identified, examined, and evaluated so that the most appropriate long-term direction may be charted. Management will then be in a position to determine the facilities and resources needed to implement the selected course or courses of action. These needs, in turn, are converted into projected income statements and balance sheets for the next five to ten years. Projected financial statements of this kind will indicate the hospital's financial needs and reveal the economic feasibility of long-range plans. The expression of future plans in financial terms thus permits the necessary coordination and reconciliation of resources with objectives.

ADVANTAGES OF BUDGETING

The preceding discussion has indicated, in general terms, the desirability of budgeting. As was noted, one fundamental purpose of budgeting is to indicate the most appropriate long-range and short-run course by which the activities of the hospital should be directed to achieve its primary service objective. Another purpose is to provide a means for assisting management in conducting the hospital activities as nearly as possible on that charted course. The benefits of budgeting, in other words, relate directly to the basic management functions of planning and control. Budgeting is THE tool by which these broad functions are more effectively accomplished.

Some of the more specific and concrete advantages of a comprehensive program of budgeting may be enumerated as follows:

1. Budgeting forces the hospital management to reconsider and evaluate its basic objectives and policies on a regular basis.
2. Budgeting requires the assembly and analysis of historical accounting data as a basis for making projections into the future. This brings to light relationships that might not otherwise be noticed.
3. Budgeting demands that assessments be made of the impact of external socioeconomic forces on hospital operations.
4. Budgeting indicates the need for desirable changes in the hospital's organizational structure. It reveals weaknesses in organization.
5. Budgeting requires that all levels of management actively participate in the establishment of objectives. It serves to enlist the assistance of the entire organization in determining appropriate courses of action.
6. Budgeting leads to the coordination of each departmental plan with all others and with the hospital's overall objectives. It provides the necessary degree of consistency and cohesiveness.
7. Budgeting forces the hospital management to quantify its plans in written form. This helps to eliminate uncertainties relative to basic objectives and policies at lower levels of management.
8. Budgeting instills in management the habit of careful investigation, research, and analysis as a basis for decision-making.
9. Budgeting leads to the establishment of plans which result in the most productive use of available facilities, personnel, and money.
10. Budgeting stimulates a high degree of cost consciousness throughout the hospital organization.
11. Budgeting reduces costs by eliminating much of the waste caused by inadequate planning and ineffective control of operations.
12. Budgeting reduces the number of supervisory personnel needed through the establishment of firm policies and clear-cut lines of authority and responsibility. This frees executives from many of the routine, day-to-day responsibilities and provides more time for creative activity.
13. Budgeting pinpoints both efficiency and inefficiency. It provides standards against which actual performance is measured to determine variances which require investigation and corrective action.

14. Budgeting aids the hospital in obtaining credit from suppliers and banks. It permits the anticipation of financial needs so that the most desirable arrangements can be made in advance for securing and repaying loans.

15. Budgeting results in more prudent planning for expansion and for procurement of plant assets.

16. Budgeting provides a continuous check on the progress being made toward the achievement of hospital objectives.

17. Budgeting permits a proper assessment of the adequacy of the hospital's rate structure. A cost-finding procedure performed on the budget is most enlightening for this purpose.

18. Budgeting affords an opportunity for periodic self-analysis by all organizational units and all personnel in the hospital.

19. Budgeting produces a team spirit among employees. It promotes an attitude of understanding and cooperation.

20. Budgeting, properly employed, can be a powerful device for motivating personnel to a high level of performance. A budget, however, should not be used only as a whip; it should be a means of giving recognition, rewards, and encouragement to people who want to give their best efforts to their assigned tasks.

Aside from the fact that budgeting is often required of hospitals by rate review commissions, planning agencies, and other external authorities, the advantages of budgeting would seem to make obvious the desirability of a budgetary program. The potentials of budgeting are impressive indeed!

It must not be assumed, however, that budgeting is a simple process, free of problems and limitations. The installation and use of a budgetary program is a highly complex undertaking; its problems and limitations are significant. Any appreciable realization of its claimed benefits requires patience, hard work, and considerable time. In budgeting, hospitals generally have the greatest difficulty with problems in the following areas:

1. Securing the serious support of management at all levels of the organization.

2. Implementing a program of budget education so as to gain the willing cooperation of employees.

3. Developing accurate revenue budgets and meaningful performance standards for departmental activities.

4. Achieving the necessary degree of flexibility in budgeting for varying levels of service.

5. Maintaining effective follow-up procedures as to the actual impact of corrective actions.

Hospital managements must also be aware of the limitations of budgets. It must be recognized that the usefulness of a budget is directly related to the quality of the estimates upon which it is almost entirely based. Even if the estimates prove reasonably accurate, however, the budget plan will not automatically execute itself. The budget will not take the place of management nor is it a substitute for individual and group effort by employees. The entire organization must be "sold" on the budget and must participate in making the program work. In budgeting, the human element is of paramount importance.

PREREQUISITES FOR EFFECTIVE BUDGETING

A number of conditions are essential to the development and operation of an effective budgetary program. Some of the fundamental prerequisites are described here briefly.

Sound Organizational Structure

Effective budgeting requires a sound organizational structure in which the lines of authority and responsibility are clearly identified and understood at all levels of management. Every job in the hospital must be carefully defined, and definite responsibility for the performance of each job must be assigned to specific individuals to avoid an overlapping of efforts. Every employee must be aware of precisely what he or she is responsible for and to whom he or she is accountable. In addition to this responsibility, each individual must be granted sufficient authority to perform the assigned job with a minimum of direction from above. A departmentalization of activities must exist in which department heads and supervisors know the scope of their responsibility and authority within the overall organizational framework of the hospital. Such relationships are best presented by formal organization charts as discussed in Chapter 1 of this book. These charts and written job descriptions should be distributed to department heads and others who are involved in the preparation of budgets.

Budgets then are developed in a manner that conforms with the existing pattern of authority and responsibility. Individual plans for the achievement of specified objectives are established for each area of responsibility so that specific individuals become responsible for carrying out each plan. In other words, the master plan is departmentalized so that each department head has a plan that can be accomplished within the scope of his or her authority and responsibility. It is also necessary that budgets relate to organizational responsibilities because control is exercised through the same individuals who are responsible for efforts to follow the agreed plan and achieve the established objectives. Were this not done, plans might be developed with no person having either the authority or responsibility for carrying them out to completion, and it would be impossible to hold anyone accountable for a failure to meet the objectives of such plans. It is in this way that the budgeting process can assist management in identifying weaknesses in the organizational structure of the hospital.

Satisfactory Chart of Accounts

Effective budgeting requires a satisfactory chart of accounts, as described in Chapter 4. In other words, the chart of accounts should be designed to conform to the plan of organization. It should provide for the accumulation, on an accrual basis, of revenues and expenses in accordance with the organizational units responsible for producing the revenues and for incurring the expenses. Hospital revenues and expenses should be recorded and reported on a **responsibility accounting** basis. Each organizational unit constitutes a responsibility center to be charged for all expenses for which it is responsible and credited for all revenues, if any, that it generates. The expense so related to each center is further classified by object of expenditure; the revenues associated with each center are classified by activity source.

An accounting system in which revenues and expenses are accumulated and reported according to responsibility centers facilitates effective budgeting in two major ways. First, such a system provides the historical data that serves as the starting point in making projections into the future. It provides that information in the form most appropriate to planning. Since plans are made for each responsibility center, historical accounting data relating to the prior activities of each center must be available. Put simply, it would be very difficult to budget departmental payroll expense for the coming year if no information were available as to departmental payrolls of prior years.

Second, a chart of accounts designed for responsibility accounting leads to effective budgeting from the standpoint of budgetary control. This is accomplished through the reporting of the actual performance, in terms of revenues and expenses, of responsibility centers in the same format in which plans were established. It then is possible to compare plans with performances in a manner that readily indicates who in the organization is responsible for variances. In this manner, significant departures from planned performance can be detected and corrective action appropriate to the situation can be taken at an early point. In all cases where corrective measures are taken, it is important for control purposes that follow-up procedures include the careful perusal of subsequent accounting reports to ascertain that such measures had the desired effect.

Thus, successful budgeting is heavily dependent upon the accounting process for both planning and control purposes. Historical accounting data are employed as a basis for projections into the future. Current accounting data, reported in comparison with budgets, are essential in controlling departmental activities so as to accomplish objectives. This requires that the chart of accounts and the classification of budgetary data be consistent.

The reports should be prepared in accordance with the principle of **management by exception.** This principle is based on the idea that the busy executive should devote attention primarily to significant exceptions or unusual matters rather than to things that are not materially "out of line." The principle may be applied to the presentation of budgeted versus actual performance by the use of simple reporting techniques that pinpoint and emphasize major variances from budgets, thereby directing the executive quickly to those areas and situations most deserving attention and time. Mangers, in fact, often say "don't tell me what's going well, tell me what isn't." In such cases, budget versus actual reports might well exclude entirely all comparisons except those which are significantly over or under budget. There is considerable truth in the adage that the insignificant tends to detract from the significant.

Appropriate Statistical Data

The availability of reliable nonmonetary statistical data relating to the volume and scope of services in prior periods is as essential to effective hospital budgeting as historical financial information. Statistical data are used in both the planning and control phases of budgeting. Studies are made of previously accumulated general statistics such as number of admissions, patient days of service, percentage of occupancy, and average length of stay as a basis for projecting the future level of activity in overall terms. Analyses are required of occasions of service statistics in order to forecast expected levels of activity in the various departments of the hospital. Statistical data are also used to develop work and performance standards by which departmental service activities may be evaluated and controlled.

As noted in Chapter 4, hospital statistics must be accurately compiled and appropriately classified in a manner parallel to and consistent with the chart of accounts and organizational structure. Only in this way can statistical and monetary measurements of departmental activity be properly related. Intelligent evaluations cannot be made of past results in dollar terms alone. The dollars must be considered in conjunction with relevant statistical measurements of service volume. Similarly, the budgeting of future operations cannot be limited to an estimation of dollar values for the various accounting classifications. Equal emphasis should be given to expected performance in terms of nonmonetary statistical standards.

Decisions must be made as to the occasions of service and other statistics to be accumulated. Statistical terms must be carefully defined in writing (see Chapter 5). Additional definitions may be found in AHA's **Uniform Hospital Definitions**. Hospitals should also develop written procedures describing the methods by which statistics are to be accumulated. These procedures should be revised periodically to assure the accumulation of reliable information. Responsibility for the gathering of statistics should be definitely assigned; it generally is placed as near to the source of activity as practicable. In those instances where it is impracticable to make complete daily records of statistics, statistical sampling methods may be used to obtain the desired information within a reasonable degree of accuracy. Responsibility for the timely preparation of summary statistical reports should be specifically assigned to an employee in the fiscal services division of the hospital.

Support of Management

To be successful, a budget program must have the full support of management at all levels, starting with the hospital's chief executive officer (hereafter referred to as the administrator). Neither the controller nor the budget officer alone can assure the success of a budget; the impetus must come from the very top level of management for the necessary cooperation and interest to be obtained at lower levels. The administrator must recognize that the ultimate responsibility for the budget and its enforcement cannot be delegated. Token support by the administrator and other members of top management is not sufficient. Management must be "sold" on budgeting.

All levels of management must have an understanding of the principles of budgeting and be convinced that the results of budgeting will be useful to them in accomplishing their planning and control functions. Formal programs of budget education are helpful for this purpose. Managerial personnel must also be willing to devote their time and considerable effort to the budgeting process. Department heads and supervisors must be given ample opportunity to participate actively in the preparation of the budgets by which their performances will be evaluated. They should be made aware that budgets are designed to give adequate recognition to outstanding individual accomplishment as well as to inefficiency.

Thus, achievement of the necessary interested and cooperative involvement in the planning phase of budgeting at the departmental level depends largely upon the importance attached to budgeting by top management. This is the critical factor. Budgets are developed by departments but enthusiastic support must come from top management. When this support is not evident, budgeting is a sterile exercise.

Formal Budgeting Procedures

Effective budgeting will not be achieved if planning is accomplished in a haphazard, disorganized manner. While the budget is a cooperative endeavor involving the active participation of many different people, a specific individual must be assigned the responsibility for developing the various inputs and integrating them into a coordinated master plan. This individual, depending upon the size of the hospital, may be the administrator, the director of fiscal affairs, the controller, or some other person of experience and ability who is highly respected within the hospital. In any event, the budget officer must be a diplomat of the first order. This person must organize the budgeting process and deal effectively with a large number of persons to ensure that established procedures are carried out smoothly. The procedures to be established and seen through to completion are described in the next two sections of this chapter. It is assumed here that the hospital controller is the budget officer.

BUDGETARY PLANNING

Details of budgetary planning differ somewhat among hospitals. There are, however, certain basic requirements that must be satisfied in one way or another. The following discussion indicates some of the procedures that are employed in the planning process by many hospitals.

Budget Committee

Most hospitals have a budget committee that serves in an advisory capacity to the budget officer who chairs the committee. The committee generally consists of a representative number of department heads with membership awarded on a rotating basis so that all major department heads eventually have one or more opportunities to serve as members. Department heads tend to leave the committee with a much greater understanding and appreciation of budgeting than they brought to it, so it becomes a valuable learning experience. Terms of office are staggered so that continuity of long-range plans is maintained. It must not be forgotten that the budget is but the current installment of the hospital's long-range plan. This objective is also achieved through appointment of the personnel director and purchasing agent to permanent membership on the committee.

Neither the budget committee nor the budget officer should attempt to actually prepare departmental budgets. This is the responsibility of the department heads. The budget officer's responsibility is that of designing the budgetary system and assisting department heads in implementing it. The budget committee has the function of advising and assisting the budget officer in discharging these responsibilities. Following are some of the areas in which the budget committee provides advice and assistance to the budget officer:

1. Determination of planning premises and formulation of the hospital's long-range plans.
2. Development and revision of the budget manual, including definitions of budgeting policies and procedures.
3. Preparation of the budget calendar with target dates for completion of each stage of the budgeting process.
4. Review of proposed departmental budgets, including recommendations for revision and change.
5. Approval of final departmental budgets and coordination of budgets into a master plan for all operations of the hospital.
6. Development and enforcement of a formal reporting and control system, including follow-up procedures.

The role of the budget committee, as described here, is advisory in nature; the committee generally should not have direct responsibility for the budget program. Authority and responsibility rest with the budget officer.

Budget Manual

Every hospital should develop a budget manual in which budgeting policies and procedures are clearly written. With respect to the planning phase of budgeting, this manual should include complete coverage of the following matters:

1. Objectives of the hospital's budgetary program.
2. Definitions of the authority and responsibilities of all personnel engaged in the preparation of budgets.
3. Instructions, in full detail, as to the mechanics of budget development and samples of standardized forms to be used.
4. Calendar of budgeting activity, with a time schedule for the completion of each stage of the program.
5. Detailed procedures for the review, revision, and approval of all budgets comprising the total program.

As will be indicated in the next section of this chapter, it is also essential that the budget manual give considerable attention to a careful description of the reporting and budgetary control system. This includes uniform report form and content, responsibility for report preparation, analysis and corrective action, and follow-up procedures.

Budgeting is a complex undertaking for which written procedures and detailed instructions are imperative. Budget manuals are necessary in order to formalize methods, to control forms and reports, to establish authority and responsibility, and to assist in budget education and training. The drafting of the manual is usually a task assigned to the budget officer working in consultation with the various department heads. Because accuracy and ease of application are particularly important considerations, the written procedures should be tested by trial runs before they are put into effect. The budget manual, of course, must be kept up to date as changes are made in the budgetary program to make it more useful to hospital management. Conditions and situations change rapidly, and the budgetary system must be reviewed and revised accordingly. An obsolete manual of budgeting procedures can be most damaging to the morale of personnel with budget responsibilities. It may easily be taken by them to mean that top management is not seriously interested in the budgetary program.

Budget Period

As noted earlier, the existence of a strategic long-range plan in hospitals is essential to the development of short-run budgets. Long-range plans look five or ten years into the future; they are concerned primarily with broad objectives and the charting of general courses of action to achieve them within that length of time. The short-range budget, on the other hand, is much more detailed and is somewhat tactical in nature; it relates to the current means by which more immediate objectives can be realized within an operating period. Traditionally, the operating or accounting period is considered to be one year, either fiscal or calendar, and therefore budgets normally are prepared for that same period. The year is the natural, basic unit of time for which highly detailed plans can be made with a reasonable degree of confidence and accuracy.

The annual budget totals should be determined by adding together the 12 monthly budgets. It is inappropriate to merely divide annual forecast data by 12 in order to arrive at monthly budgets because of the seasonal variations that occur in the activities of most hospitals. The dynamic nature of operations from month to month makes it essential that monthly budgets accurately reflect the probable pattern of high and low activity levels. In this connection, there is much to be said for continuous budgeting in hospitals rather than the widely employed periodic budgeting method.

In **periodic budgeting**, plans for the following 12-month period are developed only once each year. The **continuous budgeting** procedure, however, involves the preparation of an initial one-year plan and then, as each month passes, the addition of a budget for the corresponding month one year hence to the far end of the original 12-month plan. This process produces a continuous 12-month budget in which seasonal factors are emphasized. Each month, the budget officer is required to project the current month one year into the future. Budgets prepared by this method tend to be more accurate and useful for control purposes. An additional advantage of continuous budgeting is that, by spreading the work of budgeting evenly over the entire year, it focuses constant attention on budget problems and objectives.

Budget Calendar

In order to assure prompt completion of the various stages of budgetary planning, the budget officer should develop a **budget calendar** in which the required steps are identified and a time schedule of completion dates is established. Budgetary planning usually must begin from three to six months prior to the new budget period because initial departmental plans generally are revised one or more times before they can be finalized and approved. Hospitals with no prior budgeting experience will require a much longer lead time.

A typical budget calendar is illustrated in Figure 6-1. Note that a specific completion date is established for each step in the process. Considerable care should be given to the framing of the time schedule to avoid the frustrations and confusion that can result from delays and postponements. Department heads must be made aware that the target dates are firm and are not to be abused.

Figure 6-1.
Budget Calendar

Date	Participants	Activity
May 1	Administrator, budget officer and department heads	Specification of general assumptions and objectives; general discussion of budgetary program
May 8	Budget officer and department heads	Discussion of assumptions, departmental objectives and planning procedures
May 15 to June 15	Budget officer and department heads individually	Projection of departmental plans
June 25	Department heads and budget officer	Submission of initial drafts of departmental budgets
July 1 to July 10	Budget officer and budget committee	Coordination of departmental budgets; review and amendment of the initial drafts
July 15 to July 25	Budget officer and department heads individually	Reprojections of departmental plans
August 1	Department heads and budget officer	Submission of revised drafts of departmental budgets
August 5 to August 10	Budget officer and budget committee	Review and approval of reprojected departmental budgets
August 15	Budget officer	Submission of coordinated budget to administrator
August 20 to August 25	Administrator and budget officer	Review of budget and preparation for presentation to governing board
September 1 to September 15	Administrator, budget officer and governing board	Presentation and review of budget
September 20	Governing board	Approval of budget
October 1	All hospital personnel	Begin new fiscal year operations under approved budget

Planning Procedure

The planning phase of budgeting, often called **budget-making**, requires the cooperation of a large number of hospital personnel and the coordination of their efforts by the budget officer. It is not a simple process. Five basic steps are involved:

1. Specification of general assumptions and objectives.
2. Projection of departmental plans.
3. Review and amendment of departmental plans.
4. Review and approval of reprojected departmental plans.
5. Presentation and approval of the budget.

Following is a summarized and comprehensive view of the overall planning procedure, including a brief description of the basic steps listed.

Specification of Objectives. As indicated in the budget calendar in Figure 6-1, an initial meeting is held on May 1, about five months before the beginning of the budget period. (It is assumed here that the budget period is the coming fiscal year which commences on October 1.) The purpose of the meeting is to specify to department heads the general planning assumptions and overall objectives that will serve as a basis for the development of departmental budgets. It is important that these specifications, at least the major ones, be set forth by the hospital administrator personally. The department heads must be made to see that the budgetary program is a matter of great concern and importance to the administrator and that it has the firm support of top management. Some time should be allowed at this meeting for department heads to voice their opinions and ask questions in regard to the general premises upon which their budgets will be constructed.

The general assumptions and specifications enumerated at this meeting will have been formulated earlier by the budget officer and committee with suitable input and approval by the administrator. Projected admissions, average length of stay, occupancy, patient days, and departmental occasions of service will have been made as a result of previous formal and informal meetings and discussions, exchanges of memoranda, and studies of accounting, statistical, and other information relevant to the volume of activity to be anticipated in the budget period. Budgetary implications of changes in rate structure, reimbursement contracts, personnel policies, organization, and facilities will have been carefully evaluated. These preliminary deliberations will have produced, in clearly written form, the specifications to be presented by the administrator at the May 1 meeting.

A second meeting is held a week later on May 8. The budget officer conducts this meeting at which there is a more detailed discussion of underlying assumptions and departmental objectives. The purpose of the meeting is to translate the general guidelines laid down by the administrator into coordinated specifications at the departmental level. In addition, the budget officer will review with the department heads the budget-making procedures to be followed in the coming weeks.

Projections of Departmental Plans. A full month, May 15 to June 15, is given to a series of meetings in which the budget officer confers with department heads individually. It should be understood that the department head is fully responsible for the preparation of the departmental budget; the budget officer provides all the assistance possible and otherwise acts in an advisory capacity. In this process, the budget officer must look at each tentative departmental budget in terms of how closely it conforms to the general assumptions and objectives underlying the total budgetary program. The end result of these efforts is the submission of the initial drafts of departmental budgets to the budget officer on or before June 25.

Review and Amendment of Departmental Plans. Upon receipt of the initial drafts of departmental budgets, the budget officer develops a tentative comprehensive plan by consolidation of the individual budgets. This tentative plan is examined by the budget committee in a number of meetings starting around July 1. In this process, it is likely that the tentative plan will undergo several revisions in order to achieve the necessary degree of coordination among the many segments making up the total. As a result, amendments of the departmental budgets as initially drafted will become necessary.

Starting July 15, the budget officer will meet again with department heads individually. The department heads will be informed of needed amendments in their initial budget drafts so that they will conform with the decisions of the budget committee. Appropriate reprojections then are made by the department heads, and revised drafts of departmental budgets are submitted to the budget officer on August 1. Should department heads disagree with amendments, protests may be filed with the budget officer for further consideration by the committee.

Review and Approval of Reprojected Departmental Plans. Once again, the budget officer will pull together the various departmental plans into a fully coordinated comprehensive budget for the hospital. This budget then is given a final review and approval by the budget committee. On August 15, the coordinated budget is submitted to the administrator by the budget officer. The remainder of the month is given to preparations by the administrator and budget officer for presentation of the budget to the hospital's governing board.

Presentation and Approval of the Budget. The administrator, perhaps with the assistance of the budget officer, makes the budget presentation to the governing board in a number of meetings which begin September 1. Attitudes and procedures differ here, of course, but it generally is wise to limit the presentation to a brief narrative report in fairly broad terms — a condensed income statement with summarized schedules of departmental revenues and expenses, a summary of proposed plant and equipment acquisitions, and a monthly or quarterly cash budget. Usually, the practice is to set forth only the more significant factors considered in the development of the budgets. In this way, the attention of the board is focused upon essentials, and it is not distracted by relatively unimportant details. Nothing of major consequence is ever to be hidden from the board, and the administrator should be prepared to furnish whatever detailed information the board might request. The board's review of the proposed budget, however, is properly confined in most circumstances to a broad evaluation of the general features and implications of the budgetary program.

After the board's approval is secured, the approved budget is communicated to all department heads in the hospital. Departmental meetings may be held for the purpose of informing departmental personnel of budgetary constraints and obtaining their assistance and support as the new fiscal year begins under the approved budget.

BUDGETARY CONTROL

While a measure of control is achieved in the planning stage of budgeting, budgetary control generally refers to the executory stage where management's concern is that of keeping actual operations in conformity with previously established plans. Assuming that the budget is valid in the prevailing circumstances, the three essential steps in budgetary control are:

1. Performance appraisal
2. Corrective action
3. Follow-up

Budgetary control requires that the budget plan first be communicated to, and accepted by, those personnel responsible for carrying out the plan. No one can be held accountable for a failure to conform to a plan unless that person was made aware of the plan and has agreed to accept it as an expression of attainable goals.

Performance Appraisals

The first step in the use of budgets for control purposes is that of making appraisals of the performance of personnel charged with responsibility for specific areas of activity within the hospital. This is accomplished to a large extent through control reports in which actual and budgeted results are compared and variances are analyzed and interpreted so as to discover their causes. Much attention therefore should be given to the development of reports that provide the various levels of management with this information in the most useful manner.[1]

Effective budget reports will have certain obvious characteristics. They must be timely, they should be expressed in clear form and language familiar to the user, they should be accurate and relevant, and their preparation cost should be commensurate with their importance. To the extent possible, the **exception** principle, discussed earlier in this chapter, should be applied so as to emphasize and highlight the unusual and the important. Figures in the reports should be in the comparative form and in logical sequence. Relevant statistical data should be provided along with the monetary data.

In addition to these rather fundamental considerations, hospital budget reports should be developed in accordance with the concept of **responsibility reporting**. This means that reports of costs and revenues should be related to the individual responsibility centers. The report for each particular center should include only those costs and/or revenues which are subject to control by the center manager or which are attributable to the manager's efforts. The responsibility reporting principle is illustrated in a simplified manner in Figure 6-2.

The responsibility reporting system is based upon the organizational structure and conforms to the chart of accounts by which controllable costs are accumulated according to the centers responsible for incurring them and revenues are recorded according to the centers in which they were generated. In this way, the organizational structure and chart of accounts automatically determine the destination and content of budget reports.

Observe in Figure 6-2 that the administrator, being responsible for the entire hospital activity, receives a report in which the expenses of each division of the hospital are summarized. The administrator's report segregates expenses according to the division heads responsible for divisional activity and whom the administrator holds accountable. Division A, for example, might be the nursing services division headed by the director of nursing. The report of Division A includes a summary of expenses by departments over which the division head has effective control. The Department 1 report, in turn, includes only those expenses for which the department head can be held responsible. Should there be clearly defined subordinate organizational units within Department 1, reports may be prepared along similar lines for those lower levels of management.

There is another point to be made about responsibility reporting. It can be seen that as reports are made to higher levels of management, the reported data are increasingly summarized. While reports should provide as much detail as necessary to for

Figure 6-2.
Responsibility Reporting

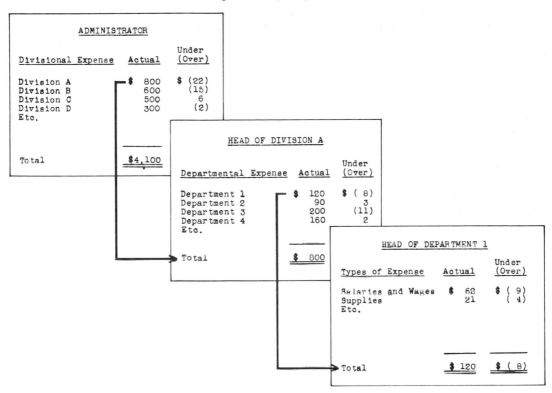

proper interpretation and decision-making, they should tend to a minimum of information. The manager, however, may request whatever amount of supporting detail he requires. The reports in Figure 6-2 are greatly simplified and do not include budget figures. When the budget figures are excluded, the readability of the report is greatly improved.

Considerably more needs to be said with respect to performance appraisal through budget reports. Accordingly, this matter will be pursued at greater length in the next three chapters.

Corrective Action

Budget reports, no matter how well conceived, will not control anything. By reflecting variances from plans, they serve to indicate the need for management action of one kind or another. Budget reports pinpoint **where** variances exist in the hospital organization and **who** is likely to be responsible. When variances arise, they must be acted upon if control is to be achieved. Appropriate action requires that the variances be investigated and analyzed so as to determine their causes. Only when the causes are known can correct responses be made.

It therefore is essential that budget reports include interpretative commentary and explanations of variances by the budget officer or controller. The reports often are supplemented by brief comments indicating **why** variances have occurred and perhaps suggesting courses of action designed to correct those situations demanding management attention. In some instances, this may be insufficient; the budget officer may be asked to make a special study of the problem and prepare a "spot" report, including recommendations for remedial action by the manager having the necessary authority.

It is worth noting that once a cost is incurred it cannot be controlled. This suggests that the first line of control lies in the development of a budget consciousness. Department heads and other hospital personnel must maintain an awareness of spending levels permitted by the budget. They must recognize that, when unauthorized variations occur, the variations will be investigated and they will have to be explained and justified. Nothing can be done to control excessive costs already incurred, but the knowledge that deviations have occurred, and the reasons why, is useful in preventing similar deviations in the future. Corrective action, then, is the second line of control. If it is to be most effective, it must be accomplished by action taken as near as possible to the source of the observed deviations, i.e., by the immediate supervisor of the particular organizational unit for which a significant budget variance is reported.

Follow-up

Once a decision has been made and implemented with regard to a particular corrective action, follow-up measures are necessary to determine whether or not the corrective action had the desired effect. The effectiveness of a corrective action tends to be reflected in subsequent budget reports relating to the area of deviation. These reports should be examined carefully to see if the variance has been eliminated or reduced. It may be found that the corrective action had little or no apparent effect in resolving the causes of the variance. In some cases, it may appear that the corrective action actually worsened the situation. Additional analysis may be necessary to determine a new and different course of action.

NEWLY EMERGING TECHNIQUES

Anyone involved in the management of hospitals is aware of the sweeping changes which are taking place in the healthcare industry. These changes are creating new problems of a serious order whose solutions challenge the adequacy of traditional financial management and accounting techniques. As the management of hospitals becomes more and more complex, an increasing use must be made of more advanced methods and techniques as a basis for decision-making. It is apparent that mathematical and statistical applications, with the assistance of computers, are replacing many of the timeworn management tools which no longer serve their purpose well.

Among the statistical and mathematical techniques with which hospital financial managers must become at least conversant are operations research (OR), sampling, probability theory, factorial analysis, game theory, linear programming, financial model building, critical path method (CPM), and program evaluation and review technique (PERT). These and other mathematical-statistical approaches to management problem solving are particularly pertinent to the hospital enterprise in which there are so many variable interrelationships. The reader is strongly urged to make an intensive study of these statistical and mathematical techniques.

THE HUMAN ELEMENT IN BUDGETING

In spite of the above comments concerning the increasing use of scientific methods in conjunction with computers, anyone who has worked with a budget or any other management tool knows that the most essential ingredient to the success of an organization is people. Nothing, no matter how sophisticated or scientific, will work unless people are willing to allow it to work. The most advanced budgetary programs will actually tend to decrease efficiency unless the human element is ranked at equal importance with the technical aspects.

The "people aspect" of budgeting—motivation, cooperation, leadership, training, education, environment, human relations—is a subject in itself. While this matter is not addressed at great length here, it is no less important to remember that a budget is merely a device to control costs through people.

CHAPTER 6 FOOTNOTES

1. Many excellent management reports are illustrated in the author's **External and Internal Reporting by Hospitals** (Chicago: HFMA, 1984)

QUESTIONS

1. Define the term **budget.** Why is budgeting essential to the successful management of today's hospital?

2. Distinguish between comprehensive and partial budgeting.

3. Distinguish between flexible budgets and fixed budgets. Which is preferable from the point of view of budgetary control?

4. Define each of the following terms: (1) fixed expense, (2) variable expense, (3) semivariable expense, (4) semifixed expense, and (5) relevant range.

5. List ten major advantages of budgeting to hospital management.

6. Name the five principal prerequisites for effective budgeting in an organization.

7. What is your understanding of the principle of management by exception? In what way is this principle related to budgeting?

8. What is the function of a hospital budget committee? Who should serve on the hospital's budget committee?

9. Why should a hospital have a budget manual? What matters should be covered in such manuals?

10. Distinguish between periodic budgeting and continuous budgeting.

11. General Hospital's fiscal year ends June 30. Prepare a budget calendar that you would recommend that the hospital follow in developing a budget for its next fiscal year.

12. What are the five major steps to be completed in the planning phase of budgeting?

13. Name and describe the three essential elements of budgetary control in hospitals.

14. What is your understanding of the term **responsibility reporting**? How is this related to budgeting?

15. Discuss the importance of the human element in budgeting.

16. You are discussing with your administrator the advantages of a budgeting program for your hospital. The administrator asks, "Why can't we just continue to compare our monthly figures with last year's monthly figures instead of going through all this trouble to set up a budget?"

    In addition to answering the administrator's specific question, present in outline form the benefits of a budgeting system.

17. Name the two basic types of operating budgets and briefly describe each of them.

18. Expenses may be classified as either direct or indirect. Name and describe another classification of expense.

19. You have been employed as the budget officer of the Memorial Hospital. In outline form, list the steps you would take in fulfilling this responsibility. Give particular emphasis to the manner in which the accounting office may be of assistance to you.

20. List the data needed to prepare a fixed budget for the dietary department. Describe the difference between a fixed budget for the dietary department and a flexible budget for the same department.

21. You have just been engaged as controller of a 350-bed hospital. This hospital has never operated on a budget system. The administrator asks that you set up the budgetary system in the hospital with particular emphasis on the payroll aspect. What controls would you set up in the budget for payroll? Explain in detail and give reasons for these controls. Your solution should include any controlling procedure relative to the employment of personnel which you would deem necessary to control payroll costs.

22. Define the following terms:
  1. Budgeting
  2. Master budget
  3. Static budget
  4. Flexible or sliding scale budget
  5. Budgetary control
  6. Budget reports
  7. Budget period
  8. Formal budget plan
  9. Budget calendar
  10. Budget committee

23. The following budget versus actual report was given to a hospital administrator.

	Actual	Budget	Variance
Dietary expense	$115,773	$119,600	$ 3,827 favorable

During this period, 92,618 meals were served, but 98,000 meals were budgeted. What conclusions might be drawn from this information?

24. Explain the importance of statistical data to budgetary planning of departmental expense dollars. Explain the importance of statistical data to budgetary control of departmental expense dollars.

PART 2

Revenues and Expenses

7
Accounting for Hospital Revenues

The **earning** of adequate amounts of revenues is a major goal of enterprises of all types. No organization can survive for long unless its revenues are sufficient to finance its current operating activities and maintain its long-run productive capacity. In an extended period of price inflation, technological advancements, and other fiscal pressures, this means that revenues must be obtained in excess of the costs of providing goods and services. The earning of reasonable amounts of profit is essential. The recently implemented prospective payment system (PPS) based on a predetermined fixed-price-per-case in itself indicates a public recognition that it is legitimate for hospitals (even those that are tax-exempt) to earn a profit on services to Medicare patients. To earn profits under this legislation, however, hospitals must be managed on cost-efficiency principles similar to those observed in other industries, and must deal successfully with competitive pressures.

Historically, however, hospitals generally were operated and managed on a nonprofit, break-even (or worse) basis. Profit in the provision of hospital services was regarded as somehow immoral or, at best, detrimental from a public relations standpoint. Because of huge and continuing donations by individual philanthropists, the making of profits seemed neither desirable nor necessary. Later, when hospital financing was secured largely through public subscription and governmental grants, a profitable financial history would have made fund-raising campaigns and efforts to obtain grants more difficult to justify.

Hospitals have now become big businesses, and general recognition is given to the fact that the solution to many of their problems lies in the adoption of businesslike methods and financial policies. Hospitals are placing an increasing emphasis upon the management of costs in an effort to reduce them to levels at which they more closely approximate revenues. Although more can be accomplished in the cost containment and reduction area, it may not be enough to relieve the financial distress with which the industry is embraced. A multitude of pressures over which the individual hospital often has little, if any, control have caused substantial increases in costs and tend to negate the many positive steps hospitals have taken to reduce costs. It is reasonable to assume that these pressures will continue unabated.

In addition to cost reduction and control measures, hospitals must give a considerable amount of attention to the revenue side of the problem. A great deal remains to be done about costs, but hospitals have been hamstrung for many decades with reimbursement systems that often failed to provide adequate amounts of revenues. While hospitals deal with millions of individual patients, more than 90 percent of patients' bills are paid by third-party contractors. Hospital revenue sources, then, are limited to a relatively few organizations having substantial economic power. These organizations can, and do, exercise that power in arranging contracts which provide for reimbursements in amounts which may not take into account all of the legitimate costs incurred in hospital operations. The definitions of "reasonable" costs and "reimburseable" costs, for example, have been matters of dispute as long as third-party contracts have existed.

The situation is confused by significant differences in the reimbursement formulas of the different third-party payers. It is a rather complicated system. In some instances, the hospital is reimbursed on the basis of its regular charges for services provided or on the basis of a fixed price established by, or negotiated with, a third-party payer. In other cases, however, the hospital is reimbursed on the basis of the "costs" of the services it provides. The reimbursed costs may be retrospectively or prospectively determined; they may be actual costs incurred by a particular hospital, or they may purport to be "average" costs for a group of hospitals in a given geographic area.

In many cases, the hospital is contractually unable to collect from patients the difference between the amount of reimbursement and its established rates for the services provided. Even where these differences may be billed to patients, the amounts may not be collectible. Nor can the hospital choose to serve only those patients who have the ability to pay the amounts billed to them for hospital services. As a result, self-responsible patients who do pay their hospital bills sometimes are paying for a disproportionate share of hospital costs.

There is every indication that substantial changes will continue to be made in the manner in which hospitals are paid for their services. Whatever these changes prove to be, the need for a high order of revenue accounting and management in hospitals will not be any less than exists at present. If anything, the importance of revenue accounting will be magnified. In the meantime, every available step must be taken to account for revenues so that they may be managed in a manner that results in maximum realization consistent with the current system by which hospitals are paid for the services they provide.

This chapter is concerned with some of the major problems of revenue accounting, including discussions of revenue recognition, measurement, and classification. This is a broad subject for a single chapter, and the reader may find it necessary to refer to periodicals and other sources for a more detailed discussion of certain aspects of the subject. Some topics related to this general area are discussed further in subsequent chapters, particularly Chapters 9 and 11.

NATURE OF REVENUES

The term **revenues** was defined in Chapter 2 as inflows or other enhancements of assets of an entity or settlements of its liabilities (or a combination of both) during a period from delivering or producing goods, rendering services, or other activities that constitute the entity's ongoing major or central operations. In other words, revenues result when an asset, usually cash or claims to receive cash, is received or a liability is extinguished in exchange for goods and services provided by the hospital to another entity, e.g., a patient.

For example, assume that a hospital provides a particular laboratory service to a patient. If the established price of the service is $30, the hospital has earned revenues of $30 which would be recorded as follows:

```
Cash (or Accounts Receivable)              $  30
     Revenues                                         $  30
     To record revenues earned from
     laboratory services.
```

This transaction involves the exchange of a service for an asset, either cash or accounts receivable. An asset was received by the hospital; a service was provided in exchange for the asset.

On the other hand, assume that a patient makes a $30 deposit with the hospital but does not receive the laboratory service until one week later. The receipt of the deposit does not result in revenue, but gives rise to a liability:

```
Cash                                       $  30
     Liability for Patients' Deposits                 $  30
     To record receipt of cash deposit from
     patient.
```

Although an asset has been received, there is no revenue at this point since the hospital has not provided any service in exchange for the asset. Nothing has been earned by the hospital. Should the patient not receive the laboratory service for some reason, the deposit would be refunded to the patient. If the service is rendered to the patient, an earnings process has been culminated, and the following entry would be made at that time:

```
Liability for Patients' Deposits           $  30
     Revenues                                         $  30
     To record revenues earned from laboratory
     services.
```

No asset was received by the hospital at the time the laboratory service was provided. Instead, a liability was extinguished. In effect, the hospital exchanged a service in return for being released from a liability.

Not all decreases in liabilities result in revenues. In fact, almost all such decreases are reflective only of the use of assets to discharge hospital obligations. Typically, a decrease in liabilities is accompanied only by a decrease in assets, usually cash, and no revenue results.

Similarly, not all increases in assets result in revenues. Many increases in particular assets are accompanied only by corresponding decreases in other assets as, for example, when accounts receivable are collected. Other increases in assets are accompanied only by an equal increase in liabilities as is the case when funds are borrowed from banks. Finally, asset increases also result from events which increase the hospital's equity without creating revenues, e.g., the receipt of cash or other assets from a donor to establish an endowment.

More often than not, then, revenue is characterized as an inflow of assets arising from an earning process and not accompanied by a corresponding increase in liabilities. It should be noted that revenue is a gross concept, i.e., it is measured in amounts undiminished by deductions for costs of goods sold or of services rendered. The term **income**, on the other hand, generally is used in a net sense as in operating income or net income for the year. Yet, in many instances of common usage, the terms revenue and income are employed interchangeably.

RECOGNITION OF REVENUES

When should hospitals recognize revenues? At what point in the stream of hospital activity is revenue to be regarded as realized so that credits to revenue accounts are required? The general rule is that accounting recognition is to be given to revenue at the earliest practical point at which the revenue is captured, measurable, and earned.

Revenue Is Captured

Revenue is regarded as captured when there is substantial certainty of an inflow of assets with which the hospital is able to do whatever it chooses, i.e., there is a severance in which the hospital comes into possession of assets whose utilization is not restricted by any external entity. This typically is the case with revenues derived from the provision of services to patients and from unrestricted gifts. Certain other asset inflows, including resources received from donors who restrict the use of the resources to specific purposes, are regarded as captured, and therefore recognized as revenues, but only when the hospital performs the particular specific purpose activities specified by the donors. In other instances, as with rent and interest, the capturing process is closely related to the passage of time.

In cases where revenues arise from a reduction of hospital liabilities, the capturing process is completed when the hospital is released from its obligation to pay the liabilities.

Revenue Is Measurable

The accounting recognition of revenue also requires that the related asset inflows (or decrease in liabilities) be reasonably measurable. Receipts of cash present no significant measurement problems. Amounts of noncash assets received generally are readily measurable at net realizable cash value (for receivables) or fair market value (for contributed properties and services). With respect to revenues arising from services to patients, it is important from a managerial standpoint that such revenues be initially measured and recorded in terms of the hospital's full, established service rates. These gross amounts are subsequently reported with appropriate reductions for revenue "losses" resulting from differences between the established prices of the services rendered and the realizable cash value of the related asset inflows, if any. Such differences arise primarily from the provision of charity service, contractual adjustments relating to third-party contracts, bad debts, and courtesy discounts. These revenue losses generally are reported in hospital income statements as direct deductions from revenues rather than as expenses. The same items are included in hospital balance sheets as an allowance for uncollectible accounts to the extent necessary to reduce the gross amount of receivables to net realizable (collectible) values.

Revenue Is Earned

Hospitals have **earned** revenue only when services have been rendered or goods have been sold to patients and others which result in either a cash receipt or a claim to the future receipt of cash (or other asset). This general rule applies to the following three situations.

Revenue Earned Before Cash Is Received. The receipt of cash subsequent to the rendering of services is the most common situation in hospitals. Patients' accounts are charged and revenue accounts are credited on a daily basis as services are provided to patients. In conformity with the accrual basis of accounting, revenue is recorded in the time period in which it is earned, whether or not cash is received at the same time. Revenue is considered realized at this point because services have been rendered in exchange for receivables, and because it is the point at which the amount of the revenue is captured and can be objectively determined. (Under the cash basis of accounting, revenue is not recorded until received in cash.)

Revenue Earned When Cash Is Received. A substantial amount of hospital services may be provided on a cash basis, i.e., there is a more or less simultaneous exchange of services for cash. Outpatients, for example, use hospital services such as laboratory and x-ray, and sometimes pay for these services as they enter or leave the hospital. In these instances, it often is possible to bypass charges to patients' accounts receivable and make debits directly to cash. Some hospitals, however, as a matter of internal control and to maintain a complete service/payment record for all patients, prefer to route all cash receipts from patients through accounts receivable.

It is important to note here that, although cash is received concurrently with the provision of services, the receipt of cash is not the determining factor in the recognition of such revenues. Nor is the amount to be recorded as revenue limited to the amount of cash received. Revenue is earned in the time period in which services are provided to patients, and the amount of revenue recorded should be the established rates for such services, irrespective of the amount of cash collected for those services.

If the hospital is to receive a bequest from the estate of a deceased benefactor, but the amount that actually may be received is not determinable with reasonable certainty, it usually is desirable to wait until the estate is settled and the funds are actually received before recognizing revenue in the accounts. In the meantime, an asset account entitled "interest in unsettled estates" is frequently established in the nominal amount of $1. The offsetting credit is made to a deferred revenue account. If preferred, disclosure may be made only in the form of an appropriate footnote to the balance sheet.

Revenue Earned After Cash Is Received. Patients may be asked to make prepayments (deposits) when they enter the hospital for treatment. The hospital, however, has no revenue until services are subsequently rendered to such patients. Prepayments of this sort often are credited to deferred revenues (Liability for Patients' Deposits) as illustrated earlier in this chapter. Upon receipt of a prepayment, however, an entry sometimes is made to debit cash and credit the patient's account receivable. The resulting credit balance in the patient's account is offset by subsequent charges for services. If material amounts of such credit balances exist at the end of a reporting period, however, they should be reflected in the balance sheet as liabilities in the manner described in Chapter 13 of this book. A similar procedure is applicable to prepayments and advances received from third-party payers.

Another problem exists with respect to the recognition of revenue arising in the form of gifts, grants, and donations. Unrestricted cash receipts of this nature are immediately credited to revenue, but where donor restrictions or contingencies are involved the treatment is necessarily different. If a grant is received in 1987, for example, with the stipulation that the money not be used until 1988, the grant should not be recorded as revenue until 1988. The receipt of such a grant is recorded by a debit to cash and a credit to deferred revenue in the Unrestricted Fund or in one of the restricted funds, depending upon whether the money will be available for general operating purposes or for donor-restricted specific purposes.

CLASSIFICATION OF REVENUES

Today's hospital obtains its revenues in a far different manner that it did several decades ago. Major changes have occurred in the number of revenue-producing activities and the in the relative importance of each source of revenues. These changes have arisen from advances in medical technology, new and different systems of third-party reimbursement, and other factors. As a result of this growing complexity, greater demands are placed on accounting for detailed information concerning the amounts of revenues generated from each of a large variety of specialized services to many types of patients in various medical and financial classifications. More attention also is being given to the application of improved procedures in accounting for gifts, grants, and other revenues not directly related to the provision of healthcare services to hospital patients.

For accounting purposes, hospital revenues are broadly classified as either (1) operating revenues or (2) nonoperating revenues. The operating revenues of the hospital consist of all revenues derived from activities necessary to the provision of healthcare services directly related to patients. The nonoperating revenue classification includes a limited number of items such as unrestricted gifts, unrestricted income from endowment funds, income and gains from investments of the Unrestricted Fund, and other miscellaneous revenues. Although the dividing line between operating and nonoperating revenues sometimes may be unclear, it is an important distinction. The following discussion is indicative of current practice in this regard.

Operating Revenues

The operating revenues of a hospital are typically classified as (1) patient service revenues, (2) deductions from patient service revenues, and (3) other operating revenues. Further breakdowns are developed within each category to the extent required for effective management of the individual revenue-producing centers.

Patient Service Revenues. Patient service revenues of the hospital are those derived from the provision of room, board, nursing, and other professional healthcare services to patients. These revenues usually are recorded in three primary classifications:

1. **Daily Patient Services.** Revenues from daily patient services arise from the provision of room, board, and general nursing services to hospital patients. The term "routine services" has often been applied to this group of patient services.

2. **Other Nursing Services.** Revenues derived from other nursing service include the patient services provided by operating rooms, recovery rooms, delivery rooms, central supply, and other units organized within the nursing services division of the hospital.

3. **Other Professional Services.** Revenues derived from other professional services, sometimes called "special" or "ancillary" services, arise from the provision of other healthcare services to patients. The classification is comprised of the services of laboratory, radiology, pharmacy, anesthesiology, physical therapy, and similar organizational units.

All revenue accounts established in these three classifications should reflect the value, at the hospital's full established rates and on an accrual basis, of all direct services rendered to patients. This principle should be rigidly observed without regard to the fact that the hospital often will receive less than established rates for these services.

Daily patient service revenues are classified in the accounts according to the sources from which the revenues were derived. The classification employed is patterned to conform with the organizational structure of the hospital in a manner somewhat as follows:

Medical
Surgical
Pediatrics
Intensive Care
Psychiatric
Obstetric
Newborn Nurseries
Other Units

A further classification may also be made on the basis of patients' financial status or on the basis of type of hospital accommodation. In this way, the accounts will reflect, in useful detail, the sources of revenues. The particular classification chosen depends upon the hospital's organizational structure and its managerial needs.

Revenues from other nursing services are also classified in accordance with the organizational structure of the hospital. The required accounts may include:

Operating Rooms
Recovery Rooms
Delivery Rooms
Central Services and Supply
Emergency Service
Other Units

As indicated with respect to daily patient services, subclassifications of these accounts on the basis of patients' financial status are also important.

Revenues from other professional (ancillary) services, like daily patient service revenues, are accumulated in accounts conforming to the hospital's organizational structure. The accounts generally maintained include:

Laboratories
Radiology
Pharmacy
Anesthesiology
Physical Therapy
Electrocardiology
Other Units

These accounts, of course, must be subclassified to provide the necessary distinction between inpatient and outpatient revenues. Further breakdowns may be made according to patients' financial status.

In summary, revenues from patient services of all three categories should be recorded, on the accrual basis and at full established rates, in accounts which associate such revenues directly with responsibility centers. This is accomplished by designing the revenue chart of accounts to conform to the organization chart of the individual hospital. As a result of this procedure, the performance of particular service units can be measured and evaluated in dollar terms as well as in statistical units. The more detailed classifications by type of patient, financial status, or hospital accommodation are also vital to a complete analysis of operations for budgeting and other financial management purposes.

Deductions From Patient Service Revenues. It was noted that patient service revenues should always be recorded at the hospital's full established rates. In many instances, however, the hospital receives less than its established rates when patients' accounts are settled. Although this situation generally can be anticipated when services are provided to patients, full rates nevertheless should be used in making initial records of revenues. The use of full rates permits a uniform measurement of the total potential earnings from all services rendered to patients during any given period of time. It also permits the measurement of revenues "lost" in those instances where full charges are not collected. Such information often points up the need for desirable revisions in hospital policies and practices. Revenue data compiled on any other basis obviously would be much less useful from a managerial standpoint.

Differences between full rates and collectible charges traditionally have been recorded as deduction from revenues. They usually are classified into four major types:

1. **Charity care.** Hospitals must provide their services to all who are in need of such services, regardless of their ability to pay. As a result, a considerable volume of service is provided to financially indigent patients. A difference therefore arises between revenues recorded at established rates and the amounts received, or to be received, from the financially indigent and from voluntary agencies or governmental units on behalf of such patients.

2. **Contractual adjustments.** The terms of contractual agreements with third-party payers often give rise to nonbillable balances representing the difference between the value of services rendered at established rates and the reimbursable amounts determined at contract rates. Such situations arise because contractual rates often are based on cost or a fixed price which falls short of the hospital's regular billing rates for its services.

3. **Courtesy discounts.** Hospitals sometimes grant special allowances or give discounts on bills incurred by their employees, members of the clergy, and others. This practice has been defended on grounds that the recipients have low income, have some special relationships with the hospital, or are otherwise deserving of such adjustments. Current attitudes, however, do not favor the giving of these types of allowances and discounts in cases where the patient, in fact, is able to pay full charges.
4. **Bad debts.** Bad debts arise from the uncollectibility of the accounts of patients who have the financial ability to meet their obligations to the hospital, but do not. Bad debts probably are inevitable, but losses in this area can be minimized through vigorous credit and collection programs, monthly analyses of receivables on an individual account basis, and in other ways (see Chapter 14).

All four categories of revenue deductions should be accounted for on the accrual basis in accordance with generally accepted accounting principles. This usually requires that, in addition to those deductions recognized during an accounting period, the revenue deductions accounts must be debited at the end of the period for the estimated amounts of such deductions to arise from current receivables. The appropriate accounting procedures are described in Chapter 13.

In the hospital's income statement, revenue deductions should be presented net of related revenue. The hospital, for example, may have received gifts or grants from donors who restrict the use of such amounts to the assistance of charity patients or to the financing of a free clinic. These amounts often are initially recorded in the Specific Purpose Fund, being subsequently transferred as revenue to the Unrestricted Fund as the donor's requirements are fulfilled. In other instances, income from investments of the Endowment Fund also may be restricted to a similar purpose. Special revenue accounts are needed in these cases so that presentations in the income statement (Figure 7-1) will be facilitated. Note, for example, the presentation of charity care as a revenue deduction.

Figure 7-1.
Any Hospital
Condensed Income Statement
Year Ended December 31, 1987

Patient Service Revenues	$415
Less Deductions from Revenues (net of related gifts of $12)	102
Net Patient Service Revenues	313
Other Operating Revenues	25
Total Operating Revenues	338
Less Operating Expenses	382
Loss from Operations	(44)
Nonoperating Revenues	61
Net Income for the Year	$ 17

*Disclosure of appropriate details is assumed to appear in supporting schedules as illustrated in Chapter 19.

While the above description of internal accounting for revenue deductions may continue, the HFMA's Principles and Practices Board has recently issued an exposure draft of a proposed position statement which contains the following conclusion:[1]

> For general purpose financial reports, revenue of institutional healthcare providers should be reported at the amount which a payer has an obligation to pay. If payment arrangements call for payment of charges, that amount is reported as revenue. If payment arrangements provide for a discount, the amount reported as revenue is net of the discount. If payment arrangements call for payment of a specific amount for a case irrespective of the services rendered, that amount is reported as revenue. This reporting of revenue is consistent with the reporting practices of other businesses. Additional information about payment arrangements should be disclosed in notes to the financial statements.
>
> Services that result in bad debts should be reported in revenue at the amount expected to be collected and this same amount should be shown as an expense. Services to patients unable to pay (charity services) is reported as revenue in an amount equivalent to that which would be reported if collection was expected and the uncollected (or uncollectible) portion is reported as an expense.

It is difficult to know whether or not this proposal will become a generally accepted reporting practice among hospitals. For this reason, the discussion and illustrations in this book will reflect the traditional methods of accounting for, and reporting, revenue deductions.

Other Operating Revenues. Other operating revenues are derived from incidental services to patients, from sales of supplies or services to persons other than hospital patients, and from other activities normal to the day-to-day operation of the hospital but not directly related to the care of patients. Following are some examples of other operating revenues:

Revenue from Educational Programs
Research and Other Specific Purpose Grants (excluding charity)
Rentals of Space to Doctors, Employees, and Others
Nonpatient Sales of Supplies
Cafeteria Sales
Revenue from Gift Shops, Snack Bars, Newsstands
Recovery of Telephone Charges
Television Rentals
Transcript Fees
Donated Commodities

These revenues should be accounted for on the accrual basis in accordance with generally accepted accounting principles. The presentation of these revenues in the hospital income statement is illustrated in Figure 7-1.

Nonoperating Revenues

Nonoperating revenue is a classification limited to a relatively few items. Among these are:

1. **Unrestricted Gifts.** Included in the category of unrestricted gifts are all gifts, grants, and legacies on which there are no donor-imposed restrictions and which are available for general operating purposes.
2. **Unrestricted Income from Endowment Funds.** Unrestricted income from Endowment Fund investments includes all income on which there are no donor-imposed restrictions (see Chapter 15).
3. **Miscellaneous.** Items such as income and gains on Unrestricted Fund investments, gains on sales of plant and equipment, and the fair market value of services donated to the hospital are included in the miscellaneous category.

It is important to note that all unrestricted gifts and income must be reported initially as nonoperating revenues regardless of the eventual purposes to which they may be designated by the hospital's governing board.

ACCOUNTING PROCEDURES

The objective of accounting for hospital revenues is to record all revenue transactions accurately and promptly in accordance with generally accepted accounting principles on a consistent basis so as to provide the information required for intelligent managerial decision-making and external reporting purposes. Revenue accounting systems vary somewhat from hospital to hospital, but, whatever the system employed, it should be designed to meet this objective fully and at a minimum cost. No particular system is described in detail here. The discussion is largely of a general nature, although some emphasis is given to certain matters of particular importance. Many of the forms and records mentioned are illustrated in the author's **Introduction to Hospital Accounting.**

Patient Service Revenues

Direct hospital services to patients may be classified into two categories: (1) daily room and board (routine) services and (2) professional (ancillary) services. These services are rendered on a virtually continuous basis to inpatients who are lodged in the hospital and to outpatients at the time of their visits to the various professional departments or clinics. In accounting for the revenue derived from these services, certain basic records must be developed and maintained. These basic records include source documents, a journal system, and a ledger system.

Inpatient Revenues. When a person enters the hospital as an inpatient, several forms are completed at the admitting office. One of these forms, often called a notice of admission, is routed to the accounting department, and an individual ledger card is prepared for the patient. The information obtained in the admitting process allows an accounting classification of the patient according to financial status, hospital accommodation, and other appropriate categories.

During the period of stay, the inpatient is charged for the services rendered to him or her and revenue accounts are credited. The accounting and control system must provide detailed written evidence of all hospital services provided to patients as well as documentation of the attending physicians' authorizations. This evidence appears in the patients' charts maintained at the nursing stations and in supporting source documents kept in the accounting department.

Room and board (routine) service revenues are compiled from information obtained from the daily census report. Forms and procedures differ, but the determination of revenue basically is a matter of multiplying occupied rooms (beds) by established daily charges for such accommodations. These revenue data are classified in various ways so that totals may be developed by type of service (e.g., medical, surgical, obstetrical, nurseries), type of financial relationship with the hospital, and type of accommodation. Procedures should be devised so that credits made to the revenue accounts are reconciled with occupancy data in the census report and are checked against charges made to patients' accounts. The objective is to secure a high degree of assurance that credits are made to the proper revenue accounts in correct amounts for all room and board services provided each day. Management decisions can be no better than the accuracy and completeness of the information on which they are based.

By studying the revenue derived from small charges for items such as adhesive bandages, lubricants, aspirins, sedatives, rubbing alcohol, and gowns, the per diem earnings from such charges can be estimated. It is practical in most instances to adjust room and board rates to absorb these small items. The procedure saves much time in both the nursing stations and in the accounting office. In addition, it saves printing and paper costs and tends to lead to better public relations.

A room charge is usually made for the day of admission but not for the day of discharge, provided the patient leaves on time. An early checkout time eliminates last minute service cancellations and enables housekeeping to make the rooms ready before new patients are admitted in the afternoon.

Credits to inpatient revenues for operating rooms, laboratory, radiology, pharmacy, and other professional services typically originate from written authorizations by attending physicians on forms generally known as **physicians' orders**. The prescribed services are requisitioned from the appropriate service departments by a nurse or a clerk working under nurses' supervision. Ward clerks can often perform many clerical details so as to relieve the nursing staff for more important duties of patient care.

The source documents for these services are usually known as **requisition** or **charge tickets**. They serve both as authorized requisitions for services and as means from which proper credits to revenues and charges to patients' accounts may be determined. Most hospitals employ different charge ticket forms for each professional service. These tickets generally are printed in different colors to facilitate the identification of the various services. They may also be prenumbered and accounted for on a serial basis when feasible.

When a nurse or ward clerk requisitions a service, usually three copies are made of the charge ticket. The original and duplicate copies may go to the service department, while the triplicate remains at the nursing station as a control copy. When the service is rendered, the service department indicates this on the charge ticket and prepares whatever report may be necessary for inclusion in the patient's medical chart.

Several times during the day, the original copies of charge tickets are collected from the service departments and are taken to the accounting department for processing.

The duplicate copy often remains on file in the service department as evidence of services performed and as a basis for compilation of various statistics. Charge tickets may be priced by the service departments, but most often this is done in the accounting department from a list of standard charges. Priced charge tickets then are sorted into various classifications so that totals may be obtained for the different categories of revenues. Again, reconciliations and proofs can be performed to assure the accuracy of the amounts credited to the various revenue accounts.

As a result of these procedures, the determined amounts of revenues are formally recorded in the accounts of the hospital. A summarized entry is as follows:

Accounts Receivable – Inpatients	$ 35,000	
Daily Patient Service Revenues		$ 18,000
Other Nursing Service Revenues		5,000
Other Professional Service Revenues		12,000
To record inpatient revenues.		

This entry is often made in an inpatient **revenue journal** or **register**. (See the author's **Introduction to Hospital Accounting.**) The revenue credits shown here are only representative of the series of credits that usually are made to the various revenue center accounts, e.g., operating rooms, pharmacy, and laboratory. In some cases, it may be feasible to maintain revenue control accounts in the general ledger supported by detailed revenue data in subsidiary ledgers.

Daily postings, of course, must be made to patients' ledger accounts, but postings of journal credits to the revenue accounts may be deferred to the end of the month when the journal columns are totaled and cross-balanced. At that time, the accumulated revenue totals are posted to the general ledger with offsetting debits being made to the appropriate general ledger accounts receivable control accounts. Nearly all hospitals find it necessary to employ accounting machines or data processing equipment of varying degrees of sophistication. With these types of equipment the journalizing and posting of revenues often is combined into a single operation. Such equipment also makes feasible the recording of revenue data in considerably more detail than otherwise.

Outpatient Revenues. When a person enters the hospital as an outpatient, he or she registers either at a central outpatient reception desk or at the particular professional department where the required service is rendered. The registration process provides the patient's name and address, indicates financial status, identifies the service(s) required, and secures other essential information. In some cases, the patient may be asked at this time to pay a registration fee. The patient may also pay for the services to be received or may make arrangements to be billed to the extent that the charges are not covered by insurance. In other situations, the patient pays the bill at a central cashier's location after he or she has received service and is leaving the hospital. Even in the case of outpatient clinics providing charity care, it is still essential that procedures be followed which provide complete and accurate records of all services rendered.

Various procedures are followed in recording revenue transactions involving services rendered to outpatients. Hospitals generally attempt to place as many outpatient services as possible on a cash basis, and, where this is done, the control of cash and the control of revenues become almost a single problem. In many cases, for example, equipment which "locks in" a copy of the outpatient visit record is utilized. This copy is used by the accounting department as a means of certifying cash receipts. Outpatient service requisitions, charge tickets, departmental service logs, and statistical records also can be employed in ways which assure the recording of complete and accurate outpatient revenue data.

Most methods relating to the recording of inpatient service revenues are also applicable to outpatient revenues. These revenues should also be recorded on the accrual basis, at full established rates, and in managerially useful classifications. Source documents, logs, and other outpatient service records typically are collected from the outpatient registration desk, cashiers' offices, and service departments, and are processed in the accounting department for daily entry in outpatient revenue journals or registers as indicated in the following summarized entry:

Cash in Bank	$ 3,000	
Accounts Receivable – Outpatients	1,500	
Revenues – Outpatients		$ 4,500
To record revenues from outpatient services.		

Outpatient revenues should be recorded in a manner that clearly separates them from inpatient revenues and provides the desired classification by departmental revenue centers and outpatient financial status. Postings are made from outpatient journals to the ledger in a manner similar to that described for inpatient revenue journals.

Revenue Deductions. As stated before, the patient service revenue accounts are credited on the accrual basis and at the hospital's full established rates for all services rendered, irrespective of whether cash has been, or ever will be, received in payment for such services. This means that amounts of revenues "lost" due to charity care, contractual adjustments, courtesy allowances, and bad debts must be recorded in revenue deductions accounts. Assuming that full rates have previously been debited to patients' accounts, the appropriate entries in summary form are:

Deductions from Patient Service Revenues –		
Charity Care	$ 2,100	
Contractual Adjustments	1,600	
Courtesy Allowances	400	
Bad Debts	900	
Allowance for Uncollectible Accounts –		
Charity Care		$ 2,100
Contractual Adjustments		1,600
Courtesy Allowances		400
Bad Debts		900
To record estimated deductions from patient service revenues.		
Allowance for Uncollectible Accounts –		
Charity Care	$ 1,800	
Contractual Adjustments	1,300	
Courtesy Allowances	290	
Bad Debts	750	
Accounts Receivable – Inpatients		$ 3,320
Accounts Receivable – Outpatients		820
To record write-off of uncollectible accounts.		

The first entry illustrates the periodic accrual of the estimated amounts of deductions; the second entry provides an example of the write-off of actual uncollectible accounts against the allowance accounts. (This procedure, including determinations of the amounts involved, is described at length in Chapter 11.) Revenue deductions are usually classified in the accounts by type of patient to provide data useful in negotiating third-party contracts and to be helpful for other managerial purposes.

Other Revenues

In addition to direct patient service revenues, hospitals also have revenues properly classified as (1) other operating revenues and (2) nonoperating revenues. The accounting procedures employed for these revenues should be no less effective and sound than those employed for healthcare services. These revenues are sometimes substantial; they can mean the difference between red or black ink in the bottom line of the hospital's income statement. Due to their diversity in source and nature, such revenues may present difficult accounting and reporting problems. In addition, because of their relatively high susceptibility to misappropriation, special internal control measures must be applied to these revenues.

Other Operating Revenues. The sources of other operating revenues were described earlier in this chapter. In assuring a proper accounting for these items, the development of adequate source documents is an essential requirement. Such documents originate at numerous locations within the hospital and at irregular intervals. It therefore is important that specific policies and procedures be established for the handling of all transactions involving services and sales to persons other than patients. The procedures should be designed to provide automatic records of these revenue transactions on prescribed forms which are promptly forwarded to the accounting department. Measures should be instituted to allow an independent verification of the completeness and accuracy of transactions reported.

Revenues from educational programs include charges to students for tuition, fees, uniforms, and supplies relating to schools of nursing, laboratory technology, and similar endeavors. Invoices for such charges are often prepared by the program administrative staff and are sent to the accounting department for processing. The following is an illustrative entry:

Accounts Receivable — Student Nurses	$ 6,000	
Deferred Revenue — Nursing School Tuition		$ 6,000
To record nursing school tuition invoiced		
for the school year.		

As the tuition is usually collected in installments, periodic entries are made to debit cash and credit accounts receivable. The revenue, however, should be recognized as it is earned, i.e., it should be allocated over the school year. Each month, a pro rata portion of the total tuition is credited to revenue with an offsetting debit to deferred revenue. The appropriate amounts can be determined by analysis of registration and enrollment statistics.

Revenues from research and other specific purpose grants should be recorded in the same period in which the research or other specific purpose activity is performed and related expenses are incurred. This provides for a proper matching of revenues and expenses. Because of donor restrictions, these grants ordinarily are recorded initially in the Specific Purpose Fund with resource transfers being made at appropriate times to the Unrestricted Fund where other operating revenue is credited. It should be noted, however, that resources that were donor-restricted to charity service are **not** reported as other operating revenues but are shown in the revenue deductions classification as indicated earlier. In any event, the accounting for these revenues should be determined by their use as indicated by donors' stipulations and terms of research contracts.

Miscellaneous revenues of the other operating revenues category include rentals of hospital-owned space, cafeteria sales, sales of supplies and services to employees, sales of scrap and waste, medical record transcript fees, and revenues from gift shops, newsstands, parking lots, and other hospital-operated enterprises. Source documents necessary to a proper recording of these revenues may be executed in many different departments, e.g., personnel, dietary, laboratory, radiology, central supply, laundry, and the medical records library. Responsibility for the handling and documentation of miscellaneous revenues should be clearly established with individuals who will carry out prescribed procedures for such transactions. The accounting department, of course, will maintain suitable files of related leases, invoices, correspondence, and memoranda.

Nonoperating Revenues. A hospital's nonoperating revenues consist principally of unrestricted gifts, unrestricted income from the investments of the Endowment Fund, and the income from all investments of unrestricted funds. It is important to note that cash gifts having no donor-imposed restrictions must be recorded as nonoperating revenues in the Unrestricted Fund. This is true regardless of any designations that may be made by the hospital's governing board. The fair market value of property and equipment contributed to the hospital, however, is recorded by a direct credit to the Unrestricted Fund balance. These gifts are not recorded as revenue (see Chapter 16). All gifts should be controlled through written gift receipts and acknowledgment procedures.

Another item of significance to certain church-sponsored hospitals is donated services. In these hospitals, a considerable amount of service in the business office, nursing service, dietary, and other areas may be provided without monetary compensation by members of religious orders. The fair market value of such services generally is charged to appropriate departmental cost centers and is credited to nonoperating revenue accounts. (For further discussion of this matter see Chapter 8.) The fair market value of donated medicines, foodstuffs, and other supplies which the hospital otherwise would purchase, however, is generally debited to operating expense and credited to "other operating revenues" (see Chapter 9).

Nonoperating revenues also properly include gains on sales of Unrestricted Fund investments, gains on dispositions of plant and equipment, net rentals of property not used in regular hospital operations, and term endowments upon termination of donor restrictions. Accounting procedures relating to these items of nonoperating revenues are discussed later in this book, particularly in Chapters 15 and 16.

INTERNAL CONTROL

The basic objective of internal control with respect to revenues is to provide assurance that all revenues earned by the hospital are promptly recorded in the proper amounts and in prescribed revenue account classifications. This is accomplished through the budgeting of revenues in dollars and in statistical units of service, the observance of sound admitting and registration procedures for inpatients and outpatients, the assignment of responsibility for the proper execution and utilization of census reports, charge tickets and other source documents, the development of a revenue account classification plan conforming to the organizational structure of the hospital, the maintenance of an adequate journal and ledger system, and the reconciliation of revenue dollars with statistical measurements of services rendered. Most of these requirements were discussed earlier in this chapter. The control of revenues is also necessarily linked with the control of cash and receivables, topics dealt with in Chapters 10 and 11.

Accounting procedures must be employed that provide for the recording of patient service revenues at full established rates, on the accrual basis and in accordance with the principle of responsibility accounting. Depending upon the requirements of the individual hospital, the admitting process should secure the information necessary to permit an appropriate classification of revenues by type of patient, service, accommodation, and financial status. In determining and recording daily patient service revenues, sound census-taking procedures should be followed which include a comparison of census data with admitting and discharge records or otherwise verify the accuracy of the daily census. Statistics of occupancy, length of stay, admissions, and patient days of service should be accumulated in conformity with uniform hospital definitions.

The system of accounting for services provided by the various professional departments must be designed to assure the proper execution of source documents so as to provide complete records of **all** services rendered. It should include appropriate safeguards to protect against the loss of revenues from overlooked charges and incorrect pricing of charge tickets. Where the use of prenumbered charge tickets accounted for on a numerical basis is not feasible, the service departments may maintain service logs against which charge tickets are compared. The pricing of charge tickets should be test-checked periodically against a current list of established service rates by a responsible person.

The effective control of outpatient revenues sometimes is complicated by the fact that the same person may make the initial record of such revenues and also handle the related cash receipts. Where these two functions are performed by the same person, the employment of special equipment designed to produce a "locked-in" copy of the revenue record and other specific safeguards is essential.

As noted before, the maintenance of sound procedures with respect to the other operating revenue and nonoperating revenue categories must not be regarded lightly. Many of these revenue items are substantial, and they may offer greater opportunities for fraudulent manipulation and honest mistakes than do patient service revenues. Appropriate steps must be taken to assure that a source document is promptly and accurately executed for all "other" revenue transactions by a responsible employee.

CHAPTER 7 FOOTNOTES

1. Principles and Practices Board, Statement No. 7, **The Presentation of Patient Service Revenue and Related Issues** (Chicago: Healthcare Financial Management Association, 1985), pp. 10-11.

QUESTIONS

1. Discuss the importance of adequate revenue accounting by hospitals.
2. Define the term **revenue**. Are all increases in assets and all decreases in liabilities sources of hospital revenue? Explain.
3. What are the three tests applied in accounting to determine whether revenue should be recognized in the accounts?
4. Revenue may be earned (1) before cash is received, (2) when cash is received, and (3) after cash is received. Give an example of each of these situations.
5. Into what major categories are revenues classified in the accounts of hospitals? Define each category and give examples of items of revenue that are included in each category.
6. What are the major objectives of accounting for the revenues of a hospital?
7. How are data relating to daily patient service revenues compiled in the hospital?
8. How are data relating to patient service revenues other than routine service revenues compiled in a hospital?
9. A hospital receives a $500,000 cash donation on which the donor places no restrictions. The hospital's governing board, however, decides to treat the $500,000 as a board-created endowment and to expend the income from the investment of the $500,000 only to acquire new plant and equipment. In this case, the $500,000 need not be reported as income in the hospital's operating statement. Do you agree? Explain.
10. Describe the major characteristics of a satisfactory system of internal control over hospital revenues.
11. The hospital administrator has asked your advice in the selection of a cost-based reimbursement formula for the state Blue Cross Plan. Two reimbursement formulas have been proposed: Per Diem and RCCAC (ratio of charges to charges applied to costs). Indicate briefly the possible advantages and disadvantages of each formula.
12. Why do hospitals have standard charges for services rendered to all patients and then treat charity and other allowances as a reduction of income?
13. Why are bad debts considered a reduction of income rather than an expense in hospital accounting?
14. Why do hospitals maintain separate accounts for each type of contractual allowance?
15. Indicate whether the following statements are true or false. If false, explain why.
    1. Board-created funds are donor-restricted specific purpose funds.
    2. In hospital accounting, bad debts are recorded as an expense.
    3. In hospital accounting, the recommended chart of accounts for revenues parallels the chart of organization.
    4. Hospital revenue consists mainly of the value at the hospital's full established rates of hospital services rendered to patients, regardless of the amounts actually paid to the hospital by or on behalf of patients.
    5. Under the cash basis system of accounting, hospital revenues are recognized when earned.
    6. Legally, revenues that are donor-restricted do not have to be used in conformance with the donors' intents.

T 7. All receipts of unrestricted funds must be recorded as operating fund income regardless of any action taken by the hospital's governing board or its administrative officers to restrict expenditure to specific purposes.

F 8. It is not a good policy to endorse all mail checks received in the business office before they are given to the cashier.

16. What does the term **third-party reimbursement** mean? Name five different third-party payers.

17. Distinguish between **operating revenues** and **nonoperating revenues** as those terms are used in hospital accounting.

EXERCISES

E1. Given the following data for the year 1987:

1. Number of days of care: 10,000.

2. Operating expenses:

Payroll	$120,000
Supplies	80,000
Depreciation	10,000
Total	$210,000

3. Classification of accounts in days:

Charity cases	600 days
Contractual cases	1,200 days
Uncollectible accounts	200 days
Full-pay patients	8,000 days
Total	10,000 days

4. Estimated collections per day:

Charity cases	None
Contractual cases	$14
Uncollectible accounts	None
Full-pay patients	Billed charges

Required. (1) Compute the minimum average billed charges per day which the hospital must experience in order to recover the total cost of care for the year. (2) After computing the minimum average billed charges, summarize the data and present the dollar amounts in the following form:

Revenue from services to patients
Less deductions from revenue
Less operating expenses
Net income

E2. Given the following information:

	12/31/87	12/31/86
Accounts receivable-patients	$346,700	$312,497
Patients' deposits (liability)	7,400	6,300

During 1987, $1,593,540 was received from patients and $21,938 of uncollectible accounts were written off the books.

Required. Compute the amount of patient service revenues for 1987.

E3. Given the following information:

	12/31/87	12/31/86
Accrued rentals receivable	$ 4,200	$ 2,800
Deferred rental income	2,600	1,900

During 1987, $14,700 of rent was received in cash.

Required. Compute the amount of rental income for 1987.

E4. Given the following information for 1987:

Operating expenses	$379,436
Patient service revenues	416,849
Nonoperating revenues	58,492
Deductions from revenues	103,476
Other operating revenues	24,695

Required. Prepare in good form an income statement for 1987.

E5. Parker Hospital completed the following transactions during the month of March:

1. Charges to patients for services rendered:

Inpatients:		
Daily patient services	$420,000	
Other professional services	510,000	$930,000
Outpatients		180,000

2. Services rendered to outpatients on a cash basis, $202,000.

3. Credits to patients' accounts:

	Inpatients	Outpatients
Charity care	$ 41,000	$ 76,000
Contractual adjustments	33,000	16,000
Courtesy discounts	2,200	
Bad debts	11,000	9,000
Cash collections	804,000	97,000

4. Estimated allowances and uncollectibles at March 31:

	Inpatients	Outpatients
Charity care	$ 4,000	$ 2,000
Contractual adjustments	5,000	1,000
Bad debts	2,000	1,500

Required. (1) Prepare journal entries to record all of the above. (2) At February 28, certain account balances were as follows:

Accounts receivable:
Inpatients	$144,000
Outpatient	36,000

Allowance for uncollectible accounts:
Charity care	$14,500
Contractual adjustments	8,200
Courtesy discounts	2,100
Bad debts	9,000

What are the balances of these accounts at March 31?

PROBLEMS

P1. Central Hospital is considering a new formula for the reimbursement of care furnished to members of the Blue Star Prepayment Plan. This new formula provides for one of the following payments:

1. A ceiling or maximum payment of 98 percent of the Blue Star's share of the billed charges on Blue Star cases.

2. A floor or minimum payment of 108 percent of Blue Star's share of the Net Operating Expense.

3. An alternate payment of Blue Star's share of the unrecovered cost resulting from noncash write-offs of accounts receivable **plus** 104 percent of Blue Star's share of the Net Operating Expense.

Required. Compute each of the three possible payments under the formula and state the amount Central Hospital would receive, based upon the following data for the year 1987:

1.	Total billed charges on the cases of all patients	$960,000
2.	Blue Star's share of the billed charges on Blue Star cases	$288,000
3.	Ratio of Blue Star's share of the charges to the charges of all patients	30%
4.	Net operating expense, i.e., cost of care	$800,000

5. Ratio of billed charges of all patients to net operating
   expense   120%

6. Total reductions in revenue, i.e., write-offs due to
   discounts, allowances, charity and bad debts $180,000

P2.   You are the controller of a 300-bed general hospital which has under
      construction a new wing, including a 15-bed intensive care unit. This will be
      your first experience with a separate intensive care facility.

      Total building contracts and equipment orders for the new wing are as follows:

General contract and architect fees	$700,000
Heating and plumbing	300,000
Electrical	200,000
Equipment	200,000

The present hospital structure contains 150,000 square feet. The new wing will
contain 30,000 square feet, of which 3,000 square feet is occupied by the
intensive care unit. Cabinet work for intensive care will cost $12,000. All other
equipment for that unit will cost $15,000. (Both items are included in the
$200,000 total). It is estimated that the following conditions will prevail in the
intensive care unit:

1.   An average daily census of 12.

2.   Staffing requirements:
     One supervisor @ $450 per month
     Seven registered nurses @ $400 per month each
     Seven licensed practical nurses @ $300 per month each

3.   It is estimated that supply usage will be proportionate to but 50 percent
     higher than that of the surgical service.

4.   Laundry and linen, housekeeping, central service, pharmacy and medical
     records costs will be proportionate to those costs on the medical service.

5.   Dietary units costs will be equivalent to one-half the dietary unit costs
     pertaining to the medical service.

   In the cost-finding study of the previous year, the following direct and indirect
costs and patient days of the medical service and the surgical service are found:

	Medical Service	Surgical Service
Direct costs:		
Salaries	$160,000	$180,000
Supplies and other expense	4,000	6,000
Allocated costs:		
Laundry and linen	16,800	20,000
Housekeeping	28,800	34,600
Dietary	72,000	90,000
Central service	5,040	6,300
Pharmacy	480	600
Medical records	11,520	14,400
Patient days	24,000	30,000

Financial statements also show these costs pertaining to the entire hospital:

Fiscal and administrative (including overhead)	$ 330,000
Operating of plant (including overhead)	150,000
Maintenance (including overhead)	75,000
Gross payroll	2,200,000
Employee benefits	154,000

Required. It is your job as controller to recommend a "routine service" charge for the intensive care unit. From the above data, determine a projected unit cost upon which the recommended charge can be based. The charge is to include the regular nursing, dietary and room cost, as well as the special nursing care cost. State any assumptions which you believe are necessary for the solution of the problem.

8
Accounting for Hospital Expenses

Annual expenditures by hospitals for the care of patients currently are in excess of $160 billion, or about 4 percent of the gross national product. While some of these expenditures represent the costs of new construction and equipment, a majority of the expenditures are recurring annual operating expenses which, due to inflation, technological advancements, and other factors, are at unprecedented levels and relentlessly increasing.

Although hospitals receive and expend huge sums of money each year in providing healthcare services, the industry currently is in a financially precarious position characterized by rising costs, competition, and declining revenues arising from a reduced demand for services and major changes in third-party reimbursement systems. The days of "wine and roses" (cost reimbursement) are largely gone, being replaced by a prospective payment system (PPS) under which hospitals are paid a predetermined fixed-price-per-case based on diagnosis-related groups (DRGs).

In these circumstances, the successful management of hospital revenues and costs is, without question, one of the major challenges of this century. A high order of expense accounting and control is essential if hospital managements are to intelligently utilize the funds made available to them and fulfill their stewardship responsibilities to the public. It is essential that hospitals be managed on cost-efficiency principles similar to those used in other industries. Productivity studies should be made on a departmental basis to develop standards that can be used to monitor costs and utilization. Hospitals also should devise a case mix management information system that (1) merges clinical and financial data on a patient-specific basis, (2) generates reports of patterns of resource consumption, and (3) measures profitability by hospital case type.[1]

This chapter is concerned with the operating expenses of the hospital enterprise. It deals with the problems of accounting for employee compensation costs, the largest single element of operating expense, and nonlabor costs such as supplies, utilities, and other purchased services. The management of these costs is considered in the following chapter. An extended discussion of depreciation expense is deferred to Chapter 16.

NATURE AND CLASSIFICATION OF EXPENSE

The term **cost** is used in a variety of ways and consequently is a source of some confusion. A number of attempts have been made to define the term generically, but these efforts have not been entirely successful. The basic idea is that a cost involves a sacrifice or foregoing of one thing for another in an exchange transaction. Thus, a cost is an expenditure, an outlay of cash or other assets or services, or the incurrence of a liability, in exchange for goods or services. It generally is measured in terms of the amount of cash disbursed or to be disbursed, or in terms of the market value of noncash assets or services given or to be given in exchange. Cost is the basis for measuring and reporting most assets.

Technically speaking, an **expense** is an expired **cost**. Expenses are costs that are directly or indirectly associated with the revenue of a given time period. The expiration of costs and the resultant recognition of expense is governed by three principles:

1. Association of cause and effect.
2. Systematic and rational allocation.
3. Immediate recognition.

Recorded costs which have not expired, and consequently have not been recognized as expense, are carried in the accounts as assets. Despite this important technical distinction, the terms **cost** and **expense** often are used interchangeably in practice.

In hospital accounting, the basic classification of expenses (costs) is a **functional** classification which conforms to the organizational structure of the particular hospital. The total hospital activity is divided into a number of separate but coordinated organizational units, each headed by a responsible person. Each unit, or **responsibility center**, performs a specific function (output) and, in so doing, incurs certain costs (input). Each organizational unit therefore is a **cost center**. As noted in Chapter 7, those organizational units whose output results in direct charges to patients are also regarded as **revenue centers**. The classification of revenue and expense accounts according to responsibility centers within the hospital was illustrated in Chapter 4.

The secondary classification of expenses is within each responsibility center — an **object of expenditure**, or **natural**, classification. Major categories of expense accumulated in this classification would include:

Salaries and Wages
Employee Benefits
Supplies — billable
Supplies — nonbillable
Purchased Services (utilities and telephone)
Rent
Insurance
Interest
Depreciation

In the normal accounting routine and for internal reporting purposes, these expenses are recorded and reported by responsibility centers only to the extent that they are **controllable** by those individuals charged with the management of the various centers. Expenses such as employee benefits, interest and depreciation, for example, generally are recorded as unassigned expenses (see Figure 4-12). They are allocated to the cost centers in the cost-finding procedure, of course, but not as a part of the routine accounting and reporting process (unless a cost accounting system is used by the hospital).

The classification of expenses is basic to the system of cost control known as **responsibility accounting**. Under this system, controllable expenses are classified in a manner designed to associate them with those individuals responsible for their incurrence. Expenses are budgeted and recorded in the same responsibility classifications so that actual performance can be directly related to planned performance in actual versus budget reports at each level of management responsibility. In this way, each supervisor's performance is judged on the basis of only those items of expense subject to his or her control. Deviations from budgeted expenses are quickly traced to the individual managers whose decision authority makes them primarily responsible for the particular costs in question.

PAYROLL ACCOUNTING

Since employee compensation costs generally represent about 50 percent of hospital operating expenses, particular emphasis should be given to the development of sound accounting methods and procedures with regard to hospital payrolls and payroll-related costs. The discussion provided here is indicative of some of the basic payroll accounting problems and practices of hospitals.

Employment Practices

Ideally, the function of screening and hiring new employees should be the responsibility of a centralized personnel department. A less desirable alternative is the hiring of employees by individual department heads and supervisors. While department heads should be allowed the final decision on hiring applicants for departmental positions, the centralization of hiring and other personnel functions is highly recommended in almost all instances. Centralization of the personnel function localizes responsibility, improves efficiency, centralizes personnel records, and facilitates internal control over payrolls.

The basic functions of a centralized personnel department include recruiting, interviewing, selecting, processing, and record-keeping. Recruitment procedures should be followed to develop and maintain adequate sources of labor supply. This effort is a continuous process and should be adapted to the differences in the types of employees required by the hospital. Job applicants are screened in a preliminary selection interview designed to sort out those persons who obviously are not qualified for the job(s) available. Those candidates approved in the preliminary interview usually complete an employment application blank designed to obtain the necessary information concerning the applicant's personal history, education, and experience. For certain types of jobs, the applicants may be given dexterity, mental ability, aptitude, and other tests to ascertain their suitability for the positions. A physical examination also may be required.

If an applicant appears to possess the required qualifications, a placement interview is arranged with the department head or supervisor to whom the applicant would be responsible if he or she is hired. This interview should take place in the department in which the job opening exists so that the prospective employee can see the physical surroundings and other conditions in which he or she would be working. As a result of the interview, the department head will indicate approval or rejection of the applicant. This decision is promptly reported to the personnel department so that the employment process can be continued without delay.

Upon final approval of the applicant for the job opening, the applicant must be fully indoctrinated as to the hospital's history, objectives, and services, and the hospital's personnel policies should be carefully explained. The applicant should be given complete information concerning the requirements and responsibilities of the job for which he or she has been hired. It is preferable that the applicant be given a written job description and statement of the hospital's policies relating to vacations, absences from work, tardiness, promotions, overtime, and other matters. It is essential that the new employee understand the importance of his or her work and where he or she fits in the hospital's organization.

Should the new employee have no social security number, he or she is required to make an appropriate application on Form SS-5 with the nearest district office of the Social Security Administration. The personnel department should keep a supply of these forms and assist new employees with the proper filing of them. In addition, each new employee must complete a Form W-4 on which the employee claims the number of income tax withholding exemptions to which he or she is entitled by federal income tax regulations. The hospital must make the new employee's social security number, Form W-4, and other information a permanent part of its payroll records. In addition to the records that must be kept for federal, state, and local tax purposes, a complete and up-to-date employment history or service file must be kept for all employees. It is also necessary to keep complete records on all applicants who are rejected.

Timekeeping

A clear-cut procedure for recording and reporting time worked must be established for all employees. Larger hospitals have used time clocks successfully for many years, and small hospitals often find them desirable. Clocks should be located at central points where their use can be supervised. Each employee is usually assigned a clock number to allow arrangement of timecards in numerical sequence so that they may be readily identified and located. The timecards may also be coded to indicate the department of employment to facilitate subsequent sorting required in payroll compilation. Since some employees may object to the use of a time clock, manual timecards may also be used.

In any case, the department head or supervisor ordinarily signs and approves the timecards and time records before they are sent to the accounting department for processing. The payroll clerk uses the cards and records in compiling the payroll for the period and in developing labor statistics of various types. It is essential that timecards and other time records be complete and accurate as to attendance and hours worked for purposes of compliance with the Fair Labor Standards Act and other laws regulating employment. Special documents may be required for overtime authorization and absence or late reports. All time-reporting records should be designed in a manner that will provide adequate data useful for subsequent analyses of payroll in terms of both dollars and hours, properly classified by cost centers.

Compilation of Gross Payrolls

The calculation of the gross payroll is not a particularly difficult process. Responsible employees independent of the timekeeping function examine all timecards for hourly employees to determine that the cards are properly executed and approved, and that the hours worked by each employee during the pay period are properly computed. These hours then are multiplied by authorized rates of pay. If overtime hours have been worked, a separate calculation is required. For salaried employees, the gross pay per period is a fixed amount which, once calculated, does not vary unless the salary is changed. The time records kept for salaried personnel should also be properly executed and signed as approved by department heads. All changes in salaries or in hourly pay rates due to promotions, merit increases, or changes in position should enter into the calculations of gross pay only when such changes are authorized in writing by department heads on change of rate notices and other prescribed documents. The payroll clerk should not act on the basis of verbal orders. Periodic audits should be made by responsible employees independent of the payroll function. These audits include the recomputation of hours worked, comparisons of pay rates with authorizations in personnel files, and other verifications of the accuracy of gross payroll determinations.

Payroll Deductions

Payroll accounting is complicated greatly by the various deductions that are required in determining the amounts in which employees' paychecks should be written. Most of these deductions are made necessary by various tax laws while others arise in connection with insurance, retirement and savings plan agreements with employees. The more common types of deductions are described here, with further discussion in Chapter 13.

FICA Taxes. The Federal Insurance Contributions Act (FICA), commonly known as social security, was originally enacted in 1935 to provide for a 1 percent tax on wages paid to each employee up to $3,000 in any one year, with a matching 1 percent tax on employers. Hospitals and their employees were at first exempt from this tax law, but the Act has been amended many times to extend its coverage to hospitals and other previously exempt organizations and to increase the tax rate, the wage base and employee benefits. The 1965 amendment included enactment of the Federal Hospital Insurance Program, popularly called Medicare.

Both the FICA tax rate and the taxable wage base have been increased frequently over the years, and it is reasonable to expect them to be higher in both the near and distant future. In any event, the reader must recognize that the matching FICA tax imposed upon the hospital represents a significant addition to labor costs. There also is the clerical expense involved in keeping the detailed payroll records required by the law. These records must include the name, birthday, address, and social security number of each employee as well as data concerning gross pay, pay dates, and taxes withheld. This information usually is maintained on forms referred to as **employees' individual earnings records.**

Income Taxes. Hospitals are required to withhold federal income taxes from employee's wages in amounts determinable from tax tables furnished by the government. Most states and many of the larger cities also levy income taxes and have similar withholding requirements. Amounts withheld are remitted periodically to the various governmental units at times specified in the laws. Additional information on the remittance of withheld taxes is provided in Chapter 13.

Other Deductions. In addition to the compulsory withholdings, a variety of other deductions may be made from salary and wage payments. Included in this category are amounts deducted for employee purchases of government savings bonds, premiums for life and hospitalization insurance, employee contributions to pension and retirement plans, and similar items. At regular intervals, these withholdings must be remitted by the hospital to appropriate agencies.

Recording the Payroll

After determination of the gross payroll and the related deductions, the payroll for the period is recorded in the appropriate accounts. A number of different systems are employed, and the one illustrated here is only indicative of the general procedure. The initial entry often is made in a **payroll journal** or **register** as summarized below:

Salaries and Wages Expense*	$50,000	
FICA Taxes Withheld		$ 3,000
Federal Income Tax Withheld		10,000
Liability for Other Withholdings		2,000
Accrued Payroll Liability		35,000
To record payroll for the period.		

*Classified by departmental cost centers in accordance with the principles of responsibility accounting.

Appropriate postings of the details of the payroll are made to the employees' individual earnings records. General ledger postings may be made on a monthly basis. Periodic reconciliations are required of the detailed records with the general ledger control accounts, usually at the time of filing payroll tax returns with the Internal Revenue Service and other taxing authorities.

At this point, a single voucher may be prepared in the amount of the net payroll, and an entry such as the following is made in the **voucher register**.

Accrued Payroll Liability	$35,000	
Vouchers Payable		$35,000
To record voucher prepared in the amount		
of the net payroll for the period.		

In some systems, a payroll journal is not used and the voucher register is designed to record the gross payroll and the various deductions.

Typically, a single check will be drawn on the hospital's general checking account in the amount of the net payroll. This check then is deposited in an imprest payroll checking account (see Chapter 10). The entry is:

Cash in Bank — Payroll Checking Account	$35,000	
Cash in Bank — General Checking Account		$35,000
To record transfer of funds for net payroll		
to the imprest payroll checking account.		

Individual employee paychecks then are prepared and drawn against the special payroll account. The individual checks are recorded separately in a payroll register or journal and a summary entry is made as follows:

Vouchers Payable	$35,000	
Cash in Bank — Payroll Checking Account		$35,000

To record summary of individual payroll
checks written in payment of the payroll
for the period.

The payroll register or journal is sometimes prepared as a carbon copy of pertinent information entered on the individual payroll checks. The payroll checks should clear the payroll account within a short time and a reconciliation of the payroll account may be unnecessary. If the account does not automatically balance to zero, then the balance in the account should equal the checks not cashed by employees.This procedure also facilitates reconciliation of the general checking account in that the clutter of the large volume of individual payroll checks has been avoided.

Donated Services

Hospitals sometimes are recipients of donated services from various organizations whose members work without monetary compensation in some area of the hospital activity. Such donated services properly are recorded at fair market value only when (1) there is the equivalent of an employer-employee relationship and (2) there is an objective basis for determining the amounts that might otherwise have been paid for such services. An objective basis for valuing donated services may in some cases be found in the contractual relationship existing with contributing organizations.

The problem of recording donated services is most likely to arise in those hospitals operated by or affiliated with a religious group. In Catholic hospitals, for example, the services of members of the religious orders should be valued at lay-equivalent salary rates for the performance of similar services. These amounts should be reported as expense (recorded in a separate salary and wage expense account classification) with an offsetting credit to nonoperating revenue. If members of a religious or other group are paid less than the fair value of their services, the difference between the nominal salaries and lay-equivalent salaries should be reported in the same manner.

Services of a nonessential nature provided by guilds, auxiliaries, and similar organizations generally should not be recorded in the accounts. It may be desirable, however, to disclose the value of such services in appropriate notes to the hospital's financial statements.

Payroll-Related Costs

In addition to the basic earnings of hourly and salaried employees, a number of other payroll-related cost elements enter into hospital labor cost considerations. These include overtime earnings, vacation and sick pay, FICA and unemployment taxes, workmen's compensation, life and hospitalization insurance, and retirement plans. The total of these and other so-called fringe benefits is a substantial cost, often 30 percent or more of total labor costs in hospitals. Certain of the more common fringe benefits are discussed here from an expense point of view; the related liabilities are dealt with in Chapter 13.

Overtime Premium Pay. The Fair Labor Standards Act of 1938, popularly known as the Wages and Hours Law, provides for a minimum hourly wage with time and a half for hours worked in a given week in excess of 40 hours. As a simplified example, assume that an employee is paid $6.10 per hour for a regular workweek of 40 hours. This employee's gross earnings for a week during which he or she worked 48 hours ordinarily would be $317.20, computed as follows:

Regular workweek (40 hours @ $6.10)	$244.00
Overtime (8 hours @ $6.10)	48.80
Overtime premium (8 hours @ $3.05)	24.40
Gross earnings	$317.20

Application of the provisions of this law to the compensation of employees can be somewhat involved, but the complicating factors are disregarded here. It is important to note, however, that good payroll accounting practice should provide for the separate recording of overtime compensation in that such information is useful in evaluating the utilization of personnel.

Vacation and Sick Pay. After a specified period of employment, hospital employees generally are entitled to an annual vacation with full pay. Assuming a two-week paid vacation annually, employees in effect are paid for 50 weeks of work over a 52-week period. The reality of the situation is that the vacation pay is earned by employees and incurred as a cost by the hospital, **during the 50 working weeks**. It therefore is incorrect to defer recognition of vacation pay as an expense until it is actually paid. Instead, vacation pay should be charged to expense in the payroll periods during which it is earned by employees. A similar accounting procedure generally is followed for sick pay and other compensated absences. A detailed discussion is provided in Chapter 13.

Payroll Taxes. As noted earlier in this chapter, the hospital is required to pay FICA taxes in amounts matching the FICA taxes withheld from employees' salaries and wages. Hospitals also may be subject to federal and state unemployment compensation tax laws, as discussed in Chapter 13. The state laws vary considerably as to rates and wage bases.

In any event, the hospital must accrue these taxes for each payroll period by entries such as the following (dollar amounts assumed):

FICA Tax Expense	$ 2,340	
Federal Unemployment Tax Expense	200	
State Unemployment Tax Expense	1,080	
FICA Taxes Payable		$ 2,340
Federal Unemployment Taxes Payable		200
State Unemployment Taxes Payable		1,080
To record payroll tax expenses.		

These expense debits, as stated previously, generally are made to unassigned expense accounts in the administrative or fiscal services classification. These expenses are allocated to the departmental cost centers in the cost-finding procedure. To charge these expenses to cost center accounts as a part of the normal accounting routine is troublesome and little value would be gained from it.

Workmen's Compensation. States have workmen's compensation laws which provide various benefits to disabled workers. in some cases, a tax is imposed on the employer in a manner similar to unemployment taxes. More frequently, the state laws establish standard benefits and allow hospital employers to provide for such benefits through the purchase of appropriate insurance form a commercial insurance company. The premiums paid are charged to expense, with no part of the cost being deducted from employees' pay.

Assume, for example, that a hospital has the usual workmen's compensation and employers' liability insurance combined in one policy for which an advance premium is required on the first of the year based upon the estimated payroll for the year as follows:

Employee Classification	Estimated Payroll	Insurance Rate (per $100)	Advance Premium
A	$ 400,000	$ .75	$ 3,000
B	240,000	.45	1,080
C	360,000	.25	900
D	100,000	.10	100
		Total	$ 5,080

Under the conditions of workmen's compensation and employers' liability insurance, workers are classified according to the degree of risk involved in the particular jobs. The greater the risk, the higher the insurance rate. This means that, in addition to the other classifications into which a hospital might accumulate gross payroll data for accounting purposes, the hospital must also maintain its records in such a manner as to be able to determine gross payroll by whatever classifications are required by the insurer.

Given the above estimates for the coming year, assume the following with respect to the actual payroll for January (the first month of the year):

Employee Classification	Payroll	Insurance Rate (per $100)	Expired Premium
A	$ 30,000	$ .75	$ 225
B	18,000	.45	81
C	28,000	.25	70
D	8,000	.10	8
		Total	$ 384

The journal entries required to record the insurance aspects of this illustration are as follows:

Prepaid Workmen's Compensation Insurance	$ 5,080	
Cash in Bank		$ 5,080
To record payment of advance premium.		
Workmen's Compensation Insurance Expense	$ 384	
Prepaid Workmen's Compensation Insurance		$ 384
To record January expiration of premium		
paid in advance.		

A similar month-end adjustment would be made throughout the year. At year-end, the prepaid insurance account will have either a debit or a credit balance. A debit balance would indicate an overpayment to the insurer and usually is used to reduce the next year's premium. A credit balance would represent a liability to the insurer for additional premiums due. In any event, representatives of the insurance company usually make periodic audits of the hospital's records to be sure that employees are properly classified and that insurable payrolls are reported correctly.

Life and Hospitalization Insurance. Life, health, accident, and hospitalization insurance plans are often established by hospitals in behalf of their employees. Participation in these programs is voluntary, but the hospital frequently pays a substantial portion of the premiums as an employee benefit. Such payments by the hospital, of course, are recorded as operating expenses. The employees' share of the cost of such plans is secured through payroll withholdings (see Chapter 13).

Pension and Retirement Plans. Increasing attention has been given in recent years to the establishment of plans to provide benefits to employees during their retirement years. Some of the advantages claimed for hospitals having pension and retirement plans are:

1. Reduction of employee turnover.
2. Improvement of the hospital's competitive position in attracting high quality personnel who might otherwise be lost to industrial firms.
3. Provision of income security to employees who have given long periods of faithful service to the hospital.

Hospitals interested in establishing a retirement program usually begin by appointing a committee consisting of the personnel director, a board member, the controller, and one or two other employees. The function of the committee is to investigate the feasibility of a retirement program, draw up a tentative plan, and make recommendations to the governing board.

Plans vary somewhat, but all full-time employees meeting minimum length of service and age requirements generally are eligible. Employees typically contribute to the plan through payroll withholdings, and the hospital assumes the remaining costs. The cost of providing future retirement benefits relating to the services of employees prior to inception of the plan, however, usually is paid totally by the hospital. Under most of these plans, the hospital makes annual payments to an insurance company or other funding agency. These resources are invested by the funding agency so that sufficient amounts will be accumulated to pay benefits to employees in their retirement years. The amounts in which annual payments are made by the hospital is an involved mathematical problem solved by actuarial methods based upon mortality tables and assumptions as to investment earnings, price levels and other matters.

Discussion of the accounting procedures and financial disclosure requirements relating to hospital pension plans appears in Chapter 18.

Internal Control

Payrolls not only account for the major portion of hospital operating expenses, but they also are particularly susceptible to fraudulent manipulations and unintentional errors. It therefore is essential that a high priority be given to the development and maintenance of an effective system of internal control over hospital payrolls. Although certain internal control practices have been mentioned in the preceding pages, it seems appropriate to repeat some of them in the following summary discussion.

The ideal control situation is characterized by a centralized personnel department that localizes responsibility for all matters relating to employment, promotion, changes in pay rates, and terminations. In smaller hospitals where a centralized personnel function may not be organizationally feasible, the administrator's office should maintain a separate record of employees and their rates of pay. These records should be independent of the records maintained in the cash handling and accounting departments so that the records can be cross-checked at regular intervals. In this way, assurances are provided that only authorized persons receive paychecks and that the approved amounts of compensation are paid to employees.

In any event, additions of persons to the hospital payroll should require administrative authorization. Many hospitals use a position control plan for this purpose. The administrator, in conference with departmental heads, should review job specifications, authorize a specific number of employees for each job classification, and establish approved rates of pay for each position. New employees, whether additions or replacements, should be hired only with administrative approval of employment requisitions submitted by department heads to the personnel department or administrator. When a new employee is hired, a notice of employment usually is prepared with copies routed to the payroll accounting unit, the appropriate department head, and the personnel records unit. A complete record of employment should be maintained by the personnel records unit for each employee. All changes in this record should be fully documented, using prescribed forms authorizing rates of pay, promotions, transfers, and terminations.

A sound procedure must be established for the accurate recording and reporting of the time worked by all personnel. Timecards and other work records should be carefully designed, and safeguards should be employed to ensure that the forms are properly executed. Steps must also be taken to make certain that proper pay rates are used in computing the gross payroll and that payroll withholdings are made in compliance with tax laws. The hospital should also have a clear policy as to prerequisites provided to employees, and procedures should be adopted to prevent the abuse of such privileges.

The employees responsible for compilation of payrolls should neither sign nor distribute payroll checks. Once prepared, the unsigned checks should be examined by the disbursing authority who should be satisfied, insofar as feasible, as to their accuracy and authenticity. This may involve a check of computations on a sample basis and a comparison of payees and pay rates with independently controlled personnel records. Particular attention must be given to (1) inclusion of nonexistent persons on the payroll, (2) issuance of checks to former employees whose names have not been removed from the payroll, (3) payment of incorrect rates of pay, and (4) payment for overtime hours when none were worked. If a mechanical check signer is required, its use should be strictly controlled.

The distribution of payroll checks should be centralized, and procedures should be employed so that employees receiving checks are properly identified. Occasionally, the method of distributing checks or the paymaster should be changed, with special attention being given to unclaimed checks. Such checks should not be returned to the payroll accounting unit but should be retained for a reasonable period of time by an independent and responsible person. Checks remaining unclaimed for long periods must be fully investigated for cause.

Separate payroll checking accounts should be maintained on an imprest basis. These accounts should be reconciled and examined periodically by someone other than an employee connected with payroll accounting and disbursement. In this process, a sample of canceled checks should be compared with the payroll journal and with employees' individual earnings records.

All employee terminations and absences should be reported without delay to the payroll accounting unit and to the payroll disbursing officer. Termination lists should be compared regularly with records maintained by the personnel department and with subsequent payrolls to assure the proper handling of resignations and dismissals. The routine of automated payroll systems sometimes results in the writing of payroll checks to individuals whose employment has been terminated.

Personnel reports are important to the internal control system. In addition to budgeted and actual dollars, these reports should include a variety of statistical data such as nursing hours per patient day classified by nursing unit. Most hospitals prepare monthly reports which also include information such as number of employees by department and job classification, ratio of employees to patients, personnel turnover by department and the reasons for this, number and value of wage increases, and statistics relating to absenteeism and overtime work.

ACCOUNTING FOR SUPPLIES AND OTHER EXPENSES

In accounting for hospital expenses, considerable attention naturally is given to salaries, wages, fees, and employee benefits because these costs added together usually represent as much as 50 percent or more of total operating expenditures. The remaining 50 percent, however, must not be regarded lightly. Very substantial amounts are expended each year for supplies, utilities, and other purchased services, and the effective management of these costs requires the use of sound accounting procedures and the maintenance of appropriate internal controls.

Purchasing

Purchasing of supplies and services is a function of major importance in hospitals. It cuts across all departmental lines and accounts for a significant percentage of the hospital's annual expenditures. Ideally, the purchasing function should be centralized and performed by an organized purchasing department headed by an experienced purchasing agent. This tends to minimize waste and duplication through standardization of buying and use of many supply items. In addition, department heads are relieved of much of the detail incidental to purchasing. Limited authority to purchase certain products and services, however, sometimes must be given to selected department heads. In small hospitals, the administrator usually does the buying personally or carefully supervises and coordinates it.

The purchasing responsibility consists of the acquisition of required supplies and services of the appropriate quality, in the proper quantity, at the times needed, and at reasonable costs. Assurance that these requirements are met is provided through a system of internal controls, including the use of purchase requisitions, purchase orders, and receiving reports. The utilization of these documents was described in Chapter 5. In the system, a copy of each purchase-related document is routed to the accounting department.

Recording Purchases

When the vendor's invoices and statements are received in the accounting department, they are compared with the related purchase orders and receiving reports. This comparison is made to ascertain the correctness of prices, quantities, extensions, and other important considerations. In many systems, this results in the preparation of vouchers authorizing subsequent disbursements for the supplies and services purchased by the hospital. Transactions evidenced by the vouchers and underlying documents are recorded as follows:

Supplies and Other Expense*	$XX,XXX	
Accounts (Vouchers) Payable		$XX,XXX
To record liability for purchased supplies, services, and other expenses.		

*Classified by departmental cost centers in accordance with the principles of responsibility accounting.

These entries typically are made in specialized journals called **voucher registers**. (See the author's **Introduction to Hospital Accounting**.)

With respect to purchased supplies, a choice must be made between the **perpetual** and **periodic** inventory accounting systems. The entry shown above assumes the use of the periodic method under which purchased supplies are charged directly to expense accounts. Under the perpetual inventory method, supplies are debited to inventory accounts when purchased. These two methods of accounting are described fully in Chapter 12.

Some hospitals record purchased supplies at **gross** invoice cost and others record purchases at **net** invoice cost. Consider, for example, the purchase of $2,000 of supplies on 2/10, EOM terms. Under the gross invoice cost method, the journal entries would be:

Supplies Expense (or Inventory)	$2,000	
Accounts Payable		$2,000
To record purchase of supplies.		
Accounts Payable	$2,000	
Purchase Discounts Earned		$ 40
Cash in Bank		1,960
To record payment of invoice.		

In other words, the supplies expense (or inventory) and the related liability are recorded at gross invoice cost without consideration of the discount opportunity. If the invoice is not paid within the discount period, the second entry would include a cash credit of $2,000. The fact that the discount was missed would not be formally recorded in the accounts.

Under the net invoice cost method, the purchased supplies would be recorded net of the two percent discount s follows:

Supplies Expense (or Inventory)	$1,960	
Accounts Payable		$1,960
To record purchase of supplies.		

If the invoice is paid promptly so that the discount may be obtained, the entry to record payment of the invoice would debit Accounts Payable and credit Cash in Bank for $1,960. No formal record is made of the discount earned. On the other hand, should the discount not be taken, the entry would be:

Accounts Payable	$1,960	
Purchase Discounts Lost	40	
Cash in Bank		$2,000
To record payment of invoice.		

Purchase discounts **lost,** rather than purchase discounts **earned,** are recorded in this manner to indicate to management the additional expense incurred due to the failure to pay invoices promptly and secure available discounts.

Thus, the gross cost method tends to conceal one of the costs of inefficiency in processing suppliers' invoices for payment. It records discounts taken as income, when it should be obvious that income cannot be earned from purchasing. The gross cost method also tends to overstate the cost of supplies used as well as the liabilities arising from purchases.

Receiving, Storing, and Issuing

Upon receipt of purchased goods from suppliers, the receiving department has the responsibility for counting, weighing, or otherwise measuring the quantities of goods received. The quality and condition of the goods is also checked. As a result of this process, a receiving report is prepared. After the incoming shipment of goods has been examined by the receiving personnel, the goods are moved into the hospital storerooms. They remain there under the control of the storekeeper until used. Meanwhile, it is essential that the goods be safeguarded against theft, fire loss, damage, and other hazards.

The issue of supplies from central storerooms usually requires execution of an authorization form called a **supplies requisition.** If the perpetual inventory system is employed, the requisitions are summarized in the accounting department as the basis for journal entries such as the following:

> Supplies Expense* $XX,XXX
>   Inventory $XX,XXX
>   To record usage of supplies.
> *Classified by departmental cost centers in accordance with the principles of responsibility accounting.

These entries usually are made in special journals called **supplies requisition journals.** The amounts involved depend upon the inventory costing method employed, e.g., average, FIFO (first-in, first-out), or LIFO (last-in, first-out). These methods are discussed at length in Chapter 12.

Internal Control

The expenditures made for supplies and other nonlabor expenses are highly significant, and internal controls should be maintained to assure accuracy in recording them. Effective controls over supplies are needed to protect against fraud and waste in purchasing and using the hundreds of different supply items required in the operation of the hospital. Supply items, because of their tangible nature and value, are susceptible to theft.

A dollar saved in supplies and other expense is as important as a dollar saved in salaries and wages. It should be recognized, however, that a balance must be achieved between the benefits that can be derived from control procedures and the cost of employing them. The desirability of adopting various methods, policies, and procedures therefore should be evaluated in terms of the needs and circumstances of the individual hospital.

The internal control of expenses other than payroll consists largely of the centralization of the purchasing authority, the employment of sound purchasing, receiving and storekeeping procedures, the maintenance of a sound system of authorization, documentation and record-keeping, and the application of effective invoice audit approval techniques. These matters were discussed in Chapter 5; additional comments relating to inventories are in Chapter 12; matters pertaining to the control of disbursements for expenses are discussed in Chapter 10.

In addition to basic procedural considerations, the internal control system must also include budgeting, reporting, and analysis. These essentials are explained in the following chapter.

CHAPTER 8 FOOTNOTES

1. These and other recommendations appear in Ernst & Whinney's 1983 publication (No. J58475) titled **The Medicare Prospective Payment System.** The document provides guidance in implementing the PPS regulations and discusses their implications for hospitals.

QUESTIONS

1. Define and distinguish the following terms as they are used in accounting: (1) cost, (2) expense, and (3) loss.

2. State the three principles by which the expiration of costs and the resultant recognition of expense are governed.

3. Distinguish between (1) a functional classification of expenses and (2) an object of expenditure, or natural, classification of expenses. Which of these types of classifications should be used by hospitals?

4. Define each of the following terms:
   1. Responsibility accounting
   2. Responsibility center
   3. Revenue center
   4. Expense (cost) center
   5. Responsibility reporting

5. Describe the operation of an imprest payroll checking account. What are the advantages of such a system?

6. List and briefly describe the major features of four typical payroll deductions.

7. Under what circumstances should donated services be recorded in the hospital's accounts? How are such services valued?

8. Describe the major features of a satisfactory system of internal control with respect to hospital payrolls.

9. What are some of the advantages claimed for hospitals having pension and retirement plans? Distinguish between (1) past service cost and (2) normal cost of pension plans.

10. Describe the major features of a satisfactory system of internal control with respect to supplies used in hospital operations.

11. You have been asked to develop a personnel report for your hospital. What information would you include in such a report?

12. What is meant by **full-time equivalents**? Describe how you would determine the number of full-time equivalent employees of a hospital.

13. How can the personnel department effectively implement the hospital budget with respect to number of employees?

14. "In hospital accounting, bad debts should be recorded as an expense." Do you agree? Explain.

15. "In responsibility accounting, hospital expenses are recorded by object of expenditure." Do you agree? Explain.

16. Your 250-bed hospital has operated without an organized salary and wage administration program. As a result, employee complaints about low salaries, favoritism, increasing cost of living, unfair treatment between groups within the hospital, and lack of merit recognition, have become alarmingly frequent. Employee turnover has increased. Certain jobs cannot be satisfactorily filled. Outline the elements of a salary and wage administration program designed to correct this situation.

17. Realistic personnel policies are a beginning of what may be a functional philosophy of hospital personnel administration and the final achievement of written personnel policies. **Realistic** and **functional** are two important words in the study of personnel policies, particularly when applied to fringe benefits.

As the controller of Hospital X you are asked to prepare:

1. An outline of the steps to be followed in the actual development and writing of personnel policies. This worksheet will serve both to help seek all the facts and be useful as a record for follow-up review and possible revision. This worksheet is for administrative use and record, and not the statement of policy presented to the employees.
2. Describe a method of determining the fringe benefit value for a particular employee.

18. As the controller of a new 250-bed hospital, you have been given the responsibility of setting up the entire payroll system, including the steps which must be taken to assure adequate internal controls. A decision to use time clocks for time reporting has previously been made by the administrator. On the assumption your assistant will be given the responsibility of actually implementing the system and indoctrinating all personnel involved, prepare a list of the steps which he should follow, relating to internal control procedures, in the course of preparing for the hospital's opening (from the reporting of employee time to the issuance of checks). Do not include any steps relative to the setting up of general ledger accounts, employee earnings records, or periodic FICA or withholding tax reports.

19. XYZ Hospital is reviewing its personnel policies and has asked you to supply the following: (1) List at least ten fringe benefits which hospitals might provide to their employees, with a short statement of the advantages of each. (2) List the economic advantages of having a sound personnel policy for a hospital.

20. Describe two methods of accounting for purchase discounts. Give the advantages and disadvantages of each method.

21. What reasons can you give for the fact that employee compensation accounts for 50 percent or more of total hospital costs?

EXERCISES

E1. A hospital employee is paid $6.00 per hour for a regular workweek of 40 hours. During the preceding week, this employee worked 50 hours. Assume that the FICA tax is 6 percent and that 18 percent of the employee's gross pay is to be withheld for federal income taxes. Assume also that the federal unemployment tax is 0.5 percent and that the state unemployment tax is 2.5 percent.

Required. Prepare journal entries to record all of the above. (Disregard any consideration of vacation pay accrual.)

E2. Assume a group of 14 hospital employees, each of whom earns $580 per week and is entitled to a two-week vacation each year.

Required. Prepare the weekly payroll entry for this group of employees. (Disregard payroll tax withholdings.)

E3. Assume that a hospital has the usual workmen's compensation and employers' liability insurance for which an advance premium is required on January 1, 1987, based upon the estimated payroll for the year as follows:

Employee Class	Estimated Payroll	Insurance Rate (per $100)
A	$ 600,000	$.80
B	400,000	.50
C	300,000	.20

The actual payroll for January 1987 was:

Employee Class	
A	$55,000
B	35,000
C	28,000

Required. Prepare the necessary entry at January 1 and at January 31.

E4. A hospital completes the following transactions:

March   21   Purchased $5,000 of supplies on 2/10, EOM terms 100
          24   Purchased $8,000 of supplies on 1/10, EOM terms 80
April   10   Paid invoice of March 21
          25   Paid invoice of March 24

Required. Prepare entries for the above transactions assuming:

1. Purchased supplies are recorded **gross.**
2. Purchased supplies are recorded **net** of discount.

PROBLEMS

P1. General Hospital employees have a 40-hour workweek. The average fulltime equivalent employee complement for the 1987 year was 1,006. The following data for 1987 are taken from the hospital's books and records:

Payroll analysis of hours:	Hours
Paid vacations	75,000
Paid holidays	44,000
Paid sick leave	40,000
Other paid absent time	1,000
Total	160,000
Hours worked	1,940,000
Hours paid	2,100,000

Leaves of absence-unpaid		20,000
Other absent time-unpaid		5,000

Annual payroll	$4,200,000
Employee contributions to tax sheltered annuity	200,000
Social security tax—employer's portion	172,000

Insurance costs:

Fire and extended coverage	2,500
General liability and professional liability	12,000
Business interruption	700
Employee fidelity bond	1,000
Health insurance	40,000
Long-term disability	10,000
Employee life insurance	9,000
Retirement (pension) program	40,000
Workmen's compensation	14,000

Deductions from patient revenue:

Charity	40,000
Contractual adjustments	60,000
Professional allowances	4,000
Employee allowances	4,000
Provision for bad debts	160,000

Cost of employee health service	12,000

Employees completed educational programs involving total tuition costs of $5,000. The hospital followed its policy of reimbursing these employees for 40 percent of tuition costs.

Miscellaneous employee benefits (parties, picnic, etc.)	$4,000

Cafeteria expense for the year:

Meals served to employees	120,000
Average income per meal	60 cents
Average cost per meal	$1.10

Laundry expense for the year:

Pounds of free laundry for employees	50,000
Total pounds of laundry processed	2,500,000
Total cost of operating laundry	$200,000

Required. The hospital administrator wishes to present in the employee newsletter a detailed analysis of the value of employee fringe benefits. For this purpose, compute the value of these benefits per hour worked.

9
Management of Revenues and Expenses

The discussion presented in the two preceding chapters was concerned mainly with a description of the essential procedures involved in accounting for hospital revenues and expenses. Through the application of these procedures, accurate and reliable information relating to the amounts and sources of revenues and the amounts and types of expenses is recorded in the hospital's accounts. This accumulation of actual revenue and expense data, in conformity with generally accepted accounting principles and managerial requirements, is a basic prerequisite to the intelligent management of operating results. Without adequate and relevant income statement information, managerial decision-making would be severely impaired.

In this chapter, the discussion turns to the reporting, analysis, and utilization of recorded revenue and expense data by management in planning and controlling hospital operating activities. If revenues and expenses are to be effectively managed, they must be budgeted. Control can be exercised only if the manager is aware of what revenues and expenses **ought** to be, as well as what they actually are. The first topic treated in this chapter therefore will be the development of an operating budget, i.e., the combined budgets of revenue and expense. As was explained in Chapter 6, historical revenue and expense records serve as a basis for the preparation of such budgets. During the ensuing budget period, the current revenues and expenses are reported in comparison with the budgeted figures. This process is illustrated and discussed in subsequent sections of this chapter. Emphasis is also given to the analysis and interpretation of operating information for internal management purposes. Although it is a directly related subject, the management of working capital is not discussed until Chapter 14.

REVENUE BUDGETING

Revenue is the very lifeblood of any organization, and it is particularly vital in the hospital enterprise. Miscalculations of anticipated revenues can result in operating losses and financial distress rather quickly. Estimates of future revenues also serve as a basis for the budgeting of cash receipts. This, in turn, has an important bearing upon the development of capital expenditure and other budgets. It therefore is evident that a considerable amount of attention must be given to the preparation of a complete and accurate budget of hospital revenues from all sources.

Patient Service Revenues

The budgeting of revenues from services to patients begins with the gathering of historical data in terms of both revenue dollars and nonmonetary statistics of volume of service. These data should be scheduled by months and should embrace a sufficient number of periods to disclose significant trends. The data should be classified according to the individual revenue centers in which it has been generated. Further classification into inpatient and outpatient totals is also necessary for many of the centers. After a thorough study and analysis of this historical information, careful consideration must be given to an evaluation of the many factors likely to have a material influence upon the volume and types of revenue-producing services to be provided during the forthcoming budget period. This procedure permits a realistic projection of statistical data which, when multiplied by the charges to be made for the various services, results in a budget of gross revenues from services to patients. A budget must also be developed for deductions from gross patient service revenues in order to obtain estimates of collectible revenues which are required in the preparation of the cash budget and in the assessment of the adequacy of service rates. This matter is discussed at a later point in this chapter.

Daily Patient Service Revenues. The revenue to be derived from room, meals, and routine nursing care obviously is dependent upon the daily rates for such services and the occupancy (by classes) of the hospital's accommodations. It follows that, given the rates to be charged, the budgeting problem is one of forecasting occupancy in terms of patient days of service for the budget period. This forecast should be developed for each month of the period to facilitate subsequent budget versus actual comparisons on a monthly basis and also to permit the preparation of the cash budget by months. Occupancy forecasts also must be formulated for each supervisory unit in accordance with the principles of responsibility accounting so that revenues may be budgeted on the same basis. Forecasts classified in this manner are also useful in planning nursing personnel requirements.

The forecast of patient days is based upon an analysis of historical data, adjusted for trends and the probable impact of variations in the factors affecting occupancy. Major factors having an influence on occupancy include changes in the characteristics (age, economic status, occupation, etc.) of the population served, in hospital capacity, in types of services offered, in medical practices, in the capabilities of other hospitals in the area, and in hospital insurance coverage. Information concerning such changes generally must be researched from hospital records and from statistics compiled by hospital associations, third-party payers, and governmental agencies. The hospital medical staff is also an important source of information for the budget committee. Major emphasis must be placed on physician involvement in the hospital's budgeting and decision-making process, including long-range strategic and program planning.

After careful consideration of the impact of predicted changes in these factors, forecasts can be developed of expected patient days by diagnosis-related groups, by patients' financial status, and by type of hospital accommodation classified by revenue centers within the nursing services division. These forecasts then are multiplied by service rates to be charged, thereby producing revenue dollar budgets in conformity with the principle of responsibility accounting. In this way, the format in which revenues are budgeted will be the same as the format in which actual revenues are recorded and reported.

If patient day statistics are not compiled by type of accommodation but by type of service, the budgeting of revenues requires a computation of an average revenue per patient day for each type of service. This average then is multiplied by estimated patient days for the budget period. The resultant figure is the revenue budget unless adjustment for rate changes is required.

Other Professional Services. The revenues to be budgeted in this category are derived from both inpatients and outpatients. Services to outpatients may originate in departments serving outpatients only or in departments providing services to both inpatients and outpatients. In any event, historical dollar and statistical occasions of service data must be divided into inpatient and outpatient classifications. These data should also be tabulated on a monthly basis and for a period of sufficient length to disclose significant trends.

After a full appraisal of the historical data and a careful evaluation of the probable effects of changes predicted in underlying factors, forecasts of activity are made for each of the professional service departments and revenue centers. These forecasts must be made in terms of occasions or units of service that will produce reliable revenue estimates and also serve as valid bases for cost analysis. The development of statistical measurements appropriate to these purposes is difficult but essential to effective planning, measurement, and evaluation of departmental activities. It is widely recognized, for example, that a lumping together of dissimilar services into a single statistical "catchall" measurement (such as number of films in radiology or number of tests in the laboratory) is unsatisfactory because of the wide variation in time, skill, materials, and equipment required between one overall statistical unit and the next. These differences generally are reflected to some extent in the hospital's rate structure, and statistics should be compiled on a corresponding basis whenever it is feasible to do so.

Refinement of general statistics into more specific or weighted units of measurement therefore permits more accurate revenue budgeting. The departmental revenue budgets are determined in such cases by multiplying the forecasted number of units of service to be rendered by the appropriate rate established for each specific or weighted unit of service. Where such refinements have not yet been developed, the forecasted number of occasions of service, stated in terms of a general statistic, may be multiplied by an average revenue per occasion of service estimated from past experience. This procedure may produce a reasonably accurate budget of total departmental revenue, but it is not particularly useful to departmental supervisors in planning personnel and equipment requirements, or in evaluating productivity.

Deductions from Patient Service Revenues. After budgeting gross revenues from services to patients, budgets must be developed for the amounts of such revenues that will not be collected due to the provision of charity care, contractual adjustments, policy discounts, and bad debts. These budgets of revenue deductions are based upon an analysis of historical data with suitable modifications being made for trends and changes in factors such as hospital policies, changes in patient groups to which charity care and allowances are given, contractual arrangements, availability of specific purpose grants and subsidies, and economic conditions in the community served by the hospital. In many cases, revenue deductions may be expressed and budgeted as percentages of budgeted gross patient service revenues. Each category of deductions should be separately budgeted and classified into inpatient and outpatient totals in conformity with the classification of gross revenues so that useful comparisons can be made by type of patient. The classification should also enable the hospital to evaluate the amount of contractual adjustments by type of third-party contractor as a basis for renegotiation of the provisions of those contracts from which disproportionate amounts of adjustments result.

Other Revenues

The budgeting of other operating and nonoperating revenues must not be regarded lightly. These revenues often are substantial and must be accurately estimated for the purpose of establishing appropriate rates for patient care services. The budgeting of many items classified as "other" revenues is difficult because related historical data either may not be available or may not be indicative of amounts to be received in the future. In any event, it generally is prudent to make conservative estimates in budgeting those items which cannot be predicted with reasonable certainty and precision.

Revenues from educational programs are budgeted on the basis of expected enrollments and tuition fees to be charged. Budgets of revenues to become available from research and other specific purpose grants may be determined from an analysis of current contracts and proposals in relation to the expected policies of granting organizations. Hospital requests for such resources generally will be included in the overall budget plan only to the extent that there is good evidence that the requests will be honored. A similar procedure usually is followed with respect to the budgeting of unrestricted gifts. An analysis of the stipulations of donors with respect to existing Specific Purpose Funds and the investments of Endowment Funds will provide estimates of revenues to be available to the Unrestricted Fund from those sources.

Rentals of space to doctors and employees may be estimated from a study of existing leases. The budget of cafeteria sales and the sales of gift shops and other hospital operated enterprises often is related to projected patient days and outpatient visits. The same relationship also may be found with respect to telephone and television service, nonpatient sales of supplies, and medical record transcript fees.

Budgets for donated services may be prepared from estimates of the hours of donated service required and committed. These hours then are multiplied by the fair market value of such services. Donated commodities also should be budgeted on the best basis available. It is important that donated services and commodities be budgeted as revenues and expenses although they have no net budgetary effect. Without the integration of accurate estimates of significant amounts of donated items with other elements of the budget, the development of an effective overall operating plan would be impaired. All costs consumed in and all revenues derived from hospital activities should be included in the budgetary plan regardless of whether such costs are paid or such revenues are received in cash.

EXPENSE BUDGETING

A primary management objective in hospitals is to keep expenses at a level equal to, or preferably less than, anticipated revenues in order to maintain a necessary financial integrity of operating results. This requires expense budgeting, and, because labor represents about 50 percent of hospital operating costs, particular attention must be given to the development of accurate budgets for salaries and wages. Supplies, purchased services, and other nonlabor costs are also significant amounts and must be budgeted with care and accuracy.

Salaries and Wages

The preparation of payroll budgets is greatly facilitated if up-to-date and carefully written **personnel manuals** are available which include clear statements of personnel policies, complete job descriptions, and expected performance standards. It is important that salary and wage budgets be developed in the classifications provided in the hospital's chart of accounts, assuming that the chart conforms to the plan of organization as required for responsibility accounting. Each departmental cost center supervisor should have responsibility for the preparation of the salary and wage budget relating to personnel over whose employment and performance the supervisor has primary control. Supervisors must be supplied with adequate information concerning forecasted levels of activity, authorized numbers of employees in each job classification, and the approved rates of pay for each position.

In effect, given a firm projection of the amount of work to be done, supervisors are asked to determine the number of personnel of each classification that will be needed to meet expected workloads in an efficient manner, taking into account established hospital policies and objectives. In this way, major emphasis is placed on the control of labor costs at the lowest levels of organization where decision authority and responsibility for the performance of personnel exists. While much of the salaries and wages paid by hospitals is fixed within wide ranges of activity, there are many areas of activity in which the quantity of labor employed and the manner in which it is utilized can vary to a considerable extent with changes in volume of activity.

Thus, salary and wage budgeting involves a determination of the expected volume of activity in meaningful work-units for each departmental cost center in the hospital. This permits a determination of the number of work hours and employees by job classes needed to perform the expected volume of work in a manner consistent with established quality standards. Then, given approved salary and wage rates, the personnel budget reflects what labor costs **ought** to be. The common practice of merely amending the previous year's payroll for expected changes in number of employees and in compensation rates is not a satisfactory labor budgeting procedure. It produces a budget of what labor costs **will be** if present policies and practices are continued, but it does not produce a budget of what labor costs **should be**. This so-called practical budgeting technique only perpetuates any existing inefficiencies.

In addition to a cost center classification, the labor budget must also be broken down by months of the year. This permits a determination of the amount and time of cash disbursements for salaries and wages that is needed for cash budgeting purposes. It also permits a better month-by-month comparison of budgeted and actual costs during the budget period. The labor **hours** budgeted for each cost center also should be classified by month for comparison with actual **hours** in subsequent budget versus actual reports. Comparisons on a dollar basis alone are not nearly as indicative of employee utilization and efficiency as are comparisons also made on the basis of hours.

If a position control plan is employed, it is particularly useful in the preparation of salary and wage budgets. A **position control plan** primarily is a management tool for controlling the number of employees on the hospital payroll and for assuring the utilization of each employee to the point of highest efficiency. Under this plan, an analysis is made of hospital personnel requirements and a job specification is prepared for each approved position in the hospital. A definite number of employees, depending upon level of activity, is authorized for each job classification, and a position control card is established for each approved position regardless of whether the job is full time or part time, permanent or temporary. (The plan provides for a supply of part-time and temporary employees when workloads require them.) The cards indicate:

1. Job title.
2. Name of incumbent employee (if any).
3. Approved salary or wage scale, and salary of the incumbent.
4. Employee turnover record.
5. Other desired information.

Control of the card file is centralized with a responsible employee who checks and reviews all employee placements against the approved roster. Increases in the authorized number of employees can be made only with the approval of the hospital administrator. Within the limits established in the position control plan, however, the departmental supervisors retain the authority to select, terminate, and recommend employees for salary adjustments or transfers. Once established and working effectively, the position control plan virtually becomes the hospital personnel budget.

In addition to salaries and wages, the personnel budget will include estimates for payroll-related costs such as FICA taxes and workmen's compensation insurance. The budgeting of these expense items is a matter of multiplying the tax or insurance rate by the budgeted amounts of salaries and wages subject to those rates. Other fringe benefits such as the hospital's share of employee insurance and pension programs are budgeted on the basis of the payroll budget and the provisions of such programs and agreements.

Supplies and Other Nonlabor Expenses

The budgeting of nonlabor costs is done in much the same manner as that described for salaries and wages. Each cost center supervisor should be supplied by the accounting department with an analysis of the major categories of supplies and other expenses that have been charged to the center in the last few years. This analysis should reflect dollars, and if applicable, units, i.e., pounds, gallons, dozens, etc. Many of these expense items will vary directly with changes in occupancy and other statistical units of service. Given the forecasted level of activity, each supervisor can determine the amounts of expense the cost center **should** incur to achieve the results desired. Dollar estimates, taking expected price changes into account, can be based partly upon historical costs per patient day or other valid units of service experience.

Repairs and routine maintenance work to be performed are estimated by the hospital engineer on the basis of his experience and knowledge of approved projects. Repairs by outside contractors may be scheduled by type of work and amount by the hospital engineer. Heat, light, power, and other utilities are budgeted in terms of past and projected usage and anticipated changes in prices or service rates.

Items such as depreciation, interest, and rentals generally are budgeted by the hospital controller's office. These budgets are prepared on the basis of plant asset records, current debt service schedules, plans for additional borrowings, and provisions of rental agreements. Because the operating budget is a comprehensive financial plan, **all** hospital expenses should be budgeted.

It should be emphasized here that the budgeting process should not interfere with the work of department or cost center supervisors. These supervisors have the responsibility for planning what is to be done and seeing that it gets done. Budgeting must not handicap them in this function. Instead, the budgeting process should assist them in planning and providing the desired services in a more efficient manner. Budgetary planning and control of expense does not mean minimizing expense; rather, it should mean spending what **ought** to be spent to achieve desired results, consistent with quality standards and commensurate with available resources.

RATE SETTING

The hospital's budget of revenues can only be regarded as tentative until expenses are budgeted and compared with budgeted revenues. Because the comparison typically reflects a deficiency of revenues, or net revenues insufficient to meet the total financial requirements of the hospital in terms of its established objectives, hard decisions must be made. Given the revenue budget, what downward adjustments might be made in the expense budget? Given the expense budget, what upward revisions might be possible in the revenue budget? Both of these possibilities should be explored as a means of balancing the hospital budget.

Forecasted deficits sometimes have been resolved by reductions on the expense side even where it has been accomplished through curtailment of desirable services and programs. On the other hand, the budgeted expenses may be wholly defensible and not subject to arbitrary curtailment. This assumption coupled with the cost-based nature of some reimbursement arrangements often leads to the adjustment of service rates as the more financially expedient solution to the budget problem. The question in such cases therefore becomes: which particular service rates should be increased and by how much?

In principle, service rates should directly reflect the costs of providing each service, thus allowing each department of the hospital to be self-sustaining. Public relations considerations and other realities of hospital financing, however, historically have resulted in the establishment of considerably below-cost rates for daily room and board services and substantially above-cost rates for certain professional services such as radiology, laboratory, and pharmacy. If a cost-finding were done on the basis of budgeted revenues and expenses, for example, the results might appear as illustrated in Figure 9-1. An analysis of this kind can be useful in determining the extent of service rate adjustments and in otherwise finalizing the operating budget.

Although there is some evidence that hospital service rates are more closely related to costs than ever before, the subsidization of the loss operations of certain departments by the profits of another continues to some extent as a hospital pricing policy. In addition, hospitals have tended to establish service rates by a consensus approach, i.e., hospitals may adopt the level and pattern of rates existing in similar hospitals located in the same general area.

Beyond this, hospital managements traditionally have used charges to self-responsible patients as the balancing factor when seeking a solution to revenue deficits. Determinations are made of (1) the amount of revenues available from third-party payers, philanthropy, and other miscellaneous sources and (2) the hospital's financial needs. The resulting revenue deficit then is resolved by establishing rates at levels sufficient to generate revenues from self-responsible patients in the amounts needed to balance financial needs and expected revenues. In effect, by paying more than the economic costs of the services they receive, self-responsible patients are subsidizing the care of third-party beneficiaries.

Figure 9-1.
Goodcare Hospital
Budgeted Departmental Income Statement
Year Ending December 31, 1987

	Net Revenues*	Direct and Indirect Expenses	Net Income (Loss) Amount	Net Income (Loss) Percent
Nursing service units	$4,100	$3,829	$ 271	+ 6.6%
Operating and recovery rooms	560	676	(116)	− 20.7
Delivery and labor rooms	150	477	(327)	−218.0
Central supply	270	315	(45)	− 16.7
Emergency service	290	386	(96)	− 33.1
Laboratory and blood bank	930	791	139	+ 14.9
Radiology	860	572	288	+ 33.5
Pharmacy	780	507	273	+ 35.0
Anesthesia	200	182	18	+ 9.0
Inhalation therapy	80	67	13	+ 16.3
Cardio-pulmonary	12	14	(2)	− 16.7
Physical therapy	116	101	15	+ 12.9
EKG/EEG	108	66	42	+ 38.9
Clinic	96	286	(190)	−197.9
Other	48	51	(3)	− 6.3
Totals	$8,600	$8,320	$ 280	
Less provision for contractual adjustments			150	
Net operating income			$ 130	
Add nonoperating revenues			230	
Budgeted net income for the year			$ 360	

*Patient service revenues after provision for bad debts and allowances but before provision for contractual adjustments.

The elimination of these inequitable and discriminatory pricing policies will require the establishment of hospital service prices on the basis of full economic costs rather than on the basis of financial expediency. Full economic costs include the basic production costs of hospital services, education, research, and community health program costs, working and plant capital needs, bad debts, and free services.

Due to their great bargaining power, third-party payers have been able to impose reimbursement arrangements upon hospitals that exclude a number of these cost elements. Third-party payers argue that as reliable volume purchasers of hospital services they are entitled to a lower price than that paid by an individual patient. While there is some validity in this position, third parties generally have demanded and gotten greater price reductions than have been justified on the basis of volume and reliability. The individual hospital, being already in a precarious financial position, has been almost powerless to do anything but accept such contracts under the terms laid down by the third-party payers.

The solution to this serious problem is largely a political one, and it probably will be solved in that arena. But until that time, hospitals have no alternatives other than going out of business or responding creatively to the financial realities of fixed-price payment systems with programs designed to improve the efficiency of hospital operations.

REPORTING OPERATING RESULTS TO MANAGEMENT

The basic requirements of a good management reporting system were set forth by one source as follows:[1]

THE BASIC
    S – Define **strategic** factors
    E – Include **external** and internal information
    C – Use **comparisons** extensively
    R – Show **relevant** data only
    E – Cover the **entire** range of operations
    T – Be **timely** in reporting
    S – Set **standards** wisely

OF EFFECTIVE
    R – Recognize and report by **responsibilities**
    E – Focus upon **exceptions** existing
    P – Follow a **pyramid** report structure
    O – Include **operating** statistics
    R – **Review** reporting needs of management
    T – Reveal significant **trends** and relationships
    S – Promote **simplicity** and clarity in reports

These elements of content and technique are essential to the effectiveness of reports prepared for internal management purposes in all types of enterprises, including hospitals. Application of these principles may be noted in the following illustrations of certain reports relating to hospital operating results; working capital reports are illustrated and discussed in Chapter 14. The reader is also referred to Chapters 10-15 of the author's **External and Internal Reporting by Hospitals** where numerous examples of internal management reports can be found.[2]

As a basis for illustration, selected portions of a monthly operating report of hypothetical Wellsville Hospital are reproduced here. The institution is a voluntary general community hospital of medium size. Its report of operations for the month of April 1987 and the four months then ended is presented mainly for illustrative and discussion purposes. While certain standard requirements should be met by all reports, many matters of format, style, terminology, and content must be decided on the basis of circumstances peculiar to the individual hospital and the desires of its management. The reader should not regard the relationships that may be observed among the figures as indicative of what is normal or desirable for any particular hospital.

Wellsville Hospital's organization chart is presented in Figure 9-2. Although certain liberties have been taken, this chart is reasonably realistic and representative of the organization plan of many hospitals. Wellsville Hospital is organized into well-defined organizational units, or responsibility centers, each having a director, department head, or supervisor specifically responsible for its activities. Each center incurs expenses, and many centers also generate revenues.

Figure 9-2.
Wellsville Hospital
Chart of Organization
(Partial)

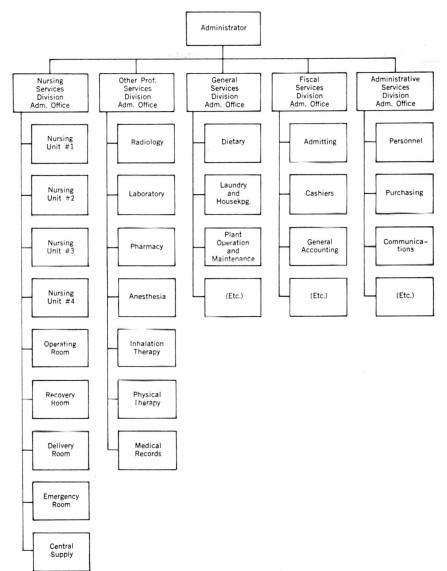

The hospital employs a system of responsibility accounting and reporting based upon this organizational structure (see Figure 4-11 and the accompanying explanation). In its accounting process, the hospital's (1) controllable expenses are accumulated in the accounts according to the centers responsible for incurring them and (2) revenues are recorded by the centers responsible for providing the services that generated them. The recorded data are **reported** in the same manner as may be seen in the following illustrations.

Summary Income Statement

The hospital's April 1987 and year-to-date report begins with a summary income statement which is presented as Exhibit 1 in Figure 9-3. This statement is prepared so that the administrator and other members of top management may be quickly informed of the highlights of operating results for the month and year to date without the distraction of a mass of detail. The illustration, of course, is only one of several possible in terms of both content and format. Most executives insist that columns showing comparisons of the prior year month and year-to-date figures also be included. Some favor a format in which the current month figures are arranged on the left and year-to-date figures on the right, with item descriptions being presented between the two. Another common practice is the inclusion of common-size and per-unit-of-service data in the summary report. Some of these alternatives are illustrated subsequently, but the exact format adopted in a particular organization depends largely on management preferences and the data-generating capability of the accounting department.

Figure 9-3.
Wellsville Hospital
Summary Income Statement
Month of April 1987 and Year to Date
(Comparisons with Budget)   EXHIBIT 1

	Detail Schedule	Month of April 1987				1987 Year to Date			
				Over (Under) Budget				Over (Under) Budget	
		Actual	Budget	Amount	Percent	Actual	Budget	Amount	Percent
Gross Patient Service Revenues:									
Inpatients	A	$ 484,149	$ 483,000	$ 1,149	0.2%	$ 2,009,218	$ 1,956,000	$ 53,218	2.7%
Outpatients	A	67,304	62,000	5,304	8.6	277,292	250,500	26,792	10.7
Total patient service revenues		$ 551,453	$ 545,000	$ 6,453	1.2	$ 2,286,510	$ 2,206,500	$ 80,010	3.6
Less revenue deductions	B	46,542	44,000	2,542	5.8	194,080	177,300	16,780	9.5
Net patient service revenues		$ 504,911	$ 501,000	$ 3,911	0.8	$ 2,092,430	$ 2,029,200	$ 63,230	3.1
Add other operating revenues	C	6,155	5,400	755	14.0	25,112	24,700	412	1.7
Total operating revenues		$ 511,066	$ 506,400	$ 4,666	0.9	$ 2,117,542	$ 2,053,900	$ 63,642	3.1
Less Operating Expenses:									
Nursing services	D	$ 220,824	$ 216,800	$ 4,024	1.9	$ 839,362	$ 820,600	$ 18,762	2.3
Other professional services	E	98,355	92,000	6,355	6.9	460,521	421,300	39,221	9.3
General services	F	94,972	101,000	(6,028)	(6.0)	383,687	378,200	5,487	1.5
Fiscal and administrative services	G	78,455	76,200	2,255	3.0	366,491	359,700	6,791	1.9
Total operating expenses		$ 492,606	$ 486,000	$ 6,606	1.4	$ 2,050,061	$ 1,979,800	$ 70,261	3.5
Net operating income		$ 18,460	$ 20,400	$ (1,940)	(9.5)	$ 67,481	$ 74,100	$ (6,619)	(8.9)
Add nonoperating revenues	H	1,090	1,600	(510)	(31.9)	5,472	6,600	(1,128)	(17.1)
Net income		$ 19,550	$ 22,000	$ (2,450)	(11.1)	$ 72,953	$ 80,700	$ (7,747)	(9.6)

The detail schedule column of Exhibit 1 is provided to identify the accompanying schedules in which may be found the major details supporting the revenue and expense totals presented in the summary statement. Eight detail schedules are indicated, but only Schedules A to G are illustrated here. It is assumed that nonoperating revenues consist principally of immaterial amounts.

Detailed Schedules of Revenues

Schedule A, illustrated in Figure 9-4, provides the major details supporting the totals of inpatient and outpatient revenues indicated in Exhibit 1. For example, in Exhibit 1, total actual inpatient revenues for April are reported to be $484,149. The components of this total are presented by functional classifications in Schedule A. It also may be noted that a subschedule column is provided to identify accompanying schedules in which may be found even greater details in support of each revenue total listed in Schedule A. Subschedule 1, for example, might provide a detailed analysis of daily patient service revenues by individual nursing unit or by type of hospital accommodation, or by both. Such subschedules, however, are not illustrated here.

Figure 9-4.

Wellsville Hospital

Gross Patient Service Revenues

Month of April 1987 and Year to Date   SCHEDULE A

	Sub-schedule	Month of April 1987		Over (Under) Budget		1987 Year to Date		Over (Under) Budget	
INPATIENTS		Actual	Budget	Amount	Percent	Actual	Budget	Amount	Percent
Nursing Services:									
Daily patient services	1	$260,587	$268,200	$ (7,613)	(2.8)%	$1,168,359	$1,151,300	$ 17,059	1.5%
Operating room	x	28,330	29,700	(1,370)	(4.6)	113,603	102,000	11,603	11.4
Recovery room	x	4,401	4,100	301	7.3	17,692	16,700	992	5.9
Delivery room	x	7,829	6,300	1,529	24.3	31,629	29,300	2,329	7.9
Emergency room	x	2,265	1,900	365	19.2	9,196	11,500	(2,304)	(20.0)
Central supply	x	23,949	24,400	(451)	(1.8)	95,077	104,900	(9,823)	(9.4)
Total		$327,361	$334,600	$ (7,239)	(2.2)	$1,435,556	$1,415,700	$ 19,856	1.4
Other Professional Services:									
Radiology	x	$ 49,871	$ 47,000	$ 2,871	6.1	$ 152,301	$ 147,800	$ 4,501	3.0
Laboratory	x	75,639	71,700	3,939	5.5	295,828	276,800	19,028	6.9
Pharmacy	x	19,085	18,000	1,085	6.0	77,294	75,700	1,594	2.1
Anesthesia	x	3,765	3,400	365	10.7	15,211	12,100	3,111	25.7
Inhalation therapy	x	4,041	4,200	(159)	(3.8)	15,436	13,000	2,436	18.7
Physical therapy	x	4,387	4,100	287	7.0	17,592	14,900	2,692	18.1
Total		$156,788	$148,400	$ 8,388	5.7	$ 573,662	$ 540,300	$ 33,362	6.2
Total inpatient revenues		$484,149	$483,000	$ 1,149	0.2	$2,009,218	$1,956,000	$ 53,218	2.7
OUTPATIENTS									
Nursing Services:									
Operating room	x	$ 2,690	$ 2,500	$ 190	7.6	$ 10,787	$ 9,500	$ 1,287	13.5
Recovery room	x	1,160	1,200	(40)	(3.3)	4,652	4,500	152	3.4
Emergency room	x	15,538	14,300	1,238	8.7	62,463	60,700	1,763	2.9
Central supply	x	2,816	2,700	116	4.3	11,348	10,200	1,148	11.3
Total		$ 22,204	$ 20,700	$ 1,504	7.3	$ 89,250	$ 84,900	$ 4,350	5.1
Other Professional Services:									
Radiology	x	$ 28,593	$ 25,700	$ 2,893	11.3	$ 121,579	$ 106,500	$ 15,079	14.2
Laboratory	x	11,230	10,800	430	4.0	45,216	39,800	5,416	13.6
Pharmacy	x	1,729	1,500	229	15.3	7,002	6,600	402	6.1
Anesthesia	x	861	700	161	23.0	3,470	3,100	370	11.9
Physical therapy	x	2,687	2,600	87	3.3	10,775	9,600	1,175	12.2
Total		$ 45,100	$ 41,300	$ 3,800	9.2	$ 188,042	$ 165,600	$ 22,442	13.6
Total outpatient revenues		$ 67,304	$ 62,000	$ 5,304	8.6	$ 277,292	$ 250,500	$ 26,792	10.7

Schedule B, illustrated in Figure 9-5, provides the major details supporting the total deductions from patient service revenues as indicated in Exhibit 1. In the schedule, these deductions are reported by major types. Subschedules, as indicated, may be developed to provide additional details of each type of revenue deduction, e.g., a classification of contractual adjustments by categories of third-party payers. Or, such deductions may be classified by type of patient. Subschedules are not illustrated here, but the reader might wish to examine Figure 19-4.

Figure 9-5.
Wellsville Hospital
Deductions from Patient Service Revenues
Month of April 1987 and Year to Date   SCHEDULE B

| | Sub-schedule | Month of April 1987 | | | | 1987 Year to Date | | | |
| | | Actual | Budget | Over (Under) Budget | | Actual | Budget | Over (Under) Budget | |
				Amount	Percent			Amount	Percent
Charity care	1	$ 11,655	$ 10,100	$ 1,555	15.4%	$ 47,786	$ 42,700	$ 5,086	11.9%
Contractual adjustments	x	29,425	28,300	1,125	4.0	124,791	115,200	9,591	8.3
Courtesy discounts	x	603	800	(197)	(24.6)	1,824	2,300	(476)	(20.7)
Bad debts	x	4,859	4,800	59	1.2	19,679	17,100	2,579	15.1
Total		$ 46,542	$ 44,000	$ 2,542	5.8	$194,080	$177,300	$ 16,780	9.5

Schedule C, illustrated in Figure 9-6, provides the major details relating to the total of other operating revenues reported in Exhibit 1. If desired, one or more subschedules may be attached to supply further details or to present an analysis of some sort.

Figure 9-6.
Wellsville Hospital
Other Operating Revenues
Month of April 1987 and Year to Date   SCHEDULE C

| | Sub-schedule | Month of April 1987 | | | | 1987 Year to Date | | | |
| | | Actual | Budget | Over (Under) Budget | | Actual | Budget | Over (Under) Budget | |
				Amount	Percent			Amount	Percent
Cafeteria sales	1	$ 4,359	$ 3,600	$ 759	21.1%	$ 17,928	$ 17,600	$ 328	1.9%
Telephone service	x	833	800	33	4.1	3,232	3,100	132	4.3
Sundry	x	963	1,000	(37)	(3.7)	3,952	4,000	(48)	1.2
Total		$ 6,155	$ 5,400	$ 755	14.0	$ 25,112	$ 24,700	$ 412	1.7

Detailed Schedules of Expenses

In Exhibit 1, the operating expenses of the hospital are reported in four totals representing the four organizational divisions of the hospital. Major details supporting each of these totals are provided in detailed schedules.

1. **Schedule D.** Schedule D (Figure 9-7) lists expenses relating to the Nursing Services Division and is designed principally for use by the Director of Nursing. It provides details of the expenses of the administrative office of the division and supplies total expense figures for each nursing unit and other cost centers for which the Director of Nursing is responsible. As indicated, subschedules are developed to support the cost center totals reported in Schedule D. Subschedule D/1 (Figure 9-8), for example, provides the details of expenses related to Nursing Unit #1. This subschedule is directed mainly to the supervisor of that unit, but the Director of Nursing also receives a copy. Although not illustrated here, the content and format of other subschedules would be very similar.

2. **Schedule E.** Schedule E (Figure 9-9) lists expenses relating to the Other Professional Services division of the hospital. It is designed primarily for use by the director of the division. This schedule provides details of the expenses of the administrative office of the division and total expense figures for each department or cost center for which the director is responsible. Detailed subschedules of expenses (not illustrated) are directed to department heads and center supervisors.

3. **Schedule F.** Schedule F (Figure 9-10) reports the expenses of the General Services Division of the hospital. It is designed for the use of the director of the division, and detailed subschedules are prepared for the dietitian, housekeeper, engineer, and other supervisors within the division.

4. **Schedule G.** Schedule G (Figure 9-11) lists the expenses of the hospital's Fiscal and Administrative Services Division. It is prepared for the Controller and for the head of administrative services. Appropriate subschedules of expenses are directed to the supervisors of cost centers organized within the division.

At each level of management responsibility, the reports include only those expenses that are relevant to each level, and only in the degree of detail that is necessary or desired. It is a pyramid report structure as indicated in Figure 9-12.

Figure 9-7.
Wellsville Hospital
Nursing Services Division Expenses
Month of April 1987 and Year to Date   SCHEDULE D

	Sub-schedule	Month of April 1987				1987 Year to Date			
		Actual	Budget	Over (Under) Budget		Actual	Budget	Over (Under) Budget	
				Amount	Percent			Amount	Percent
Administrative Office:									
Salaries and wages		$ 2,100	$ 2,000	$ 100	5.0%	$ 8,300	$ 8,100	$ 200	2.5%
Supplies and other expenses		886	800	86	10.8	3,644	3,500	144	4.1
Total		$ 2,986	$ 2,800	$ 186	6.6	$ 11,944	$ 11,600	$ 344	3.0
Nursing Units:									
# 1	1	$ 67,957	$ 66,900	$ 1,057	1.6	$244,048	$240,500	$ 3,548	1.5
# 2	2	42,971	44,200	(1,229)	(2.8)	151,438	149,700	1,738	1.2
# 3	3	22,886	22,800	86	.4	91,086	89,800	1,286	1.4
# 4	4	16,437	15,600	837	5.4	59,761	61,000	(1,239)	(2.0)
Total		$150,251	$149,500	$ 751	.5	$546,333	$541,000	$ 5,333	1.0
Other Centers:									
Operating room	5	$ 26,463	$ 24,400	$ 2,063	8.5	$106,118	$104,200	$ 1,918	1.8
Recovery room	6	1,969	1,800	169	9.4	7,915	7,100	815	11.5
Delivery room	7	6,748	6,200	548	8.8	26,857	26,300	557	2.1
Emergency room	8	18,299	18,400	(101)	(.5)	73,745	74,200	(455)	(.6)
Central supply	9	14,108	13,700	408	3.0	66,450	56,200	10,250	18.2
Total		$ 67,587	$ 64,500	$ 3,087	4.8	$281,085	$268,000	$ 13,085	4.9
Total expenses		$220,824	$216,800	$ 4,024	1.9	$839,362	$820,600	$ 18,762	2.3

Figure 9-8.
Wellsville Hospital
Expenses – Nursing Unit #1
Month of April 1987 and Year to Date   SCHEDULE D/1

	Month of April 1987				1987 Year to Date			
			Over (Under) Budget				Over (Under) Budget	
	Actual	Budget	Amount	Percent	Actual	Budget	Amount	Percent
Salaries and Wages:								
Staff nurses	$ 36,735	$ 36,000	$ 735	2.0%	$120,360	$118,000	$ 2,360	2.0%
Nursing assistants	3,398	3,100	298	9.6	13,692	13,500	192	1.4
Orderlies	8,834	8,700	134	1.5	36,336	36,000	336	0.9
Nurses' aides	14,951	15,000	(49)	(0.3)	57,804	58,100	(296)	(0.5)
Total salaries and wages	$ 63,918	$ 62,800	$ 1,118	1.8	$228,192	$225,600	$ 2,592	1.1
Supplies (detailed)	2,863	3,100	(237)	(7.6)	11,252	10,500	752	7.2
Other expenses (detailed)	1,176	1,000	176	17.6	4,604	4,400	204	4.6
Total expenses	$ 67,957	$ 66,900	$ 1,057	1.6	$244,048	$240,500	$ 3,548	1.5

Figure 9-9.
Wellsville Hospital
Other Professional Services Division Expenses
Month of April 1987 and Year to Date   SCHEDULE E

	Sub-schedule	Month of April 1987				1987 Year to Date			
				Over (Under) Budget				Over (Under) Budget	
		Actual	Budget	Amount	Percent	Actual	Budget	Amount	Percent
Administrative Office:									
Salaries and wages		$ 3,300	$ 3,200	$ 100	3.1%	$ 13,200	$ 12,900	$ 300	2.3%
Supplies and other expenses		791	600	191	31.8	2,864	2,900	(36)	(1.2)
Total		$ 4,091	$ 3,800	$ 291	7.7	$ 16,064	$ 15,800	$ 264	1.7
Cost Centers:									
Radiology	1	$ 29,599	$ 27,600	$ 1,999	7.2	$144,131	$132,800	$ 11,331	8.5
Laboratory	2	36,618	34,900	1,718	4.9	186,472	162,900	23,572	14.5
Pharmacy	3	14,685	13,700	985	7.2	60,208	58,700	1,508	2.6
Anesthesia	4	2,056	1,800	256	14.2	8,306	8,200	106	1.3
Inhalation therapy	5	1,847	1,700	147	8.6	7,369	7,100	269	3.8
Physical therapy	6	4,183	3,600	583	16.2	16,857	15,500	1,357	8.8
Medical records	7	5,276	4,900	376	7.7	21,114	20,300	814	4.0
Total		$ 94,264	$ 88,200	$ 6,064	6.9	$444,457	$405,500	$ 38,957	9.6
Total expenses		$ 98,355	$ 92,000	$ 6,355	6.9	$460,521	$421,300	$ 39,221	9.3

Figure 9-10.
Wellsville Hospital
General Services Division Expenses
Month of April 1987 and Year to Date   SCHEDULE F

	Sub-schedule	Month of April 1987				1987 Year to Date			
				Over (Under) Budget				Over (Under) Budget	
		Actual	Budget	Amount	Percent	Actual	Budget	Amount	Percent
Administrative Office:									
Salaries and wages		$ 1,700	$ 1,700	$ - - -	- - - %	$ 6,800	$ 6,800	$ - - -	- - - %
Supplies and other expenses		406	300	106	35.3	1,792	1,500	292	19.5
Total		$ 2,106	$ 2,000	$ 106	5.3	$ 8,592	$ 8,300	$ 292	3.5
Cost Centers:									
Dietary	1	$ 41,632	$ 43,100	$ (1,468)	(3.4)	$159,159	$162,800	$ (3,641)	(2.2)
Laundry and housekeeping	2	27,491	29,700	(2,209)	(7.4)	119,964	114,500	5,464	4.8
Plant operation and maintenance	3	23,743	26,200	(2,457)	(9.4)	95,972	92,600	3,372	3.6
Total		$ 92,866	$ 99,000	$ (6,134)	(6.2)	$375,095	$369,900	$ 5,195	1.4
Total expenses		$ 94,972	$101,000	$ (6,028)	(6.0)	$383,687	$378,200	$ 5,487	1.5

Figure 9-11.

Wellsville Hospital

Fiscal and Administrative Services Division Expenses

Month of April 1987 and Year to Date   SCHEDULE G

	Sub-schedule	Month of April 1987		Over (Under) Budget		1987 Year to Date		Over (Under) Budget	
		Actual	Budget	Amount	Percent	Actual	Budget	Amount	Percent
Fiscal Services:									
Administrative office									
Salaries and wages		$ 2,600	$ 2,600	$ ---	---%	$ 10,400	$ 10,400	$ ---	---%
Supplies and other expenses		280	300	(20)	(6.7)	1,020	1,200	(180)	(15.0)
Total		$ 2,880	$ 2,900	$ (20)	(0.7)	$ 11,420	$ 11,600	$ (180)	(1.6)
Cost centers (detailed)	xx	23,418	22,800	618	2.7	130,075	128,100	1,975	1.5
Total		$ 26,298	$ 25,700	$ 598	2.3	$141,495	$139,700	$ 1,795	1.3
Administrative Services:									
Administrative office									
Salaries and wages		$ 3,400	$ 3,400	$ ---	---	$ 13,600	$ 13,600	$ ---	---
Supplies and other expenses		600	700	(100)	(14.3)	2,510	2,400	110	4.6
Total		$ 4,000	$ 4,100	$ (100)	(2.4)	$ 16,110	$ 16,000	$ 110	0.7
Cost centers (detailed)	xx	12,985	12,500	485	3.9	68,769	67,300	1,469	2.2
Total		$ 16,985	$ 16,600	$ 385	2.3	$ 84,879	$ 83,300	$ 1,579	1.9
Unassigned Expenses:									
Employee benefits		$ 17,734	$ 16,900	$ 834	4.9	$ 73,802	$ 71,900	$ 1,902	2.6
Depreciation		12,240	12,000	240	2.0	47,491	46,500	991	2.1
Interest		3,930	3,900	30	0.8	15,720	15,400	320	2.1
Other		1,268	1,100	168	15.3	3,104	2,900	204	7.0
Total		$ 35,172	$ 33,900	$ 1,272	3.8	$140,117	$136,700	$ 3,417	2.5
Total expenses		$ 78,455	$ 76,200	$ 2,255	3.0	$366,491	$359,700	$ 6,791	1.9

Figure 9-12.

Pyramid Report Structure

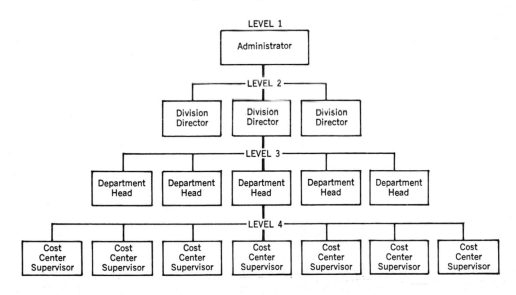

At Level 1, the basic report of operating results is the summary income statement previously illustrated (Figure 9-3) in which expenses are presented in totals classified by organizational division. This focuses attention on the overall actual versus budget performance of those individuals directly responsible to the administrator, i.e., the divisional directors. By reference to appropriate schedules and subschedules, the administrator can secure more detailed information concerning the operations of each division and its component departments. The amount of attention given to such details by the administrator will depend upon interest, experience, and other attendant circumstances.

The divisional directors at Level 2 will consider Schedules D to G (Figures 9-7, 9-9, 9-10, 9-11) as their basic reports for purposes of expense control. Each of these schedules presents (1) a detailed **object of expenditure** analysis of the expenses of the director's administrative office and (2) totals of expenses classified by departments, or **primary** cost centers, organized within the division. The latter information directs attention to the overall actual versus budget performance of those individuals who are directly responsible to the director, i.e., the department heads. Various subschedules may be examined by the directors to obtain more detailed information relating to the operations of particular departments and **secondary** cost centers.

At Level 3, the basic expense report is the subschedule such as was illustrated in Figure 9-8. In the subschedule, the department head usually is given a detailed analysis of departmental expenses by object of expenditure, i.e., salaries and wages, supplies, purchased services, etc. If the department is large, multifunctioned, and organized into several subordinate (secondary) cost centers, the subschedule takes the format of a Level 2 report and will reflect expense totals classified by such centers. The Laboratory Department, for example, may be organized into subordinate centers such as Pathology, Chemistry, Hematology, Bacteriology and other subdepartments, each having a supervisor. When this organizational structure exists, a fourth level of reporting is required. The Level 4 reports should present center expenses classified by object of expenditure in detail and should support the center expense totals listed in the Level 3 reports.

It is important to note that the manager at each level is supplied with copies of all reports directed to all subordinate managers at every lower level. It should also be recognized that not all hospitals will have four reporting levels as described. The large hospital may have more than four levels; smaller hospitals may have only two or three levels. The reporting system must follow the organization plan of the individual hospital.

OTHER REPORTS AND ANALYSES

The most significant analysis of operating results available to hospital management is the comparison of actual against budgeted performance as illustrated in the preceding pages. If budgeting is done properly, it may be assumed that the budget figures present what revenues and expenses **should be**. And, given sound accounting procedures and effective internal controls, the accuracy and reliability of **actual** revenue and expense figures reported by the accountant also may be assumed. It therefore follows that the variances observed in the actual versus budget comparison should be indicative of areas worthy of management attention. Budget variances, however, are only indicators of **where** trouble spots may exist and **who** may be responsible. The really difficult problem facing management is the determination of **why** such variances occur and **what action**, if any, should be taken to correct them. The variances merely pinpoint areas in which further investigation and analysis may prove fruitful.

As discussed in Chapter 6, the significance of budget variances depends largely upon the validity of the actual versus budget comparison. Actual and budgeted **dollars** should always be evaluated in conjunction with related non-monetary statistical measurements of activity levels. Unless the budgeted volume of service and the actual volume of service are approximately the same, variances may easily be misleading and improper conclusions may be drawn from them. Flexible budgeting (see Chapter 6) may be the solution to this problem, at least for many departments of the hospital. If this technique is not employed, however, the proper interpretation of budget variances is considerably more difficult. When there is a material difference between actual and budgeted activity and budgeted dollars are not adjusted to the actual activity level, intelligent analysis of the budget variance requires an understanding of cost behavior in response to changes in activity volume. The manager's ability to recognize fixed and variable costs, as pointed out in Chapter 6, is of critical importance in the interpretation of budget variances and in the management of hospital costs. It must be recognized that a variance, either over or under budget, is not automatically nor necessarily good or bad. Further discussion of this matter is provided in a subsequent section of this chapter.

Certain reports and analyses other than those involving a comparison of actual and budgeted dollars are illustrated first. These additional reports and analytical techniques may provide insights helpful to the interpretation of budget variances and also may bring to light conditions which might otherwise go unnoticed.

Comparisons with Prior Periods

In addition to the actual versus budget comparison, management generally wants reports in which the actual revenue and expense data of current and prior periods are compared. Columns providing data for the previous year may simply be added to the reports already illustrated, but this tends to detract from the more important budget comparison and places an excessive amount of information on a single page. The preferable practice is to provide comparisons for the prior period in separate, supplementary reports such as the one illustrated in Figure 9-13. Should it be desired, a similar presentation could be made in the detailed schedules. Annual comparisons may also be made for periods of several years, and trend percentages (see Figure 20-3) may be computed for use in budgeting and long-range planning.

Comparisons of actual performance in succeeding periods are useful for certain purposes, but the manger must recognize that conditions differ from one year to the next. No two years are the same and, unless the important differences are taken into account, comparisons of "this" year with "last" year can be highly misleading. One major drawback of such comparisons is, for example, the effect of changes in the purchasing power of the dollar.

Figure 9-13.
Wellsville Hospital
Summary Income Statement
Month of April 1987 and Year to Date
(Comparisons with Prior Year)

	Month of April				Year to Date			
			Increase (Decrease)				Increase (Decrease)	
	1987	1986	Amount	Percent	1987	1986	Amount	Percent
Gross Patient Service Revenues:								
Inpatients	$484,149	$450,003	$ 34,146	7.6%	$2,009,218	$1,804,512	$204,706	11.3%
Outpatients	67,304	60,011	7,293	12.2	277,292	241,844	35,448	14.7
Total patient service revenues	$551,453	$510,014	$ 41,439	8.1	$2,286,510	$2,046,356	$240,154	11.7
Less revenue deductions	46,542	40,618	5,924	14.6	194,080	164,097	29,983	18.3
Net patient service revenues	$504,911	$469,396	$ 35,515	7.6	$2,092,430	$1,882,259	$210,171	11.2
Add other operating revenues	6,155	6,011	144	2.4	25,112	24,044	1,068	4.4
Total operating revenues	$511,066	$475,407	$ 35,659	7.5	$2,117,542	$1,906,303	$211,239	11.1
Less Operating Expenses:								
Nursing services	$220,824	$203,511	$ 17,313	8.5	$ 839,362	$ 815,570	$ 23,792	2.9
Other professional services	98,355	103,175	(4,820)	(4.7)	460,521	421,986	38,535	9.1
General services	94,972	85,395	9,577	11.2	383,687	347,287	36,400	10.5
Fiscal and administrative services	78,455	67,373	11,082	16.4	366,491	270,839	95,652	35.3
Total operating expenses	$492,606	$459,454	$ 33,152	7.2	$2,050,061	$1,855,682	$194,379	10.5
Net operating income	$ 18,460	$ 15,953	$ 2,507	15.7	$ 67,481	$ 50,621	$ 16,860	33.3
Add nonoperating revenues	1,090	8,147	(7,057)	(86.6)	5,472	14,175	(8,703)	(61.4)
Net income	$ 19,550	$ 24,100	$ (4,550)	(18.9)	$ 72,953	$ 64,796	$ 8,157	12.6

Common-Size Analysis

Another analytical technique of particular value in the managerial interpretation of operating results is the development and reporting of component percentages within the income statement as illustrated in Figure 9-14. (Additional illustrations and an explanation of the mathematics involved are provided in Chapter 22.) In Figure 9-14, the actual and budgeted dollars are expressed as percentages of a single figure, i.e., total operating revenues. Revenue deductions, however, are reported as a percentage of gross patient service revenues as this is a more meaningful relationship.

The analysis in the first half of the statement indicates the relative importance of inpatient as opposed to outpatient revenues. In addition, the impact of revenue deductions is clearly revealed, i.e., about 8.5 cents of each dollar of charges prove to be uncollectible. Taking this into account, the relative importance of collectible patient service revenues and other operating revenues is shown. Application of this common-size technique to the data in Schedule A (Figure 9-4) would be even more enlightening as to the sources of hospital revenues.

In the second half of Figure 9-14, the disposition of revenues to the coverage of hospital expenses by organizational division is set forth in a useful manner. In April of 1987, for example, nursing services took 43.2 cents of each dollar of operating revenues. It also may be noted that, in April of 1987, the hospital's **operating ratio** (total operating expenses divided by total operating revenues) was 96.4 percent. In other words, operating expenses consumed 96.4 cents of each dollar of operating revenues. The operating ratio is commonly interpreted as an indicator of operating efficiency.

Figure 9-14.
Wellsville Hospital
Summary Income Statement
Month of April 1987 and Year to Date
(Common-Size Analysis)

Month of April				Year to Date		
1987		1986		1987		1986
Actual	Budget	Actual		Actual	Budget	Actual
			Gross Patient Service Revenues:			
87.8%	88.6%	88.2%	Inpatients	87.9%	88.6%	88.2%
12.2	11.4	11.8	Outpatients	12.1	11.4	11.8
100.0%	100.0%	100.0%	Total patient service revenues	100.0%	100.0%	100.0%
8.4	8.1	8.0	Less revenue deductions	8.5	8.0	8.0
91.6%	91.9%	92.0%	Net patient service revenues	91.5%	92.0%	92.0%
98.8%	98.9%	98.7%	Net patient service revenues	98.8%	98.8%	98.7%
1.2	1.1	1.3	Add other operating revenues	1.2	1.2	1.3
100.0%	100.0%	100.0%	Total operating revenues	100.0%	100.0%	100.0%
			Less Operating Expenses:			
43.2%	42.8%	42.8%	Nursing services	39.6%	40.0%	42.8%
19.2	18.2	21.7	Other professional services	21.7	20.5	22.1
18.6	19.9	18.0	General	18.2	18.4	18.2
15.4	15.0	14.1	Fiscal and administrative	17.3	17.5	14.2
96.4%	95.9%	96.6%	Total operating expenses	96.8%	96.4%	97.3%
3.6%	4.1%	3.4%	Net operating income	3.2%	3.6%	2.7%
.2	.3	1.7	Add nonoperating revenues	.2	.3	.7
3.8%	4.4%	5.1%	Net income	3.4%	3.9%	3.4%

The last line of the statement presents the **net income ratio** (net income divided by total operating revenues). In April of 1987, for example, the net income ratio was 3.8 percent; Wellsville Hospital was able to generate only 3.8 cents of net income from each dollar of operating revenue. This was less than was budgeted (4.4%) and lower than was earned in April of the prior year (5.1%). While generalizations are dangerous, it can safely be said that many large American business firms would consider a net income ratio in the range of 6 to 8 percent as indicative of an adequate performance. Most business corporations, however, are more concerned with the ratio of net income to stockholders' equity and to total assets. These ratios are discussed further in Chapter 22.

Statistics and Units-of-Service Analysis

As discussed in Chapter 4, hospital service statistics have many important management uses. They are as essential to effective management and to the appraisal of operating results as are the dollar data in hospital financial statements. Consequently, a monthly statistical summary report should always be included in presentations of the results of operations. Wellsville Hospital's statistical summary report for April and the year to date is reproduced in part in Figure 9-15. Although not shown here, the budgeted statistics also may be included in the summary.

Figure 9-15.
Wellsville Hospital
Statistical Summary
Month of April and Year to Date

	April		Year to Date	
	1987	1986	1987	1986
General Statistics				
Adult and Pediatric:				
Admissions	589	577	2,376	2,298
Discharges and deaths	581	573	2,357	2,283
Patient days of care	3,937	3,891	15,781	15,573
Average daily census	131.2	129.7	131.5	129.8
Percentage of occupancy	87.5	86.5	87.7	86.5
Average length of stay	6.8	7.0	7.0	6.8
Newborn:				
Births	182	176	731	709
Discharges and deaths	179	174	726	701
Newborn days of care	698	704	2,787	2,818
Average daily census	23.3	23.5	23.2	23.5
Percentage of occupancy	83.1	83.8	82.9	83.9
Average length of stay	3.9	4.0	3.8	4.0
Total patient days of service	4,635	4,595	18,568	18,391
Outpatient visits	1,116	1,097	4,486	4,399
Average number of employees (full-time equivalent)	406	395	404	397
Departmental Statistics				
Operating room (hours)	561	557	2,246	2,238
Radiology (procedures)	2,143	1,987	8,578	7,981
Laboratory (examinations)	8,212	8,079	32,848	32,316
Dietary (meals served)	34,765	33,903	139,060	135,608
Etc.				

The statistics provided in summary reports are often combined with the financial data of the period to produce supplementary unit-of-service measurements, e.g., the dollar data in the income statement may be divided by patient days of service to obtain revenues or expenses per patient day. It should be recognized, however, that patient-day unit-of-service figures may be somewhat distorted because outpatient services are included in the operating revenue and expense figures. For this reason, some hospitals use a combined statistic consisting of a **weighted** total of adult, pediatric, and newborn days and outpatient visits. Another common practice is to report unit-of-service data in the detailed schedules of revenues and expenses where departmental statistical occasions of service are divided into revenue and direct cost dollars. Consider, for example, the following unit-of-service analysis applied to laboratory revenues and direct expenses:

	April	
	1987	1986
Average Revenue per Examination:		
1987 ($86,869/8,212)	$10.58	
1986 ($82,486/8,079)		$10.21
Average Direct Expense per Examination:		
1987 ($36,618/8,212)	4.46	
1986 ($32,765/8,079)		4.06
Average Operating Income per Examination	$ 6.12	$ 6.15

Similar analyses may be made for other revenue-producing departments of the hospital. In all cases, however, it must be emphasized that the expense figures in these computations are **direct** departmental expenses **before** indirect or overhead cost allocations are made as a result of a cost-finding procedure. Careful note should also be made of the fact that the unit-of-service figures are **averages**; they may be distorted by changes in "product mix" (see the following section).

Departmental Margin Analysis

A useful variation of the unit-of-service technique is the analysis of departmental margins, i.e., revenues minus direct expenses. To illustrate, examine the following data from Wellsville Hospital's report:

	April 1987			
			Over Budget	
	Actual	Budget	Amount	Percent
Laboratory:				
Revenues	$86,869	$82,500	$ 4,369	5.3%
Direct Expenses	36,618	34,900	1,718	4.9
Margin	$50,251	$47,600	$ 2,651	5.6
Number of Examinations	8,212	8,100	112	1.4

In attempting to interpret the budget variances, several important questions must be answered. How much of the $4,369 variance in revenues was due to (1) the difference in service volume and (2) differences, if any, in service rates? How much of the $1,718 variance in expenses was due to (1) the difference in volume and (2) a difference, if any, in operating efficiency? In short, what are the causes of the $2,651 difference between actual and budgeted margin?

The difference between the actual and budgeted margin is due to one or a combination of the following:

1. Differences between actual and budgeted service rates billed to patients for laboratory examinations.
2. Differences between the actual and budgeted volume of services, i.e., the total number of examinations.
3. Differences between the actual and budgeted "product (service) mix," i.e., the relative number of **each type** of examination.
4. Differences between the actual and budgeted elements of direct expenses.

In margin analysis, it is possible to compute the dollar amount of variation attributable to each of the above factors. The laboratory department, however, performs many kinds of examinations, each having a different service rate and cost. For this reason and because revenues may not be budgeted in detail by type of examination, computations of product mix variances usually are not feasible and will not be illustrated here. Instead, a "volume variance" will be computed which reflects the combined effects of the differences between the actual and budgeted volume of services and differences between the actual and budgeted product mix.

Margin analysis begins with the development of unit-of-service revenue and expense figures as follows:

| | Per Examination | |
	Actual	Budget
Revenues	$10.58	$10.19
Direct Expenses	4.46	4.31
Margin	$ 6.12	$ 5.88

With this information, the $2,651 difference between the actual and budgeted margin can be accounted for as shown in Figure 9-16.

As may be observed, the analysis indicates that the $4,369 excess of actual over budgeted revenues arose because of (1) the higher than budgeted volume of service and (2) the higher than budgeted average revenue per examination. The excess of actual expenses over budgeted expenses was due to (1) the higher than budgeted volume of service and (2) the higher than budgeted average cost per examination. Thus, the technique of margin analysis can be of considerable value to management in interpretations of budget variances.

Figure 9-16.
Wellsville Hospital
Laboratory Department
Margin Analysis

1. *Factors causing difference between actual and budgeted revenues:*

Actual revenues	$86,869		
Actual number of exams × budgeted revenue per exam (8,212 × $10.19)	83,680		
Favorable service rate variance		$ 3,189	
Actual number of exams × budgeted revenue per exam (above)	$83,680		
Budgeted revenues	82,500		
Favorable revenue volume variance		1,180	
Revenue budget variance			$ 4,369

2. *Factors causing difference between actual and budgeted expenses:*

Actual expenses	$36,618		
Actual number of exams × budgeted expense per exam (8,212 × $4.31)	35,393		
Unfavorable service cost variance		$ 1,225	
Actual number of exams × budgeted expense per exam (above)	$35,393		
Budgeted expenses	34,900		
Unfavorable cost volume variance		493	
Expense budget variance			1,718
Difference in departmental operating margin			$ 2,651

Cost-Volume-Profit Relationships

All persons in hospital management positions should acquire a thorough understanding of cost-volume-profit relationships, sometimes called **break-even analysis**. While a full discussion of this highly important topic is not provided here the basic principles involved will be outlined briefly because of their fundamental relevance to the management of hospital revenues and expenses.[3]

In hospitals, as in other economic enterprises, operating costs may be classified into four types according to their behavior (increase or decrease) in response to changes in volume of activity. These cost behavior patterns are illustrated graphically in Figure 9-17.

Type A costs, called **variable costs**, vary in total in proportion to changes in activity volume, e.g., raw food cost in the dietary department. Type B costs, called **fixed costs**, are relatively fixed in total, regardless of changes in volume of activity, e.g., salary of the chief dietitian. Certain other costs tend to change in total in the direction of changes in volume of activity, but such changes are not proportionate. For example, Type C costs, called **semifixed costs**, are fixed in total within given ranges of activity, e.g., 10 food service employees may be required within a 10,000 to 20,000 meals-served range, but 15 may be needed in the 20,000 to 30,000 range. Type D costs, called

Figure 9-17.
Cost Behavior Patterns

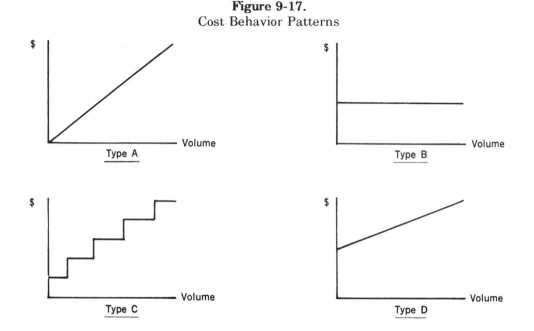

semivariable costs, are fixed amounts at zero output, but increase proportionately with increases in volume beyond the zero point, e.g., a food service contract calling for a fixed minimum payment plus a premium of a certain amount per meal served. Costs of Type C and Type D are difficult to deal with and, for purpose of discussion, it is assumed that all costs are either **purely** variable or **purely** fixed. Regression analysis and other mathematical techniques are available which permit the resolution of Type C and Type D costs into their fixed and variable components.

To illustrate the application of these cost concepts, assume some hospital department that sells a single product, or provides a single service, at a price of $10 per unit. The department's estimated costs are:

Variable, $4 per unit
Fixed, $6,000 per year

It is assumed that these costs are valid in an activity range of zero to 1,500 units of product, or service.

The cost-volume-profit relationships existing in this hypothetical department can be depicted graphically as shown in Figure 9-18. This is referred to as the **break-even chart.** It reflects what revenues, costs, and profit (loss) will be at any level of activity from zero to 1,500 units of product (service). The chart, of course, is based upon an assumption of linearity and has a number of important limitations. It also is true that such charts cannot be drawn with absolute precision in actual practice. Nevertheless, it is an extremely useful model, having many applications to management problems in hospitals.

Figure 9-18.
Break-Even Chart

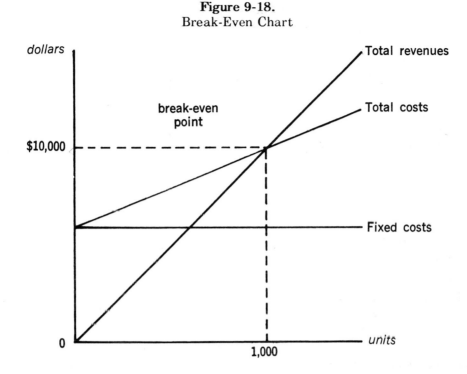

As may be seen from the graph, the department must "sell" 1,000 units of its product (service) per year in order to break even, i.e., to reach the point where total revenues equal total costs. If volume is greater than 1,000 units, profits will result in amounts that may be measured by the vertical distance between the total revenues and total costs lines. On the other hand, if volume is less than 1,000, a loss will be incurred, which is also measured by the vertical distance between the total revenues and total costs lines.

In addition to graphic presentation, break-even analysis may also be done algebraically. The formula is:

$$R = FC + VC + P$$

In this question, R is total revenue, FC is fixed cost, VC is variable cost, and P is profit. Because variable costs per unit are $4 and the unit sales price is $10, VC = .4R, i.e., variable costs are 40 percent of revenues. With this in mind, the break-even formula may be used to obtain approximate answers to a number of questions of major significance to management. For example:

1. How many units must be sold for the department to break even?

    $S = FC + VC + P$
    $S = \$6,000 + .4R + 0$
    $S = \$10,000$
       $\$10,000/\$10$ sales price = <u>1,000 units</u>

2. What profit will be earned if 1,200 units are sold?

    S = FC + VC + P
    P = S - FC - VC
    P = ($1,200 X $10) − $6,000 − .4(1,200 x $10)
    P = $1,200

3. If only 800 units can be sold, what must the unit sales price be in order for the department to break even?

    S = FC + VC + P
    S = $6,000 + ($4 x 800) + 0
    S = $9,200
        $9,200/800 units = $11.50 sales price

Many other applications of break-even analysis are possible. A major stumbling block in actual practice, of course, is the classification of costs into fixed and variable categories. Nevertheless, the break-even formula is indicative of a useful way of thinking about revenue and expense management problems.

CHAPTER 9 FOOTNOTES

1. B. Joplin and J. Pattillo, **Effective Accounting Reports** (Englewood Cliffs, New Jersey: Prentice-Hall, Inc., 1969), p. 55.

2. L. Vann Seawell, **External and Internal Reporting by Hospitals** (Oak Brook, Illinois: HFMA, 1984).

3. James D. Suver and Bruce R. Neumann, **Management Accounting for Health Care Organizations** (Oak Brook, Illinois: HFMA, 1981), Chapter 4.

QUESTIONS

1. You have just been engaged as controller of a 350-bed hospital. This hospital has never operated on a budget system. The administrator asks you to set up a budgetary system for the hospital with particular emphasis on the payroll aspect. What controls would you set up in the budget for payroll? Explain and give reasons for these controls. Your solution should include any controlling procedures relative to the employment of personnel which you would deem necessary to control payroll costs.

2. What, in your opinion, should be the objectives of hospital service pricing policy?

3. What is a **position control plan?** Of what value is such a plan in the budgeting of hospital payroll costs?

4. Distinguish between a **functional** and an **object of expenditure** classification of expenses. Which is preferable in budget reports?

5. State the break-even formula and define each of the components of the formula.

6. A knowledge of cost behavior patterns is important to a hospital financial manager. Identify four different types of hospital costs in terms of how they change in response to a change in volume of service.

7. What is common-size analysis and how is it used in the interpretation of financial statements?

8. The Board of Directors of Community Hospital has asked you to aid in a review of their rate structure. They have inquired as to whether the following items should be included in costs to be recovered from patients:

   1. Research programs
   2. Educational programs
   3. Charity care
   4. Inflation and technological change

   Prepare a memorandum to the Board explaining the principal arguments for and against the inclusion of the above items in the hospital's rates and your recommendation as to whether they should or should not be included.

9. Explain the difference between (1) average cost per patient day, (2) actual cost per patient day for services rendered to patients under specific contracts, and (3) marginal cost per patient day.

10. Given the following actual vs. budget report for Department X:

	Actual	Budget	Variance
Salaries and wages	$121,400	$115,000	$ (6,400)
Supplies	46,780	42,000	(4,780)

What additional information would you require before concluding that the above variance were "bad"? Explain how such information would affect your interpretation of the figures.

EXERCISES

E1.   City Hospital has estimated that pharmacy operations during the coming year will be as follows:

Cost of drugs	$68,000
Payroll, supplies, and overhead cost	22,000
Number of prescriptions to be filled:	
Compounded	2,000
Dispensed	9,000
Ratio of labor involved in compounding as opposed to dispensing	5:1
Estimated drugs which will not be billed to patients	12.5%

Required. Compute the pharmacy surcharge to be added to drug cost as (1) a percentage of drug cost and (2) a charge per prescription compounded or dispensed.

E2.   The administrator of Beldon Hospital is approached by a representative of a local charitable organization. The charitable organization wishes to know whether the hospital would be willing to accept approximately 20 patients per year, each requiring approximately 10 days hospitalization (minor, if any, surgery). The charitable organization would be willing to reimburse the hospital at the rate of $20 per patient day. The following data are available:

Beds 10%	200
Patient days ≠200 days	54,750 (excluding newborn)
Total income≠ 4000	$1,320,375
Total expenses	1,341,375
Outpatient income	20,000
Outpatient expenses	31,375
Outpatient visits	10,121

Required. The administrator asks you: "Assuming our other third-party contractors do not object, can we accept this contract for the coming year, considering economic factors only?"

E3.   A hospital department sells a single product at a price of $16 per unit. The department's estimated costs are:

Variable, $4 per unit
Fixed, $15,000 per year

It is unlikely that the department will sell more than 2,000 units per year.

Required. Construct a break-even chart, indicating the number of units which must be sold in order to break even.

E4.   Refer to the data provided in Exercise 3.

Required. Using the algebraic break-even formula, answer the following questions:

1.   What profit will be earned if:
     a. 1,500 units are sold?
     b. 1,000 units are sold?

2.   If only 1,000 units are sold, what must the unit sales price be in order for the department to break even?

3.   If 1,500 units are sold, what will the profit be if:
     a. The sales price is $20?
     b. The sales price is $12?

     $1500 \times 20 = 30,000$ (30,000)

     $15,000 \times 12 - 18,000$ (2,000) loss $= 18,000$

4.   Assuming that 1,500 units will be sold at $16 per unit, what would be the effect on profit if:
     a. Variable costs increased by 60 percent?
     b. Fixed costs increased by $15,000?

E5.   Given the following information concerning diagnostic radiology for the month of March:

	Actual	Budget	Variance Amount	Percent
Revenues	$166,750	$150,000	$ 16,750	11.2%
Direct expenses	146,625	120,000	26,625	22.2
Margin	$ 20,125	$ 30,000	$ (9,875)	32.9
Number of examinations	11,500	10,000	1,500	15.0

Required. Prepare an analysis indicating the factors causing the difference between budgeted and actual margin.

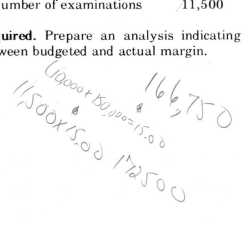

E6.   Lakeside Hospital provides you with the following information concerning its
       operating results for the year ended December 31, 1987:

	Actual	Budget
Nursing service expense	$218,572	$210,000
Gross patient service revenue – outpatient	71,345	74,000
General service expense	90,463	88,000
Revenue deductions	44,168	42,000
Non operating revenue	2,046	1,600
Other professional service expense	100,689	99,000
Gross patient service revenue – inpatient	479,362	475,400
Fiscal and administrative service expense	87,546	84,000
Other operating revenue	18,573	17,000

   The hospital's unrestricted fund had total assets of $600,000 at December 31,
   1987.

   Required. 1.   Prepare a summary income statement for 1987, showing:
                       a. Actual vs. budget
                       b. Amount and percent over or under budget
                       c. Common-size data

                 2.   Compute the net income ratio, the operating ratio, and the return
                      on total assets.

                                   PROBLEMS

P1.   Various information relating to the Laboratory Department of Community
       Hospital is provided below:

       1.   Community Hospital establishes charges for services at an amount that will
            approximate costs as nearly as possible. Total budgeted income for a
            department should be within a range of $1,000 of total budgeted expenses.
            A relative unit system is used in the Laboratory Department. During the
            fiscal year ended June 30, 1987, the average charge per unit was $1.02.

       2.   Contractual adjustments and other revenue deductions should be assumed to
            be 10 percent of gross revenues.

       3.   In preparing the budget, assume that the Laboratory Department will
            continue to grow at the same rate, as far as the number of relative units
            of service is concerned, as it has in the past two years.

       4.   The two pathologists are guaranteed a base salary of $20,000 each, plus a
            pool of 10 percent of net revenue (gross charges less deductions) which is
            divided equally.

5. The budget committee of the hospital has instructed you to allow for a 5 percent salary increase to all eligible personnel except the pathologists. These increases are to become effective for each employee on the first of the month following the anniversary of each employee's employment data.

6. Because of an increased workload, the budget committee has approved the addition of one new technologist to begin at the approved starting rate.

7. Overtime, vacation and holiday relief and on-call pay should be computed at 15 percent of the technologists' and aides' salary.

8. The indirect cost ratio for the Laboratory Department is 25 percent of direct expenses.

9. The nonsalary direct expenses for the Laboratory Department in the year ended June 30, 1987, amount to $50,000. It is expected that the 1987-88 nonsalary direct expenses will continue at approximately 25 cents per unit.

	Year Ended June 30		
	1985	1986	1987
Units of service	165,300	181,820	200,000
Gross charges	$175,218	$189,093	$204,000
Deductions	17,500	18,900	170,193
Net charges	157,718	20,300	183,700

Selected wage range for year ending 6/30/88:

Job Code	Title	Range in Dollars Per Month
23	Secretary	$325-$450
44	Laboratory Technologists	375- 525
67	Aides	300- 400

Analysis of personnel, 7/1/87:

Authorized Position

Job Code	Name	Current Annual Rate	Monthly Rate	Employment Date
01	J. Brown, Pathologist	$20,000		7/1/79
01	T. Smith, Pathologist	20,000		9/1/78
23	J. Rocket	4,800	$400	1/15/83
44	A. Dick	6,120	510	8/5/76
44	B. Searle	6,000	500	7/9/75
44	C. Noonan	5,520	460	9/14/80
44	O. White	4,680	390	12/13/83
67	N. Dupree	4,560	380	6/12/79
67	L. Jones	4,080	340	7/13/83

Required. Prepare an annual income and expense budget for the Laboratory Department of Community Hospital for the year ending June 30, 1988. Indicate what you would do if, at the end of six months, the actual increase in the number of units of service for the department is only 50 percent of that anticipated in preparing the budget.

P2. Following is information relating to the Radiology Department of Bingham Hospital relating to the preparation of a budget of revenue and expense for the year ending December 31, 1987.

1. A relative unit value system has been adopted to account for the activities of the Radiology Department. Below is a schedule of these relative unit values:

	1985 Actual	1986 Actual	1987 Budget
January	10,500	11,000	11,500
February	10,000	10,500	11,000
March	12,500	12,500	13,500
April	11,500	12,000	13,000
May	13,500	14,500	15,000
June	14,500	14,500	15,500
July	10,500	11,000	12,000
August	13,000	13,500	14,000
September	15,500	16,000	16,500
October	14,500	15,500	16,500
November	12,500	14,000	14,500
December	10,000	11,000	11,500
	148,500	156,000	164,500

2. A review of management's overall plans does not indicate any changes which will affect the Radiology Department in the coming year.

3. The average revenue per relative unit value for the budget year is estimated to be 85 cents.

4. Past experience indicates that a 2 percent of gross revenue combined bad debt and allowance rate will prevail during 1987.

5. Salary increase in accordance with approved personnel policies are indicated below:

Position	Name	Present Salary	Date of Increase	Monthly Increase
Supervisor	Nolan	$ 7,680	2/1/87	$ 40
Sr. Technician	Phillips	7,020	7/1/87	30
Sr. Technician	Baker	5,820	7/1/87	30
Jr. Technician	Witt	4,320	3/1/87	20
Jr. Technician	Mann	4,440	10/1/87	20
Jr. Technician	Orville	4,080	1/1/87	10
Student Technician	James	3,840	7/1/87	10
Student Technician	Williams	3,780	1/1/87	10

6. An allowance of 5 percent of each monthly budgeted salary should be provided for on-call and overtime pay.

7. Supplies and expenses for the budget year have been determined to be 15 cents per relative unit value.

8. Radiologists' fees are determined at 40 percent of net income. Indirect expenses have been determined to be 8 percent of direct expenses excluding the radiologist's fee.

Required. Prepare a revenue and expense budget for the Radiology Department in annual form, but entering only the dollar detail for the first three months of 1987. Show all computations; round all figures to the nearest dollar.

P3.   The Board of Trustees of Memorial Hospital has adopted the following policy as recorded in the minutes:

> The primary fiscal obligation of Memorial Hospital is to operate on a sound and conservative basis thus assuring uninterrupted and undiminished service to the community. Toward fulfilling this obligation, it is the policy of this Board that rates charged for services rendered to patients shall be based on current costs plus 5 percent of current cost at an occupancy level 4 percent below that of the preceding year but not to exceed 80 percent.

Income and expense figures in summary forms and related statistics for the years ended June 30, 1986 and 1987 and for the nine months ended March 31, 1988, are as follows:

	Nine Months 1988	Year Ended June 30 1987	1986
Gross revenue from services to patients	$3,104,542	$3,795,500	$3,396,600
Allowances	22,400	32,100	26,800
Bad debts	13,600	18,000	16,500
Deductions from revenue	36,000	50,100	43,300
Net revenue from services to patients	3,068,542	3,745,400	3,353,300
Operating expenses (80% fixed)	2,940,942	3,566,500	3,219,300
Net operating revenue	127,600	178,900	134,000
Other revenue	15,400	14,100	16,000
Net income	$ 143,000	$ 193,000	$ 150,000
Normal bed capacity	300	300	300
Patient days	70,950	95,265	91,980

Required. (1) Outline the steps that you would follow in computing the gross revenue per patient day that would be required in order to carry out the Board's policy. (2) Compute the required amount (gross revenue per patient day) for fiscal year ending June 30, 1989, following the steps outlined.

P4.   In connection with your work on an income and expense budget for the Department of Radiology for Community Hospital for the year ending June 30, 1987, you are supplied with the following information:

1. The hospital establishes gross charges for services at an amount that will approximate costs as nearly as possible. Total budgeted income for a department should be within a range of $1,000 of total budgeted expenses. A relative unit system for its Department of Radiology is used. During the fiscal year ended June 30, 1986, the average charge per unit was $1.

Year Ended	Units of Service	Gross Charges	Deductions	Net Charges
6/30/84	247,933	$210,743	$ 21,074	$189,669
6/30/85	272,727	259,090	25,909	233,181
6/30/86	300,000	300,000	27,000	273,000

2. Deductions from gross income, such as free care, contractual allowances, and provision for uncollectible accounts, should be assumed to be 10 percent of gross income.

3. In preparing the budget, assume that the Radiology Department will continue to grow at the same rate, as far as the number of relative units of service is concerned, as it has in the past two years.

4. The radiologists are guaranteed a base salary of $10,000 each plus a pool of 20 percent of the net revenue (gross charges less deduction) which is divided equally among the four radiologists.

5. The budget committee of the hospital has instructed you to allow for a 5 percent salary increase to all eligible personnel except the radiologists. These increases are to become effective for each employee on the first of the month following the anniversary of each employee's employment date.

6. Because of an increased workload, the budget committee has approved the addition of two new technicians to begin at the approved starting rate.

   Schedule of selected wage ranges:

Job Code	Title	Range in Dollars Per Month
23	Secretary	$325-$450
44	Radiology Technician	375- 525
67	Aides	300- 400

7. Premium pay, vacation, holiday relief and on-call pay should be computed at 15 percent of the technicians' salary.

8. The indirect cost ratio for the hospital is 25 percent of direct expenses.

9. The nonsalary direct expenses for the Department of Radiology for the fiscal year ended June 30, 1986, amounted to $75,000. It is expected that the 1986-87 nonsalary direct expenses will continue at approximately 25 cents per unit.

Analysis of personnel, 7/1/86:

Authorized Position

Job Code	Name	Current Annual Rate	Monthly Rate	Employment Date
01	J. Brown, Radiologist	$10,000		7/1/80
01	T. Smith, Radiologist	10,000		9/1/79
01	J. Green, Radiologist	10,000		10/1/76
01	P. Russe, Radiologist	10,000		10/1/75
23	J. Rocker	4,800	$400	1/15/84
23	M. Plane	4,080	340	4/11/85
23	R. Sansome	5,100	425	9/6/80
44	A. Dick	6,120	510	8/5/77
44	B. Searle	6,000	500	7/9/76
44	C. Noonan	5,520	460	9/14/81
44	M. Brown	4,800	400	8/12/82
44	N. Frank	4,800	400	7/10/82
44	O. White	4,680	390	12/13/84
44	V. Flite	4,680	390	10/16/83
44	T. Goode	4,800	400	3/15/82
67	N. Dupre	4,560	380	6/12/80
67	Z. Baker	4,560	380	6/18/81
67	L. Jones	4,080	340	7/13/84

Required. Prepare an income and expense budget for the year ending June 30, 1987. Indicate what you would do, if at the end of six months, the anticipated increase in the number of units of service for the department is only 50 percent of that used in preparing the budget.

P5.   Manufax Hospital has prepared the following budget for 1988 for one of its major departments:

Variable cost per unit of service, $25.
Fixed costs for the year, $30,000.
Price per unit of service, $100.
Normal activity level per year, 1,000 units of service.

Required. Answer each of the following questions:

1. What net income (or net loss) will result if:

    a. 1,000 units of service are billed during 1988?
    b. 800 units of service are billed during 1988?
    c. 200 units of service are billed during 1988?

2. How many units of service must be billed during 1988 to earn a net income of: *FC + Income ÷ S-V = units*

    a. $7,500?
    b. 15% of gross revenue?
    c. $15 per unit of service?

3. At what price per unit must the service be billed for the department to earn a net income of $70,000, assuming 1,000 units of service are billed during the year?

4. Assume that the service is billed at $62.50 per unit.

    a. How many units of service must be billed to break even?
    b. How much profit will be made if 900 units of service are billed during the year?

5. If the service is billed at $125 per unit, how many units of service must be billed to earn a profit of $12.50 per unit?

6. Assume that the department expects to bill only 900 units of service at $100 per unit. A third-party payer wishes to enter into a contract for 100 units of service at a discount price. What unit price should the hospital charge for this special contract in order to increase total profits by $5,000?

PART 3

Current Resources and Obligations

10
Cash and Temporary Investments

There is perhaps a natural tendency on the part of some managers to equate the accumulation of large cash balances with good cash management when, in fact, it is the exact opposite of effective cash management. The modern concept of the proper objective and result of cash management has been dramatized as follows:[1]

"Frisby, what's our cash position?"

"Well . . . er . . . uh . . . you see, boss . . . well, right now we haven't got any cash."

"Wonderful, Frisby! You're the best treasurer this company ever had."

It was with this imagined dialogue that a **Wall Street Journal** writer began an article describing the increased sophistication with which business firms are managing their cash resources. Hospitals, like their commercial cousins, also must recognize that the accumulation of excessive cash balances is unproductive and that appropriate accounting and administrative controls must be exercised to minimize the amount of idle cash holdings. There are, of course, other objectives in accounting for and managing hospital cash receipts, disbursements, and balances. The purpose of this chapter is to examine these objectives and to describe methods and procedures by which they may be achieved.

IMPORTANCE OF CASH

The importance of cash stems largely from its high activity characteristic, its susceptibility to misappropriation, and its rather obvious value as the means of financing hospital activities. The cash transaction occurs frequently; nearly every rendered service eventually leads to a cash receipt and most expenses sooner or later require a cash disbursement. The daily activities of the hospital produce a more or less continuous flow of cash. This inward and outward movement of cash completes substantially all of the transactions entered into by hospitals. Cash is both the beginning and the end of the operating cycle:

Cash → Inventory and Payroll → Revenue and Receivables → Cash

As cash is the most active asset, the accountant gives special attention to the development of procedures for processing the great mass of transactions in an efficient and accurate manner. In a sense, cash is the other side of the coin of liabilities, revenues, expenses, and noncash assets. If the flow of cash is controlled, a degree of control is obtained over the offsetting account or accounts in the double-entry system.

Cash is also the asset most susceptible to fraudulent misappropriation by employees and others. Because is has small bulk, it is easily transported and concealed. It lacks owner identification so that its ownership is established mainly by possession, and it can be exchanged readily for other kinds of assets. Irregularities in cash are very difficult to detect because of the high activity characteristic of cash. Considerable effort must be given to the design and maintenance of a system of internal control to safeguard the movement of cash from the time it is received until it is expended so as to protect the hospital's cash resources from honest error and dishonest employees.

Cash, of course, is a necessity in the operation of any enterprise. In the hospital, an adequate cash balance is essential to high standards of patient care in that a sufficient amount of cash must be available at the time needed to meet financial obligations to employees and creditors. The hospital's credit standing depends, to a large extent, upon the promptness with which its debts are paid. A supplier naturally will look unfavorably upon a history of untimely payments and may react with higher prices, credit limits, and removal of discount terms. An inability to take advantage of discount opportunities can result in significantly higher costs for supplies and purchased services.

Yet, when held idle in excessive amounts, cash is unproductive, earning nothing of benefit to the hospital. The earning power of cash, in fact, is negative; it actually earns less than nothing. Consider, for example, the maintenance of a minimum cash balance of, say, $100,000 during a year when the general purchasing power of money declines 4 percent due to price inflation. The $4,000 ($100,000X 4%) price-level loss is quite real although not directly measured and reported in the hospital's financial statements. Thus, since cash as the medium of exchange and the measure of value is subject to inflationary depreciation, the balance of cash that is maintained should be regulated so that neither too little nor too much is held. Effective cash management requires that all available cash be continuously at work as part of the operating cycle or as a temporary investment.

In addition, cash presents formidable problems for the hospital accountant from the standpoint of basic bookkeeping procedure alone. Every day, almost every few minutes, cash is moving into and out of the hospital bank accounts. Apart from other considerations, the accounting routine itself must be carefully devised and executed to provide assurance that each cash receipt and disbursement is recorded promptly and accurately. A proper work procedure and effectively designed accounting records are required for the efficient processing of the enormous mass of cash transactions into a controlled flow of reliable information. It is upon such information that cash management decisions rest.

COMPOSITION OF CASH

What is **cash**? Cash may be defined as consisting of actual money and other immediately available resources or credit instruments generally accepted as a medium of exchange and used as money equivalents. The definition includes coin and paper currency, demand deposits in banks, checks, money orders, and other nonmonetary forms of cash which are readily accepted in exchange for goods or services and in settlement of obligations. The very essence of cash is its availability as a medium of exchange, i.e., as purchasing power.

Postage stamps are supplies, not cash. Postdated checks should be considered as receivables until the time they can be presented to a bank for payment. IOUs from hospital employees also are properly treated as receivables, and not as cash. Patients' notes given to a bank for collection should not be considered as cash until they are collected. Expense advances to employees, funds in closed banks, and dishonored checks also should be excluded from the cash classification. Time deposits and temporary investments in bank savings accounts or treasury bills should be carried in the accounts as investments rather than as cash. Cash that has been designated by the governing board for plant replacement and expansion or, for retirement of long-term debt, should be labeled clearly and reported separately in a noncurrent asset section of the balance sheet. It is extremely important, of course, that donor-restricted cash balances be segregated from unrestricted cash balances.

CASH ACCOUNTS

Even the smallest hospital will find it desirable to maintain two or more different cash accounts. Consider, for example, the following listing representative of the types of unrestricted fund cash accounts generally employed by hospitals:

110.00 Cash in Banks

      110.10 General Checking Account
      110.20 Payroll Checking Account
      110.30 Payroll Tax Checking Account
      110.40 Patient Refunds Checking Account

110.50 Imprest Cash Funds

      110.51 Petty Cash Fund A
      110.52 Petty Cash Fund B
      110.55 Change Fund No. 1
      110.56 Change Fund No. 2
      110.59 Check Cashing Fund

Where circumstances make it feasible, checking accounts may be located with different banks to maintain broader financial contacts and to avoid the confusion that might arise in having all accounts at the same bank. This also applies to checking accounts kept for the cash resources of the restricted funds.

Note that separate checking accounts are provided for each specific major type of disbursement. In addition to a general checking account into which all receipts are deposited, it is desirable to set up one or more payroll checking accounts. An amount equal to the periodic net payroll is transferred into the payroll account by the deposit of a single check drawn on the general account. Payroll checks totaling this same amount then are drawn on the payroll checking account. This not only facilitates the reconciliation of checking accounts, but it also provides a measure of control over the amount that can be disbursed from the payroll account. The basic idea is that, if the total amount entering an account is controlled, the total amount leaving the account can be more easily controlled. A similar procedure can be employed with respect to payroll taxes, patient refunds, and other disbursements.

Bank Reconciliations

The bank reconciliation should be regarded as one of the more important internal cash control procedures. It will aid in the prevention and detection of fraud, the discovery of errors in the accounting records, and the determination of the accuracy of the bank statement. Bank statements, of course, should be delivered unopened to the person who is to perform the reconciliation, and should remain in his or her possession until the reconciliation is completed. Reconciliations should be supervised by the controller or his delegate, and should be performed by someone who does not handle cash or cash records. Irregularities always should be reported directly to the controller or internal auditor.

Practice varies somewhat, but the reconciliation process should include, at least on a sample basis, most of the following procedures if the greatest value is to be obtained from the reconciliation:

1. Arrange checks returned by the bank in numerical sequence and compare them with the list of checks outstanding from the prior month's reconciliation and with cash disbursement journal entries of the current month.
2. Prepare a list of checks outstanding by date, payee, check number, and amount. Investigate all checks that remain outstanding from the prior month's reconciliation and determine if payment should be stopped on such checks.
3. Examine endorsements on canceled checks for irregularities.
4. Compare deposits as shown on the bank statement with entries in the cash receipts journal. If a deposit was listed as in transit on the prior month's reconciliation, ascertain that it appears on the current month's bank statement.
5. Prepare a list of deposits in transit at the end of the current month by date and amount.
6. Ascertain that adjustments required by the reconciliation of the prior month were correctly entered in the accounting records.

When the reconciliation is completed, it should be reviewed and approved by the controller who will authorize the necessary adjusting entries to correct errors, record bank service charges, book bad checks, and otherwise bring the book and bank balances of cash into agreement.

A bank reconciliation is primarily a matter of adjusting two incorrect cash balances to a correct amount representing the actual amount of cash over which the hospital has control, i.e., the balance sheet figure for cash. Ordinarily, the book balance will be incorrect for two reasons: (1) items may have been subtracted from the bank balance but not from the book balance, e.g., bank service charges and bad checks, and (2) items may have been added to the bank balance but not to the book balance, e.g., collection of patients' notes by the bank. On the other hand, the bank balance normally will be incorrect because (1) items may have been added to the book balance but not to the bank balance, e.g., deposits in transit, and (2) items may have been subtracted from the book balance but not from the bank balance, e.g., outstanding checks.

Sometimes bank reconciliations are accomplished by adjusting the bank balance to agree with the book balance or by adjusting the book balance to agree with the bank balance. While either of these methods will produce a satisfactory reconciliation, many accountants prefer the method illustrated in Figure 10-1 where each of the two incorrect balances is adjusted to a correct balance. A preference is given to this procedure because it produces the proper balance sheet figure for cash and because it organizes all the necessary adjustments in one place, i.e., in the "books" columns. Neither of the other two methods of reconciliation necessarily provides these two advantages.

Figure 10-1.
Hoosier Hospital
Bank Reconciliation—General Checking Account
March 31, 1987

	Books Dr.	Books Cr.	Bank Dr.	Bank Cr.
Balances, 3/31	$ 9,478			$17,093

Deposits in transit, 3/31:

Date	Amount				
3/30	$1,427				
3/31	1,681				
Total	$3,108				3,108

Checks outstanding, 3/31:

Date	Ck.#	Amount				
2/14	236	$ 124				
3/27	342	57				
3/29	348	285				
3/30	354	863				
3/31	355	112				
3/31	356	75				
Total		$1,516			$1,516	

	Books Dr.	Books Cr.	Bank Dr.	Bank Cr.
Bank service charges		$ 12		
NSF check returned with March bank statement		106		
Proceeds from sale of U.S. Treasury bonds by bank	10,200			
Book error in recording check #327, correctly drawn for $306, as $603	297			
Bank error in failing to credit for March 24 deposit for $1,172				1,172
Totals	19,975	118	1,516	21,373
Offsets	118			1,516
Correct balances, 3/31	$19,857			$19,857

   To illustrate the preparation of a bank reconciliation, the following information concerning a general checking account maintained by Hoosier Hospital during March is assumed (cents are omitted for ease of exposition):

1. The March 31 ledger balance of the general checking account is $9,478.
2. The March 31 balance of the general checking account on the March bank statement is $17,093.
3. The deposits in transit at March 31 total $3,108.
4. The checks outstanding at March 31 total $1,516.
5. Bank service charges for March are $12.
6. Hoosier Hospital owned $10,000, face value, of U.S. Treasury bonds as a short-term investment. The bank sold these bonds for Hoosier Hospital on March 28, crediting the proceeds of $10,200 to Hoosier Hospital on that date.
7. A Hoosier Hospital accountant journalized check #327 as $603 in error; the check was corrected drawn for $306. The error had the effect of understating the ledger balance of cash by $297 ($603 - $306).
8. The bank made an error by failing to credit Hoosier Hospital for its $1,172 bank deposit of March 24.

The deposits in transit at March 31 consist of late-March deposits that did not reach the bank in time to appear as deposits on the bank statement for March. The checks outstanding at March 31 consist of checks written and recorded by Hoosier Hospital that have not yet cleared the banking system. Both deposits in transit and checks outstanding are determined by comparing Hoosier Hospital's cash records with the information on the March bank statement.

   Hoosier Hospital's accounting records indicate a March 31 cash balance of $9,478; the March 31 cash balance according to the bank is $17,093. Neither of these balances, however, is the correct amount of cash to be reported in Hoosier Hospital's March 31 balance sheet. The balances shown by the accounting records and by the bank statement are incorrect for several reasons:

1. Certain cash items, such as deposits in transit, have been properly added to the book, but not to the bank, balance of cash.
2. Certain cash items, such as outstanding checks, have been properly deducted from the book, but not from the bank, balance of cash.
3. Certain cash items, such as bank service charges and NSF (not sufficient funds) checks, have been properly deducted from the bank, but not from the book, balance of cash.
4. Certain cash items, such as the proceeds from the sale of the investment in U.S. Treasury bonds, have been properly added to the bank, but not to the book, balance of cash.
5. Errors have been made in the accounting records of Hoosier Hospital and in the accounting records of the bank.

Observe the treatment of these reconciling items in the bank reconciliation presented in Figure 10-1. Deposits in transit are added to, and outstanding checks are deducted from, the bank balance of cash. Bank service charges and the NSF check are deducted from, and the proceeds from the sale of the investment in U.S. Treasury bonds are added to, the book balance of cash. Adjustments for errors vary, depending on the nature of the errors.

Based on the bank reconciliation, the following adjusting entry is required at March 31 on the books of Hoosier Hospital:

Cash In Bank	$ 10,379	
Banking Expense	12	
Accounts Receivable	106	
Temporary Investments		$ 10,000
Investment Income		200
Accounts Payable		297
Adjustments of accounts per March 31		
bank reconciliation.		

The debit to Cash In Bank adjusts the ledger balance of cash to the correct balance at March 31 ($19,857 - $9,478 = $10,379). Bank service charges for March are debited to expense. The NSF check represents a patient's personal check that was deposited by Hoosier Hospital, but return uncollected by the bank. It is recorded as an account receivable. Assuming that the investment in U.S. Treasury bonds cost $10,000, the adjusting entry credits the Temporary Investments account for $10,000, and records the balance of the sales proceeds as Investment Income. The credit to Accounts Payable corrects the understatement arising in this account from the error made in journalizing check #327.

As noted earlier, the use of special checking accounts for different types of disbursements facilitates the bank reconciliation process. The reconciliation just illustrated, for example, would be rather cumbersome if all hospital checks were drawn against that one account. By establishing a payroll checking account, the large volume of payroll checks can be removed from the general checking account reconciliation. The payroll checking account ordinarily will require minimal work for reconciliation; it tends to reconcile itself, i.e., balance to zero. This is true because the deposit of the net payroll amount in the account is exactly offset by the total of the individual payroll checks clearing the account. Should employees not cash their payroll checks promptly, the checks may be printed to read "void if not presented for payment within 30 days." Of course, checks will be placed in numerical order, endorsements examined, deposits in transit and checks outstanding identified, and a reconciliation prepared.

The bank reconciliation can be expanded to include a reconciliation of cash receipts and cash disbursements, or a **proof of cash** as it is sometimes called. This procedure, illustrated in Figure 10-2, consists of a more thorough analysis of the bank statement in comparison with the cash receipts and disbursements as shown by the accounting records. It aids in the location of errors and is used by independent auditors as a standard procedure to detect discrepancies in the handling of cash. There is no reason why it should not also be equally useful to the hospital internal auditor.

Figure 10-2.
Hoosier Hospital
Reconciliation of Cash Receipts and Disbursements
General Checking Account
Month Ended March 31, 1987

	Balance 2/28	Receipts	Disbursements	Balance 3/31
Per March bank statement	$10,397	$98,195	$91,499	$17,093
Deposits in transit:				
2/28	2,934	(2,934)		
3/31		3,108		3,108
Check outstanding:				
2/28	(2,109)		(2,109)	
3/31			1,516	1,516
Bank error – failure to credit for March 24 deposit for $1,172		1,172		1,172
NSF check returned with March bank statement		(106)	(106)	
Correct balances	$11,222	$99,435	$90,800	$19,857
Per books	$11,222	$89,341	$91,085	$9,478
Bank service charges for March			12	(12)
NSF check returned with March bank statement		(106)		(106)
Proceeds from sale of U.S. Treasury bonds by bank		10,200		10,200
Book error in recording check #327, correctly drawn for #306, as $603			(297)	297
Correct balances	$11,222	$99,435	$90,800	$19,857

Imprest Cash Funds

No hospital should keep cash on hand unnecessarily. All cash receipts should be deposited promptly and intact, i.e., disbursements should never be made directly from cash receipts. Disbursements, as a general rule, should be made only by checks, properly authorized and executed. Violations of these basic control principles are open invitations to confusion, error, and fraud.

As a practical matter, however, provision usually must be made for the maintenance of cash funds in limited amounts from which cash disbursements can be made for items for which the writing of checks is not feasible. Hospitals, for example, typically maintain several so-called petty cash funds, change funds, and check cashing funds. The need for such funds should be evaluated regularly so that their number and amount will be neither excessive nor inadequate. All such funds should be accounted for on an imprest basis, i.e., each fund should be established in a fixed amount to which it is replenished periodically when exhausted. Responsibility for each imprest fund should be assigned to a specific employee who, as the fund custodian, has sole control over it.

Petty Cash Funds. When a petty cash fund is initially established, a check for the imprest amount of the fund is drawn payable to the fund custodian who cashes the check and places the money for safekeeping in a locked petty cash drawer or box. An entry should be made as follows:

Petty Cash Fund	$ 500	
Cash in Bank		$ 500
To record establishment of a		
petty cash fund.		

Disbursements from the fund are made only by the fund custodian and only in return for signed receipts, petty cash slips or vouchers, and other supporting documents. When the fund is nearly exhausted, a reimbursement check is drawn to replenish the fund to its imprest amount. The entry might be:

Sundry Expense Accounts	$ 482	
Cash Over and Short	2	
Cash in Bank		$ 484
To record reimbursement of the		
petty cash fund.		

It is assumed here that the fund contained $16 in coin and currency, thus requiring a $484 reimbursement, but that documentation for only $482 of expenditures was available. The $2 shortage, charged to a special cash over and short account, is perhaps due to a failure to obtain and retain documentation or to simple errors in making change from the fund. Continual and sizable shortages may indicate the need to appoint a different custodian.

Reimbursements of petty cash funds are made at the end of each accounting period and whenever the fund is depleted. Infrequent reimbursements may indicate that the funds have been established in excessive amounts; the opposite may be true if reimbursements are required so often as to become bothersome. Through an appraisal of reimbursement experience, the optimum size of these funds can be ascertained. This is important because excessive petty cash funds represent a nonproductive use of cash and also increase the danger of fraud.

It should be noted that nowhere in the reimbursement process is the petty cash account debited or credited. This is done only when the fund is originally established, or its imprest amount is increased or decreased. Suppose, for example, that the imprest amount of the above fund ($500) is increased to $750. A check is drawn for $250 and debited to the petty cash account. On the other hand, if the fund is to be decreased from $500 to, say, $400, one would remove $100 from petty cash and deposit it to the general checking account. An entry would be made to debit $100 to Cash in Bank and credit the petty cash account.

Change Funds. Change funds are established in nominal amounts at cash receiving locations **only** for the purpose of providing change to patients, employees, and hospital visitors. These funds should be balanced daily to the total of recorded cash receipts at each location plus the imprest amount of the change fund. In depositing cash receipts, over and short variances are considered to be in the day's receipts and not in the change fund which is retained in its imprest amount. Such variances, of course, are recorded in the cash over and short account which should be monitored as a means of checking the effectiveness of the cash receiving function.

Check Cashing Funds. While hospital policy should be that of not cashing any checks, personal or payroll, for anyone, check cashing funds often are established as a convenience to employees who wish to cash their paychecks at the hospital. This practice is not particularly desirable, but it is difficult to discontinue once it has been started. Where check cashing funds are used, the custodian should be independent of any of the payroll functions.

INTERNAL CASH CONTROLS

For the several reasons stated in Chapter 5 and earlier in this chapter, internal cash controls are essential in the hospital's business offices and at all other locations where cash is received or disbursed. Effective safeguards must be built into the accounting system if hospital cash resources are to be accurately recorded and adequately protected from error and misappropriation. The following discussion expands the introductory considerations presented in Chapter 5.

General Principles

Some of the general principles typically incorporated into internal control systems with respect to cash are:

1. All hospital employees who handle or have access to cash should be adequately bonded.
2. Petty cash and change funds should be limited in number and should be established in minimum imprest amounts.
3. Bank accounts should be reconciled regularly by persons other than those who handle cash receipts, sign checks, or maintain cash records.
4. There must be a distinct segregation of duties between cash handling and cash accounting, e.g., persons who handle incoming cash should not have control of the accounts receivable records.
5. All cash record forms, such as checks, bank deposit tickets, cash receipt slips, and petty cash vouchers, should be prenumbered and accounted for by numerical sequence.
6. Definite responsibility for cash handling functions and for custody of cash funds should be assigned.
7. A minimum number of employees should be given access to cash.
8. Internal audits and surprise cash counts should be made by a responsible employee at irregular intervals.
9. Vacations should be mandatory and business office positions should be rotated among employees.
10. The work of the business office personnel should be made complementary so that an error by one automatically will be discovered by another.
11. Physical protection should be provided through the use of vaults, bank facilities, cashier's cages, locked cash drawers, and similar devices.

12. Definite procedures should be established in writing for the handling of all routine cash transactions; decisions as to the handling of nonroutine cash transactions should be made by the controller or chief accountant.
13. Office procedures should be so arranged that misappropriations are unlikely to go undetected without the collusion of two or more employees.
14. The system of internal cash control should be reviewed periodically for adequacy and effectiveness by the internal auditor.

While the listing is not exhaustive, it does indicate the major principles to be considered in developing and maintaining adequate internal cash controls.

An evaluation of internal control processes and the verification of cash by surprise counts and other means is a primary task of the external auditor. The time spent by the auditor in an examination of the cash accounts is directly related to the effectiveness and completeness of the internal control program employed by the hospital client. Substantial savings in audit fees can be realized by the hospital that follows sound internal control procedures. Obviously, the less the chance for error or theft, the less time will be required by the outside auditor in detail checking and investigation of the accounting records. In addition, many audit procedures often performed by the auditors can be done just as well, and less expensively, by hospital employees. It is not necessary to pay a professional auditor $50 an hour to prepare a bank reconciliation, for example, when it can be performed at a fraction of that cost by a hospital employee. The auditors, of course, will wish to review such work, but this review will consume considerably less of their time. The audit and reconciliation of petty cash funds is another example of an area in which much preliminary work can be done by hospital employees. Schedules can be prepared and adding machine tapes of subsidiary records can be kept ready for the auditors when they start the audit. The auditors, in fact, should supply on request a listing of schedules and tapes that can be prepared to reduce audit time.

Besides the savings in audit fees, observance of sound internal controls promotes efficiency in the business office. Daily and monthly reports are more timely and accurate in that errors and out-of-balance situations are minimized. Even more important is the fact that employee theft and error prevention is clearly more desirable than any measure of detection. Thus, the primary objectives of internal control systems should always relate to prevention and determent. Governing boards, administrators, and controllers who close their eyes to a faulty system of internal control cannot avoid blame for an embezzlement by an employee who could not resist the temptation placed before him. No system is foolproof, but even the simplest of systems can be discouraging to the potential thief. The hospital management has an obligation to employees, as well as to the community, to install and maintain the best available methods of internal cash controls consistent with the circumstances.

It has been said that 25 percent of all people are honest, 25 percent are dishonest, and 50 percent are as honest as they are forced to be by the controls under which they work. If this is true, hospital internal cash controls must be such as to provide sufficient discouragement to about half of the hospital's employees. The 25 percent who are honest will not steal in any event, but the 25 percent who are dishonest may attempt to steal regardless of the quality of the internal control system. Some of the usual method of cash misappropriation are:

1. Paying bills to nonexistent companies, then forging signatures and cashing the checks.
2. Altering the dollar amounts of checks, invoices, vouchers, or other documents.
3. Collecting patients' accounts, but listing them as uncollectible.
4. Adding "ghosts" to the payroll or padding payrolls by misstating time records and rates of pay.
5. Lapping, wherein an employee diverts payments on one patient's account to himself and subsequently covers the defalcation by applying payments received from another patient to the first account.

It is important that hospital controllers and internal auditors be aware of the manner in which defalcations are generally accomplished. In this way, the control system can at least be designed to force the peculator to devise entirely new methods.

A high degree of sophistication in internal control systems is sometimes difficult to obtain in smaller hospitals since it may be impossible to provide for an entirely satisfactory division of all duties, e.g., the cashier often may also be the accounts receivable bookkeeper. In such cases, increased attention and importance must be given to the application of other internal control principles and procedures. The administrator should strive to put into effect as many additional internal controls as are workable and feasible in the particular circumstances. Bonding, job rotation, surprise cash counts, and similar practices are highly desirable in such instances. The external auditor also should have suggestions relating to this matter.

Cash Receipt Controls

Hospital cash receipts fall into two main classifications: (1) mail receipts and (2) counter receipts. To be effective, the internal control system must be designed to meet the unique requirements of each source of receipts.

Mail Receipts. The control of mail receipts begins with the preparation of a mail remittance report by a bonded employee independent of the cashier and of the accounting department. This person may be a responsible clerk in the mail room in a large hospital or an employee in the administrator's office in a small hospital. Some hospitals have two employees work together for opening mail and preparing mail remittance reports. Checks received in the mail should be immediately endorsed "for deposit only" and entered by amount and payer name on the remittance report. It may also be advisable at times to make photocopies of checks to assist in the subsequent identification of payments by the accounting department. In some systems, the person who opens the mail also prepares prenumbered cash receipt slips, sending one copy to payers as a receipt.

The report of mail receipts, signed by the mail opener, often is prepared in triplicate, with disposition of copies as follows:

1. The original, with correspondence and related papers attached, is forwarded to the accounting department where it is used as the media for appropriate entries in cash, accounts receivable, and other records. At the end of the day, an accounting department employee will also compare the mail remittance list with a copy of the bank deposit ticket to verify the prompt banking of all receipts intact.

2. The duplicate copy, with the cash items, is given to the general cashier who compares the cash items with the report to see that they are correctly listed.
3. The triplicate, signed by the cashier and perhaps certified through a cash register, is retained as a receipt by the mail opener.

The cashier, of course, will record the receipts in the cash register. Either the cashier or an independent employee subsequently makes up the daily bank deposit, sending a copy of the deposit ticket to the accounting department for the purpose already noted. The deposit should include all receipts, including those as yet unidentified and unmatched with receivable records. Such receipts, until a proper determination is made, may be credited to a special "unidentified credits" account.

If this system is employed, a successful misappropriation of funds is difficult in the absence of collusion. The mail opener cannot appropriate mail receipts without omitting such receipts from the mail remittance report. If this is done, the patients' accounts will not be credited by the accounting department and subsequent billings to these patients will be met with considerable complaint. Mail receipts cannot be abstracted by the cashier since the accounting department will verify the deposit of all mail receipts by an independent comparison of the mail remittance list with authenticated bank deposit tickets. Accounting department personnel obviously are unable to make defalcations of receipts because they have no access to them. This is an example of how systems can be designed so as to make the work of one employee subject to automatic check by the work of another.

Counter Receipts. Over-the-counter receipts present more serious internal control problems than do mail receipts. This is the case because a major portion of hospital cash receipts typically is collected by cashiers and receptionists at various departmental locations, e.g., cafeteria, pharmacy, laboratory, radiology, and other outpatient centers. Employees may also be receiving cash in hospital-operated snack bars, gift shops, newsstands, etc. In some hospitals, 25 or more cash collection locations may exist. The number of such locations, however, must be minimized; cash receiving should be centralized to the degree practicable in the circumstances.

As cash is received across the counter at each location, an immediate record of some type should be made. This record may be prepared manually in the form of cash receipt slips and pegboards or by cash registers and machines which lock a record copy within the devices. In addition, departmental locations often are required to submit daily cash receipt and service records, distributed as follows:

1. The original is presented as a receipt to the payer.
2. The duplicate is routed to the accounting department where it is used as the media for appropriate entries in cash, accounts receivable, and revenue records. At the end of the day, a comparison is made of these records with a copy of the bank deposit ticket to verify the banking of the day's receipts at each location.
3. The triplicate copy, along with the cash items, is given to a central cashier who compares the cash items with the listing and certifies the receipts in the cash register, issuing a receipt for the total amount to the departmental cashier.

It is important that cash received at different locations not be commingled; a separate report of, and accounting for, cash receipts should be required of each subcashier or cashier-receptionist.

Cash registers and other receipting devices should be positioned so that the person making payment can easily observe the amounts recorded by the cashiers. These registers, of course, should provide for a locked-in tape or other record which cannot be subsequently altered or destroyed by the cashier. Periodically, accounting department personnel should reconcile the accounting records of receipts with the locked-in controls at the various cash receiving locations.

Cash Disbursement Controls

As noted before, the key to disbursement control is the determination of the authenticity of hospital liabilities and the correctness of their amounts at the time they are initially recorded. There is a tendency to accept as authentic, and pay, liabilities if they have been established in the accounts. Properly recorded liabilities generally lead to proper disbursements, but improperly recorded liabilities also are likely to be paid as recorded unless additional safeguards are observed. Procedures for determining and recording liabilities for payrolls, for supplies, and for purchased services were described in Chapters 7-9. The following is a discussion of the procedures and controls involved in the remainder of the disbursement cycle.

With the exception of expenditures from imprest cash funds, all disbursements should be made by prenumbered checks printed on protective paper to prevent alterations of payee names. The use of a check protector, which imprints the amount of the check in an unalterable manner, also is useful. Definite authority and responsibility for signing checks should be given to only a few persons, and it may be appropriate to require two signatures in certain instances. There should be a proper division of duties among (1) approving liabilities for payment, (2) preparing checks, (3) signing checks,(4) mailing or distribution of checks to payees, and (5) reconciliation of bank statements.

The central control document in many disbursement systems is the voucher, or the combined voucher-check, as described in Chapter 5. This document is the authorization to make a disbursement of hospital funds; no disbursement can be made without a properly executed voucher. It requires the assembly and examination of all supporting evidence such as purchase orders, receiving reports, and invoices. The voucher bears signatures and initials indicating that the proper checks have been made of authorizations, quantities, prices, accounting distributions, mathematical accuracy, and other matters. In short, it is a declaration by the accounting department that the proposed disbursement, insofar as can be determined by the existing system, is valid and that the disbursement therefore should be made in the manner indicated.

The voucher and attached papers are presented along with a check to the disbursing authority. The check signer should ascertain that the check is properly drawn in accordance with the voucher. A review also is made of the underlying documents. If satisfied as to the propriety of the disbursement, the disbursing officer signs the checks either manually or mechanically. Where check signing equipment is used, the signature die must always be kept under the control of the disbursing authority. The signed checks should be mailed to payees directly from the disbursing office; signed checks should never be returned to the accounting department for mailing. Finally, the voucher and supporting documents are indelibly stamped PAID, so that they cannot be again presented for payment, and are then returned to the accounting department where the disbursement is recorded in the check register or cash disbursements journal.

With respect to disbursements for payrolls, the person responsible for signing payroll checks should have nothing to do with the compilation or recording of the payrolls. Before signing payroll checks, the disbursing officer should be satisfied from a review of underlying documentation that the checks are properly drawn. This may be done on a sample basis. Check signing equipment usually is required because of the large volume of checks associated with payrolls.

Signed payroll checks should not be returned to the accounting department but should be given to someone independent of accounting for and approving payrolls. In smaller hospitals, the person who distributes payroll checks may be an individual who knows most employees by sight whereas in large hospitals reliance must be placed upon identification cards or badges. The practice of having payroll checks distributed by department heads is not particularly desirable in that nonexistent persons might be included on departmental payrolls. However paychecks are distributed, the usual procedure should be changed occasionally without prior warning and a different person should distribute the paychecks. Unclaimed checks should be carefully investigated.

The maintenance of special payroll checking accounts on an imprest basis is a highly desirable internal control practice. These accounts should be reconciled by a person not involved in payroll functions. In the course of such reconciliations, a sample of payroll checks can be compared with payroll records and endorsements might be compared with employee signatures found in employment records. Much work of this nature is often done by the internal auditor due to the significance of payroll costs in hospitals.

CASH FLOW AND NET INCOME

The adequacy of internal cash controls sometimes may be questioned by management when hospital cash balances decline severely during periods in which successful operating results are reported in the income statement. Governing board members and administrators having little understanding of accounting may ask questions such as: Why did the cash balance decrease by $100,000 when the income statement for the period shows a $150,000 excess of revenues over expenses? Where did our cash go? Are all our cash receipts getting to the bank? Is there a breakdown in our cash receiving and disbursing procedures? Non-accountants often are puzzled when a favorable operating performance is not immediately reflected in increased cash resources. If a net income is reported but the cash balance declines, they wonder where the net income went. They have difficulty understanding how it is possible to have a net income at all for a period in which a substantial portion of the cash balance apparently disappears. Doubts may arise as to the effectiveness of the internal control system.

It must be recognized that no direct short-run relationship exists between the net income of a period and the change which occurs in the cash balance during the same period. The net income of a period, as shown by the income statement, is the excess of revenues over expenses as determined by the accrual basis of accounting. This means that revenues are reported in the time period **earned** and expenses are recognized in the time period **incurred**, irrespective of the flow of cash. The revenues and cash receipts of a given period therefore are not identical, nor are expenses synonymous with cash disbursements. In other words, the income statement is **not** a report of cash receipts and disbursements, nor is the net income (or loss) the net change in the cash balance.

While successful operations, reported as revenues in excess of expenses, tend to increase cash resources in the long run, the net income of a particular period is not necessarily accompanied by an increase in cash during the same period. Similarly, the net loss of a period will not always be matched by a corresponding decrease in cash. Successive periods of operating losses, however, will rather quickly erode the hospital's cash resources.

Some healthcare organizations still determine their operating results on a cash basis accounting method rather than on an accrual basis. Under the cash basis, revenues are recorded only when received in cash and expenses are recognized only when paid. A hospital employing this method therefore would have no accounts receivable or payable in its balance sheet. Its income statement would be incomplete at best in that it would include only those revenues collected and only those expenses that actually have been paid. The use of the cash basis of accounting is likely to produce some rather bizarre results.

Assume, for example, that two hospitals begin operations on January 1 of a given year with identical balance sheets as shown below. These hospitals are similar in all respects except that Hospital A employs the accrual basis of accounting while Hospital B is on the cash basis.

	Hospital A	Hospital B
Cash	$ 50	$ 50
Plant Assets	750	750
Total	$800	$800
Hospital Equity	$800	$800

During the ensuing fiscal year, the two hospitals complete the following identical transactions:

1. Services rendered to patients on account, $395.
2. Collections on patients' accounts, $350.
3. Supplies purchased on account, $100.
4. Supplies used in operating activities, $90.
5. Cash disbursements:

Payroll	$290
Accounts Payable	85
Total	$375

Hospital A, on the accrual basis, would record all these transactions, but Hospital B, being on the cash basis, would record transactions 2 and 5 only. For accounting purposes, Hospital B would ignore transactions 1, 3 and 4 as these do not involve cash during the fiscal year. Comparative financial statements for the two hospitals are presented in Figure 10-3.

Figure 10-3.
Financial Statements
Accrual Basis vs. Cash Basis

	Hospital A	Hospital B
Income Statement:		
Revenues	$395	$350
Less Expenses:		
Payroll	$290	$290
Supplies	90	85
Total Expenses	$380	$375
Net Income (loss)	$ 15	$(25)
Balance Sheet:		
Cash	$ 25	$ 25
Accounts Receivable	45	..
Inventories	10	..
Plant Assets	750	750
Total	$830	$775
Accounts Payable	$ 15	$ ..
Hospital Capital	815	775
Total	$830	$775

Which set of statements is correct? Which is most complete and useful? The $25 net loss that Hospital B reports actually is nothing more than the decrease in the cash balance for the year. The $15 net income reported by Hospital A is a much superior measure of operating results. Hospital B's balance sheet includes no receivables, inventories, or liabilities when, in fact, patients owe the hospital $45, an inventory of $10 exists, and the hospital owes $15 to suppliers. Thus it is that the cash basis of accounting can produce rather strange and misleading results.

For many years, the HFMA and the AHA have recommended the adoption of accrual basis accounting by all hospitals. It is generally agreed that the accrual basis produces the most managerially useful financial statements. Accrual basis statements, however, do have one serious drawback—they do not reflect the flow of cash that is so vital in the operations of a hospital enterprise. Hospital A's income statement, for example, reflects a $15 excess of revenues over expenses, but the cash balance declined by $25 in the same period. Some managers would have difficulty understanding this seemingly contradictory situation.

From what sources and in what amounts was cash received during the period? For what purposes and in what amounts was cash disbursed? These are critical questions, but answers are not readily obtained from accrual basis financial statements. Due to the importance of directing managerial attention to the movement of cash, it is necessary to supplement the usual financial statements with a **statement of cash receipts and disbursements**. In this way, information is provided about the flow of cash as well as about operating results and financial position. A condensed illustration of a statement of cash receipts and disbursements is provided in Figure 10-4. Such a report often is referred to as a **cash-flow statement**. It lists the cash receipts and disbursements in meaningful classifications and accounts for the change which occurred in the cash balance during the period.

Figure 10-4.
Hypothetical Hospital
Statement of Cash Receipts and Disbursements
Unrestricted Fund
Year Ended June 30, 1987

Cash Balance, July 1, 1986		$ 43
Cash Receipts:		
Inpatient Accounts	$600	
Outpatient Services	120	
Other Operating Revenues	55	
Nonoperating Revenues	30	
Proceeds from Sale of Plant Assets	20	
Short-Term Borrowings from Bank	40	
Total Cash Receipts	$865	
Cash Disbursements:		
Payrolls	$500	
Supplies and Other Expenses	204	
Purchase of Plant Assets	55	
Payments on Mortgage	46	
Purchase of Investment Securities	35	
Total Cash Disbursements	$840	
Excess of Cash Receipts over Cash Disbursements		25
Cash Balance, June 30, 1987		$ 68

CASH BUDGETING

The financial manager of a hospital enterprise has the responsibility for managing the hospital's cash resources so that money will be available in the amounts and at the times needed for meeting obligations. It is imperative that a hospital maintain the ability to meet its payrolls and pay creditors' claims promptly and in full. If cash resources prove inadequate, the hospital may find itself in serious financial distress. Yet, the financial executive must not permit the holding of cash balances in excess of actual needs.

The manager's dilemma of liquidity versus productivity is discussed in Chapter 14. A degree of liquidity (cash) necessarily must be maintained; a hospital must carry cash balances adequate to meet obligations as they become payable. Resources held in the form of cash, however, are nonproductive. To be productive, cash balances must be invested in income-producing assets of one kind or another. A reasonable balance between the two objectives must be found.

It also should be recognized that growth in service volume increases a hospital's cash requirements. At higher levels of activity, it is likely that considerably more money will be tied up in patient service receivables and in inventories. Since personnel and purchasing requirements are increased, the amount of liabilities to employees and suppliers also will be larger. To meet these expanded obligations, greater amounts of cash resources must be available.

Good cash management is necessary if a hospital is to avoid expensive short-term borrowing and the financial embarrassment caused by inadequate cash balances. At the same time, it leads to the maximum utilization of resources by permitting a determination of the amount of excess cash that can prudently be released for investment in productive assets. Finally, careful management of cash may enable a hospital to support a higher volume of service without a corresponding increase in cash requirements. It is in these ways that financial management can make a significant contribution to securing optimum resource utilization in the achievement of patient care objectives.

Nature of the Cash Budget

The preparation of a cash budget is basic to effective cash management. A cash budget is a detailed estimate for future cash receipts from all sources and cash disbursements for all purposes. It is a forecast, based on past experience and anticipated future conditions, of the flow of cash through the hospital's bank accounts. By the cash budgeting process, the financial manager can predict the cash balance at various future points in time in a reasonably accurate manner. Knowing the approximate cash balance at future dates, the need for additional funds can be foreseen and plans can be made for the investment of excess funds, if any. In many instances, the development of a cash budget will indicate the necessity for substantial adjustments in plans for acquisition of plant assets or for retirement of bank loans, mortgages, and other debts.

The basic time period covered by the cash budget ordinarily is one year. Anticipated cash receipts and disbursements are developed and classified by months, and a forecast is made of the probable cash balance at the end of each month of the year. Where volume of service and the working capital position fluctuate to a considerable degree from month to month, however, good cash management may require weekly or even daily breakdowns of projected cash flow data. It is not at all uncommon to find hospital cash budgets refined to day-to-day projections for the current month. As the year transpires, the monthly totals in the coming month's budget are recast in daily terms as described at a later point in this chapter.

Construction of the Cash Budget

The construction of the cash budget is largely an arithmetical matter of converting previously prepared budgets of revenues, salaries and wages, supplies expense, and purchased services from the accrual basis to cash basis terms. Also to be considered are the budgets for capital expenditures and debt retirement. To illustrate the procedure of making a cash budget, the balance sheet presented in Figure 10-5 is assumed in order to provide a starting point. The balance sheet, as well as some of the other information, has been simplified somewhat to allow a clearer exposition of the fundamentals involved. The key requirement for cash budgeting is the existence of a well-conceived operating budget. Without it, reliable cash budgeting is extremely difficult.

Cash Receipts. It is assumed that the January 1, 1987, accounts receivable of $235 originate from charges made to patients for services during the previous three months as follows:

1986	Total Charges	1/1/87 Receivables
December	$200	$140
November	240	72
October	230	23
		$235

Figure 10-5.
Metropolitan Hospital
Balance Sheet—Unrestricted Fund
January 1, 1987

Cash		$ 60
Accounts Receivable		235
Inventories		40
Plant and Equipment	$950	
Less Accumulated Depreciation	360	590
Total Assets		$925
Accounts Payable		$ 55
Mortgage Payable		400
Total Liabilities		$455
Fund Balance		470
Total Liabilities and Fund Balance		$925

A study must be made of the hospital's collection experience in order to determine the pattern by which its receivables generally are collected in cash. Assume that such an analysis shows that about 30 percent of a given month's charges are collected in the same month, 40 percent are collected in the first following month, 20 percent are collected in the second following month, and the remaining 10 percent are collected in the month after that. For the purpose of this illustration, the matter of allowances and the possibility of bad debts are disregarded. Such factors, of course, must be considered in an actual situation and should be treated as reductions in the estimates of receipts. Special consideration must be given to the expected timing of cash inflows governed by the particular terms of various third-party reimbursement contracts. Anticipated cash transfers from restricted funds to the Unrestricted Fund also must be taken into account.

Assume also that the hospital's revenue budget for January 1987 indicates that the month's charges to patients' accounts will total some $220 and that outpatient services provided on a cash basis, not recorded through accounts receivable, will be approximately $33. Using this and the information relating to the usual collection pattern, January cash receipts from patient services can be estimated as follows:

Collection of accounts originating from charges made in:	
January (30% of $220)	$ 66
December (40% of $200)	80
November (20% of $240)	48
October (10% of $230)	23
Total collections on accounts receivable	217
Cash receipts from outpatient services	33
January cash receipts	$250

Cash receipts from inpatient and outpatient services can be projected for subsequent months in the same manner. In February, for example, collections of patients' accounts should be 30 percent of February charges, 40 percent of January charges, 20 percent of

December charges, and 10 percent of November charges. To this total would be added the February budget of outpatient services to be provided on a cash basis.

While the primary source of a hospital's cash receipts is services to its patients, many hospitals have a substantial inflow of cash from other sources such as cafeteria sales, investment income, and contributions. There also may be cash receipts from bank loans and from the sale of plant assets and investments. When the occasional cash inflows from these sources can be anticipated, they should be included in the estimates of cash receipts. All sources of cash receipts should be included in the cash budget. However, these estimates should be developed in a somewhat conservative manner.

Cash Disbursements. The estimates for cash disbursements are derived from previously established budgets for departmental salaries and wages, supplies and other expenses, and capital expenditures. With a knowledge of payroll periods, the monthly cash requirements for salaries and wages are easily determined. The budgeted amount of a month's payroll plus the estimated accrued payroll at the beginning of the month minus the accrued payroll at the end of the month produces the necessary figures. Taxes and other payroll deductions are excluded from the monthly payroll budget but are included in cash disbursements of the month in which such withholdings are to be remitted to governmental and other agencies.

Cash requirements also must be estimated by months with regard to the purchase of supplies and payments for insurance, interest, and purchased services such as utilities and telephone. (Depreciation expense, of course, is omitted from the budget of expenditures unless it is being "funded" as described in Chapter 16.) These determinations are based on budgets for purchasing, insurance expiration and debt retirement schedules, and other relevant data provided by the operating budget. Requirements also must be determined with respect to scheduled principal payments on borrowings and planned investments in new equipment.

With assumptions as to dollar amounts, the estimated January cash disbursements may be summarized as follows:

Payrolls and Deductions	$154
Supplies and Other Expenses*	76
Principal Payments on Mortgage	10
Purchase of New Plant and Equipment	32
Total	$272

*Including 1/1/87 accounts payable (net of applicable discounts), insurance, interest, payroll taxes, utilities and telephone and other operating costs.

Cash disbursements for subsequent months of the year can be estimated in a similar manner. Essentially, it is a matter of converting to a cash basis the previously developed operating expense budgets and the plans for capital expenditures and debt retirement.

Summary. A summary illustration of a cash budget for Metropolitan Hospital is presented in Figure 10-6. As is often the practice, the hospital's cash budget is detailed by months for the first quarter of the year and by quarters only for the balance of the year. It sometimes may be impractical to try to prepare a detailed monthly cash budget beyond, say, three months into the future. As the year progresses, however, these quarterly budgets are adjusted to more current expectations and are converted into detailed monthly budgets.

Figure 10-6.
Metropolitan Hospital
Cash Budget — Unrestricted Fund
Year Ended December 31, 1987

	Total	January	February	March	2nd Quarter	3rd Quarter	4th Quarter
Cash balance — beginning	60	60	27	12	34	18	104
Estimated Cash Receipts:							
Collections on patients' accounts receivable	3054	217	226	251	720	830	810
Receipts from outpatient services	517	33	41	49	126	138	130
Other operating revenues	167	12	11	15	45	49	35
Nonoperating revenues	82	9	4	6	17	26	20
Other receipts	119	3	75*	4	12	15	10
Total cash receipts	3939	274	357	325	920	1058	1005
Total cash available	3999	334	384	367	954	1076	1109
Estimated Cash Disbursements:							
Payrolls and deductions	2673	187	219	225	680	672	690
Supplies and other expenses	813	76	88	93	205	181	170
Principal payments on mortgage	120	10	10	10	30	30	30
Purchase of new plant and equipment	228	32	27	5	21	14	129
Other disbursements	75					25*	
Total cash disbursements	3909	305	344	333	936	972	1019
Cash balance — ending	90	27	12	34	18	104	90

*Includes 180-day, $75 bank loan.

In unusual circumstances, some hospitals may find it possible and useful to budget cash on a daily basis for one month into the future. As each new month begins, the major receipt and disbursement items budgeted for the month are entered in the appropriate column on a wall chart in the financial manager's office. The format for a general checking account is illustrated in Figure 10-7. The chart provides a continuous comparison of cash budget data with actual cash receipts and disbursements, as a daily report. This serves as a constant reminder of the significant elements of cash flow anticipated for the month and is useful in the day-to-day management of cash balances. Actual receipts and disbursements, along with the new balances, are added to the chart each day as they are determined by the accounting department. In this way, cash balances can be constantly monitored so that both additional requirements and idle balances for even a few days can be foreseen. The lead time thus provided permits better decisions for dealing with deficiencies and for taking advantage of temporary investment opportunities.

Figure 10-7.
Metropolitan Hospital
Daily Cash Report – Unrestricted Fund
Month of XXXX, 19XX

Date	Item	Budget			Actual		
		Inflow	Outflow	Balance	Inflow	Outflow	Balance
1	Balance						
1							
2	Payroll						
3							
4							
5							
6	Blue Cross						
7							
8							
9							
10	Accounts Payable						
11							
12	County Welfare						
13							
14							
15	S.P.F. Transfer						
16	Payroll						
17							
18							
19	Blue Cross						
20	H.E.W.						
21							
22	Notes Payable						
23							
24							
25	Mortgage Payable						
26							
27							
28	Plant Fund						
29							
30	Payroll						
31							
	Totals						

Managerial Use of the Cash Budget

The importance of the cash budget in the management of working capital is emphasized in Chapter 14, but some of the managerial uses of the cash budget are noted here. Observe, for example, that Metropolitan Hospital (Figure 10-6) plans to borrow $75 from a bank in February. Without this loan, a deficiency in cash would have arisen and continued into the next several months. This deficiency, and the need to secure funds to cover it, might not otherwise have been foreseen. Through the process of cash budgeting, the coming difficulty is recognized well in advance. Management thereby is given lead time to make the most advantageous arrangements for obtaining the bank loan. Also, banks often will require prospective borrowers to submit a cash budget as a part of the loan application. The cash budget indicates that the hospital should be able to pay the loan in the third quarter, and this is what the bank wants to know.

Instead of borrowing, the hospital might be able to resolve its cash problems in some other manner. It may be possible to make certain adjustments in the projected cash flow so as to eliminate or minimize the need to borrow additional funds. The scheduled purchases of new plant and equipment in January and February, for instance, might be postponed. Or, perhaps special arrangements could be made with suppliers so that payments on accounts payable might be deferred for a time. Although difficult, means might be found to accelerate the inflow of cash.

The preparation of the cash budget also has the advantage of forcing someone in the hospital to direct close attention to the flow of cash. This person must recast the operating and other budgets into a form indicating the impact of such plans on the hospital's cash position. Operating revenues and expenses, proposed plant asset acquisitions, and debt retirement schedules must be considered in the light of available cash. In the absence of cash planning, the hospital might embark upon an ambitious program which it might not be able to pay for and which might lead to serious embarrassment. It is possible to "go broke while making a profit." For this reason, operating budgets generally are not finalized until their impact upon cash flows is ascertained through the preparation of a tentative cash budget.

On the other hand, a hospital's cash budget may show that a more than adequate cash balance will exist for some period of time. The financial executive then is faced with the problem of putting the excess cash to productive use. It may be decided, for example, to invest such funds in short-term marketable securities such as treasury bills and notes. Or, if purchase prices of supplies are expected to rise substantially in the near future, the excess cash may be used to purchase inventory items at the currently lower costs. These matters are discussed in Chapter 14.

Students of accounting and finance often ask how much cash a hospital should have. Ideally, the cash balance of any enterprise should be maintained at exactly zero. As a practical matter, however, the ideal is impossible to attain because a precise matching of cash inflows and outflows requires perfect planning. Thus, it is prudent to maintain precautionary cash balances as a margin of safety to meet unanticipated emergencies. Cash balances may also be maintained for speculative motives, e.g., to take advantage of special investment opportunities. The objective, then, becomes that of determining and maintaining minimum cash balances. Cash budgets and cash reports are useful tools for this purpose.

TEMPORARY INVESTMENTS

The well-managed hospital will place all excess cash funds in productive employment. Temporarily excess funds are usually used for various forms of short-term, highly marketable investment outlets. Although cash balances may be idle for a period as short as 30 days, or perhaps even less, temporary investments often may be worthwhile. The principal outlets for excess funds are commercial bank savings accounts or certificates of deposit, high-grade commercial paper such as the 30-day notes of leading American corporations, and U.S. Treasury bills, notes, and bonds. Investments such as these produce income that would not be earned if excess cash funds were left idle in bank checking accounts.

The short-term investment objectives should be (1) safety and immediate availability of principal and (2) reasonable investment income. From this standpoint, securities of the

U.S. Treasury are generally superior short-term investment outlets. Widely favored for temporary investment are treasury bills which are issued weekly and mature in 91 or 182 days. While the original maturity of treasury notes and bills is one year or longer, there are so many different issues outstanding so that the needs of the short-term investor are nicely served. Should a hospital incorrectly estimate its cash flows and be forced to sell these securities before the maturity dates, little difficulty would be encountered. The prices of government securities tend to be relatively stable, there is a ready market and, the income yield is adequate.

In some instances, however, hospitals may have temporary or short-term investments in marketable **equity** securities, e.g., the capital stocks of industrial corporations. The accounting and reporting requirements for investments in equity securities are much more complex than for debt securities. Accounting for temporary investments in both debt and equity securities is discussed in the following sections of this chapter.

Temporary Investments in Debt Securities

Suppose, for example, that a projection of a hospital's cash position indicates that $90,000 of cash will not be needed for approximately three months. A decision therefore is made on March 1 to invest the $90,000 in 8% securities of some type that pay interest semiannually on October 1 and April 1. An entry such as the following may be made:

Temporary Investments	$ 89,500	
Accrued Interest Receivable	3,000	
Cash		$ 92,500

To record purchase of marketable securities for temporary investment purposes as follows:

Purchase price ($90,000 @ 99 1/4)	$89,325
Brokerage and other costs	175
Total	89,500
Accrued interest:	
$90,000 X 8% X 5/12	3,000
Cash disbursement	$92,500

The "cost" of such investments is the quoted price paid plus brokerage and other acquisition costs. It is assumed here that the quoted price is 99.25% of par or face value, and that acquisition costs total $175. For accounting purposes, the cost of the investment is $89,500.

Because these bonds were acquired between interest payment dates, the seller must be paid the accrued interest on the bonds since the last interest payment date, i.e., from October 1 to March 1, or five months. This $3,000 will be recovered by the hospital on April 1 when the issuer of the bonds pays six months' interest to bondholders. Accrued interest settlements are made in this manner between investors who trade in bonds; it would not be convenient for the issuer to attempt to make these adjustments.

Where temporary investments are acquired at a price that is more or less than their par or face value, amortization of the premium or discount is generally not necessary.

proceeds and the acquisition cost is reported as a gain or loss. The amortization procedure, however, should be followed with respect to long-term investments (see Chapter 15).

At the end of each monthly reporting period, an entry is required to record the accrued income on the investment. The entry at the end of March, for instance, would be:

Accrued Interest Receivable	$ 600	
Investment Income		$ 600
To record accrued interest on investment		
in marketable securities, as follows:		
$90,000 X 8% X 1/12 = $600		

The amount of this entry is an approximation of interest for one month; precise computations to exact cents can be made but are not really necessary in recording most accruals. Similar entries would be made at the end of each month until the maturity date of the securities.

On April 1, the next interest payment date, the following entry would be in order to record the receipt of six months' interest on the bonds:

Cash	$ 3,600	
Accrued Interest Receivable		$ 3,600
To record receipt of semiannual interest		
on temporary investment, as follows:		
$90,000 X 8% X 6/12 = $3,600		

The procedure described here would be continued as long as the hospital holds the securities. In the balance sheet, the bonds are reported at original cost, but it often is the practice to show their market value parenthetically. Only in rare circumstances would it be appropriate to adjust temporary investments in debt securities to current market value.

To complete the illustration of short-term investments in debt securities, assume that the investments are sold at 101 on June 1, with brokerage fees and other expenses of sale amounting to $190. The necessary entry is:

Cash	$91,910	
Accrued Interest Receivable		$ 1,200
Temporary Investments		89,500
Gain on Sale of Investments		1,210
To record sale of temporary investments		
as follows:		

Sale price ($90,000 @ 101)	$90,900	
Less brokerage and other expenses	190	
Net	90,710	
Accrued interest:		
$90,000 X 8% X 2/12	1,200	
Total cash received	$91,910	

The credit to Accrued Interest Receivable is necessary to eliminate the balance of that account as established by the income accruals at the end of April and May. A gain of $1,210 was realized on the sale; it is computed as the difference between the net proceeds ($90,710) and the carrying value of the bonds ($89,500).

Temporary Investments in Marketable Equity Securities

The term **marketable equity securities** refers to any readily tradeable security that represents ownership shares or the right to acquire ownership shares in an enterprise at fixed or determinable prices. This definition includes common and preferred stocks, warrants, and options, but excludes securities such as convertible bonds and redeemable preferred stocks. The following discussion is based on the relevant provisions of the **Hospital Audit Guide.**[2]

Acquisition. Assume that a hospital purchased the common stock of three different corporations on April 1, 1987:

Short-Term Investments	$ 41,000	
Cash In Bank		$ 41,000

Purchase of corporate common stocks, as follows:

Company	Shares	Cost
A	200	$ 6,000
B	500	20,000
C	300	15,000
Total		$41,000

Investments in marketable equity securities are recorded at cost. The cost of purchased securities is the amount paid, including acquisition costs such as brokerage fees and taxes. The cost of securities acquired by donation is the fair value of the securities at date of donation.

Investment Income. During the last nine months of 1987, $3,500 of cash dividends were received on the stock investments:

Cash In Bank	$ 3,500	
Dividend Income		$ 3,500

Receipt of cash dividends on investments in corporate stocks.

A detailed treatment of accounting for dividends and other types of investment income is presented in Chapter 15.

Balance Sheet Valuation. The current portfolio of marketable equity securities had the following market value at December 31, 1987:

Company	Shares	Cost	Market Value
A	200	$ 6,000	$ 6,600
B	500	20,000	18,400
C	300	15,000	14,100
		$41,000	$39,100

Investments in marketable equity securities should be reported at the lower of aggregate cost or market at the balance sheet date. Since the aggregate market in this example ($39,100) is lower than aggregate cost ($41,000), the current investment portfolio must be reported at market value in the hospital's balance sheet at December 31, 1987. The necessary December 31, 1987, entry is:

Unrealized Loss on Investments	$ 1,900	
Allowance for Decline in Market		
Value of Investments		$ 1,900
Reduction of short-term investments to		
lower of aggregate cost or market.		

The unrealized loss is reported as nonoperating expense in the 1987 income statement. The marketable equity securities are presented in the December 31, 1987, balance sheet as follows:

Current assets:
    Marketable equity securities, at the lower of
    aggregate cost ($41,000) or market value $39,100

Had the aggregate market value been greater than aggregate cost, no entry would have been necessary at December 31, 1987, and the investments would have been reported at cost, with market value shown parenthetically.

Sale and Purchase Transactions. Assume that the investment in Company C stock was sold on May 1, 1988, for $14,400, and that 400 shares of Company D stock were purchased on September 1, 1988:

Cash In Bank		$ 14,400	
Loss on Sale of Investments		600	
Short-Term Investments			$ 15,000
Sale of Company C stock:			
Cost	$15,000		
Sales price	14,400		
Loss on sale	$ 600		
Short-Term Investments		$ 18,000	
Cash In Bank			$ 18,000
Purchase of Company D stock.			

The realized loss on the sale of Company C stock is determined on the basis of its acquisition cost ($15,000). The carrying amount for the stock was not changed by application of the lower of aggregate cost or market rule at the end of 1987. The valuation allowance applies to the investment portfolio as a whole, and not to the individual securities in the portfolio.

The $600 loss should be reported in the 1988 income statement as an item of nonoperating expense. Had the Company C stock been sold at a gain, the gain would have been reported in the 1988 income statement as an item of nonoperating revenue.

Subsequent Year Valuation. Assume that the current marketable equity securities investment portfolio had the following market value at December 31, 1988:

Company	Shares	Cost	Market Value
A	200	$ 6,000	$ 6,800
B	500	20,000	18,300
C	400	18,000	17,700
		$44,000	$42,800

Because aggregate market value is less than aggregate cost, the investment portfolio must be reported at market value. A valuation allowance of $1,200 ($44,000 − $42,800) is required, but an allowance account of $1,900 already exists (it was carried over from 1987). This means that the valuation allowance account must be reduced by $700, with the $700 recovery of market value being treated as nonoperating revenue in the 1988 income statement:

Allowance for Decline in Market Value of Investments	$ 700	
Unrealized Gain on Investments		$ 700
Adjustment of valuation allowance for market value recovery in 1988.		

The presentation of the marketable equity securities in the balance sheet at December 31, 1988, would be as follows:

Current assets:	
Marketable equity securities, at the lower of cost ($44,000) or market	$42,800

Had the December 31, 1988, market value of the portfolio been in excess of cost, the allowance account would have been totally eliminated, and the securities would have been reported in the December 31, 1988, balance sheet at cost (with the higher market value being shown parenthetically). Had the December 31, 1988, market value been less than cost by, say, $2,400, an entry would have been made to record an unrealized loss of $500 ($2,400 − $1,900) and increase the valuation allowance to $2,400. In other words, mark to market down or up but not up in excess of acquisition cost.

Reclassifications. On occasion, it may be appropriate to transfer certain marketable equity securities from the current to the noncurrent portfolio, perhaps due to a management intent as to the conversion of the securities to cash. Assume, for example, that a particular security carried in the current investment portfolio has a cost of $4,500 and a current market value of $4,000. If this security is transferred from the current to the noncurrent portfolio, the appropriate entry is:

Long-Term Investments *value*	$ 4,000	
Realized Loss on Investments	500	
Short-Term Investments *cash*		$ 4,500
Reclassification and transfer of a security		
from the current to the noncurrent investment		
portfolio.		

Such reclassifications or transfers are recorded at the lower of cost or market at the transfer date. The loss, if any, is reported as an item of nonoperating expense in the income statement of the period of transfer.

Required Supplementary Disclosures. Various supplementary disclosures relating to investments in marketable equity securities are required by the **Hospital Audit Guide.** These disclosures are discussed in Chapter 15.

BALANCE SHEET PRESENTATION

The balance sheet presentation of temporary or short-term investments has been described earlier in this chapter. To summarize, temporary investments in debt securities are valued at cost; temporary investments in stocks or other marketable equity securities are stated at the lower of aggregate cost or market.

Since cash is the standard of value, there is no problem of cash valuation in the financial statements. The hospital accountant, however, must be careful not to misstate the cash balance by improper exclusions from or inclusions in the cash category. The composition of cash was discussed earlier in this chapter. Cash presentation in the hospital balance sheet is primarily a matter of adequate classification and description. Cash, as a completely liquid asset representing immediately available purchasing power, normally is shown first among the assets of each fund maintained by the hospital. Restrictions on the expenditure of cash balances must be clearly indicated.

While the cash item in monthly and annual balance sheets prepared for the governing board or outside agencies may be labeled simply "cash on hand and in banks," internal administrative reports should make a clear distinction between petty cash and change funds, undeposited cash on hand, cash in general checking accounts, and cash in special purpose checking accounts. Managerial control of cash, as well as of receivables and inventory, requires detail reporting. Inadequacies and excesses may be readily hidden in a lump-sum figure, and irregularities or undesirable trends may go unobserved and uncorrected.

Suppose, for example, that comparative unrestricted fund balance sheets indicated the following situation:

	June 30	
	1987	1986
Cash on hand and in banks	$184,000	$184,000

All is well? No irregularities or undesirable situations are noticeable. Looking beyond these lump-sum figures, however, some rather disturbing details might be found about which some questions should be asked:

	June 30	
	1987	1986
Cash on hand and in banks:		
Petty cash funds	$ 5,000	$ 500
Change funds	4,000	700
Undeposited cash on hand	22,000	-0-
Cash in first bank	162,000	120,000
Cash in second bank	(35,000)	37,800
Payroll checking account	26,000	-0-
Board-designated checking account	-0-	25,000
Totals	$184,000	$184,000

What makes it necessary to maintain substantially larger petty cash and change funds in 1987? Were these increases approved? Why was $22,000 of cash on hand undeposited at June 30, 1987? How did the overdraft in the second bank occur? If the payroll account is maintained on an imprest basis, why does the account have a $26,000 balance? What happened to the $25,000 balance in the board designated checking account? These important questions might never have been asked had the underlying details not been disclosed.

Incidentally, the above presentation of the overdraft in the second bank is an incorrect one. When an account in one bank has been overdrawn, the amount of the overdraft should not be netted against positive cash balances in other banks. Such overdrafts must be shown among the liabilities of the hospital. Although deposits may be made before the outstanding checks actually clear the bank, a liability situation exists and the balance sheet should reflect it clearly.

The window dressing of cash is not an unknown practice. Through the device of holding open the cash records until several days after the close of a reporting period, it may be possible to arrange for a balance sheet cash figure which is larger (or smaller) than would otherwise be the case. The cash receipts journal, for example, may be kept open in order to record the cash receipts of the first few days of the next accounting period as if they had occurred before the balance sheet date. Such a procedure would result in the balance sheet presentation of a stronger cash position than actually existed at the balance sheet date. Needless to say, this is a distortion of fact which cannot be condoned.

THE AUDIT OF CASH

In the performance of the annual hospital audit, the external auditor spends a considerable portion of audit time in an examination of cash transactions and in verification of cash balances. This is done because cash is most susceptible to fraud and error, cash transactions are closely related to the balances and activity in other accounts, and internal control procedures can be evaluated concurrently. The auditor usually begins the examination with a more or less standard audit program which will be expanded or contracted as the auditor forms an opinion of the degree of internal control in effect at the hospital. If internal cash control is satisfactory, less time is spent than might otherwise be the case. Audit fees also can be reduced, without diminishing the value or completeness of the audit, if hospital personnel will prepare certain schedules and perform many of the detailed procedures which the auditor would otherwise be forced to do.

In order to properly assist the independent auditor and derive the greatest benefit from the audit, it is important that the hospital controller and internal auditor have at least a general understanding of what the independent auditor does and how he does it. Information can be obtained from auditing textbooks and directly from the independent auditors as to objectives and general procedures. A number of specifics, however, will not be divulged by the external auditor.

Governing boards, administrators, and controllers should understand that the standard cash audit by an independent accountant is no guarantee that any and all instances of fraud will be detected. Audits by certified public accountants often **may** uncover fraud, but they are not specifically designed to do so. The auditor cannot examine each and every cash transaction. The cost of such an audit would be prohibitive. Auditors necessarily must rely upon an examination of a random sample of cash transactions. If no irregularities are discovered in such test of the accounting records, it generally is assumed that the remaining cash transactions are substantially error – and fraud-free. Where some suspicion of fraud exists, the governing board should specifically ask the auditor to include the detection of fraud in the scope of the audit. Nevertheless, the responsibility for safeguarding the assets of the hospital remains with the governing board and the administrator. It cannot be delegated to the independent auditors.

CHAPTER 10 FOOTNOTES

1. Albert R. Kerr, "Stretching the Cash," **Wall Street Journal**, October 6, 1966, p. 1.

2. Subcommittee on Health Care Matters, **Hospital Audit Guide** (New York: AICPA, 1982), pp. 75-79.

QUESTIONS

1. Define **cash** in terms of its inclusion among the current assets of the Unrestricted Fund in the hospital balance sheet.

2. Southland Hospital included the following items in cash among the current assets of the Unrestricted Fund in its April 30 balance sheet. How do you think each of these items should have been reported?

   a. Travel advance to employee.
   b. Balance in bank savings account (time deposit).
   c. Patient's check returned by bank marked NSF.
   d. Undeposited cash receipts on hand at April 30.
   e. Patient's postdated check.
   f. Cash on deposit with trustee for retirement of bonds.
   g. Unused postage stamps.
   h. U.S. Treasury bills temporarily held until cash is needed to pay for construction costs on new wing.
   i. A petty cash fund of $500, composed of the following:

Coin and currency	$387
Expense vouchers	86
Employee IOU	25

   j. Cash on deposit in escrow on purchase of real estate.
   k. Change funds in cash registers.
   l. Balance in special payroll checking account.

3. Give some important reasons why particular attention should be given to cash by the hospital accountant and financial manager.

4. The cash in bank account of Northerly Hospital shows a balance of $97,429 at June 30. The June bank statement, however, shows a balance of $121,483 at the same date. List four types of factors which may cause such a difference and give an example of each type.

5. How should the following situations be handled for the purposes of balance sheet reporting?

   a. Overdraft in the hospital's only bank account.
   b. Overdraft in account in Bank A when the hospital has a larger positive balance in Bank B.
   c. Overdraft in one account and a larger positive balance in another account in the same bank.
   d. Overdraft in account with Bank A and a smaller positive balance in another account in the same bank.

6. What purposes are served by the preparation of bank reconciliations? Describe the two methods by which bank reconciliations may be performed. Which method do you prefer?

7. Briefly describe the imprest system for operating a cash fund and state the principal advantages of the imprest system from the standpoint of internal control.

8. Prepare a questionnaire to be used in internal auditing in evaluating internal control over a petty cash fund.

9.   With respect to cash receipts, what questions might the internal auditor ask to determine the effectiveness of the internal control system?

10.   The following auditing procedures are customary in connection with the verification of cash balance or the testing of cash transactions:

    a.   Verification of the composition of deposit slips.

    b.   Comparison of deposits as shown by the bank statement for several days prior to the end of the period under examination with receipts as shown by the cashbook.

    c.   Comparison of checks returned with the next subsequent bank statement and with the list of checks outstanding at the date of the reconciliation.

    d.   Reconcilement of cash receipts by months as shown by the cashbook with deposits as shown by bank statements.

Indicate the type of irregularity which could be expected to be disclosed by the application of each procedure and explain how the procedure would disclose the irregularity.

11.   List the major requirements for a good system of internal control over cash receipts.

12.   What is meant by the terms **lapping** and **kiting?** Name five other practices that might result in cash misappropriations in the absence of a good system of internal control.

13.   Explain how it is possible for a hospital to have an excess of revenues over expenses in a year during which the cash balance **declines** by a substantial amount.

14.   Distinguish between the cash basis and the **accrual basis** of accounting. What is a **cash-flow statement,** and what useful information might it contain for management purposes? Would a cash-flow statement be useful in external reporting by hospitals?

15.   What is the **responsibility** of hospital management with respect to cash? Indicate some techniques that are useful to management in carrying out this responsibility.

16.   What is a reconciliation of cash receipts and disbursements? How does it differ from a bank reconciliation? Why is a so-called cash proof performed by the hospital's auditors?

17.   Define the term **temporary investments.** Distinguish between marketable securities and temporary investments. List some common types of temporary investments available to hospitals.

18.   In the Unrestricted Fund of a hospital balance sheet, at what amount should current investments in marketable equity securities be reported?

EXERCISES

E 1.   On September 1, 1987, Community Hospital purchased $100,000 of 6% bonds at 97 and accrued interest, with brokerage and other acquisition costs amounting to $250. Interest is payable semiannually on April 1 and October 1. The maturity date of the bonds is April 1, 1990, but the hospital intends to hold these securities as a short-term investment. The hospital closes its books annually on September 30. At September 30, 1987, the securities have a quoted market value of $98,250. On December 1, 1987, the securities are sold at 99 1/2 and accrued interest, with brokerage costs amounting to $280.

Required. Assuming 30-day months and that discount is **not** to be amortized:

1. Prepare the necessary journal entries at:

    a.   September 1
    b.   September 30
    c.   October 1
    d.   October 31
    e.   November 30
    f.   December 1

2. Indicate fully how all matters relating to this investment should be reflected in the hospital's financial statements for the year ended September 30, 1987.

E2.   On March 1, Memorial Hospital established a petty cash fund in he imprest amount of $500. On March 12, the contents of the petty cash box were as follows and the fund was reimbursed.

Coin and currency	$124
Petty cash expense vouchers	152
IOU from employee	20
Envelope marked "basketball betting pool" and containing	18
Check of another employee made payable to Memorial Hospital	200

It was decided to reduce the imprest amount of the fund to $225, and this was done on March 14.

Required. (1) Prepare the necessary entries at March 1, 12, and 14. (2) Comment, from an internal auditing standpoint, on the contents of the petty cash fund as of March 12.

E3.   Midcity Hospital's general ledger showed a balance of $12,642.15 on June 30. The bank statement for June showed a month-end balance of $13,253.01, but the bank erroneously charged Midcity's account for a check drawn by Uptown Hospital in the amount of $267.50. Bank service charges for June were $5.20, and the bank also made a charge of $15.46 for printing of checks. Analysis revealed that checks outstanding totaled $2,326.62 and that a deposit of $1,427.60 was in transit at June 30.

Required. (1) Prepare a bank reconciliation at June 30. (2) Prepare the necessary adjusting journal entry.

E4.   The January 1 accounts receivable of Williams Hospital originate from charges
       made to patients during the previous three months as follows:

Month	Charges	Accounts Receivable
December	$100,000	$100,000
November	90,000	27,000
October	85,000	8,500
		$135,500

The hospital's past experience shows that about 70 percent of charges in any
month are collected in the following month. An additional 20 percent are
collected in the second following month, 8 percent are received in the third
month, and the remaining 2 percent prove to be uncollectible.

Required. Calculate the probable collections on accounts receivable during
January for purposes of cash budgeting.

E5.   Given the following data for Marlene Hospital:

	Nov.	Dec.	Jan.	Feb.	Mar.
Revenues	$100,000	$10,000 *120,000*	$90,000	$80,000	$110,000
Purchases of supplies	10,000	15,000	12,000	12,000	20,000
Other expenses	80,000	93,000	69,000	64,000	79,000

Eighty percent of revenues are collected in the month following the month in
which services are rendered. The remaining 20 percent are collected in the
second following month. Fifty percent of purchases are made for cash. The
remainder are paid, net of a 1 percent discount, in the month following the
month of purchase. Other expenses are paid in cash in the month incurred.
(Depreciation of $5,000 per month is included in expenses above.)

A short-term bank loan of $40,000 falls due on March 1, and the hospital plan to
purchase new equipment for $75,000 cash on February 1. The cash balance at
December 31 is $25,000.

Required. Prepare a cash budget for January, February, and March, showing the
projected cash balance at the end of each month.

E6.   According to its books, Case Hospital has a cash balance of $438,104 at June 30.
       The June bank statement, however, shows a June 30 balance of $486,681. An
       investigation produces the following information:

       1. The bank credited, in error, Pace Hospital for a deposit of $28,417 made by
          Case Hospital on June 22.

2. Bank service charges for June amounted to $27.

3. Outstanding checks at June 30 were $107,092.

4. A deposit of $39,865 was in transit at June 30.

5. The June bank statement shows a credit of $10,600 representing the proceeds of a patient's note collected for Case Hospital by the bank.

6. The bank returned patients' checks marked "not sufficient funds" in the amount of $2,606.

7. Check number 1791 issued in payment of an account payable of $200 was recorded in error by a Case Hospital bookkeeper as $2,000 even though the check was drawn in the correct amount.

Required. (1) Prepare a bank reconciliation at June 30. (2) Prepare the necessary adjusting journal entry at June 30.

E7.   On May 1, 1987, Cashwise Hospital purchases 100, $1,000 par value, 6% bonds. These bonds mature on September 1, 1993, with semi-annual interest payable on March 1 and September 1. The bonds were purchased at 100 7/8 plus accrued interest and costs (brokerage commission, taxes, postage) of $125. The bonds are sold in October 1, 1987, at 101 3/8 plus accrued interest, with costs of sale amounting to $135. It was the intent of management to hold these securities as temporary investments. Market quotations on the bonds were:

May 31	101
June 30	101 1/8
July 31	101 1/8
August 31	100
September 30	101 3/8

Cashwise Hospital prepares monthly financial statements.

Required. Prepare journal entries to record all transactions and adjustments relating to the bonds.

E8.   Cash Hospital decided to establish a petty cash fund on June 1 in the imprest amount of $1,000. The following transactions relating to the fund took place during June:

1. The fund was established on June 1.

2. The fund was replenished on June 15 at a time when the contents of the funded were as follows:

Currency and coin	$725
Expense vouchers	215
Employee IOU	50

3. On June 20, it was decided to reduce the imprest amount of the fund by $400.

4. The fund was replenished on June 30 at a time when the contents of the fund were as follows:

Currency and coin	$407
Expense vouchers	196

Required. Prepare journal entries to record all of the above.

E9. Select the best answer for each of the following multiple-choice questions.

1. Houchens Hospital held the following current investments in corporate stocks in its Unrestricted Fund at 12/31/87:

	Cost	Market
Company X stock	$ 30,000	$ 35,000
Company Y stock	50,000	40,000
Company Z stock	120,000	115,000
	200,000	190,000

On 6/1/88, the Company B stock was sold for $36,000. Cash dividends of $4,000 were received during 1988. The market values of Company X and Z stock investments at 12/31/88 were $38,000 and $109,000, respectively. If Houchens Hospital has a 1988 net income of $100,000 before investment transactions, the net income for the year including investment transactions should be

a. $104,000
b. $ 97,000
c. $ 90,000
d. $ 87,000

2. In its 12/31/87 Unrestricted Fund balance sheet, McNabb Hospital reported the following current investments in marketable equity securities:

Marketable equity securities, at cost	$300,000
Less allowance to reduce marketable equity securities to market value	28,000

At 12/31/88, the market value of the current investment portfolio was $298,000. What should McNabb report in its 1988 income statement?

a. $-0-$
b.   Unrealized loss of $2,000.
c.   Realized gain of $26,000.
d.   Unrealized gain of $26,000.

3. Brunson Hospital has decided to reclassify its Unrestricted Fund investment
    in the marketable equity securities of Brock Company from current to
    noncurrent assets. On the date of the decision, the Brock securities (which
    had originally cost $50,000) have a current market value of $44,000. Proper
    accounting treatment of this transfer requires

    a.   A cost basis of $44,000 within a realized loss of $6,000.
    b.   A cost basis of $50,000 with a realized loss of $6,000.
    c.   A cost basis of $44,000 with an unrealized loss of $6,000.
    d.   A cost basis of $50,000 with an unrealized loss of $6,000.

4. When the market value of a hospital's current marketable equity securities
    investment portfolio in the Unrestricted Fund is lower than its cost, the
    difference should be

    a.   Accounted for as a realized loss in the income statement.
    b.   Disclosed and described in a footnote to the hospital's financial
          statements.
    c.   Accounted for as a valuation allowance deducted from the asset to
          which it relates.
    d.   Accounted for as a negative element in the fund balance section of
          the Unrestricted Fund balance sheet.

5. Carson Hospital's current marketable equity securities portfolio in the
    Unrestricted Fund is as follows:

	12/31/87		12/31/86	
	Cost	Market	Cost	Market
Archer stock	$100,000	$100,000	$100,000	$120,000
Kelly stock	200,000	150,000	300,000	260,000
Pelt stock	250,000	260,000	200,000	240,000

What amount should be reported as a charge against income in Carson's
1987 income statement?

    a. $-0-$
    b. $10,000
    c. $40,000
    d. $60,000

PROBLEMS

P1.   Roper Hospital's bank account shows a book balance of $346,920 at April 30. An examination of the April bank statement in comparison with the cash records of the hospital, however, discloses the following information:

1. April 30 balance per bank statement, $465,900.

2. Deposit in transit at April 30, $12,800.

3. Checks outstanding at April 30, $89,300.

4. Patient's NSF check returned by bank with April statement, $5,100.

5. Bank service charges for April, $120.

6. The bank inadvertently credited another of its depositors for the Roper Hospital's April 22 bank deposit of $10,600.

7. Matured certificates of deposit of $50,000, plus interest of $2,000, were cashed and credited by the bank to the hospital's checking account on April 29.

8. A hospital employee journalized a properly drawn check for $700 as $7,000 on April 9 in settlement of an account payable.

Required. Prepare (1) a bank reconciliation at April 30 for Roper Hospital and (2) the necessary April 30 adjusting entry.

P2.   The cash in bank ledger account of Bankroll Hospital shows a debit balance of $11,471 on October 31, but the October bank statement indicates a balance of $14,792. The cash receipts of October 31 in the amount of $1,650 were deposited that evening in the night depository but were not included on the statement for October. The October statement included a debit memo for $12 of service charges for the month. A credit memo included with the bank statement indicated that a 9%, 180-day, $4,000 note receivable left with the bank for collection at maturity had been collected and credited to the hospital. A debit memo showed a $20 collection charge for this service. Comparison of the cancelled checks with the hospital's disbursement journal indicated that a check for $341 for the purchase of office equipment was journalized in error on October 21 as $314. Also included with the bank statement was an NSF check of $300 which had been deposited by the hospital on September 30. Checks outstanding at October 31 totaled $1,150.

The following additional information is available:

1. The October cash receipts journal shows total cash receipts of $33,360, and the cash disbursements journal shows total cash disbursements of $31,711.

2. The October bank statement includes debits which total $31,780 and credits of $37,090.

3. At September 30, the following bank reconciliation was prepared:

Balance per bank	$9,482
Deposits in transit	1,200
Checks outstanding	(860)
Balance per books	$9,822

Required. (1) Prepare a reconciliation of cash receipts and disbursements for the month ended October 31. (2) Prepare the necessary adjusting journal entry at October 31.

P3. A comparison of Rayco Hospital's cash records and its November bank statement provides the following information:

1. General information:

	Book	Bank
Balances, 10/31	$ 15,810	$ 15,862
Receipts	14,331	17,495
Disbursements	14,754	16,087
Balances, 11/30	15,387	17,270

2. Deposits in transit:

10/31	$ 1,375
11/30	946

3. Checks outstanding:

10/31	$ 2,482
11/30	1,949

4. Bank service charges on November statement, $16.

5. NSF check of a Rayco Hospital patient returned by bank with November bank statement, $479.

6. On November 30, the bank collected a Rayco Hospital patient's note of $2,000 plus $40 interest. The bank debited the hospital $7 for this service.

7. A hospital bookkeeper on November 12 journalized a $487 deposit as $847. This money came from the outpatient registration desk.

8. On November 27, one of the hospital's bookkeepers journalized a $10 check as $100. This check was issued in settlement of an account payable.

9. On November 22, the bank charged the hospital's account with a $388 check of another of the bank's depositors. Bank indicated that this mistake would be corrected on the December statement.

10. On October 29, the bank failed to give the hospital credit for a $1,055 deposit of that date. When notified of the error on November 4, the bank made the necessary correction (which appeared on the November statement).

Required. (1) Prepare a bank reconciliation at October 31. (2) Prepare a bank reconciliation at November 30. (3) Prepare a reconciliation of cash receipts and disbursements (a proof of cash) for November. (4) Prepare the necessary adjusting entry at November 30.

P4. Cashful Hospital has developed the following budgets of revenues and supplies purchases for the first three months of 1987:

	Jan.	Feb.	Mar.
Revenues:			
Charges to patients	$250,000	$350,000	$300,000
Cash	40,000	50,000	45,000
Purchases:			
Charge	70,000	60,000	90,000
Cash	24,000	32,000	28,000

Billings are made to patients on the last day of each month. Past experience shows that 90 percent of a month's billings are collected in the following month and 10 percent are collected in the next following month. Purchases on account in any month are paid on the tenth of the following month in order to obtain a 1 percent discount. Purchase discount opportunities are never missed.

Operating expenses (other than mentioned above) are paid as incurred and are budgeted as follows:

Fixed, $18,000 per month
Variable, 52 percent of monthly gross revenues

Depreciation expense is estimated at $3,500 per month and is included in the above fixed expenses. Selected balances taken from the general ledger of the hospital at December 31, 1986, are given below:

Cash		$150,000
6%, 90-day notes receivable,		
dated 11/10/86		8,000
Accounts receivable from:		
November billings	$ 18,000	
December billings	200,000	218,000
8%, 180-day bank loan, due		
1/20/87		75,000
Accounts payable		80,000

In addition, Cashful Hospital plans to purchase certain equipment which will require a cash outlay of $110,000 on March 10, 1987.

Required. (1) Prepare in good form a cash budget for the first quarter of 1987, showing the projected cash position at the end of each month. (2) On the basis of the budgeted cash flow, what recommendations would you make to the management of Cashful Hospital?

P5.   You are provided with the following balance sheet and various other information relating to Futura Hospital:

Futura Hospital
Balance Sheet
December 31, 1986

Cash		$ 25,000
Accounts receivable	$ 70,000	
Less allowance for bad debts	10,500	
Accounts receivable (net)		59,500
Plant and equipment	$360,000	
Less accumulated depreciation	20,000	340,000
Total		$424,500
Note payable		$ 65,000
Accounts payable		28,000
Hospital equity		331,500
Total		$424,500

1986 billings to patients were:

December	$58,000
November	60,000
October	62,000
September	57,000
August	58,000
July	65,000
June	62,000

The hospital's collection experience has been as follows:

40% collected in month billed (month of service)
30% collected in first following month
15% in second month
7% in third month
5% in fourth month
3% uncollectible

Budgeted billings to patients in 1987 are:

January	$55,000	April	$50,000
February	50,000	May	58,000
March	60,000	June	65,000

Budgeted disbursements for expenses in 1987 are:

January	$45,500	April	$39,800
February	36,700	May	40,900
March	41,650	June	45,150

Required. (1) Prepare a cash budget by months, January through June 1987. (2) Comment on the hospital's ability to retire the note payable on June 30, 1987. (3) What is your recommendation for maintaining an adequate cash balance at Futura Hospital?

P6. Valley Community Hospital had completed its budget of operations for the new fiscal year ending September 30, 1987, as shown:

	Year Ended 9/30 1986*	Year Ended 9/30 1987+	Increase (Decrease)
Patient days (excluding newborn)	66,029	69,000	2,971
Newborn days	3,870	3,870	...
Operating income:			
Routine services	$3,152,616	$3,286,322	$ 133,706
Professional services	2,970,628	3,012,600	41,972
Gross earnings from patients	6,123,244	6,298,922	175,678
Less deductions	622,136		(622,136)
Net earnings	5,501,108	6,298,922	797,814
Auxiliary services	98,286	114,359	16,073
Total operating income	5,599,394	6,413,281	813,887
Less operating expenses	5,467,750	6,655,623	1,187,873
Operating gain (loss)	131,644	(242,342)	(373,986)
Other income	78,809	64,400	(14,409)
Net gain (loss)	$ 210,453	$(177,942)	$(388,395)

*Actual for nine months plus last quarter estimated.
+Budget (preliminary).

The controller must make a recommendation to the executive committee in September of 1986 regarding the hospital's cash objectives as shown below:

Capital budget		$173,974
Estimate due to third-party payers for 9/30/84 and 9/30/85 audits		76,000
Bond amortization:		
2/1/87	$43,000	
8/1/87	44,000	87,000
Property A note payment		15,603
Property B note payment		6,777
Cash transfer to Building Fund		150,000
Total cash objectives for year ending 9/30/87		$509,354

The controller also must do a cash flow analysis to see if these cash objectives can be met. The following additional information is available:

1. Included in operating expenses for the year ending September 30, 1987, is depreciation of $361,720.

2. The hospital selected an accelerated method of depreciation for third-party reimbursement, and the amount for depreciation is $496,720 for the new fiscal year. Third-party patients account for one-third of the total patient days.

3. The third-party contract within the hospital provides a 5 percent plus factor superimposed over the basic reimbursement cost of $2,040,000 for the fiscal year ending September 30, 1987.

4. Before any rate increases, the cost/charge ratio for the third-party contractual relationship is over 100 percent.

5. Inpatient accounts receivable for patients not under a reimbursement program is expected to affect cash flow. The utilization of the hospital for the fiscal year ending September 30, 1987, will increase patient days and cause an increase of 5 percent in receivables. Only 20 percent of such receivables are not under a cost reimbursement program. The inpatient accounts receivable total, as of September 30, 1986, is $850,000.

6. The hospital is also expecting an increase in outpatient activity of 20 percent, and the accounts receivable in this classification at September 30, 1986, are $100,000.

Required. Prepare a cash flow analysis and compare the results of the analysis to the hospital's cash objectives.

P7.   Use the data provided for Problem 6. Since the cash flow analysis shows that cash flow is substantially under the cash objectives, a recommendation for both routine service and professional service rate adjustments must be made by the controller to the executive committee for implementation on October 1, 1986. The following additional information is available:

1. Projected patient days for the year ending September 30, 1987, are 72,870, of which 3,870 are applicable to newborn. The room rate adjustment per day is $6 for both categories. Additional income from patient day utilization can be obtained from the budget of operations.

2. Special professional service rate adjustment is $5 per day. Additional income from patient day utilization can be obtained from the budget of operations.

3. All deductions from earnings represent allowances resulting from cost reimbursed contractual arrangements with third parties. After the various rate adjustments and reimbursement calculations, the cost/charge relationship is 94.4 percent.

4. The rate adjustments will have an effect on both inpatient and outpatient accounts receivable and will cause an increase of $50,000 and $20,000 respectively.

Required. (1) Prepare a projected statement of operations for the year ending September 30, 1987, (after the rate adjustments have been in effect for one year) in comparison with the actual results of the year ended September 30, 1986, and showing variances in dollars. (2) Prepare a cash-flow statement resulting from rate adjustments and compare the statement to the cash objectives for the coming year. (3) Will the rate adjustments, as proposed, meet all objectives of the hospital? Do you have any comments regarding either the proposed rate adjustments or the cash objectives of the hospital?

P8. Following is information relating to current investments in marketable equity securities by Realcare Hospital:

1. 10/31/86: Purchased the following corporate stocks:

Company A	$1,000
Company B	2,000
Company C	3,000

2. 12/31/87: Quoted market values were:

Company A	$1,200
Company B	1,700
Company C	2,500

3. 10/31/88: Sold Company C stock for $2,200.

4. 11/30/88: Purchased Company D stock for $4,000.

5. 12/31/88: Quoted market values were:

Company A	$1,300
Company B	1,800
Company D	3,400

6. 10/31/89: Sold Company D stock for $4,300.

7. 11/30/89: Purchased Company E stock for $2,500.

8. 12/31/89: Quoted market values were:

Company A	$1,200
Company B	1,300
Company E	2,300

9.   11/30/90: Transferred Company B stock to noncurrent investment portfolio when Company B stock had a quoted market value of $1,400.

10.   12/31/90: Quoted market values were:
     Company A $ 900
     Company E   2,700

Required. Make all necessary entries for the 1987-1990 period, assuming the fiscal year ends December 31.

11
Receivables

The hospital's basic objective is to provide the health care services needed by the community it serves. These services typically are provided to all members of the community without regard to ability to pay. Legally, and as a matter of public relations, the hospital ordinarily cannot refuse its services to those in need. Some patients may never pay for the services provided to them, or they may pay only a portion of established charges. Other patients eventually pay their hospital bills, but it often takes some time. Even in cases where patients are covered by hospitalization insurance, there is a significant time-lag between the provision of services and collections from third-party payers.

As a result, hospitals are unable to operate on a cash basis in collecting for their services either from self-paying patients or from third parties. Hospitals literally are forced into the credit business; the extension of credit is largely an unavoidable operational necessity. Even the best-managed hospital may have as much as 75 percent of its current assets tied up in receivables.

Because of the magnitude of receivables in the hospital asset structure and the somewhat unique manner in which the hospital is paid for its services, it is most imperative that effective accounting procedures and administrative controls be developed and maintained for the investment in receivables. This chapter deals with a number of accounting and financial management matters relating to hospital receivables; certain other considerations relating to the management of this asset are discussed in Chapter 14.

NATURE AND COMPOSITION

The term **receivables**, as employed in hospital accounting, refers to the realizable cash value of the hospital's legal claims against patients, third-party payers, and others. Receivables arise primarily from the provision of healthcare services on a credit basis. Indeed, the hospital industry is one of the largest single grantors of credit in the economy of the United States. Collections on patients' accounts ordinarily are not received until some considerable time has elapsed after the related hospital services are rendered. In the meantime, the hospital has legal claims against patients and their sponsors for such services. These receivables, due to the nature and cost of hospital services as well as the third-party payment system, generally constitute the largest single hospital asset with the exception of the investment in property, plant, and equipment. It also must be recognized that the cost of extending credit is substantial. Even where interest is charged on patients' accounts, it is unlikely that interest charges would be adequate to cover the hospital's credit-granting, carrying, and collection costs.

In view of these facts, it seems obvious that considerable attention must be given to the management of the hospital investment in receivables. The basic objective is that of minimizing, insofar as feasible, the amount of that investment. To attain this objective, the adoption of sound accounting procedures and internal controls for receivables is an essential requirement. Hospital receivables may be classified as (1) those arising from the provision of hospital services to patients and (2) those arising from miscellaneous sources only indirectly related to the provision of health care services. A large majority of hospital receivables are of the first type, and they appear as current assets in the balance sheet of the hospital's Unrestricted Fund. The latter category of receivables also appears in the Unrestricted Fund, but they may be found in one or more of the restricted funds as well. Each of the two categories of receivables is discussed here.

Receivables from Patient Services

The major portion of hospital receivables arises directly from the provision of healthcare services to patients. In effect, the hospital exchanges its services, including goods and supplies, for the patient's and/or the third party's promise to pay for such services in the near future. It is an economic exchange measured in terms of the hospital's **full established** rates irrespective of expectations as to eventual collectibility. The entry basically is:

Receivables (appropriately classified) $XX,XXX
   Revenues (appropriately classified) $XX,XXX
  To record charges to patients' accounts for
services rendered.

As noted in Chapter 7, the recognition of revenues and the related assets must conform to the accrual basis of accounting. Revenues are recorded in the time period in which they are earned regardless of when, if ever, the associated cash inflows occur. Typically, there is a time-lag of varying duration between the rendering of services and the receipt of payment for such services, and this gives rise to legal claims against patients and third parties. These claims are called **receivables**.

In addition to an appropriate classification of revenue accounts on a responsibility accounting basis, debits to patients' accounts receivable should also be classified in a managerially useful manner. In view of the fact that patients' accounts typically are collected in part from patients and in part from third-party payers, hospitals usually require separate control accounts in three primary classifications somewhat as follows:

1. Inpatients Not Discharged ("in-house" accounts).
2. Inpatients Discharged.
3. Outpatients.

Each of these categories generally is subclassified according to the financial status of the patient, i.e., Blue Cross, Medicare, Medicaid, compensation and liability, self-pay, and indigent. These control accounts are supported by subsidiary ledger cards or other records that are frequently reconciled.

When a patient is discharged, or earlier, amounts initially charged to a particular control account often must be transferred to another control account, depending upon determinations of payer responsibilities and other considerations. In certain instances, patients may be asked to execute promissory notes to the hospital for the self-responsible portion of their unpaid accounts. It may be desirable in such cases to maintain a separate "notes receivable" control account, particularly where there is a large number of notes and they are of the interest-bearing type. This matter is considered further at a later point in this chapter.

A somewhat unique characteristic of hospital receivables, as compared with the receivables of other organizations, is that the full rates charged to patients' accounts very often are not collected. Charges incurred by patients usually are settled at amounts less than full rates by reason of contractual arrangements, charity service, policy discounts, and bad debts. As a result, the proper valuation of accounts receivable for balance sheet presentation requires special attention. This matter also has important implications with respect to the income statement.

Receivables from Miscellaneous Sources

Hospital receivables may also arise in relatively small amounts from transactions that are only indirectly related to the provision of services to patients. Included in this category are accruals for interest, dividends, and rental income earned but not yet received in cash. Advances to employees, unpaid tuition charges to students enrolled in hospital-operated educational programs, pledges receivable from donors, claims against insurance companies resulting from insured losses, and reasonably certain prospective refunds are also examples of miscellaneous receivables. Where collection of these receivables within one year is a normal expectation, they are classified as current assets; otherwise, if material in amount, they should be reported under a noncurrent caption in the balance sheet. Full and separate disclosure should be made of the nature of all material amounts of miscellaneous receivables.

Significant debit balances in accounts payable, because of the accounting rule against offsetting assets and liabilities, also should be classified as receivables. Similarly, material credit balances in accounts receivable resulting from patients' deposits or overpayments should be reported as liabilities.

Advance payments to suppliers on merchandise purchase contracts are properly reported as current assets. Advances to vendors for the purchase of plant and equipment items, however, should be classified as noncurrent assets.

VALUATION OF RECEIVABLES

Theoretically, notes and accounts receivable should be reported in the hospital balance sheet at their net realizable or cash value. In other words, the gross amount of receivables recorded at full service rates in the accounts should be reduced to the net amount that can be reasonably estimated to be actually collectible in cash. Appropriate estimates, as described below, should be made of the amounts uncollectible due to charity service, contractual adjustments, courtesy discounts, bad debts, and administrative adjustments. Such amounts should be treated as reductions of gross receivables in the balance sheet by the use of suitable "allowance" accounts. These amounts should also be included as "revenue deductions" in the income statement of the period in which the receivables arose. This procedure is required to obtain a proper matching of revenues and revenue deductions on an accrual basis as well as to secure a proper balance sheet valuation of receivables.

In addition to uncollectible amounts that are susceptible to reasonable estimation, accounting theory also requires that receivables be reduced by any unearned interest charges included in their face amounts. Even where specific interest charges are not made on patients' notes and accounts, the AICPA suggests that (theoretically) receivables be reduced by any interest **implicit** in their face amount, i.e., that receivables be discounted to **present value** by an **imputed** rate of interest appropriate under the circumstances.[1] If a noninterest-bearing note receivable of $2,160 will not be collected until one year hence, for example, and money is worth 8 percent, the receivable, and the related service revenue, should be recorded at $2,000 ($2,160/1.08) with the $160 being accrued as interest income over the period the note receivable remains outstanding. Or, if the receivable is recorded at $2,160, the difference between the recorded amount and the present value should be recorded as a discount to be amortized as interest income over the collection period.

While this procedure is theoretically sound, it generally is not feasible with respect to receivables arising from transactions with patients and their sponsors in the normal course of hospital business and due within approximately one year. Since the Accounting Principles Board specifically provided for such exceptions, it is assumed here that ordinary short-term receivables need not be discounted to present value. Hospitals that arrange patient payment terms that result in material amounts of receivables which extend over a longer period, however, may need to apply the present value procedure to such receivables. A similar need may arise where a hospital's accounts include long-term pledges receivable in connection with a construction program.

Valuation Allowance—Bad Debts

It is reasonable to expect that a certain amount of receivables arising from services provided to self-responsible patients will prove to be uncollectible. At the time of admission, or as soon thereafter as practicable, the financial status of each patient should be determined so that an appropriate classification and distinction can be made between uncollectible amounts arising from patients' unwillingness to pay (bad debts) and those arising from patients' inability to pay (charity service). Bad debts also may arise from the uninsured portion of the accounts of patients covered by Blue Cross or other hospitalization insurance. The commercial business will not extend credit unless collection is reasonably assured, but the hospital is not permitted this luxury. This is not to say, however, that the hospital's credit and collection procedures need not be seriously regarded or that a high percentage of bad debt losses should be accepted as inevitable and beyond control. To the contrary, the hospital must work as hard, or harder, than the commercial enterprise in its efforts to reduce such losses to a minimum.

Estimation of Bad Debts. At the end of the accounting period, an estimate must be made of the amount of receivables which ultimately will prove to be bad debts. This is necessary in order to prevent an overstatement of assets in the balance sheet and to provide for a proper matching of revenues and deductions from revenues in the income statement of the period in which the receivables arose. It is a procedure required under the accrual basis of accounting.

Assume, for example, that a hospital charges patients $900,000 for services provided during a given year and that $400,000 of this amount is collected. At the end of the year, then, accounts receivable amount to $500,000. Also assume that operating expenses for the period total $850,000. If nothing is done with respect to potential bad debts, the hospital balance sheet will include accounts receivable of $500,000 among the assets, and the hospital's income statement will report a net income of $50,000 ($900,000 − $850,000).

Suppose, however, that $50,000 of the accounts receivable prove to be uncollectible in the ensuing year. As these accounts were deemed worthless by the credit manager, they were at that time recognized as losses (revenue deductions). Such a procedure obviously results in placement of the bad debt losses in the wrong year! The $50,000 of bad debts should have been given accounting recognition in the first year, the year in which the related revenue was recorded. There is a serious mismatching of revenues and revenue "losses" here. The reported net income of the first year should have been **zero**, not $50,000. In addition, there was an overstatement of assets (accounts receivable) in the balance sheet at the end of the first year. The accounts should have been reflected in the balance sheet at net realizable cash value, or $450,000.

The difficulty, of course, is that it is impossible to predict precisely which **specific** accounts will prove to be bad debts. It also is impossible to estimate, with exactitude, the **total** dollar amount of accounts that will prove to be uncollectible in the future. Nevertheless, reasonable estimates can be made so that the degree of misstatement in the financial statements will be minimized to an acceptable level.

As discussed in the author's **Introduction to Hospital Accounting**, there are three methods by which bad debts may be estimated for accrual basis accounting purposes. These methods are:

1. Application of a percentage, based on past experience, to the balance of accounts receivable at the end of the accounting period.
2. Application of a percentage, based on past experience, to the total of charges to patients' accounts during the accounting period.
3. Determination through an analysis of individual accounts in the patients' ledger taking into account the length of time each account has remained unpaid. This method is called **aging** the accounts receivable.

As a matter of actual practice, hospitals generally employ all three methods, comparing the results of each so as to arrive at the most accurate estimate possible of probable bad debts.

The percentage used in these methods is usually an average percentage based upon several prior years' experience and tempered by expectations of conditions that might exist in the subsequent collection period. It may be found, for example, that in recent years about 10 percent of the accounts outstanding at year-end became worthless. If factors influencing collections of receivables are not expected to be materially different, then one could estimate that 10 percent of accounts receivable at the end of the current year might prove to be worthless.

The **aging** procedure is likely to provide the most accurate estimate of the amount of bad debts that might arise from current receivables in the next accounting period. It also is the most managerially useful method in that it requires a detailed examination of patients' accounts on an individual account basis. As is shown in Figure 11-1, account balances are classified into "age" groups, depending upon the number of days that have elapsed since the date of discharge. (The **aging** also may be made on the basis of time elapsed since the date of the last payment received on each account.) Totals are obtained for each group, and appropriate percentages based on past experience are applied to these totals to obtain an estimate of probable bad debts. As might be expected, the percentage that is applied increases with the age of the accounts. The older the account, the less likely it is to be collected. Collectibility, in fact, decreases with age at an increasing rate.

Figure 11-1.
Accounts Receivable Aging Schedule
December 31, 1986

Patient Name	Account Balance	In-House	1–30	31–60	61–90	91–180	Over 180
Able, James W. (etc.)	1482			1482			
Totals	500000	150000	120000	140000	30000	40000	20000
Percentage		.02	.05	.10	.20	.25	.50
Estimated Bad Debts (Total: $49000)		3000	6000	14000	6000	10000	10000

Referring to the data of the previous illustration and assuming that bad debts are estimated at $49,000, the appropriate entry at the end of 1986 is:

Provision for Bad Debts	$49,000	
Allowance for Bad Debts		$49,000

   To record required provision for bad debts as
estimated by accounts receivable aging schedule.

It should be noted that no specific accounts are written off because, at this time, it is not known which specific accounts will prove uncollectible. Instead, the estimated total amount of bad debts is credited to a so-called valuation account. The balance sheet presentation at December 31, 1986, is:

Accounts Receivable	$500,000	
Less Allowance for Bad Debts	49,000	$451,000

Thus, the allowance account serves to reduce the valuation of accounts receivable to net realizable value ($451,000) for balance sheet presentation purposes. The allowance account is sometimes titled **reserve for bad debts**, but that is unfortunate terminology. The term **reserve** often is interpreted by the layman to mean a fund of money set aside for some rainy day. There is, of course, no money in the account. For this reason, the use of the word **reserve** should be avoided in financial reporting.

The **provision for bad debts** account, sometimes called **bad debts expense** or **provision for doubtful accounts**, generally is presented in the income statement as a deduction from revenues, as follows:

Gross Patient Service Revenues	$900,000	
Less Deductions from Revenues:		
Provision for Bad Debts	49,000	
Net Patient Service Revenues		$851,000
Less Operating Expenses		850,000
1986 Net Income		$ 1,000

It has been argued that estimated bad debts should be presented in the income statement as an operating expense rather than as a revenue deduction. In fact, the HFMA's Principles and Practices Board recently issued an exposure draft in which it is proposed that the provision for bad debts be reported as an expense.[2] There is theoretical merit in this point of view, but current practice tends to favor the presentation indicated above.

Write-Off of Uncollectible Accounts. Assume that during the ensuing year (1987), a total of $850,000 is collected on the December 31, 1986, receivables. A summary entry is given below:

Cash in Bank	$850,000	
Accounts Receivable		$850,000
To record collections on accounts receivable during 1987.		

Assume also that the hospital credit manager notifies the accountant that the remaining $50,000 of receivables are uncollectible and should be written off as bad debts. As a result, the following entry is required:

Allowance for Bad Debts	$ 50,000	
Accounts Receivable		$ 50,000

   To record the write-off of uncollectible
accounts receivable deemed to be bad debts.

The specific accounts written off at this time are removed or otherwise eliminated from the active section of the patients' subsidiary ledger. Records of accounts written off are placed in an inactive file and are retained under the control of a responsible employee who does not have access to incoming cash receipts. This is an important internal control requirement designed to prevent the theft of subsequent cash collections, if any, on written-off accounts.

If payments are received on accounts previously written off, the accounting procedure often followed is to debit Cash in Bank and credit a Recovery of Accounts Written Off account. The recovery is reflected in the income statement of the period as a reduction of the Provision for Bad Debts. Appropriate notation of such payments should be made on the patients' ledger cards so that an accurate credit history is maintained.

    Subsequent-Year Procedure. Assume that the required Provision for Bad Debts at the end of 1987 is $57,000, determined in the manner previously described. A problem arises in that the Allowance for Bad Debts account at this date has a debit balance of $1,000 ($50,000 − $49,000). In other words, actual bad debts arising from the December 31, 1986, accounts receivable were $1,000 greater than was estimated. This means that the reported net income for 1986 was overstated by $1,000; the net income should have been zero. In addition, the December 31, 1986, accounts receivable were overstated in the balance sheet of that date by $1,000. Relatively small misstatements of this sort cannot be avoided, and it should not be a cause for concern. The misstatement might well have been in the other direction. In any event, a $1,000 misstatement is preferable to a $50,000 error which would have resulted had no estimate been made at all.

No revision or adjustment of the reported data for 1986 is necessary. In earlier years, a correction of the prior year's net income might have been recognized in some way, but that is no longer acceptable accounting procedure in ordinary circumstances. Instead, as provided in APB Opinion No. 20, normally recurring adjustments of the type illustrated here should be made in the income statement of the current period.[3]

Thus, if an Allowance for Bad Debts of $57,000 is required at the end of 1987 when the account has a debit balance of $1,000, the necessary entry is:

Provision for Bad Debts	$ 58,000	
Allowance for Bad Debts		$ 58,000

   To record required provision for bad debts at
December 31, 1987, as follows:

Required allowance	$57,000
Present balance (debit)	1,000
Required provision for bad debts	$58,000

In a sense, this is tantamount to saying that two wrongs make a right. The **under**statement of bad debts in 1986 is countered by a purposeful **over**statement of the provision for bad debts for 1987. While a slight misstatement is made in each year, the two years taken together are correct. The errors are counterbalancing.

Direct Write-Off Method. In contrast to the **allowance** (accrual basis) method, some organizations choose to account for bad debts by the direct write-off method. No allowance account is established or maintained, and uncollectible accounts are charged off against the revenues of the period in which the accounts are deemed to be worthless. Although this method has the advantage of greater objectivity and eliminates the necessity for estimating probable bad debts, it clearly overstates receivables and may not properly match bad debts against the revenues to which they are related. The allowance method previously described would appear to be much more appropriate for hospital accounting and financial (credit) management purposes.

Valuation Allowances—Other

It was shown in Chapter 7 that operating revenues should be credited and receivables should be debited, on the accrual basis, for **all** hospital services rendered to **all** patients, regardless of financial status, at the hospital's **full** established rates. The hospital, however, often will not collect these full-rate charges. A certain amount of "revenue losses" can be expected because of bad debts. Additional revenue losses may occur because of contractual agreements with third parties under which the hospital receives less than its full rates but is prohibited from recovering the difference directly from the patients involved. Other significant revenue losses are experienced in connection with the provision of free (charity) service to the medically indigent who are unable to pay more than a fraction, if any, of normal charges. Finally, hospitals sometimes grant courtesy discounts or allowances to members of religious orders and to employees.

Because operating revenues are recorded on the accrual basis, the **matching principle** of accounting requires that revenue losses (revenue deductions) also be recognized and recorded on the accrual basis. Misstatements of reported assets and operating results will occur when this requirement is not observed.

To illustrate, assume that gross revenues from services to patients amount to $800,000 during 1986. Operating expenses for the year are $747,000. Assume also that $650,000 of the gross revenues are collected, leaving $150,000 of accounts receivable at December 31, 1986. If potential revenue losses in year-end accounts receivable are ignored, the income statement for 1986 would report a net income of $53,000 ($800,000 − $747,000), and the assets in the year-end balance sheet would include $150,000 of receivables. Suppose, however, that only $102,000 of the receivables are actually collected in the ensuing year and that the uncollected balance of $48,000 is attributable to:

Bad Debts	$ 9,000
Charity Service	21,000
Contractual Adjustments	15,000
Courtesy Discounts	3,000
Total Revenue Losses	$48,000

Clearly, when potential revenue losses included in year-end receivables are not properly anticipated, the financial statements for the year will be incorrect.

It therefore is necessary to make an analysis of receivables at the end of the reporting period to determine whether a significant portion is likely to be uncollectible for the reasons stated above. This may be done by a direct analysis of individual accounts or on a percentage basis developed from a sample of the accounts or from past experience. An entry somewhat as follows then can be made in the accounts:

Deductions from Revenues —		
Provision for Bad Debts	$ 9,000	
Charity Service	21,000	
Contractual Adjustments	15,000	
Courtesy Discounts	3,000	
Allowance for Uncollectible Accounts —		
Bad Debts		$ 9,000
Charity Service		21,000
Contractual Adjustments		15,000
Courtesy Discounts		3,000
To record estimated revenue deductions included in December 31, 1986, accounts receivable of $150,000, as follows:		
Bad debts (6%)	$ 9,000	
Charity service (14%)	21,000	
Contractual adjustments (10%)	15,000	
Courtesy discounts (2%)	3,000	
Total	$48,000	

Where the precise amounts of the revenue deductions can be determined for each individual patient's account, credits may be made directly to accounts receivable rather than to the allowance accounts. This procedure, however, generally is not feasible.

The effect of the above entry on the reported results of operations for the year 1986 is noted below:

Gross Revenues		$800,000
Less Deductions from Revenues:		
Provision for Bad Debts	$ 9,000	
Charity Service	21,000	
Contractual Adjustments	15,000	
Courtesy Discounts	3,000	48,000
Net Revenues		752,000
Less Operating Expense		747,000
Net Income		$ 5,000

Thus, the 1986 net income is reported as $5,000 rather than the $53,000 that would have been reported had revenue losses not been anticipated. In addition, the December 31, 1986, balance sheet should reflect $150,000 of receivables reduced by an Allowance for Uncollectible Accounts of $48,000, i.e., at the net realizable value of $102,000.

ACCOUNTING FOR NOTES RECEIVABLE

It is not uncommon for hospitals to accept promissory notes from patients who, faced with a substantial bill for hospital services, require some extended period of time to accumulate the resources with which to pay their accounts. In some cases, the face amount of such notes is payable in a single amount at a specified maturity date. Under other arrangements, the face amount may be payable in equal periodic (weekly or monthly) installments over a specified period of time. These notes may or may not bear interest. Although hospital managements historically have regarded the charging of interest as morally wrong or unwise from a public relations standpoint, the charging of interest by hospitals is currently viewed as both necessary and justifiable.

Term Notes Receivable

Assume, for example, that a patient signs an 8%, 90-day promissory note on September 1, 1987, in settlement of a $4,500 hospital bill. The interest on this note is $90 ($4,500 x .08 x 90/360). It should be recognized on the basis of the passage of time, and should be recorded by the hospital as earned income through monthly accruals as shown in Figure 11-2. In this illustration, the interest income is $1 per day. Elapsed days between two dates are computed by counting the first day or the last day, but not both, i.e., the number of days from September 1 to September 30 is 29. At the maturity date of the above note, November 30, 1987, the hospital will collect $4,590. Journal entries to record all matters pertaining to this note are presented in Figure 11-2.

Figure 11-2.
Accounting for Notes Receivable
Summary of Journal Entries

Notes Receivable	$4,500	
Accounts Receivable		$4,500
To record receipt of 8%, 90-day note for $4,500 on September 1, 1987		
Accrued Interest Receivable	$ 29	
Interest Income		$ 29
To record interest income earned in September.		
Accrued Interest Receivable	$ 31	
Interest Income		$ 31
To record interest income earned in October.		
Accrued Interest Receivable	$ 30	
Interest Income		$ 30
To record interest income earned in November.		
Cash in Bank	$4,590	
Accrued Interest Receivable		$ 90
Notes Receivable		4,500
To record collection of note and accrued interest on November 30, 1987		

Should the patient fail to pay the note at maturity, a debit of $4,590 is made to Dishonored Notes Receivable rather than to Cash in Bank. The failure of the patient to honor the note in no way changes the fact that interest income of $90 was earned. If further collection efforts are unsuccessful, the $4,590 may be written off as a bad debt.

Installment Notes Receivable

Where the principal amount of a note receivable is collected in periodic installments, the accounting procedure is more complicated than for term notes as illustrated above. Arrangements vary, and it is not possible to describe all of them here. Consider, however, an arrangement under which the patient agrees to pay an account balance of $500 in five equal monthly installments commencing in one month. Interest is to be charged at the rate of 1 percent per month.

The first step is to determine the amount of the required monthly payments. This is best accomplished by reference to standard compound interest tables (see Table 4 in Appendix A) from which a factor (4.8534) representing the present value of an ordinary annuity of $1 per period for 5 periods at 1% per period can be located. The required monthly payment is computed by dividing the principal amount to be paid ($500) by the appropriate factor (4.8534). In this case, the monthly payment is $103.02, and collections of these payments would be recorded as indicated by the schedule shown in Figure 11-3.

Figure 11-3.
Installment Notes Receivable
Schedule of Collections

Month	Monthly Payments			Balance
	Amount	Interest*	Principal	
				$500.00
1	$103.02	$ 5.00	$ 98.02	401.98
2	103.02	4.02	99.00	302.98
3	103.02	3.03	99.99	202.99
4	103.02	2.03	100.99	102.00
5	103.02	1.02	102.00	. . .
	$515.10	$ 15.10	$500.00	

*1% of unpaid balance.

Consider, for instance, the receipt of the first monthly installment payment of $103.02. The necessary entry is:

Cash in Bank	$103.02	
Interest Income		$ 5.00
Installment Notes Receivable		98.02
To record receipt of initial installment		
payment on patient's note.		

As each subsequent payment is received, a decreasing portion is credited to interest income; an increasing portion is applied to the reduction of principal.

In all cases where interest charges are made, either on notes or on accounts, the hospital must exercise extreme care in complying fully with the requirements of the Truth in Lending laws. The patient must be fully informed of the actual or effective interest rate being charged, the total amount to be paid (interest and principal) under the arrangement, and all other significant matters. It is also essential that the necessity for charging interest be explained in terms understandable to patients.

FINANCING WITH RECEIVABLES

Much of the cash resources required in the normal operating activities of a hospital arise from the collection of receivables. When the volume of activity increases and larger investments in receivables result, or when the collection process slows, hospitals sometimes find themselves in a "tight" cash position where cash requirements exceed the amounts currently available from the usual inflow sources. In such cases, it may be possible to alleviate the situation temporarily by using current receivables to obtain needed cash immediately rather than waiting out the normal collection cycle. This may be accomplished by (1) selling receivables, (2) using receivables as collateral for borrowing, and (3) discounting patients' notes receivable. These steps generally are taken only in times of serious financial distress, but satisfactory continuing arrangements of these types have been worked out by many hospitals in cooperation with local financial institutions.

Sale of Receivables

The early conversion of receivables into cash may be effected by selling the receivables outright to a financial institution. The procedure is known as **factoring**. The credit risk, collection effort, and waiting period typically are transferred to the factor for a fee which includes a commission as well as interest. While the amount of the fee invariably is substantial, it does vary according to the size of the transaction, the quality of the accounts involved, and the particular obligations assumed by the factor. Patients usually are notified of the arrangement and are instructed to make future payments on account directly to the factor. If the factoring is arranged on a "non-notification basis," however, the hospital receives patients' remittances and is required to turn them over to the factor. No special accounting problems arise in connection with ordinary factoring arrangements. It is important that the factor be chosen according to the same criteria that one would use in selecting a collection agency.

Assignment of Receivables

The use of receivables as collateral for short-term borrowings is much more common than is the sale of receivables by hospitals. In many instances, this involves a relatively simple pledge of accounts receivable under an agreement to apply collections on such accounts exclusively to the retirement of a loan from a bank or other financial institution. No special accounting problems arise in such arrangements, but full disclosure must be made in the hospital's financial statements of all significant details of the pledging and loan agreement.

Under a more formal arrangement called **assignment**, the hospital may assign (pledge) all or some portion of its receivables to an assignee (lender) in return for an immediate cash advance on the receivables. The cash advance typically is less than 100 percent of the face amount of receivables assigned and is evidenced by an interest-bearing promissory note executed by the hospital to the assignee. The hospital usually retains the credit risk and continues its usual collection efforts. Patients generally are not aware of the assignment of their accounts; they make payments on account to the hospital which, in turn, remits such collections to the assignee at agreed times.

To illustrate, assume that on March 1 a hospital assigns $150,000 of its accounts receivable and receives a cash advance of $135,000 less a financing fee of a flat 2.5%. A note for $135,000 is executed that requires interest of 1.5% per month on the unpaid balance. Assume also that during March the hospital collects $86,025 on the assigned accounts and remits this amount to the assignee on March 31. The appropriate entries are:

March 1

Assigned Accounts Receivable	$150,000	
Financing Expense ($2.5% of $135,000)	3,375	
Cash in Bank ($135,000−$3,375)	131,625	
Accounts Receivable		$150,000
Notes Payable to Assignee		135,000
To record assignment of $150,000 of		
patients' accounts receivable.		

During March

Cash in Bank	$ 86,025	
Assigned Accounts Receivable		$ 86,025
To record collections on assigned accounts.		

March 31

Notes Payable to Assignee	$ 84,000	
Interest Expense	2,025	
Cash in Bank		$ 86,025
To record remittance of March collections on		
assigned accounts to assignee, including		
interest of $2,025 (1.5% of $135,000).		

Matters pertaining to this assignment may be shown in the hospital's March 31 balance sheet in the following manner:

Accounts Receivable

Unassigned		$424,763
Assigned	$ 63,975	
Less note payable to assignee	51,000	
Equity in assigned accounts		12,975
Total		$437,738

The general accounting rule against the offsetting of assets and liabilities is not applicable in this situation in that collections on the assigned accounts are legally earmarked to liquidation of the note.

Now assume that April collections on the assigned accounts total $54,475. On April 30, the amount owed to the assignee is paid, and the assignment agreement is terminated. The entries are:

<u>During April</u>

Cash in Bank	$ 54,475	
Assigned Accounts Receivable		$ 54,475
To record collections on assigned accounts.		

<u>April 30</u>

Notes Payable to Assignee	$ 51,000	
Interest Expense (1.5% of $51,000)	765	
Cash in Bank		$ 51,765
To record final remittance to assignee.		

Accounts Receivable	$ 9,500	
Assigned Accounts Receivable		$ 9,500
To transfer uncollected balance of previously assigned accounts back to accounts receivable.		

Discounting of Notes Receivable

Another method of financing with receivables involves the discounting of patients' notes receivable with a bank or other financial institution. In other words, the hospital transfers patients' notes to a bank in exchange for cash in an amount equal to the discounted present value of the maturity amount (interest and principal) of the notes. Assume, for example, that a 120-day, 6% note for $3,000 is received from a patient upon discharge from the hospital. If the note is immediately discounted at 9% at a bank, the proceeds to the hospital would be $2,968.20, determined as follows:

Face Value	$3,000.00
Add Interest to Maturity ($3,000 x .06 x 120/360)	60.00
Maturity Value	3,060.00
Less Bank Discount ($3,060 x .09 x 120/360)	91.80
Proceeds of Note	$2,968.20

Thus, the hospital obtains for 120 days the use of $2,968.20 which would not otherwise be available for meeting operating requirements. Should the patient dishonor the note at maturity, the hospital must pay the bank the maturity value of the note, plus a service charge, unless the note was discounted **without** recourse. Because notes customarily are discounted **with** recourse, the hospital is contingently liable to the bank until the maturity date. This contingent liability must be fully disclosed either parenthetically or by footnote in the hospital's balance sheet.

INTERNAL CONTROL

The control of the hospital investment in receivables is inextricably linked with the control of revenues. Methods and procedures differ greatly from one hospital to another, and specific systems are beyond the scope of discussion in this book. Certain observations of a general nature, however, can be made.

Receivables control begins in the admitting process where complete and accurate information must be secured so that an initial determination can be made of each patient's financial status and unnecessary delays may be avoided in subsequent collection efforts. Patients typically are concerned about the amount of the obligation they may incur to the hospital and, where it is feasible, they should be informed of established hospital charges, the extent to which these charges may be covered by their insurance, and the hospital's credit and collection policies. In some instances, deposits or advance payments may be requested. These matters can be handled in a tactful manner in preadmission procedures and often in the admitting interview itself. Much depends upon impressions created by the admitting personnel, the efficiency of the admitting process, and even the physical characteristics of the admitting office itself. Readers having a special interest in this subject should examine the AHA's **Manual of Admitting Practices and Procedures.**

Once patients are admitted, the accounting system should be such as to provide a high degree of assurance that **all** billable services rendered to patients are promptly and accurately charged to patients' accounts. Here again is the inseparable relationship between receivables and revenues. Unrecorded revenues are unlikely to be charged; if not charged, they will not be billed and, therefore, will not be collected. On the other hand, incorrect charges and "late" charges also are damaging, although for different reasons. In any event, the first phase of receivables control is that of establishing appropriate **debits** in patients' accounts. Internal controls over charges are as important as internal controls over credits.

Assuming that complete and accurate charges are made to patients' accounts, the objective becomes that of maximum collection of such charges either from the patients directly or from third parties. Appropriate determinations must be made promptly as to the portion of charges recoverable from each payer, and suitable billings must be prepared on a timely basis. Follow up procedures are particularly important so as to avoid tying up the hospital's working capital in unnecessarily large unpaid balances of receivables. Studies clearly indicate that the degree of collectibility is inversely related to the length of time an account remains unpaid.

The billing function usually should be performed by someone other than cashiers or those who maintain the patients' subsidiary ledger records. Patients' complaints concerning incorrect billings should be investigated and resolved by a responsible employee working independently of billing, cash receipts, and receivables accounting. As collections are received, sound procedures should be followed to assure that patients' accounts are promptly and properly credited. Noncash credits made to accounts receivable deserve particular attention as such credits often are used to hide errors and defalcations. Some hospitals, for example, do not actually write off bad debt accounts but continue to carry them indefinitely in a special control account against which a 100 percent allowance is maintained. Sound credit and collection systems are vital to the control and management of the huge investment hospitals have in receivables. A considerable volume of literature is available in this important area to the interested reader.

A basic requirement for effective internal control over receivables is a regular reconciliation of subsidiary ledgers with related general ledger control accounts. This process is facilitated through the maintenance of several control accounts along the lines suggested earlier in this chapter. Continued and significant differences disclosed by the reconciliation process should always be examined carefully. Control accounts and subsidiary ledgers also provide the information required for managerial reports and analyses relating to the investment in receivables. Some of these reports are described in Chapter 14, which deals with the management of working capital.

CHAPTER 11 FOOTNOTES

1. APB Opinion No. 21, **Interest on Receivables and Payables** (New York: AICPA, 1972).

2. Principles and Practices Board, **The Presentation of Patient Service Revenue and Related Issues** (Oak Brook, Illinois: HFMA, 1985), p. 11.

3. APB Opinion No. 20, **Accounting Changes** (New York: AICPA, 1971).

QUESTIONS

1. Soon after Peerless Hospital had mailed statements to patients on the first of the month, three complaints were received stating that credit had not been given for checks mailed at least a week before the end of the previous month. Upon investigation, the proper credits were found to have been made to the patients' accounts as of the second and third of the month. Is there any need for further investigation? Explain.

2. With respect to accounts receivable, what questions might be asked to determine the extent of internal control in effect?

3. You have just recently been appointed controller of a 300-bed general hospital with inpatient receivables averaging about $380,000, of which some $300,000 is receivable from discharged patients. The accounts receivable are handled by machine. You find that no effort has been made to balance the accounts receivable detail against the general ledger control account during the past several years. What steps would you take to establish and maintain good internal controls receivable?

4. Why do hospitals have standard charges for services rendered to all patients and then treat charity and other allowances as reductions of income? Should bad debts be considered as a reduction of income or as an expense? Why?

5. What are the advantages, if any, of accepting notes receivable from patients in temporary settlement of their accounts?

6. List what you believe to be some of the more important features of a good credit and collection program in a hospital.

7. What are the objectives of an audit of hospital receivables? Name some of the procedures completed by the auditor in the audit of patients' unpaid accounts.

8. Describe three methods of estimating the required provision for bad debts. Which method is preferable for hospitals?

9. Why is it necessary to provide for an allowance for bad debts prior to the time specific accounts receivable are deemed uncollectible?

10. Why is the collection of an account receivable written off in a previous year not a direct adjustment to the Unrestricted Fund balance?

11. Describe three methods of "financing with receivables" that are available to hospitals.

12. Identify and explain the nature of four deductions that are made in arriving at a balance sheet valuation for accounts receivable.

13. Distinguish between the **allowance** and the **direct charge-off** methods of accounting for bad debts.

EXERCISES

E1. On September 1, Amtex Hospital accepted a 90-day, 6% note for $1,600 from each of three patients in settlement of their past due accounts. Concerning these notes:

Note 1: Collected note and accrued interest at maturity.

Note 2: Patient prepaid interest on September 1. Principal amount collected at maturity.

Note 3: Discounted note on October 1 at First National Bank (discount rate, 8%). Patient honored note at maturity.

Required. Prepare all entries necessary to record properly all matters relating to the above promissory notes.

E2. The Aberdeen Hospital received from a patient a 60-day, 6% note for $3,000, dated November 6. Thirty days later the hospital discounted the note at the bank at 6% and recorded the contingent liability. At maturity the bank protested nonpayment of the note by the patient and charged the hospital with protest fees of $10 in addition to the amount due on the note. Sixty days later the hospital collected the amount due, with interest at 8% on $3,000 charged from the due date to date of collection.

Required. Prepare entries for all of the above transactions.

E3. Lacey Hospital employs the accrual system of accounting. On June 30, just before the annual closing of the books, the balance of patients' accounts receivable was $645,600 and the allowance for uncollectible accounts had a debit balance of $3,250.

Required. (1) Prepare the entry to make provision for the estimated uncollectible accounts at June 30, assuming that it is estimated that 10 percent of the June 30 receivables will prove to be uncollectible. (2) Prepare the entry on September 1 to write off the $1,400 account of George Patient as uncollectible. (3) Prepare the entry to record the collection of George Patient's account on November 1.

E4. On March 1, Alpha Hospital assigned $100,000 of its accounts receivable to Zero Finance Company, receiving an 80 percent advance net of a finance charge of 2 percent on the advance. Collections are to be made by the assignor and remitted to the assignee monthly with interest at 1% per month. The following additional transactions were completed:

1. During March, Alpha collected $48,000 on the assigned accounts.

2. On March 31, Alpha remitted the March collections with interest to Zero.

3. On April 30, Alpha remitted the balance due to the assignee, thereby terminating the assignment contract.

Required. (1) Prepare the entries on the books of Alpha Hospital to record all of the above. (2) Indicate how the situation at March 31 would be reflected in Alpha Hospital's balance sheet.

E5. During 1987, Bloom Hospital charged patients' accounts for a total of $2,450,000. Its general ledger at December 31, 1987 (the end of the fiscal year), shows the following balances:

Patients' accounts receivable	$316,000 Dr.
Allowance for uncollectible accounts	1,750 Cr.

Required. Prepare the necessary adjusting entries for estimated doubtful accounts under each of the following assumptions: (1) doubtful accounts are estimated at 2 percent of charges, (2) doubtful accounts are estimated at 15 percent of the accounts receivable and (3) doubtful accounts, based upon an aging of the receivables, are estimated at $51,400.

E6. Bradley Healthcare Center provides an allowance for its doubtful accounts receivable. At 12/31/87, the allowance account had a credit balance of $4,000. Each month, Bradley accrues bad debts in an amount equal to one percent of gross revenues. Gross revenues for 1988 were $1,000,000. During 1988, uncollectible accounts of $16,000 were written off against the allowance account. An aging of accounts receivable at 12/31/88, indicates that an allowance of $20,000 should be provided for doubtful accounts at that date.

Required. By how much should bad debts previously accrued during 1988 be increased at 12/31/88?

PROBLEMS

P1. Carson Hospital has been in operation for five years but its balance sheet does not carry an allowance for bad accounts; bad accounts having been written off when deemed uncollectible and recoveries credited to income as collected. The hospital's policy has been to write off at December 31 of each year those accounts on which no collections have been received for three months. The hospital wishes to revise its accounts for 1987 to give effect to bad account treatment on the allowance basis. The allowance is to be based on a percentage of charges derived from the experience of prior years. Statistics for the past five years are as follows:

		Accounts Written Off		Recoveries	
	Charges	Year of Origin	Amount	Year of Origin	Amount
1983	$100,000	1983	$ 550		
1984	250,000	1983	1,500	1983	$ 100
		1984	1,000		
1985	300,000	1983	500	1984	400
		1984	4,000		
		1985	1,300		
1986	325,000	1984	1,200	1985	500
		1985	4,500		
		1986	1,500		
1987	275,000	1985	2,700	1986	600
		1987	5,000		
		1987	1,400		

Accounts receivable at December 31, 1987, were as follows:

1986 accounts	$ 15,000	3%
1987 accounts	135,000	5%
Total	$150,000	

Required. Prepare the adjusting entry (with an appropriate explanation) to set up the Allowance of Uncollectible Accounts. Show all computations.

P2. The following data are taken from the accounts of the Unrestricted Fund of Community Hospital at December 31, 1986, (after closing) and at December 31, 1987, (before closing):

		December 31, 1986		December 31, 1987	
101.01	Cash		$ 73,566		$114,048
103.01	Accounts receivable		418,470		500,824
104.01	Allowance for uncollectibles	$(25,107)		$ (195,625)	
104.11	Accounts written off			166,068	
104.21	Recovery of write-offs		(25,107)	(21,477)	(51,004)
105.01	Other receivables		15,672		19,465
107.01	Inventory		62,725		101,660
108.01	Prepaid expenses		1,119		2,009
109.01	Due from other funds				89,529
			$546,446		$776,531
111.01	Accounts payable		$ 7,936		$ 24,747
112.01	Accrued salaries and wages		50,952		57,251
113.01	Withholdings payable				18,597
			58,888		100,595
191.01	Fund balance		487,558		487,558
193.01	Summary-Revenue from services to patients			$3,407,320	
194.01	Summary-Deductions from patient revenue			(349,942)	
195.01	Summary-Nonpatient revenue			137,431	
196.01	Summary-Expense			(3,006,431)	188,378
			487,558		675,936
			$546,446		$776,531

1. There are no material differences in the type of accounts (Blue Cross, liability, compensation, etc.) which make up the accounts receivable at each date. There has been no material change in either revenue from services to patients or in deductions from patient revenue from 1986 to 1987.

2. The provision for bad debts is included in summary account #194.01-deductions from patient revenue. The provision for bad debts is recorded monthly by the following entry:

690.01	Provision for bad debts	$xx,xxx	
104.01	Allowance for uncollectibles		$xx,xxx

No other entries have been made to account 104.01 during the year.

3. Accounts determined to be uncollectible are written off monthly by the following entry:

104.11	Accounts written off	$xx,xxx	
103.01	Accounts receivable		$xx,xxx

4. Collections on accounts previously written off are recorded monthly by the following entry:

101.01	Cash	$xx,xxx	
104.21	Recovery of write-offs		$xx,xxx

5. Accounts 104.11 and 104.21 are closed to account 104.01 at the end of the year.

Required. Compute the following and comment on the adequacy of the provision for bad debts:

1. Analyze deductions from revenue.

2. Compute collectible services rendered.

3. Compute collections from patients.

4. Compute percentage of collections.

5. Compute percentage bad debts provision.

6. Comment on adequacy of provision.

P3.   The following information is made available to you:

Accounts Receivable Balances
By Financial Groups and Time of Discharge
September 30, 19--

	Blue Cross	Other Group Insurance	Notes and Individual Insurance	Open Accounts	Total Accounts Receivable	Percent of Total
Grand totals	$283,100	$144,300	$104,000	$142,100	$673,500	
In-house	72,200	32,800		15,000	120,000	17.8%
Discharge total	210,900	111,500	104,000	127,100	553,500	82.2
Time since discharge:						
30 days	170,000	68,100	14,000	41,700	293,800	43.6
30–60 days	16,200	19,900	13,900	16,600	66,600	9.9
60–90 days	6,700	10,100	8,500	15,000	40,300	6.0
90 days and over	18,000	13,400	67,600	53,800	152,800	22.7
Percent of total	42.0%	21.4%	15.5%	21.1%	100.0%	

Accounts Receivable Allowances
September 30, 19--
(End of Fiscal Year)

	Bad Debts	Charity	Total
Beginning of month	$115,600	$ 28,600	$144,200
Provision for month	14,000	4,665	18,665
Charges for month	9,300	600	9,900
End of month balance	$120,300	$ 32,665	$152,965

Required. The Finance Committee is questioning the amounts of receivables carried as well as allowances, charity and bad debt write-off policies. The balance of accounts receivable at September 30 represents about 50 days business. Average monthly gross income is fairly stable. As the new controller, you are asked to give your opinion on these figures and to present a course of action to investigate and correct or improve the accounts receivable picture.

P4.   The controller of Murphy Hospital has recently resigned and you have been appointed to fill the vacancy. The administrator furnishes you with the comparative reports shown below and tells you that he is concerned with the cash position of the hospital. The reports cover inpatients only and were prepared from audited hospital records. The administrator asks you to analyze the data and report to him regarding the credit and collection situation of the hospital.

Schedule I:	1983	1984	1985	1986	1987
Gross charges	$2,000,000	$2,100,000	$2,200,000	$2,420,000	$2,430,000
Contractual adjustments:					
City and county	70,000	77,000	60,000	74,000	75,000
Other agencies	50,000	43,000	45,000	51,000	50,000
Blue Cross	80,000	90,000	95,000	115,000	120,000
Net charges before					
bad debts	1,800,000	1,890,000	2,000,000	2,180,000	2,185,000
Bad debt write-offs	90,000	100,000	110,000	123,000	125,000
Collections	1,660,000	1,760,000	1,880,000	1,952,000	2,065,000
Accounts receivable, 12/31	450,000	480,000	490,000	595,000	590,000
Schedule II:					
Total patient days	100,000	102,000	107,000	110,000	115,000
Percent increase of patient					
days over previous year	5.0%	2.0%	4.9%	2.8%	4.5%
Percent patient days by					
type of patient:					
City and county	10.0	10.5	7.0	7.5	7.6
Other agency	15.1	16.6	16.8	18.3	18.8
Blue Cross	40.0	39.5	40.1	41.0	40.5
Other patients	34.9	33.4	36.1	33.2	33.1
Schedule III:					
Percent of net charges:					
Accounts receivable	25.0%	25.4%	24.5%	27.3%	27.0%
Bad debts	5.0	5.3	5.5	5.6	5.7
Collections	92.2	93.1	94.0	89.6	94.5
Schedule IV:					
Percent increase over					
previous year:					
Gross charges	5.26%	5.00%	4.76%	10.00%	.41%
Net charges	4.96	5.00	5.82	9.00	.23
Collections	4.27	6.02	6.82	3.83	5.76
Accounts receivable	12.50	6.67	2.08	21.43	−(0.84)
Schedule V:					
Contractual adjustments					
Percent of gross charges:					
City and county	3.50%	3.67%	2.73%	3.06%	3.09%
Other agency	2.50	2.05	2.05	2.11	2.06
Blue Cross	4.00	4.29	4.32	4.75	4.94

Required. (1) Prepare the report requested based on the information given. Discuss each problem area within a separate paragraph in the answer, indicating your recommendations to improve or correct each problem area. (2) Outline any additional information which you would like to have or need in order to make a more complete analysis.

12
Inventories and Prepaid Expenses

A substantial portion of the resources reported in the balance sheet of a hospital's Unrestricted Fund appears in the current asset classification. The majority of these resources are so-called **quick assets**, i.e., cash and other assets that may be quickly converted into cash. Accounting and financial management matters relating to quick assets (cash, short-term investments, and receivables) were discussed in the two preceding chapters. Consideration is given here to the financial accounting aspects of hospital inventories and prepaid expenses, the remaining assets included in the current category. While the resources of restricted funds generally include a small amount of quick assets, inventories and prepaid expenses usually are found only in the hospital's Unrestricted Fund.

Purchasing, receiving, and other matters pertaining to the acquisition of inventoriable supplies were treated in Chapter 8. The present chapter is concerned largely with accounting procedures relating to hospital inventories, but an appreciable amount of material having direct managerial significance is also included. A fair knowledge of this material is necessary to a full comprehension of certain major issues in inventory management which are presented in Chapter 14.

NATURE AND IMPORTANCE OF INVENTORIES

Because the operations of a hospital enterprise require the ownership of a stock of goods and consumable supplies, it is necessary for accounting purposes that proper determinations be made of the cost of such goods and supplies used, and of the goods and supplies remaining unused in the hospital inventory. The term **inventory** has been defined as:[1]

> . . . the aggregate of those items of tangible personal property which (1) are held for sale in the ordinary course of business, (2) are in process of production for such sale, or (3) are to be currently consumed in the production of goods or services to be available for sale.

In a hospital, inventories include the drugs and pharmaceuticals shelved in the pharmacy, the foodstuffs located in the dietary storerooms, the trays and packs assembled in central services and supply, and numerous other items ranging from cleaning supplies used in housekeeping to laboratory chemicals and radiological film. Some of these inventory items are in continuous use whereas others are used infrequently. Many of these items have an extremely high unit cost, while other items are purchased at relatively insignificant prices. This suggests the advisability of employing different methods of accounting and management control for different types of inventories.

Theoretically, the cost of an inventory item should include all direct and indirect expenditures relating to its acquisition, preparation, and placement for use or sale:[2]

> The primary basis of accounting for inventories is cost, which has been defined generally as the price paid or consideration given to acquire an asset. As applied to inventories, cost means in principle the sum of the applicable expenditures and charges directly or indirectly incurred in bringing an article to its existing condition and location.

It generally is not practicable, however, to attempt to allocate to inventory such indirect costs as purchasing, handling, and storing. Theory is tempered by practical considerations and in actual practice an inventory cost is usually regarded as list price less any trade discounts to which the hospital may be entitled, i.e., the invoiced price. Where feasible, however, it is preferred practice to **include** freight charges and **exclude** available cash discounts in determining **net invoice cost**. This matter was discussed in Chapter 8.

The hospital should include in its inventory all purchased merchandise in transit at the balance sheet date when the terms of purchase are "f.o.b. shipping point." In such cases, title to the goods passes to the hospital with the loading of the goods at the shipping point. The hospital inventory should not include merchandise in transit at the balance sheet date if the terms of purchase are "f.o.b. destination." Hospitals may also receive various goods on a consignment basis, but such goods should be excluded from inventory in that title to items held on consignment is retained by the consignor.

While the inventory of a hospital generally is not substantial relative to other assets, inventory accounting and management is of critical importance. It must be recognized that as much as 12 to 15 percent of hospital costs may be represented by supplies expense. Only a fraction of this may be on hand and in the inventory at any particular time, but the dollar value of the annual usage of supplies from inventory is a significant cost. Inventory is an active element in hospital activity, being continuously acquired, issued, and consumed. Whenever an account reflects a high activity characteristic, the possibility of error is magnified. Inventory errors are particularly important because of their direct impact on reported expense and assets. If, for example, the inventory is understated by $5,000, hospital expense will be overstated by the same amount. On the other hand, if the inventory is overstated by $5,000, expenses will be understated by $5,000. The inventory asset, in either case, will be misstated in the hospital's balance sheet.

Like cash and investment securities, the hospital inventory also is highly susceptible to misappropriation by hospital personnel and others. Losses arising from employee theft and waste can be substantial. It is essential, then, that suitable internal controls be developed to safeguard inventories from these hazards.

Studies have shown that the cost of maintaining an inventory is quite significant. Some authorities place this cost as high as 25 percent of acquisition cost. In other words, a $4 inventory item is likely to have cost $5 by the time it has been used. The additional $1 cost consists of the "hidden" costs of purchasing, receiving, storing, handling, insurance, and imputed interest. To the extent that inventory levels are excessive, avoidable costs are incurred. Yet, because of its mission, a hospital must never allow inventories to become depleted to the point of endangering patients' lives. Thus, there is the need to maintain adequate, but not excessive, inventories. The determination of an optimum inventory level can be rather difficult (see Chapter 14).

Finally, certain inventory items are billable through specific charges to patients; many other supplies are not directly billed. Inventory management and accounting procedures therefore are needed which provide assurance that all billable supplies are, in fact, properly billed. In the absence of adequate procedures, revenues may be lost in substantial amounts. Whether supplies are billable or not, however, a proper accounting for the costs of supplies consumed is essential for control, rate setting, and reimbursement purposes.

PERIODIC AND PERPETUAL SYSTEMS

Most hospitals will, and should, employ two basic inventory accounting systems concurrently. Certain supplies may be accounted for by the periodic inventory method, while other supply items should be maintained on a perpetual inventory basis. Supplies should be stratified according to dollar value of annual usage and susceptibility to theft, with the choice of inventory system for particular types of supply items depending mainly upon these characteristics. If the dollar value of annual usage is substantial and if the supplies are highly susceptible to theft, the perpetual system generally should be employed. The perpetual system is expensive to employ, however, and compromises sometimes must be made.

To illustrate the two inventory accounting methods, assume the following information with respect to a particular supply item:

Inventory, March 1	20 units @ $5 =	$100
Purchase, March 10	_80_ units @ $5 =	_400_
Total	100	500
Usage, March 20	−70 units @ $5 =	−350
Inventory, March 31	_30_ units @ $5 =	$150

The month begins with $100 in an inventory account. What entry should be made on March 10 when 80 additional units were purchased? What entry should be made to record the usage of 70 units on March 20? By what procedure is the March 31 inventory determined? The latter question would be complicated somewhat if the March 10 purchase was made at a unit cost other than $5, but this matter is deferred to a later point.

Periodic Inventory System

Under the periodic inventory system, no day-to-day record of supplies in inventory is maintained in the accounting records. Supplies are charged either to inventory or directly to expense when purchased:

Inventory (or Supplies Expense)	$ 400	
Accounts Payable		$ 400
To record purchase of supplies.		

If the department that will use the supplies is known, the above debit may be made to the appropriate departmental supplies expense account. Otherwise, the debit must be made to an inventory account.

No journal entry is made on March 20 when 70 units of these supplies are requisitioned and used in departmental activities. At intervals, then, a physical inventory must be taken as a basis for determining the quantity of supplies that remains unused in inventory. In the absence of error or theft, this quantity is found to be 30 units. Cost prices then are assigned to these units, and the accounts are adjusted accordingly.

Assume, for example, that the March 10 purchase was debited to supplies expense. In such case, the general ledger accounts would reflect the following balances at March 31:

Inventory, March 1	$100
Supplies expense	400

Since the March 31 physical inventory indicates a 30-unit inventory priced at $150 (30 units @ $5), the following adjustment is required:

Inventory	$ 50	
Supplies Expense		$ 50
To record increase in inventory and reduction in departmental expense for unused supplies.		

The entry restates the inventory to $150 and reduces the departmental supplies expense for the month to $350 (70 units @ $5).

The periodic inventory system has the advantage of simplicity; it is clerically inexpensive. Because monthly physical inventories usually are not practical, however, the accounts will be somewhat distorted until physical counts are taken and appropriate adjustments are made. The degree of misstatement usually is not serious for interim reporting purposes, but adjustments should be made at least once each year, generally at the end of the fiscal period. The major disadvantage of the periodic inventory system is that the accounting records do not provide a means for control. The physical inventory indicates what the inventory **is**, of course, but the accounting records do not indicate what the inventory of supplies **should be**. Significant shortages may go undetected. There is also no indication in the accounting records as to **where** the inventory is located or **who** is responsible for it. These are the significant weaknesses of the periodic inventory system.

Perpetual Inventory System

Under the perpetual inventory system, records are maintained to provide a continuous record of supplies purchased, used, and on hand. Supplies accounted for in this way are always charged to inventory accounts when purchased. The March 10 entry is:

Inventory	$ 400	
Accounts Payable		$ 400
To record purchase of supplies.		

An entry is also made in the subsidiary inventory records to reflect this inventory addition, raising the inventory balance to 100 units. Perpetual inventory ledger cards (see the author's **Introduction to Hospital Accounting**) may be used, or the subsidiary records may be maintained by electronic equipment.

As the supplies are requisitioned from inventory and used in departmental activities, journal entries are made to credit the inventory accounts and charge the appropriate supplies expense accounts for the cost of such supplies:

Supplies Expense	$ 350	
Inventory		$ 350
To record the requisition from inventory		
70 units of supplies priced at $5 per unit.		

An entry is also made in the subsidiary inventory records to reflect a reduction of 70 units in the inventory, thus lowering the inventory balance to 30 units of the supply item. These subsidiary records may be kept in terms of quantities only or in both quantities and costs. At least once each year, a physical inventory is taken and the perpetual records are adjusted, if necessary, to reflect the actual count. The point is that the perpetual records indicate precisely what the inventory **should** be at any time.

As noted earlier, the choice of inventory system depends mainly upon the characteristics of particular supply items. If the dollar value of annual usage is substantial, if the supplies are highly susceptible to theft, and if the supplies are directly billable to patients, use of the perpetual inventory system generally is desirable. The perpetual system provides a continuous control over the inventory in that information is immediately available as to inventory levels. Purchasing is facilitated, the adequacy of supplies on hand is more assured, and any shortages are readily determined. Perpetual records are also useful for insurance purposes in connection with monthly reporting policies and documentation of losses. While the method is costly to employ, some hospitals probably should have a greater portion of their inventories under perpetual controls than they do at present. The tendency in hospitals is to standardize the quantities of supplies ordered and requisitioned irrespective of inventory levels, and to give more attention to the standardization and optimization of quantities of supplies maintained in inventory. In this regard, perpetual inventory systems can be of considerable assistance. Careful studies should be made to determine the value of the benefits to be derived from perpetual records in comparison with the costs of installing and maintaining them.

TRADITIONAL INVENTORY COST PROCEDURES

Typically, supplies are purchased during a given time period at different unit costs. A problem therefore arises in determining which costs relate to the supply items that have been used during the period and which apply to the units remaining in inventory at the end of the period. Such determinations are quite important because they have a direct effect upon the reported operating expense of both the current and subsequent period as well as upon the balance sheet asset valuation of the inventory. In making these determinations, primary consideration should be given to the computation of the cost of supplies used:[3]

In accounting for the goods in the inventory at any point of time, the major objective is the matching of appropriate costs against revenues in order that there may be a proper determination of the realized income. Thus, the inventory at any given date is the balance of costs applicable to goods on hand remaining after the matching of absorbed costs with concurrent revenues.

The effect of any inventory costing procedure upon the resultant asset valuation for balance sheet purposes is important, but it is a secondary consideration. A preference should be given to the method which most clearly provides an appropriate measurement of the cost of supplies used and, consequently, the periodic net income of the hospital.

As a basis for subsequent illustrations, assume the following data with respect to a particular item of supplies used in hospital operations on a fairly frequent basis:

				Costs	
Date			Units	Unit	Total
April	1	Inventory	100	$5.00	$ 500
	5	Purchase	100	6.00	600
	10	Usage	150		
	15	Purchase	250	6.40	1,600
	20	Usage	200		
	25	Purchase	100	6.80	680
	30	Usage	50		
					$3,380

As can be seen, the April 1 inventory consisted of 100 units which had cost $5 each. During April, a total of 450 units was purchased at steadily increasing unit prices, and 400 units of this supply item were used during the month. The April 30 inventory therefore is comprised of 150 units. In this illustration, the total "pool of costs" is $3,380. What part of this total cost is the cost of the 400 units issued from the inventory in April? What part of the $3,380 of total cost should be assigned to the 150 units remaining in the inventory at the end of the month? The answers to these questions are not obvious.

Specific Identification

It may be possible to make a specific identification of purchase costs with individual units of inventory. If the units are packaged in cartons, boxes, or other types of containers, the containers may be marked or tagged in some manner to indicate the actual unit costs of the supply items. Should it be desirable to avoid the general disclosure of such costs, the cost figures may be expressed in an alphabetical code. A community general hospital, for example, might code purchase costs in this way:

COST	1	2	3	4	5	6	7	8	9	0
CODE	C	G	H	O	S	P	I	T	A	L

For example, an item of supplies which cost $24.50 could therefore be crayon-marked or tagged with a cost code of GOSL. A record is kept of the letter codes of items issued from inventory. When translated and totaled, this provides the costs of supplies used. The inventory at any time may be determined by the same process.

The specific identification method, however, does not necessarily result in an appropriate matching of costs and revenues. The selection of units removed from inventory, and consequently the expense of the period, may be contrived or purely accidental. Beyond this objection, of course, is the fact that the specific identification of cost flows may be simply impractical, if not impossible, because of the multiplicity of products found in hospital inventories. Therefore, it usually is necessary to turn to some **assumed** flow of inventory costs. Any one of a number of different assumptions can be made which, in the circumstances, may be in conformity with generally accepted accounting principles. Different assumptions, in fact, may be made for different classifications of inventory.

Average Costing

Hospitals may employ the weighted average cost method for determining the cost of supplies used and for valuing inventories. The assumption is that the units issued from inventory are drawn more or less equally from each acquisition of supplies. It is not necessary, however, that the physical flow of the units in inventory be such as to actually correspond with the assumption.

Periodic Inventory System. If the periodic inventory system is employed, a weighted average cost for the month of April would be computed as indicated in Figure 12-1. Similar calculations could be developed in terms of data for a quarter or even for a year, depending upon how often the cost information is required.

Figure 12-1.
Computation of Weighted Average Cost
Periodic Inventory System

<u>April</u>

1	Inventory	100 units @ $5.00 =	$ 500
5	Purchase	100 units @ $6.00 =	600
15	Purchase	250 units @ $6.40 =	1,600
25	Purchase	<u>100</u> units @ $6.80 =	<u>680</u>
	Total	<u>550</u>	<u>$3,380</u>

Weighted Average Cost ($3,380/550) = <u>$6.14</u>

In this example, the April 30 inventory is computed as $921 (150 units @ $6.14), and the cost of supplies used during the month therefore would be $2,459 ($3,380−$921).

Perpetual Inventory System. If the perpetual inventory system is employed but the cost of units issued is recorded only at the end of each month or other convenient period, the weighted average cost can be computed as shown above. On the other hand, it may be desirable to compute and record costs as supplies are issued from the inventory. This requires the computation of a new weighted average cost after each purchase of supplies at a unit cost different from the current average cost of the inventory. In other words, a "moving" weighted average cost involving successive recalculations is necessary. The method is shown in Figure 12-2 as it might appear on a subsidiary inventory ledger card.

Figure 12-2.
Computation of Weighted Average Cost
Perpetual Inventory System

	Purchases			Issues			Balance		
		Cost			Cost			Cost	
Date	Units	Unit	Total	Units	Unit	Total	Units	Unit	Total
4/1							100	$5.00	$ 500
4/5	100	$6.00	$ 600				200	5.50	1,100
4/10				150	$5.50	$ 825	50	5.50	275
4/15	250	6.40	1,600				300	6.25	1,875
4/20				200	6.25	1,250	100	6.25	625
4/25	100	6.80	680				200	6.52	1,305
4/30				50	6.52	326	150	6.52	979
	Cost of Supplies Used					$2,401			

A new weighted average cost is determined after each additional purchase at a unit cost different from the existing average inventory cost. After the purchase of April 5, for instance, the recomputed average cost is $5.50, determined by a division of $1,100 by 200 units. As a result of this moving average, the cost associated with the units issued (2,401) and the ending inventory ($979) is somewhat different than the costs obtained earlier ($2,459 and $921) where a periodic inventory system was used.

First-In, First-Out (FIFO) Costing

The first-in, first-out (FIFO) costing method is based on the assumption that the supplies issued from inventory are drawn from the oldest stock, i.e., the units are charged out of inventory in the order in which they were acquired. This means that the remaining units in inventory are stated in terms of the most recently incurred costs. That is, the ending inventory is valued at the latest invoice prices. The assumption seems natural and logical in that some effort ordinarily is made to use up the oldest stock first. Nevertheless, the actual physical flow of the units need not conform exactly with the underlying assumption for the use of this method to be acceptable.

Periodic Inventory System. Under the periodic inventory system, the 150-unit inventory at April 30 may be computed as follows:

100 units @ $6.80	=	$ 680 Most recent (April 25) invoice price
50 units @ $6.40	=	320 Next most recent (April 15) invoice price
150 units		$1,000 April 30 inventory valuation

As the inventory is composed of the most recently incurred costs, the cost of supplies issued during the month is $2,380 ($3,380 - $1,000), i.e., the "oldest" costs. A variation of this procedure, referred to as the latest invoice price (LIP) method, applies the most recent invoice price to **all** units in the ending inventory, disregarding quantities. That is, the ending inventory might be stated at $1,020 (150 units @ $6.80) in order to avoid searching invoice files for purchased quantities equal to the quantity in the inventory at the end of the period. It is a shortcut and should be applied with care.

Perpetual Inventory System. Under the perpetual inventory system, it is possible to compute and record the cost of units used at the time they are issued from the inventory. The procedure is illustrated in Figure 12-3 as it might appear on a subsidiary inventory ledger record. It should be noted that the periodic and perpetual inventory systems produce identical results when the FIFO procedure is employed. The cost of supplies issued is $2,380 and the April 30 inventory is $1,000, as previously computed under the periodic inventory system.

Figure 12-3.
Computation of FIFO Cost
Perpetual Inventory System

Computation of FIFO Cost
Perpetual Inventory System

	Purchases			Issues			Balance		
		Cost			Cost			Cost	
Date	Units	Unit	Total	Units	Unit	Total	Units	Unit	Total
4/1							100	$ 5.00	$ 500
4/5	100	$ 6.00	$ 600				100	$ 5.00	$ 500
							100	6.00	600
4/10				100	$5.00	$500			
				50	6.00	300	50	$ 6.00	$ 300
4/15	250	6.40	1,600				50	$ 6.00	$ 300
							250	6.40	1,600
4/20				50	6.00	300			
				150	6.40	960	100	$ 6.40	$ 640
4/25	100	6.80	680				100	$ 6.40	$ 640
							100	6.80	680
4/30				50	6.40	320	50	$ 6.40	$ 320
							100	6.80	680
	Cost of Supplies Used					$2,380			

Last-In, First-Out (LIFO) Costing

The last-in, first-out (LIFO) costing method is based on the assumption that the supplies issued from inventory are drawn from the most recently purchased stock, i.e., the units are charged out of inventory at the most recently incurred costs. This means that the remaining units in inventory are stated in terms of the earliest costs experienced.

Periodic Inventory System. Under the periodic inventory system, the physical inventory of 150 units at April 30 would have a cost computed as follows:

100 units @ $5.00 = $500 Earliest costs (April 1 inventory)
 50 units @ $6.00 =   300 Next earliest costs (April 5 purchase)

150                       $800 April 30 inventory valuation

As the inventory is assumed to be composed of the earliest costs incurred, the cost of supplies issued during the month is $2,580 ($3,380 − $800), i.e., the most recently incurred costs. While it is unlikely that the oldest physical units comprise the inventory, the validity of the FIFO method does not depend upon the actual physical flow of the units of inventory.

Perpetual Inventory System. Under the perpetual inventory system, the cost of units used may be computed and recorded as they are issued from the inventory. The procedure is illustrated in Figure 12-4 as it might appear on a subsidiary inventory ledger record. The perpetual LIFO cost of supplies used is $2,470 and the month-end inventory is $910 ($250 + $320 + $340). It should be noted that the periodic and perpetual inventory systems ordinarily do not produce the same results when the LIFO method is employed.

Figure 12-4.
Computation of LIFO Cost
Perpetual Inventory System

Computation of LIFO Cost
Perpetual Inventory System

	Purchases			Issues			Balance		
		Cost			Cost			Cost	
Date	Units	Unit	Total	Units	Unit	Total	Units	Unit	Total
4/1							100	$ 5.00	$ 500
4/5	100	$ 6.00	$ 600				100	$ 5.00	$ 500
							100	6.00	600
4/10				100	$ 6.00	$ 600			
				50	5.00	250	50	$ 5.00	$ 250
4/15	250	6.40	1,600				50	$ 5.00	$ 250
							250	6.40	1,600
4/20				200	6.40	1,280	50	$ 5.00	$ 250
							50	6.40	320
4/25	100	6.80	680				50	$ 5.00	$ 250
							50	6.40	320
							100	6.80	680
4/30				50	6.80	340	50	$ 5.00	$ 250
							50	6.40	320
							50	6.80	340

Cost of Supplies Used $2,470

Evaluation of Traditional Costing Methods

A summary of the three traditional inventory costing procedures is presented in Figure 12-5. As the hospital management usually has a choice of methods, which one should be adopted? The method that is chosen should, of course, be theoretically sound and clerically feasible. Managers must also consider the probable effect of the method on the reported financial position and the results of operations. Consideration also might be given to the implications of each method with respect to cost reimbursement contracts.

Figure 12-5.
Summary of Traditional Inventory Costing Procedures
Perpetual Inventory System

	Costing Method		
	FIFO	Average	LIFO
Inventory, April 1	$ 500	$ 500	$ 500
Purchases	2,880	2,880	2,880
Total	3,380	3,380	3,380
Less Inventory, April 30	1,000	979	910
Cost of Supplies Used in April	$2,380	$2,401	$2,470

The three methods produce three different amounts of supplies expense for the month. There also are three different inventory valuations for the month-end balance sheet. Which of the methods is "best" or "correct"? All are generally accepted methods: [4]

Cost for inventory purposes may be determined under any one of several assumptions as to the flow of cost factors (such as first-in, first-out, average, and last-in, first-out); the major objective in selecting a method should be to choose the one which, under the circumstances, most clearly reflects periodic income.

Accountants and other interested groups, however, tend to disagree as to which cost flow assumption most clearly reflects a hospital's periodic income (or expense). The controversy has been centered mainly on FIFO versus LIFO in periods of rising prices such as have been experienced in the United States in recent years. Under such conditions:

1. The use of FIFO tends to produce smaller charges to expense, larger net income, and larger inventory valuation for balance sheet purposes.

2. The use of LIFO tends to produce larger charges to expense, smaller net income, and smaller inventory valuation for balance sheet purposes.

In periods of steadily declining prices the effects would be reversed. As can be seen in Figure 12-5, the use of the average cost method produces results that fall somewhere between those obtained under the FIFO and LIFO methods.

Advocates of the FIFO procedure argue that it produces the most meaningful inventory valuation for balance sheet presentation. By inventorying the most recently incurred costs, the FIFO inventory approximates current replacement cost. Under LIFO costing where the inventory consists of "old" costs, the inventory figure generally is considerably below current replacement cost. LIFO supporters admit this but argue that the advantage attributed to FIFO inventory is gained at the expense of a proper determination of the charges against periodic revenues. In other words, the major objective of inventory accounting should be to secure a proper determination of income; balance sheet considerations are of secondary importance.

Adherents of FIFO point out that the LIFO assumption is not in accord with the actual physical flow of units of product into and out of the hospital inventory. It is more logical, they say, to assume that the "older" units are the first units to be issued and used. Those who advocate LIFO costing reply that it is the flow of cost factors, not the physical movement of the goods, that is most important for costing purposes. They show that, by assigning the most recently incurred cots to units used, LIFO results in the proper matching of the most **current** costs with **current** revenue. It is contended that FIFO fails to do so.

Putting aside theoretical considerations, LIFO adoptions by many business firms probably are due in part to income tax minimization efforts. It is often stated that the use of FIFO in periods of rising prices results in the reporting of fictitious profits and in the overpayment of income taxes. LIFO tends to eliminate some of the undesirable effects of inflation. Similarly, hospitals may find that LIFO costing will produce larger reimbursements than might otherwise be obtained under cost-based third-party contracts. The increased cash flow generated by LIFO costing could assist the hospital in the replenishment of inventories at ever increasing replacement costs.

Whatever method of inventory valuation a hospital happens to select, it should be logically defensible, managerially useful, clerically feasible, and consistently followed from period to period. This is not to say, however, that desirable changes in inventory costing methods are precluded. The position of the AICPA is:[5]

> The basis of stating inventories must be consistently applied and should be disclosed in the financial statements; whenever a significant change is made therein, there should be disclosure of the nature of the change and, if material, the effect on income.

If there were complete freedom to change indiscriminately from one method of inventory costing to another and back again, the expenses and net income of the hospital could be manipulated to some degree to suit the purposes of the management.

A change in the inventory costing method is considered to be a change in accounting principle. All such changes should be reported in conformity with the requirements of APB Opinion No. 20.[6] In general, a change in accounting principle requires a computation of the cumulative effect of the change on the net income of all prior years, i.e., the amount by which the net income of all prior years would have been greater or smaller had the newly adopted principle been employed in those years. The cumulative effect usually is reported as a special item in the income statement of the year of change, and the financial statements of prior periods are not retroactively restated. Special rules, however, apply to changes to or from the LIFO method.

THE LOWER OF COST OR MARKET RULE

Inventories in the hospital balance sheet should be stated at the lower of cost, however determined, or "market." In this context, "market" means replacement cost at the balance sheet date. This is a generally accepted practice that has been carried over from the early days of accounting when the dominant consideration was conservatism: "Anticipate no income but provide for all possible losses." In other words, if the inventory can be replaced at an amount that is less than its determined cost, the inventory generally should be written down to that lower figure. The amount by which the inventory is written down is treated as an addition to the expense of the period.

For example, assume that the 150-unit inventory in the preceding illustration could be replaced at April 30 at a cost of only $6.60 per unit, or at a total cost of $990. No adjustment of the inventory would be required if its cost had been determined by the weighted average or LIFO methods as such costs ($979 and $910, respectively) are lower than replacement cost ($990). Typically, a write-down may be required in cases where inventory cost is determined on a FIFO basis. The FIFO inventory of $1,000 may be adjusted to the lower "market" by an adjusting entry debiting supplies expense and crediting the inventory for $10 ($1,000 − $990).

The application of the cost or market rule, however, is not always as simple as might be implied above. Note the following:[7]

As used in the phrase **lower or cost or market**, the term **market** means current replacement cost (by purchase or by reproduction, as the case may be) except that:
(1) Market should not exceed the net realizable value (i.e., estimated selling price in the ordinary course of business less reasonably predictable costs of completion and disposal); and
(2) Market should not be less than net realizable value reduced by an allowance for an approximately normal profit margin.

Thus, there is a "ceiling" and a "floor" to be considered in applying the rule. These and other complications, however, are of interest mainly to the independent auditor, and the matter is not pursued further in this book.

When inventory write-downs are made because of price declines, obsolescence, damage, or deterioration, it may be desirable to credit the reduction to an inventory valuation account rather than directly to the inventory account. This eliminates the necessity of adjusting the detailed perpetual inventory records where such records are kept. Assume, for example, that a $68,000 inventory is to be written down by $5,000. The journal entry is:

Loss on Reduction of Inventory	$ 5,000	
Allowance for Reduction of Inventory		$ 5,000
To record write-down of inventory to reflect		
loss due to price declines.		

If material, the loss is shown as a separate item in the income statement. The inventory is reported on the balance sheet at $63,000 ($68,000 − $5,000). When the inventory is sold or consumed during the subsequent period, the allowance account is no longer needed. It is eliminated as follows:

Supplies Expense	$ 63,000	
Allowance for Reduction of Inventory	5,000	
Inventory		$ 68,000
To record the adjusted cost of supplies used		
and eliminate the allowance account established		
at the end of the previous period.		

Under no circumstances should the inventory valuation account be eliminated in this subsequent period by transfer to a revenue account.

LOSSES ON PURCHASE COMMITMENTS

A hospital may contract to purchase goods for a given future period at a fixed price per unit in an effort to assure an adequate supply of such goods as they are needed. If the current market price of the goods declines below the agreed price in noncancelable purchase contracts, the loss should be recorded in the period during which the price decline occurred. Assume, for instance, a noncancelable purchase agreement of $40,000 where a 10 percent price decline occurs before any purchase orders are placed. The necessary entry is:

Loss on Purchase Commitments	$ 4,000	
Liability on Purchase Commitments		$ 4,000
To record loss on purchase commitment of the		
difference between contract and market price.		

The loss, if material, is shown in the income statement as a separate item. The liability is reflected among the current liabilities in the balance sheet.

In a subsequent period when purchase orders are placed for the goods covered by the agreement, the appropriate entry is:

Inventory	$ 36,000	
Liability on Purchase Commitments	4,000	
Accounts Payable		$ 40,000
To record purchase of supplies for inventory		
under purchase contract on which loss was		
recorded in previous period.		

The procedure is an application of the lower of cost or market rule. In no case are gains on purchase commitments anticipated in the accounts.

GROSS MARGIN METHOD

A physical count of inventories should be made at least once each year. In many instances, employees may work in teams of two with one making the actual count and the other making a written record of the inventory item and quantities counted. When the count is completed, unit costs are assigned to the counts and a dollar valuation is obtained for the inventory. The physical count indicates, of course, what the inventory **is**; the perpetual inventory records will indicate what the inventory **should be**. The two independently developed records then are compared, and significant differences are investigated. In this process, errors and shortages due to misappropriation can be detected.

A good portion of the hospital inventory, however, may not be maintained on a perpetual inventory system. In such cases, how can determinations be made as to what the inventory **should be** so that errors and shortages may be uncovered?

With respect to billable supplies in the inventory, it may be feasible to apply the gross margin method as a means of obtaining an estimate of the amount that should be in the inventory.

To illustrate, assume the following data with respect to a particular type of billable supplies whose price is determined through a standard markup of 50 percent on cost:

Inventory, January 1	$ 7,000
Year ended December 31:	
Purchases	42,000
Billings to patients	60,000

These supply items are marked up 50 percent on cost to determine the prices to be billed to patients. If, for example, an item cost $10, the patient would be charged $15 for the item. This means that the billed price includes a one-third "profit" margin, i.e., the markup is 33 1/3 percent of billed price. When the rate of markup is not uniform for a particular category of supplies, a weighted average markup may be computed for inventory estimation purposes.

The estimated inventory, by application of the gross margin method, is shown as $9,000 at December 31 in Figure 12-6. This ordinarily will be a fairly close approximation of the ending inventory figure that would result from maintenance of inventory ledger cards on a continuous basis. As shown here, it generally will be close enough to permit the detection of significant shortages when compared with the physical inventory. Indicated shortages may be due to employee theft or to accounting errors, or both. Such shortages might also arise from errors in the determination of the physical inventory. Before judgments of these types are made, however, there should be proper assurance that the application of the gross margin method produces reliable results.

The gross margin method of estimating inventories has other important uses in hospitals where perpetual inventory records are not kept:

1. When an inventory has been destroyed by fire or other casualty, the gross margin method often may be used to determine the amount of the loss to be claimed for insurance purposes.

Figure 12-6.
Estimation of Inventory
Gross Margin Method

Inventory, January 1	$ 7,000	
Add purchases for the year	42,000	
Total cost of goods available		$49,000
Billings to patients for the year	$60,000	
Less estimated gross margin (33⅓%)	20,000	
Estimated cost of goods billed		40,000
Estimated inventory, December 31		$ 9,000
Less physical inventory (assumed)		6,800
Apparent inventory shortage		$ 2,200

2. Fire insurance policies on inventories may call for the hospital to report approximate inventories at the end of each month. As monthly physical inventories are impractical, the gross margin method may be applied to calculate month-end inventories more accurately than by mere observation. Insurance premiums might be reduced in this way.

3. The preparation of accurate monthly financial reports to management requires inventory figures, and the gross margin method often can be employed for this purpose.

RETAIL INVENTORY METHOD

A variation of the gross margin method sometimes can be applied to advantage in the pharmacy and in "retail" shops operated by the hospital. It is called the **retail inventory method.** Under this method, the goods placed in inventory are priced at retail, using a uniform markup rate. Records must be kept of inventory acquisitions at cost and at retail, although not on an item-by-item basis. If selling prices initially established are changed, records must also be kept of the retail value of such changes with respect to the goods in inventory at the time such markups and markdowns are made.

To illustrate the application of the retail inventory method, assume the following data concerning the 1987 operations of a retail shop in a hospital:

	Cost	Retail
Inventory, January 1	$10,000	$15,000
Purchases for 1987	60,000	90,000
Markups		5,000
Markdowns		10,000
Sales		80,000

The retail value of the purchases is based upon the sales prices at which the goods were initially priced to be sold. During the year, unsold goods in inventory were marked up an additional $5,000, and other goods were marked down by $10,000 below the original sales price assigned to them. No perpetual inventory records need be maintained of inventory quantities.

Figure 12-7 shows the determination of the estimated inventory at December 31 by application of the retail inventory method. Markdowns may be excluded in the determination of the cost to retail percentage. If that is done, it is said that the method produces an inventory figure which conforms most closely with the **lower of cost or market** rule. In any event, the physical inventory is compiled on the basis of sales prices rather than cost. Should the December 31 physical inventory be determined as, say, $17,500, then the indicated shortage in the inventory would be $2,500 ($20,000 − $17,000) at sales value or $1,750 ($2,500 x 70%) at cost.

Figure 12-7.
Estimation of Inventory
Retail Inventory Method

	Cost	Retail
Inventory, January 1	$ 10,000	$ 15,000
Add purchases	60,000	90,000
Add markups		5,000
Less markdowns		(10,000)
Totals (cost percentage = 70%)	$ 70,000	$100,000
Less sales		80,000
December 31 inventory, at retail		$ 20,000
Cost percentage (above)		70%
December 31 inventory, at estimated cost		$ 14,000

STANDARD COSTS

Hospitals might also give consideration to the feasibility of using standard costs in connection with certain inventories. To illustrate, assume a particular inventory classification for which a standard cost of $5 per unit is established at the beginning of the year. This standard unit cost is based upon anticipated purchase prices for the year and established purchasing policies. It also assumes a desired degree of efficiency in the purchasing function. In other words, the standard cost is representative of what the unit cost **should be** for the coming year after giving due consideration to all relevant factors.

In order to demonstrate the standard cost procedure, assume the following data for a year's activity in the inventory item mentioned above:

Date	Units	Unit Cost
1/1 Inventory	100	$5.00
3/1 Purchase	300	4.80
6/1 Usage	280	
9/1 Purchase	250	5.40
11/1 Usage	260	

Inventory acquisitions are recorded at standard cost. A purchase price variance account is used to record differences between standard and actual costs. Issues from inventory also are recorded at the predetermined standard cost. The entries for the year are:

<u>March 1</u>

Inventory	$ 1,500	
Purchase Price Variance		$ 60
Accounts Payable		1,440
To record purchase of 300 units @ $4.80		

<u>June 1</u>

Supplies Expense	$ 1,400	
Inventory		$ 1,400
To record usage of 280 units.		

<u>September 1</u>

Inventory	$ 1,250	
Purchase Price Variance	100	
Accounts Payable		$ 1,350
To record purchase of 250 units @ $5.40.		

<u>November 1</u>

Supplies Expense	$ 1,300	
Inventory		$ 1,300
To record usage of 260 units.		

The net purchase price variance for the year is $40 ($100 − $60), the standard cost charged to supplies expense is $2,700 (540 units @ $5) and the December 31 inventory is $550 (110 units @ $5).

Since charges and credits to inventory during the year are made at a single standard unit cost figure, the maintenance of the subsidiary inventory records is greatly simplified. Perpetual inventory records may be kept in terms of quantities only. The need to compute average costs or to apply FIFO or LIFO procedures is eliminated. The net purchase price variance for the year may be treated as an item of expense (or income). If the variance is substantial, however, an appropriate portion of it should be allocated to the year-end inventory to approximate the inventory at actual cost. Finally, if the standard cost is properly determined, the purchase price variance may be indicative of the effectiveness of the purchasing function.

INTERNAL CONTROL

Matters pertaining to internal controls over the purchase and receipt of supplies for inventory were discussed in Chapter 8. Once supplies are acquired, the internal control objective largely is that of protecting the inventories from theft, damage, obsolescence, and waste as they remain in storage and then are consumed in hospital operations. The perpetual inventory system is likely to be most effective for these purposes, but the use of this system for all hospital inventories cannot be justified on a cost-benefit basis. Which items of supply should be accounted for by the perpetual system and which by the periodical system is an important matter to be determined by the individual hospital on the basis of its particular circumstances and needs.

A major requirement for adequate inventory control is the assignment of responsibility to specific individuals for inventories at each location in the hospital. These personnel must have a clear understanding of the policies and prescribed procedures with respect to purchase requisitions, safekeeping procedures, and authorizations for issues from inventory. Periodic investigations should be made, perhaps by the internal auditing staff, to ascertain the degree of adherence with established policies and procedures.

The number of inventory locations should be minimized so that centralized control may be achieved to the degree feasible. The inventory storage areas must be clean, well lighted, and large enough to permit a suitable organization and arrangement of the stock so that desired items can be easily located and identified. Supplies should be stored in a manner to provide protection from damage. Where possible, inventories should be kept in locked rooms or other enclosures, with access strictly limited to responsible employees. Supplies should be released from inventory storerooms only upon presentation of properly authorized supply requisition forms. Preprinted standard requisition forms may be used for supplies frequently requisitioned. Where floor stocks for nursing stations are requisitioned from inventory, however, emphasis should be placed on a standardization of the size of the floor stock rather than on a standardization of the amounts requisitioned. A greater degree of control is obtained when floor stocks are maintained on an imprest (or replenishment) basis.

Maximum-minimum controls should be established over inventories so that inventories are maintained in amounts that are neither inadequate nor excessive. Studies should be made to determine optimum order size for additions to inventory, and periodic reports should be developed as to supplies usage and inventory status. To avoid spoilage and obsolescence, color-coded stickers are often affixed to inventory items to indicate their age.

Where perpetual inventory records are kept, comparison of inventories indicated by the accounts should be made with physical inventories taken at least on an annual basis. Many hospitals have adopted a cycle physical inventory system under which portions of the inventory are verified by count at intervals during the year. Since a degree of control is lost when the periodic inventory system is employed, additional procedures should be developed to provide the necessary safeguards against theft and waste. Whatever the inventory method used, material differences between physical inventories and "book" or estimated inventories should be investigated and resolved. Suitable adjustments for such differences should be made in the accounts when these differences are found to exist.

PREPAID EXPENSES

In addition to cash, marketable securities, receivables, and inventories, the current asset classification in the hospital's Unrestricted Fund will also include prepayments for such items as insurance, rent, and interest. These prepayments qualify as assets in that they represent rights to future services, i.e., insurance protection, use of space or equipment, and use of money. They are presented in the hospital balance sheet as **prepaid expenses.** The general presumption is that the service represented by the prepayment will be consumed during the ensuing operating cycle. If material amounts have been prepaid for a period longer than one year, it may be necessary to report such amounts in a noncurrent asset category.

Premiums on policies for insurance against fire and other hazards usually are paid in advance. In most instances, it is necessary to maintain a subsidiary record called an **insurance register** which provides the details of each insurance policy. This information permits a determination at the end of each reporting period of premiums chargeable against current revenues and the amounts that are related to future periods. The latter amounts are reported in the balance sheet as prepaid or unexpired insurance. Similar analyses are required for prepaid rent, prepaid interest and other items. (These matters are treated at length in the author's **Introduction to Hospital Accounting.**)

CHAPTER 12 FOOTNOTES

1. "Restatement and Revision of Accounting Research Bulletins," Accounting Research Bulletin No. 43 (New York: AICPA, 1953), Chapter 4, Statement 1.

2. Ibid, Statement 3.

3. Ibid, par. 4.

4. Ibid, Statement 4.

5. Ibid, Statement 8.

6. "Accounting Changes," APB Opinion No. 20 (New York: AICPA, 1971).

7. "Restatement and Revision of Accounting Research Bulletins," Accounting Research Bulletin No. 43 (New York: AICPA, 1953), Chapter 4, Statement 6.

QUESTIONS

1. Distinguish between the periodic inventory system and the perpetual inventory system. What are the advantages and disadvantages of each system? Which system should be used in hospitals?

2. Define the term **inventory.** Name some of the major types of supplies that are maintained in hospital inventories.

3. Due to an error, Braxton Hospital's December 31, 1987, inventory was understated by $8,000. What is the effect of this error on the hospital's reported operating results for 1987 and its reported financial position at December 31, 1987? What effect, if any, will this error have on the hospital's 1988 operating results?

4. As chief fiscal officer of a 300-bed hospital, you and the purchasing agent are exploring the possibility of using disposable medical and surgical products in lieu of certain conventional reusable items. List the various considerations which should be explored in arriving at a decision.

5. State the reasons why a considerable amount of importance should be assigned to inventory accounting by hospital managements.

6. What is your understanding of the **lower of cost or market rule** as applied to hospital inventories?

7. Describe the **gross margin method** of estimating inventories. For what purposes might this method be employed by hospitals?

8. Distinguish between the FIFO and LIFO inventory costing methods. In a period of rising prices, which method would tend to result in the recording of the highest cost for supplies used? For end-of-period inventories?

9. During 1987, Westside Hospital entered into a noncancellable purchase agreement with a supplier. Under this agreement, the hospital contracts to purchase 1,000 units of a particular product at $10 per unit in 1988. At the end of 1987 before any purchase orders are placed, the price at which this product can be purchased has declined to $8.50 per unit. What entry, if any, should be made by the hospital's accountant?

10. A hospital marks up certain billable supplies 25 percent on cost to determine price. During a given time period, patients are billed $10,000 for these supply items. What is the estimated cost of the supplies billed to patients?

11. What are some of the major features of a satisfactory system of internal control over inventories in hospitals?

12. Motter Hospital had a 1987 net income of $30,000. Cost of supplies used during the year totaled $150,000. This hospital's inventory of supplies increased by $10,000 and accounts payable to suppliers increased by $13,800 during the year. What was the amount of cash paid to suppliers during 1987?

13. Hospital K establishes a print shop which eventually will do about 80 percent of the printing needs for all departments of the hospital. There are three full-time employees in the shop. Paper stock as well as various quantities of printed forms are stored in the print shop. Describe a simple and practical way of accounting by which departments may be charged with a reasonable value of the supplies and forms furnished through the print shop.

14.   At December 31, 1987, Memorial Hospital has on hand 144 cartons of Item Z which had cost $1.50 per carton. On December 15, 1987, the manufacturer of Item Z sends a notice to the hospital that effective immediately the price of Item Z is reduced to $1.25 per carton. This price is guaranteed for a period of 18 months. Memorial Hospital's administrator directs that the existing sales price to patients of $2.50 per carton be continued. What is the proper inventory valuation of Item Z at December 31, 1987?

EXERCISES

E1.   On March 1, a fire destroyed 60 percent of the inventory (all billable supplies) of Department A at Merkey Hospital. The following data are available:

Sales, 1/1-2/28	$72,000
Inventory, 1/1	10,000
Purchases, 1/1-2/28	70,000
Markup on cost	20%

Required. Compute the cost of the inventory lost in the fire.

E2.   Matovina Hospital provides you with the following information concerning the operations of one of its departments in which the retail inventory method is employed:

	Cost	Retail
Inventory, 1/1	$ 7,500	$ 20,000
1987 purchases	58,500	91,000
Net markups		9,000
Net markdowns		10,000
1987 sales		80,000

Required. Compute the cost of inventory sold and the cost of the December 31 inventory, assuming the retail inventory method is applied so as to obtain a lower of cost or market approximation.

E3.   Starcevich Hospital began operating a new department on March 1. This department purchased and issued a single supply item as follows:

March	1	Purchased 500 units @ $5
	5	Issued 300 units
	10	Purchased 200 units @ $6
	15	Purchased 300 units @ $7
	25	Issued 400 units

Required. Compute the cost of the March 31 inventory assuming (1) perpetual LIFO costing, (2) periodical FIFO costing, and (3) periodical weighted average costing.

E4. Holsten Hospital provides you with the following information concerning a single supply item it purchases and uses:

2/1 Inventory	400 units @ $7
2/7 Usage	300 units
2/14 Purchase	200 units @ $8
2/21 Purchase	200 units @ $9
2/28 Usage	200 units

At 2/28, suppliers quoted the supply item at a price of $8.50 per unit.

Required. Compute the cost of supplies used in February assuming (1) periodical costing, (2) perpetual FIFO costing and (3) perpetual weighted average costing.

E5. Monthly purchases and sales of billable supplies at Currytown Hospital are listed below. The hospital began the year with an inventory of $44,500. All supplies have been priced to patients at a uniform markup of 33 1/3 percent on cost.

	Purchases	Sales
January	$30,520	$38,600
February	30,900	51,620
March	50,200	58,300

Required. Compute the estimated amount of the inventory at February 28.

E6. Matson Hospital's December 31, 1986, inventory of Supply Item X was 10 units which had cost 89 cents per unit. During 1987, purchases of Supply Item X were:

January	10 units @ 90 cents
April	15 units @ 92 cents
July	15 units @ 90 cents
September	10 units @ 92 cents
November	10 units @ 93 cents

There were 14 units of Item X on hand at December 31, 1987. During 1988, purchases of Supply Item X were as follows:

January	10 units @ 93 cents
May	25 units @ 95 cents
August	15 units @ 96 cents
November	10 units @ 97 cents

There were 13 units of Item X on hand at December 31, 1988.

Required. Compute the cost of Supply Item X used in 1987 and 1988 assuming (1) LIFO costing and (2) FIFO costing.

PROBLEMS

P1.   Stockup Hospital maintains a sizable inventory of foodstuffs, dietary supplies, pharmaceuticals, and other items. Assume, however, that the inventory consists of a single supply item. Transactions in this item for the month of May are as follows:

	Units	Unit Cost
Inventory, May 1	3,000	$1.00
Purchase, May 5	2,000	1.20
Usage, May 10	1,500	?
Purchase, May 20	1,000	1.40
Usage, May 25	2,100	?

The hospital prices this item to patients at $2 per unit.

Required. Prepare journal entries to record all of the above assuming (1) the perpetual LIFO costing method and (2) the periodical weighted average method.

P2.   Given the following data relating to a single billable supply item purchased and sold by Ducton Hospital:

	Units	Unit Cost	Total Cost
Inventory, 3/1	200	$1.00	$ 200
Purchases:			
3/5	200	2.00	400
3/15	400	3.00	1,200
3/25	200		900
Total	1,000		$2,700
Sales:			
3/10	300		
3/20	400		
Total	700		
Inventory, 3/31	300		

Required. Compute the cost of supplies sold to patients during March and the inventory at March 31, assuming:

1. Periodic inventory system:
   a. Weighted average costing
   b. FIFO costing
   c. LIFO costing

2. Perpetual inventory system:
   a. Weighted average costing
   b. FIFO costing
   c. LIFO costing

P3. The following data were available from the records of a department of Johlson's Hospital for the current year:

	Cost	Retail
Inventory, January 1	$ 90,000	$130,000
Purchases	330,000	460,000
Markups		10,000
Markdowns		40,000
Gross revenues		480,000

Required. Using the retail method, what is the estimated amount of the December 31 inventory, valued at the lower of cost or market?

13
Current Liabilities

Liabilities, as defined in Chapter 2, are probable future sacrifices of economic benefits arising from present obligations of a particular entity to transfer assets or provide services to other entities in the future as a result of past transactions or events. More simply stated, the liabilities of a hospital are its economic obligations, based upon past transactions, to pay cash or convey other assets, or to perform certain services at some time in the future. Due to the credit-based economic system within which the hospital operates, its balance sheet will include a wide variety of debts representing goods and services purchased on account, borrowings from financial institutions, bond issues, and accruals for payrolls, payroll-related obligations, interest, and other expenses. All cash disbursements made by the hospital ordinarily require debits to previously established liability accounts of one kind or another.

Certain of these obligations are current liabilities of the hospital, and others are properly classified as noncurrent, or long-term, liabilities. This distinction is an important one for purposes of determining the current and long-term financial position of the hospital and in evaluating its ability to meet currently maturing commitments to banks, suppliers, employees, and other creditors. Long-term liabilities are discussed in Chapters 17 and 18; the present chapter deals with the problems of accounting for current liabilities; the management of current debt is a topic treated in the following chapter.

NATURE AND COMPOSITION

The traditional working definition of current liabilities commonly employed identifies them as those obligations which mature and normally will be paid within one year from the balance sheet date. While this definition is simple to apply and fairly satisfactory in many situations, it is arbitrary, incomplete, and fails to take into account the essential relationship between current assets and current liabilities. A strict **one year** interpretation of current liabilities is much too narrow. Accordingly, a more sophisticated and useful definition has been developed:[1]

The term **current liabilities** is used principally to designate obligations whose liquidation is reasonably expected to require the use of existing resources properly classifiable as current assets, or the creation of other current liabilities.

The latter part of the definition refers to the substitution of one current liability for another, such as executing a note to a supplier in settlement of an account payable. In short, current liabilities are those liabilities which are expected to be satisfied by either the use of assets classified as current in the same balance sheet or the creation of other current liabilities. Ordinarily, current liabilities are liquidated within a relatively short period of time, usually one year.

The current liability classification includes legally enforceable debts resulting from past (not future) transactions which will require future outlays in amounts that can be measured or estimated with reasonable accuracy. Yet, in somewhat unusual instances, legal obligations may arise that are so uncertain in amount that they defy measurement; thus, they may not be formally recorded in the accounts. Their existence nevertheless must be disclosed by footnote or in some other appropriate manner. On the other hand, there may be future outlays arising from past transactions that can be measured and should be recorded as current liabilities although they are not legally enforceable debts at present. Thus, the element of uncertainty is a significant factor in dealing with the problem of accounting for current liabilities. Most of these liabilities are definitely determinable, but the amounts of others must be estimated.

Theoretically, current liabilities should be measured in terms of the present values of the future outlays of money their liquidation will require. (A similar valuation basis for receivables was noted in Chapter 11.) Since current debts remain unpaid only for relatively short periods of time, the difference between their face amounts and their present values ordinarily is immaterial. In actual practice, therefore, current liabilities generally are recorded at their face amounts as a compromise of a relatively small degree of accuracy for convenience and simplicity. The omission or understatement of current liabilities, however, must be avoided. Such errors necessarily are accompanied by equal misstatements of assets, long-term liabilities, or fund balances, and may seriously affect the development of accurate cash budgets and estimates of short-term financial requirements.

In the hospital balance sheet, current liabilities usually are listed in a sequence that results in the best compromise between the amounts (largest to smallest) involved and the order of their maturities. Both objectives generally cannot be met, and the order of size often is followed except where there are significant differences in maturity. It is theoretically preferable, however, to list liabilities in the order of maturity. The extent of detail to be provided will depend largely upon the purposes for which the balance sheet is to be used. For general purposes, it usually is sufficient to disclose broad totals by major class of liability as indicated in the following discussion.

NOTES PAYABLE

Notes payable are obligations in the form of promissory notes issued to trade creditors for the purchase of goods and services, to banks and other financial institutions for loans of a short-term character, and to other organizations for the purchase of plant assets. Whereas trade accounts payable generally fall due within a month, notes may be outstanding for periods of 90, 180, or more days from the balance sheet date. If a note's maturity date is more than one year into the future, it should be classified in the balance sheet as a noncurrent liability. In the case of certain installment notes payable, a portion of the note may be current with the remainder being properly shown in a noncurrent section.

Liabilities in the form of notes payable are sometimes secured by the pledge of certain assets such as marketable securities or accounts receivable. In such instances, it is desirable to disclose the amount of the pledged asset either parenthetically or by footnote. The reader of the balance sheet is entitled to know that the use or disposition of the proceeds of such assets is restricted until the related obligation is liquidated. In addition to disclosing the extent to which notes payable may be secured by liens on assets, it also is useful to classify notes in terms of their origin. This provides important information concerning the extent to which the hospital has relied upon various sources of funds in financing its activities.

Although there are numerous types of promissory notes, the accounting procedures described in the author's **Introduction to Hospital Accounting** are fully applicable to most types. These procedures are not discussed here. An opinion of the Accounting Principles Board, however, requires a present value procedure where the hospital acquires assets on terms involving the issue of a noninterest-bearing note.[2] Assume, for example, that equipment is acquired in exchange for a one-year note of $16,200 without any reference being made to an interest rate. If money is worth 8% per year, the asset should be recorded at the cash equivalent or present value of the note, as follows:

Equipment	$ 15,000	
Discount on Notes Payable	1,200	
Notes Payable		$ 16,200

    To record acquisition of equipment and related
    liability at present value ($16,200/1.08).

The cost of the equipment for purposes of computing depreciation is $15,000, and the discount is amortized to interest expense through monthly amortization over the term of the note. In the balance sheet, the unamortized balance of the discount is deducted from the face amount of the note. The discount should not be shown as a prepaid expense on the asset side. If this procedure is not applied, the hospital's assets, liabilities, and expense would be misstated, possibly to a significant degree.

ACCOUNTS PAYABLE

Trade accounts payable originate from the purchase of supplies and services on account. As indicated in Chapter 8, the accounting procedures in this area should be systemized so that the existence, amount, and due date of these liabilities can be easily determined. Particular attention should be given to purchase transactions which take place near the end of the reporting period to ascertain that all accounts payable are properly reflected in the accounting records. If goods have arrived in the latter part of the period but the related invoice is not received until later, the goods might easily be included in inventory with the corresponding liability being overlooked.

Material amounts of debit balances in accounts payable sometimes arise due to overpayments or allowances granted by suppliers. For balance sheet presentation purposes, such amounts should be reclassified as receivables. Material credit balances in patients' accounts receivable, on the other hand, should be classified as accounts payable, deposits received from patients, or deferred income, depending upon the particular circumstances.

Where cash discounts in significant amounts will be taken in subsequent payment of accounts payable, such discounts should be anticipated. An entry is required debiting an Allowance for Purchase Discounts and crediting Purchase Discounts. The allowance account then is subtracted from accounts payable in the balance sheet presentation of current liabilities. When the accounts are paid, the allowance account is eliminated by credits. If, of course, accounts payable are initially recorded net of discounts as described in Chapter 8, this entry is unnecessary in that the valuation problem is resolved in the transaction entries.

The contingent liability created by purchase commitments for future delivery of supplies or services is not formally recorded in the accounts under ordinary circumstances. An entry may, however, be required to recognize a loss caused by a material decline in the market price of supplies or services ordered for resale. Recognition of such a loss necessitates the recording of a corresponding liability (see Chapter 12).

CURRENT MATURITIES OF LONG-TERM LIABILITIES

Mortgages, bond issues, and other long-term obligations of the hospital should be reported as current liabilities to the extent that they are to be paid within one year from current assets. In many instances, such as with mortgage notes and bonds that mature in annual installments, a portion of the particular obligation is presented as a current liability and the balance of the debt remains in a long-term classification. The amount that is current is usually called **current maturities of long-term debt.** If the maturing obligation is to be paid from a noncurrent asset such as a debt retirement fund or is to be retired from the proceeds of a new debt issue (as in the case of bond refunding), the obligation should continue to be listed as a long-term liability.

A short-term obligation, however, should be excluded from current liabilities only if both of the following criteria are met:[3]

1. The hospital must intend to refinance the obligation on a long-term basis, and
2. The hospital must demonstrate an ability to consummate the refinancing.

In this context, the term "refinance" means replacing the short-term obligation with a long-term obligation (or with equity securities), or renewing, extending, or replacing the short-term obligation with another short-term obligation for a period beyond one year from the balance sheet date. In other words, the short-term obligation will not require the use of working capital within one year.

The ability to consummate a refinancing is evidenced (1) by actually refinancing the short-term obligation after the balance sheet date but before the balance sheet is issued or (2) by entering into a financing agreement that clearly enables the hospital to accomplish the refinancing on a long-term basis. The financing agreement must be noncancellable, it must extend beyond one year from the balance sheet date, and it must not be in default. In addition, the lender or investor must be capable of honoring the agreement.

The amount of short-term obligations excluded from current liabilities may not exceed the proceeds from the issue of the new long-term obligations or equity securities. In the case of a financing agreement, the amount of short-term obligations so excluded cannot exceed the amount available for refinancing under the agreement.

To illustrate, assume that a hospital has a short-term obligation of $250,000 at December 31, 1987, that matures on April 1, 1988. Subsequent to the balance sheet date (December 31, 1987) but before the balance sheet was issued, the hospital issued long-term notes payable, intending to use the proceeds to pay the short-term debt at its maturity. If the proceeds from the issue of the long-term notes are $250,000 or more, the entire amount of the short-term obligation may be excluded from current liabilities at December 31, 1987. Should the proceeds be only $200,000, for example, then only $200,000 of the short-term obligation could be excluded from current liabilities at December 31, 1987.

On the other hand, the current liability section of the balance sheet should include obligations that, by their terms, are due on demand or will be due on demand within one year (or operating cycle, if longer), even though liquidation may not be expected within that period. Under certain circumstances, long-term obligations that are or will be callable by the creditor also should be included in current liabilities.[4]

ACCRUED LIABILITIES

Accrued liabilities, sometimes called accrued expenses payable, consist of obligations that arise as a result of past operations involving contractual commitments or tax legislation. In reporting accrued liabilities, the usual practice is to report accrued payroll and payroll-related liabilities separate from interest, rentals, and other miscellaneous accruals because of their materiality.

Accrued Payroll

Employees ordinarily are paid subsequent to their performance of services, and the end of pay periods may not coincide with the end of the reporting period. It therefore is likely that a hospital balance sheet at a given date will include an obligation for unpaid salaries and wages. A two-week pay period, for example, may have begun on a Monday, but the accounting period may end on Friday, five days later. The balance sheet must therefore include a current liability for the five days of unpaid salaries and wages that have been earned by employees. The accrual should include the salaries and wages of all hospital personnel, whether paid on an hourly, weekly, or monthly basis.

In most instances, accruals for salaries and wages are made on the basis of "gross" compensation, i.e., without reduction for taxes and other withholdings. (Governmental regulations and cost reimbursement contracts, however, may require this breakdown on the expense side.) The separation of withholdings is unnecessary and can be postponed until the payroll for the complete period is vouchered for payment. The determination of the amount of the accrual, particularly for hourly employees, can be a laborious process. It ordinarily is sufficient to estimate the amount of the accrual by some reasonably accurate method. A commonly used method is to estimate on the basis of historical data the payroll cost per day and multiply it by the number of days involved in the accrual period. The entry is:

Salaries and Wages Expense*	$xxx,xxx	
Accrued Salaries and Wages Payable		$xxx,xxx
To record accrued payroll.		

*Classified by department or cost center.

At the beginning of the following accounting period, the entry is reversed. This procedure is required under the accrual basis of accounting in order to give recognition to the expense in the period in which it is incurred rather than in the period in which it is paid. In this way, there is a proper matching of expenses with revenues for purposes of measuring periodic operating results.

Vacation Pay and Other Compensated Absences

Employees are given vacations with pay usually after a specified period of employment, and the length of the vacation period often increases with the completion of a certain number of years of continued service. Assume, for example, that an employee who earns $300 per week has a right to a two-week vacation each year. This employee, in effect, is paid $15,600 for 50 weeks of actual productive service, or $312 per week. When should the $12 per week of vacation pay be recorded as an expense? When should the liability for the vacation pay of $600 be recorded for accounting purposes?

Although the **legal** liability depends upon the terms of the employment contract, there would appear to be no question of the **economic** liability, particularly where the amount can be closely estimated on a composite basis in terms of the hospital's employee turnover experience. Both the liability for vacation pay and the related compensation expense should be recorded in the year in which earned by employees. The accrual basis of accounting for expenses therefore suggests an entry at each pay period as follows (using the above example):

Salaries and Wages Expense*	$12	
Accrued Vacation Pay Liability		$12
To record accrued liability for employee's		
vacation pay.		

*Classified by department or cost center.

This accrual usually is based on the employee's current wage or salary rate rather than an estimate of the pay rate that may exist during the actual period of compensated absence. There may be considerable uncertainty as to the future rate of pay.

When individual employees actually take their vacations, the accrued liability account is debited; cash and the withholding accounts are credited. Any excess of actual vacation pay over the amounts previously accrued should be charged to expense in the period of payment.

The matter of compensated absences arising from vacations, holidays, and illness is addressed in FASB Statement No. 43 which requires the accrual of a liability for the cost of compensated future absences when all four of the following conditions exist:[5]

1. The employer's obligation relating to employees' rights to receive compensation for future absences is attributable to employees' services already rendered.
2. The obligation relates to the rights that vest or accumulate.
3. Payment of the compensation is probable, and
4. The amount can be reasonably estimated.

An employee has vested rights when the employer is obligated to pay for future absences even if employment is terminated. Accumulated rights are those which accumulate and may be carried forward to future periods if not used in the period in which earned by the employee.

Special treatment is given to the cost of compensated absences arising from illness. An accrual must be made for sick pay benefits that are vested rights. If such benefits accumulate but do not vest, the employer may make an accrual but it is not required.

Payroll Withholdings and Tax Accruals

Legislation enacted by the federal, state, and local governments imposes a number of taxes on salaries and wages paid to hospital personnel. The principal features of some of these laws were described earlier in Chapter 8. Provisions of the legislation require that the hospital and other employers maintain detailed records concerning individual employees' hours, earnings, tax deductions, etc. A large volume of clerical effort and expense is involved in the keeping of payroll records in compliance with these laws. The hospital employer, of course, is not reimbursed by any governmental agency for this record-keeping and tax collection function. This aspect of the paycheck is not widely appreciated by employees. The hospital is also required to match the employee's social security tax and this alone amounts to a significant element of hospital operating costs.

Tax Withholdings. The federal income tax has been collected on a pay-as-you-go basis for more than forty years. This payment system requires employers to withhold from employees' wages an amount approximating the income tax due on such wages. The amount, generally determined from tables furnished by the government, varies according to the amount of taxable wages, the length of the payroll period, the employee's marital status, and the number of dependents claimed by the employee. Withholding is required only where a legal employer-employee relationship exists, thus excluding the compensation paid to independent contractors.

The amounts so withheld by the hospital must be paid to the government on a quarterly, monthly, or other specified basis, depending upon the amount of tax involved. For most hospitals, remittance must be made within three days following the close of each quarter-monthly period, depending upon the amount of tax involved. This is accomplished by a deposit of the withheld amounts, plus FICA tax accrued, in an authorized government depository. In addition, a quarterly statement must be filed to provide a summary of all wages paid during each quarter. Rather severe penalties and interest charges are imposed on employers who fail to deposit withheld taxes or file payroll tax returns in the prescribed manner and at prescribed times. Most states and many large cities also levy income taxes. In such cases, hospitals often must withhold these taxes also. Amounts withheld, determined by formulas or tables, are remitted periodically to the governmental units as required by law.

The Federal Insurance Contributions Act (FICA), more popularly called Social Security, provides for a tax on employees' earnings to finance a federal program of old age, survivors, disability, and hospital insurance benefits for employees and members of their families. As is true of income tax, the FICA tax is required to be withheld by the hospital from taxable wage payments to employees. The tax rates and base earnings (maximum annual earnings subject to this tax) have increased often and substantially in recent years, and it is reasonable to assume that this trend will continue. Currently, the FICA tax is 7.05 percent of the first $39,600 of taxable wages paid to each employee.

Provisions of the FICA tax legislation require an equal contribution by the hospital of the amount paid by employees through the withholding procedure. Both the employer's and employee's FICA taxes are remitted by the hospital at the same time as, and together with, federal income tax withholdings.

Tax Accruals. As FICA taxes are withheld from employees' salaries and wages, the hospital must accrue, as an expense and a liability, its matching FICA tax contributions. It is important that **taxable** salaries and wages be determined accurately (some payments to employees may be exempt) and that FICA withholdings be properly computed. The employer required to withhold income and FICA taxes is liable for the timely payment of the correct amount of such taxes **whether or not** it actually is collected from employees.

In addition to FICA tax accruals, many hospitals must also accrue federal and state unemployment taxes. The Federal Unemployment Tax Act (FUTA) provides for a tax, currently 6.2 percent of the first $7,000 of taxable wages paid to each employee, to finance the administration of the federal/state unemployment compensation program. This law does not provide for the payment of unemployment benefits; that is the function of the state programs. The federal tax is levied entirely on the employer who generally is allowed a credit of up to 90 percent against the federal tax for contributions made by the employer to an accredited state unemployment fund. An additional credit may sometimes be granted under a "merit rating" provision of the law.

State unemployment compensation laws vary widely in rates and other details. In almost all cases, however, the tax is levied exclusively on the employer.

The hospital therefore must accrue federal and state unemployment taxes during each reporting period by a debit to expense and a credit to a tax liability account. While FUTA taxes are payable on an annual basis each January 31, the state tax (SUTA) generally is remitted on a quarterly basis. Payroll tax return forms, of course, must be filed for both federal and state unemployment taxes.

Other Withholdings and Accruals. In addition to the compulsory withholdings related to income and FICA tax laws, a large variety of other deductions may be withheld from salary and wage payments. These withholdings usually require the consent of the employee. Included in this category are deductions for government savings bonds, premiums for health, accident, hospital, and life insurance, deductions for union membership dues, deductions in connection with employee pension and retirement plans, withholdings related to employee credit unions, and withholdings representing employees' contributions to community chests or other charitable organizations. At regular intervals, the hospital must summarize the withholdings for the period in suitable reports and remit the amounts withheld to the appropriate agencies.

In the case of certain so-called fringe benefits such as insurance and pension plans, it is common for hospitals to share the cost with their employees. The employee's agreed share is withheld from earnings, and the hospital's share is accrued by debiting an expense and crediting a liability account.

Summary. To illustrate the accounting procedure for payroll withholdings and accruals, assume a taxable payroll of $100,000 for a given time period. The entry to record the payroll might appear as shown below:

Salaries and Wages Expense	$100,000	
Federal Income Taxes Withheld		$ 18,000
FICA Taxes Payable		7,050
Noncompulsory Withholdings Liability		1,150
Accrued Salaries and Wages Payable		73,800
To record payroll for the period.		

The debit in this entry, of course, represents a series of debits to appropriate departmental cost centers on a responsibility accounting basis. The single credit to Noncompulsory Withholdings represents the several credits that typically are necessary to properly record the various items for which such withholdings are made.

At the time the payroll is recorded, or at the end of the monthly reporting period, appropriate tax accruals such as the following are made:

FICA Tax Expense	$ 7,050	
FUTA Tax Expense	620	
SUTA Tax Expense	5,580	
FICA Taxes Payable		$ 7,050
FUTA Taxes Payable		620
SUTA Taxes Payable		5,580
To record accrued liabilities for hospital's share of payroll taxes.		

The expense debits shown above ordinarily should be charged to an unassigned expense category within the administrative services classification. As discussed in Chapter 8, employee benefits often are not allocated to cost centers in the formal accounting routine (unless, of course, the hospital employs a cost accounting system). It can be a laborious process and it accomplishes little or nothing of value, except in some cases where it might affect the amount of cost reimbursement to the hospital. In the absence of a cost accounting system, the allocation of employee benefits to cost centers generally is best deferred to the cost-finding procedure.

In addition to payroll tax accruals, the hospital must also accrue all other employee benefits which it has agreed to pay. These benefits would include such items as the hospital's agreed share of employees' insurance and pension plan costs. Debits are made to appropriate employee benefit expense accounts and credits are established in suitable liability accounts.

Periodically, in accordance with tax laws and contractual requirements, the liabilities established in the above entries are paid. At those times, of course, the liability accounts are debited and credits are made to Cash in Bank for the amounts remitted. Sight must not be lost of the fact that the hospital is acting as the employee's agent in making withholdings, and the amounts withheld must be considered as being held in trust for the employee until such time as they are remitted to the proper authority.

Property Taxes

Hospitals that are subject to state and local property taxes generally must accrue such taxes on a monthly basis during the taxing authority's fiscal year for which the taxes are levied.[6] To illustrate, assume that the fiscal year of a hospital ends on

December 31, but that the fiscal year of the governmental unit in which the hospital is located ends on June 30. The governmental unit assesses property taxes in its jurisdiction in the Spring of each year, and places a lien against these properties on July 1. Property taxes are billed to property owners on October 1, and payment in full is due by December 31.

In this situation, the hospital must estimate on July 1, 1987, the amount of its tax liability for the year ending June 30, 1988 (the fiscal year of taxing authority). Assume that the property tax is estimated at $8,400 (based on assessed valuation and anticipated tax rates). On October 1, 1987, however, the tax bill indicates a total tax of $8,940. The tax is paid by the hospital on December 31, 1987. Assuming that monthly financial statements are prepared, what entries for property taxes should be made by the hospital?

The most commonly employed procedure is to recognize property tax expense and accrue the tax liability on a monthly basis. On July 31, August 31, and September 30, 1987, the following entry would be made:

Property Tax Expense	$ 700	
Property Taxes Payable		$ 700
Monthly property tax accrual, based on		
estimated taxes of $8,400 for the 12		
months ending June 30, 1988.		

On October 1, 1987, when the tax bill is received, the actual property tax for the year is known to be $8,940. Since property tax expense of $2,100 ($700 X 3 months) has previously been recorded, the remaining $6,840 should be allocated over the remaining nine months (October, 1987, through June, 1988) at the rate of $760 per month. Thus, the following entry should be made at October 31 and November 30:

Property Tax Expense	$ 760	
Property Taxes Payable		$ 760
Monthly property tax accrual, computed as		
follows:		
Total taxes	$8,940	
Previously accrued	2,100	
Balance, allocable over nine		
months	$6,840	
Monthly allocation ($6,840/9)	$ 760	

When the property taxes are paid on December 31, 1987, the appropriate entry would be:

Property Taxes Payable	$ 3,620	
Deferred Property Tax Expense	5,320	
Cash		$ 8,940

Payment of 1987-1988 property taxes:

Taxes paid	$8,940
Previously accrued ($700 for 3 months and $760 for 2 months)	3,620
Deferred (prepaid) taxes	$5,320

Starting on December 31, 1987, and extending through June 30, 1988, the monthly adjustment for property taxes would be:

Property Tax Expense	$ 760	
Deferred Property Tax Expense		$ 760

Monthly adjustment for property tax expense ($5,320/7 months).

An alternative practice is to record the full amount of the estimated tax liability on the lien date (July 1, in the above illustration), with a debit to Deferred Property Tax Expense. While the monthly expense will be the same as above, the balances of the deferred tax and tax liability accounts will be somewhat different until the tax is paid.

Other Accrued Liabilities

While most accrued liabilities usually are payroll-related, accruals also may be necessary for various expense items such as interest and rent. Immaterial amounts of these liabilities generally are combined in a single category such as "interest, rent, and other accrued liabilities" or, simply, "other accrued liabilities." In some cases, accrued interest expense may be combined with the amount of the note payable liability to which it relates, assuming that both are current obligations. Interest currently payable on a long-term liability is properly classified as a current liability. Accruals for interest and rent ordinarily are made on the basis of the passage of time. Entries for such accruals are illustrated in the author's **Introduction to Hospital Accounting**.

DEFERRED REVENUES

Hospitals sometimes receive cash advances from patients, third-party payers, and others for services that are to be provided in the future. Prepayments of this kind are recorded as liabilities when they are received. If the provision of such future services will involve significant costs to be financed from the hospital's current resources, the advances should be classified as current liabilities.

The hospital, for example, may operate an educational program for which students pay tuition in advance of the period during which the program will be conducted. Tuition receipts, then, should be credited to a deferred revenue account. As the educational program progresses through the school year or other term, the tuition payments are earned by the hospital. And, as this occurs, entries should be made to transfer the earned amounts from deferred revenues to tuition income. This procedure gives appropriate recognition to the hospital liability to provide the educational services and also results in a proper matching of revenues and expenses.

Advances may also be received from third-party payers in connection with certain reimbursement programs. Such advances ordinarily are made in anticipation of hospital services to be provided to patients in the near future. They are intended to assist the hospital with the problem of financing such services on a current basis. Where this is the case, these advances properly are classified as current liabilities. As the services are rendered, the obligation is liquidated and appropriate amounts of the advances should be recognized as revenues. Thus, a suitable matching of revenues and expenses is obtained.

Amounts received on a tentative basis prior to a final settlement of claims against third parties arising from services **already** provided by the hospital to patients should be credited to accounts receivable.

Deferred revenue may also arise when third-party reimbursements received are based upon costs determined by an accelerated depreciation method while, at the same time, smaller amounts of depreciation are being taken for financial accounting purposes. These deferred revenue amounts may be classified to some extent as current liabilities, with the balance being properly shown as a noncurrent liability.[7] Similar deferrals may also be required in connection with pension costs and vacation pay where they are accounted for in different periods for reimbursement and for financial reporting purposes. In all these cases, the objective is to place the revenues in the same reporting period in which the related cost and expenses are recognized so as to secure a proper determination of periodic net income or loss.

It sometimes has been the practice to report all deferred revenues in a separate balance sheet classification located between current liabilities and long-term liabilities. Use of a special classification of this kind should be avoided. A failure to properly identify deferred revenues as either current or noncurrent obligations may lead to serious misinterpretations, although the practice is often defended on grounds of conservatism.

CONDITIONAL OBLIGATIONS

The amounts of certain current liabilities that are accrued on a monthly basis are dependent upon annual operating results. Examples of such liabilities include income taxes payable and amounts due to employees under bonus and profit-sharing plans. Liabilities of this type are estimates subject to a future final determination of their actual amounts.

Income Taxes Payable

Income tax payable is a conditional liability because the computation of taxable income and the related tax is subject to subsequent review and approval by the taxing authorities. Should taxes be assessed in excess of the estimate for a prior year, the additional taxes should be accounted for as a change in an accounting estimate as required by APB Opinion No. 20.[8] In other words, the additional taxes should be recognized as an expense and as a liability in the current year, with no retroactive restatement of prior periods. When there are timing differences between accounting income before tax and taxable income, a deferred income tax liability arises. In some cases, the deferred taxes are reported as current liabilities.

Bonus and Profit-Sharing Plans

Officers, physicians, and employees sometimes may be given compensation in the form of a bonus, profit-sharing, or other conditional payments that are dependent upon the performance of a department or the hospital as a whole. Performance may be measured in terms of attaining established revenue, expense, or income objectives.

To illustrate, assume that an employee bonus plan provides for a bonus of 25% of net income after deducting the bonus as an expense. If the net income before consideration of the bonus is, say, $62,500, then the bonus is computed as follows:

Let X equal the net income after deducting the bonus. Therefore, $62,500 equals 1.25X, and X equals $50,000. The bonus is 25% of $50,000, or $12,500.

The entry to record the bonus would be one debiting Employee Bonus Expense and crediting Accrued Employee Bonus Payable. The bonus may be recorded monthly on an estimated basis, with an appropriate adjustment being made at year-end when the net income for the year is determined.

CONTINGENT LIABILITIES

FASB Statement No. 5 defines a **contingency** as an existing condition, situation, or set of circumstances involving uncertainty as to possible gain or loss to an enterprise that will ultimately be resolved when one or more future events occur or fail to occur.[9] A **contingent liability** is one that arises from the existence of a loss contingency. For example, assume that a hospital is being sued by a supplier because of a dispute relating to a purchase of inventory items. The lawsuit is pending at the balance sheet date, but a decision will not be rendered by the courts for several months. Should the hospital record an estimated loss and report a contingent liability at the balance sheet date?

An important factor to be considered in the likelihood that the future event (the decision of the courts, for instance) will confirm the loss and the incurrence of a liability. The FASB employs the terms "probable," "reasonably possible," and "remote" to characterize this likelihood:

1. **Probable** means that the future event is likely to occur.
2. **Reasonably** possible means that the chance of the future event occurring is greater than remote, but less than likely.
3. **Remote** means that the chance of the future event occurring is slight.

The second critical consideration is whether or not the amount of loss is subject to reasonable estimate.

FASB Statement No. 5 requires that the estimated loss from a loss contingency be accrued by a charge against income if both of the following conditions are met:

1. It is probable that a liability has been incurred at the balance sheet date, and
2. The amount of the loss can be reasonably estimated.

When no accrual is made because one or both of these conditions are not met, but there is at least a reasonable possibility that a liability may have been incurred, a footnote is required to disclose the nature of the contingency and an estimate of the possible loss or range of loss (or the fact that an estimate cannot be made). Where the possibility that a liability may have been incurred is remote, disclosure generally is not necessary.

The **Hospital Audit Guide** requires that the estimated loss contingency resulting from malpractice risks be accrued and disclosed in conformity with the above provisions of FASB Statement No. 5 and FASB Interpretation No. 14.[10] Unasserted claims require disclosure only if it is probable that a claim will be asserted and there is a reasonable possibility that the outcome will be unfavorable. Because of the significance of malpractice risks to hospitals, however, it is recommended that hospitals also disclose in their financial statements the possibility of losses from unasserted claims that do not meet these criteria. Following is an example of appropriate financial statement disclosure:[11]

Malpractice claims in excess of insurance coverage have been asserted against the hospital by various claimants. The claims are in various stages of processing and some may ultimately be brought to trial. Counsel is unable to conclude about the ultimate outcome of the actions. There are known incidents occurring through [balance sheet date] that may result in the assertion of additional claims, and other claims may be asserted arising from services provided to patients in the past. The hospital is unable to estimate the ultimate cost, if any, of the settlement of such potential claims and, accordingly, no accrual has been made for them.

Disclosure of contingent liabilities arising from the discounting of patients' notes with recourse may be made by parenthetical comment, by footnote, or by a fund balance appropriation:

1.   Parenthetical comment.

     Notes receivable from patients (net of $50,000 of notes which have been discounted and for which the hospital is contingently liable) $120,000

2.   Footnote.
     Note B—The hospital is contingently liable with respect to $50,000 of patients' notes receivable which have been discounted with recourse.

3.   Appropriation of fund balance.

     Unrestricted Fund Balance:
        Appropriated for contingent liability with
        regard to patients' notes receivable which
        have been discounted $ 50,000
        Unappropriated balance   680,145

     Total Unrestricted Fund Balance $730,145

BALANCE SHEET PRESENTATION

Current liabilities are presented as the first section on the "liabilities and fund balances (equity)" side of the balance sheet. It is important that descriptive titles or captions be used for the current liability items. Sufficient detail and supplementary information should be provided in parenthetical notations and footnotes to meet disclosure requirements. Disclosure should be made of all secured liabilities, and the assets pledged to their payment should be identified. The offsetting of current liabilities against assets is not an acceptable practice unless a right of setoff exists. Existing commitments of material amounts, although not formally recorded in the accounts, should be disclosed by appropriate footnotes. Accounting policies having a significant effect on the measurement or presentation of current liability items also should be described in the "Summary of Significant Accounting Policies."[12] An excerpt from an actual balance sheet that is representative of the presentation of current liabilities by hospitals is provided in Figure 13-1.

Figure 13-1.
Balance Sheet Presentation of Current Liabilities

Current liabilities:	
Notes payable	$ 30,000
Accounts payable	234,322
Accrued salaries and related liabilities	147,710
Accrued interest payable	19,750
Other accrued expenses payable	29,555
Medical professional fees	78,799
Third-party settlements (Note 5)	255,000
Due to restricted funds	12,636
Current maturities of long-term debt	95,863
Total current liabilities	$903,635

INTERNAL CONTROL

The key to effective internal control over liabilities lies in (1) the approval of purchase, borrowing, payroll, or other transactions giving rise to hospital liabilities and (2) the proper determination of the amounts in which such liabilities are recorded. This means that all necessary steps should be taken to provide assurances that only bona fide liabilities are established in the accounts and that they are recorded in correct amounts. The vouchering system should require that appropriate authorizations and approvals be fully evidenced in writing before any liabilities are recorded and before disbursements are made to discharge them. On the other hand, it is important that procedures be followed which reduce the possibility that actual liabilities will be overlooked and omitted from the accounting records. Open purchase orders, unmatching receiving reports, and unprocessed invoices should be reviewed to ascertain whether or not unrecorded commitments exist (see Chapters 5, 8 and 10).

Subsidiary ledger records must be maintained for accounts payable. Detailed records of a supportive nature must also be kept available for balances of notes payable, payroll withholdings, and other accrued liabilities. Employees who maintain these detailed records should be independent of the general ledger accounting function. The individual creditor balances provided in the detailed records should be reconciled with the related control accounts at the end of each monthly reporting period. Reconciliations should be reviewed periodically by a responsible employee independent of the approval and payment of liabilities.

Accounting procedures must also exist to assure timely payment of accounts and notes payable in proper amounts. While liabilities need not be paid earlier than necessary, substantial losses can arise from the failure to pay maturing obligations in time to take advantage of discount opportunities. A reputation for delayed payment of its obligations may also damage the hospital's credit standing with suppliers and bankers.

All borrowings by the hospital should have the approval of the governing board or an executive finance committee. Notes and other evidences of debt should be executed in the corporate name of the hospital and be signed by designated hospital officials. Copies of these instruments should be provided to the accounting department for comparison with related cash receipt and disbursement transactions.

CHAPTER 13 FOOTNOTES

1. **"Restatement and Revision of Accounting Research Bulletins,"** Accounting Research Bulletin No. 43 (New York: AICPA, 1953), Chapter 3A, Par. 7.
2. **"Interest on Receivables and Payables,"** APB Opinion No. 21 (New York: AICPA, 1971), par. 12.
3. **"Classification of Short-Term Obligations Expected to Be Refinanced,"** Statement of Financial Accounting Standards No. 6 (Stamford, Connecticut: FASB, 1975), par. 10-11.
4. **"Classifications of Obligations That Are Callable by the Creditor,"** Statement of Financial Accounting Standards No. 78 (Stamford, Connecticut: FASB, 1983), par. 5.
5. **"Accounting for Compensated Absences,"** Statement of Financial Accounting Standards No. 43 (Stamford, Connecticut: FASB, 1980), par. 6.
6. **"Restatement and Revision of Accounting Research Bulletins,"** Accounting Research Bulletin No. 43 (New York: AICPA, 1953), Chapter 10A, par. 14.
7. **"Balance Sheet Classification of Deferred Income Taxes,"** Statement of Financial Accounting Standards No. 37 (Stamford, Connecticut: FASB, 1980), par. 4.
8. **"Accounting Changes,"** APB Opinion No. 20 (New York: AICPA, 1971), par. 31.
9. **"Accounting for Contingencies,"** Statement of Financial Accounting Standards No. 5 (Stamford, Connecticut: FASB, 1975), par. 1.
10. **"Reasonable Estimation of the Amount of a Loss,"** Interpretation No. 14 (Stamford, Connecticut: FASB, 1976).
11. **"Clarification of Accounting, Auditing, and Reporting Practices Relating to Hospital Malpractice Loss Contingencies,"** Hospital Audit Guide — Fourth Edition (New York: AICPA, 1982), Appendix B, p. 68.
12. **"Disclosure of Accounting Policies,"** APB Opinion No. 22 (New York: AICPA, 1972), par. 8.

QUESTIONS

1.   Define the term **liability.** Distinguish between current and noncurrent liabilities.
2.   Zipp Hospital's liabilities include a $50,000 note payable to a bank. This liability is secured by the pledge of $75,000 of accounts receivable. It has been suggested that the note be shown in the hospital's balance sheet as a deduction from accounts receivable. Would you agree with such a presentation? If not, how would you recommend that these matters be presented in the hospital's balance sheet?
3.   Tripp Hospital acquired an item of equipment in exchange for a one-year note of $26,750 with no reference being made to interest. At what **cost** should the equipment be recorded in the accounts of the hospital if money is worth 7% per year? Explain.
4.   Kent Hospital purchased supplies of $8,000 in late 1987. These supplies were received on December 29, 1987, and were included in the December 31 inventory. The related invoice, however, was not received until January 10, 1988, when an entry was made debiting supplies expense and crediting accounts payable. What misstatements existed in the hospital's 1987 financial statements?
5.   Phipp Hospital's December 31, 1987, balance sheet includes gross accounts payable of $65,000 in the current liabilities. All these accounts are subject to a 2 percent discount if paid by January 10, 1988, and Phipp Hospital has a policy of taking all available discounts. What adjusting entry, if any, would you recommend at December 31, 1987?
6.   Dipp Hospital obtains a $100,000, 8% mortgage loan from a bank on January 1, 1987. The mortgage is to be repaid in ten equal annual installments of $10,000 (plus interest), commencing December 31, 1987. Indicate how these matters should be presented in the hospital's December 31, 1987, balance sheet.
7.   Explain why it is necessary to make adjusting entries at the end of each accounting period for accrued payroll.
8.   It was noted in the text of this chapter that the FICA tax rates and base earnings have increased substantially in recent years. What is the current FICA tax rate? What is the current amount of a hospital employee's annual earnings subject to FICA taxes?
9.   What are **deferred revenues?** Why are they classified in the hospital balance sheet as liabilities? Give three examples of items that may be shown as deferred revenues in a hospital's balance sheet.
10. Define the term **contingent liability.** Give two examples of contingent liabilities and state how these items might be reflected in the hospital's balance sheet.
11. Describe the major features of a satisfactory system of internal control over current liabilities.

EXERCISES

E1.   Bonny Hospital issued its $60,000, 90-day, 8% note to a bank on August 1. Interest on the note was not prepaid by the hospital. The note, with interest for the 90 days, was repaid on the maturity date.

Required. Prepare the necessary journal entry at (1) August 1, (2) August 31, (3) September 30, and (4) the maturity date. Indicate how all matters relating to the note should be presented in the hospital's financial statements prepared on September 30.

E2. Bennett Hospital acquired an item of depreciable equipment on April 1 in exchange for a noninterest-bearing note of $53,750 due in one year. The equipment has a 10 percent salvage value and an estimated useful life of five years. Money is worth 7.5% per year.

Required. Prepare the necessary journal entries at April 1 and April 30, including depreciation expense for April. Indicate how all matters relating to the above should be presented in the hospital's April 30 balance sheet and in its income statement for April.

E3. Bagley Hospital purchased $45,000 of supplies for inventory in the month of March. The invoices are subject to 2 percent discount if paid by April 10. All the invoices, except one of $5,000, are paid within the discount period. The $5,000 invoice is not paid until April 20.

Required. Prepare journal entries to record all of the above, assuming that Bagley Hospital employs an Allowance for Purchase Discounts account.

E4. Bellamy Hospital's general ledger at September 30 (the end of its fiscal year) shows a preadjusted balance of salaries and wages expense in the amount of $875,000. At September 30, however, accrued salaries and wages total $15,400. The first pay date of the next fiscal year is October 11 at which time a total of $36,700 of salaries and wages is paid. Payroll taxes may be ignored for the purposes of this problem.

Required. Prepare entries to record the accrued payroll at September 30 and to record the payroll disbursement of October 11.

E5. Bagwell Hospital has 50 employees, each of whom earns $350 per week and is entitled to a two-week vacation each year. Assume that the FICA tax rate is 6% and that 16% federal income tax withholdings are to be made.

Required. Prepare a summary journal entry to record all matters relating to the hospital payroll for a single weekly pay period.

E6. Boswell Hospital operates an educational program in which 22 students have been enrolled for the nine-month school year which begins on September 1. The $225 tuition for the school is collected in advance from each student on September 1 (a total of $4,950).

Required. Prepare the necessary journal entries at September 1 and September 30. Indicate how these matters should be presented in the hospital's income statement for September and in its September 30 balance sheet.

E7. Blank Hospital accepts notes from patients in settlement of their accounts but immediately discounts these notes with a local bank. At June 30, for example, the hospital's accounting records indicate active notes receivable of $95,000, all of which have been discounted (with recourse) at the local bank. All notes bear interest at 8% and were discounted at 8%. Experience has shown that approximately 10 percent of patients' notes are discounted at maturity.

$7,600

Required. Indicate fully how you would recommend that all of the above matters be reflected in Blank Hospital's June 30 balance sheet.

E8. Bliss Hospital began operations on January 1. The payroll period is monthly with payroll disbursements being made on the first of each month. In the first quarter of the year, salaries and wages were as follows:

January	$100,000
February	140,000
March	120,000

360

All salaries and wages are fully taxable and are subject to the following assumed tax rates:

FICA taxes	6.0%
Federal income tax withholdings	15.0 — 54,000
FUTA taxes	.5
SUTA taxes	2.7

FICA taxes and income tax withholdings are remitted on February 15 and March 15, with the balance of such taxes for the quarter being remitted on April 30. The SUTA taxes are payable quarterly on the last day of the month following each calendar quarter. The FUTA taxes are payable annually on January 31.

Required. Prepare journal entries for all of the above for the four months ended April 30. Indicate how these matters should be presented in the hospital's financial statements for the quarter.

E10. The following multiple-choice items relate to liabilities.

1. Estimated liabilities are disclosed in hospital financial statements by

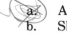

   a. A footnote to the statements.
   b. Showing the amount among the liabilities but not extending it to the liability total.
   c. An appropriation of the Unrestricted Fund balance.
   d. Appropriately classifying them as regular liabilities in the balance sheet.

2. On September 1, 1987, a hospital borrowed cash and signed a one-year, interest-bearing note on which both the principal and interest are payable on September 1, 1988. How will the note payable and the related interest be classified in the December 31, 1987, balance sheet?

	Note Payable	Accrued Interest
a.	Current liability	Noncurrent liability
b.	Noncurrent liability	Current liability
c.	Current liability	Current liability
d.	Noncurrent liability	No entry

3. Which of the following sets of conditions would give rise to the accrual of a contingency under current generally accepted accounting principles?

   a. Amount of loss is reasonably estimable and event occurs infrequently.
   b. Amount of loss is reasonably estimable and occurrence of event is probable.
   c. Event is unusual in nature and occurrence of event is probable.
   d. Event is unusual in nature and event occurs infrequently.

4. An estimated loss from a loss contingency that is probable and for which the amount of the loss can be reasonably estimated should

   a. Not be accrued but should be disclosed in the notes to the financial statements.
   b. Be accrued by debiting an appropriated fund balance account and crediting a liability account or an asset account.
   c. Be accrued by debiting an expense account and crediting an appropriated fund balance account.
   d. Be accrued by debiting an expense account and crediting a liability or an asset account.

5. How should a loss contingency that is reasonably possible and for which the amount can be reasonably estimated be reported?

	Accrued	Disclosed
a.	Yes	No
b.	No	Yes
c.	Yes	Yes
d.	No	No

6. In determining whether to accrue employees' compensation for future absences, one of the conditions that must be met is that the employer has an obligation to make payment even if an employee terminates. This is an example of a (an)

    a.   Vested right.
    b.   Accumulated right.
    c.   Contingent right.
    d.   Estimable right.

7. Morgan Hospital determined that: (1) it has a material obligation relating to employees' rights to receive compensation for future absences attributable to employees' services already rendered, (2) the obligation relates to rights that vest, and (3) payment of the compensation is probable. The amount of Morgan's obligation at 12/31/87 is reasonably estimated for the following employee benefits:

Vacation pay, $100,000
Holiday pay, $25,000

What total amount should Morgan report as its liability for compensated absences in its 12/31/87 balance sheet?

    a. $--0--
    b. $25,000
    c. $100,000
    d. $125,000

8. Gain contingencies are usually recognized in the income statement when

    a.   Realized.
    b.   Occurrence is reasonably possible and the amount can be reasonably estimated.
    c.   Occurrence is probable and the amount can be reasonably estimated.
    d.   The amount can be reasonably estimated.

Required. Select the best answer for each of the above multiple-choice items.

14
Working Capital Management

The four preceding chapters described generally accepted accounting methods and procedures employed to develop accurate and reliable information concerning the current assets and current liabilities of the hospital as reported in the Unrestricted Fund. In this chapter, the emphasis is on the uses of such information in the management of the hospital's current financial position, i.e., the optimization of the level and composition of current assets, and the manner in which they are financed. Included is a description of the hospital's operating cycle, an analysis of the investment of current resources, the development of control reports, the determination of the appropriate sources of current financing, and the use of other tools and techniques in the effective administration of working capital.

An appraisal of working capital position requires the use of certain income statement information. For purposes of illustration, references will be made in this chapter to financial data which are assumed for a hypothetical Finecare Hospital. The hospital's condensed balance sheet is presented in Figure 14-1; this statement is supplemented by a schedule of changes in working capital in Figure 14-2. The hospital's condensed income statement is illustrated in Figure 14-3. It should be noted that the balance sheet and working capital schedule presentations include a common-size analysis as well as an analysis of changes in terms of both dollar amounts and percentages. For a full discussion of these basic analytical techniques, see Chapter 22.)

NATURE AND IMPORTANCE OF WORKING CAPITAL

An appreciation of the nature and importance of working capital requires an understanding of the accounting concepts of current assets and current liabilities, a definition of working capital, and an explanation of the operating cycle in a hospital enterprise.

Current Assets

The generally accepted definition of current assets is the one formulated by the American Institute of Certified Public Accountants:[1]

> For accounting purposes, the term **current assets** is used to designate cash and other assets or resources commonly identified as those which are reasonably expected to be realized in cash or sold or consumed during the normal operating cycle of the business.

Figure 14-1.
Finecare Hospital
Condensed Balance Sheet — Unrestricted Fund
December 31, 1987 and 1986

	December 31, 1987		December 31, 1986		Increase (Decrease)	
	Amount	Percent	Amount	Percent	Amount	Percent
Current Assets:						
Cash	$ 180	2.2%	$ 140	2.0%	$ 40	28.6%
Temporary investments	44	0.5	99	1.4	(55)	(55.6)
Receivables (net)	660	8.3	470	6.7	190	40.4
Inventories	102	1.3	79	1.1	23	29.1
Prepaid expenses	14	0.2	12	0.2	2	16.7
Total current assets	$1,000	12.5%	$ 800	11.4%	$ 200	25.0
Property, plant and equipment (net)	7,000	87.5	6,200	88.6	800	12.9
Total assets	$8,000	100.0%	$7,000	100.0%	$1,000	14.3
Current Liabilities:						
Notes payable	$ 175	2.2%	$ 75	1.1%	$ 100	133.3
Accounts payable	108	1.4	82	1.2	26	31.7
Accrued expenses payable	144	1.8	103	1.5	41	39.8
Other	73	0.9	60	0.8	13	21.7
Total current liabilities	$ 500	6.3%	$ 320	4.6%	$ 180	56.3
Noncurrent liabilities	2,281	28.5	1,680	24.0	601	35.8
Total liabilities	$2,781	34.8%	$2,000	28.6%	$ 781	39.0
Fund balance	5,219	65.2	5,000	71.4	219	4.4
Total liabilities and fund balance	$8,000	100.0%	$7,000	100.0%	$1,000	14.3

Figure 14-2.
Finecare Hospital
Schedule of Changes in Working Capital
Year Ended December 31, 1987

	December 31, 1987		December 31, 1986		Increase (Decrease)	
	Amount	Percent	Amount	Percent	Amount	Percent
Current Assets:						
Cash	$ 180	18.0%	$ 140	17.5%	$ 40	28.6%
Temporary investments	44	4.4	99	12.4	(55)	(55.6)
Receivables (net)	660	66.0	470	58.7	190	40.4
Inventories	102	10.2	79	9.9	23	29.1
Prepaid expenses	14	1.4	12	1.5	2	16.7
Total current assets	$1,000	100.0%	$ 800	100.0%	$ 200	25.0
Current Liabilities:						
Notes payable	$ 175	35.0%	$ 75	23.4%	$ 100	133.3
Accounts payable	108	21.6	82	25.6	26	31.7
Accrued expenses payable	144	28.8	103	32.2	41	39.8
Other	73	14.6	60	18.8	13	21.7
Total current liabilities	$ 500	100.0%	$ 320	100.0%	$ 180	56.3
Working capital	$ 500		$ 480		$ 20	4.2

Figure 14-3.
Finecare Hospital
Condensed Income Statement
Years Ended December 31, 1987 and 1986

	1987	1986
Net patient service revenues	$4,600	$3,840
Other operating revenues	120	100
Total revenues	$4,720	$3,940
Less Operating Expenses:		
Salaries and wages	$2,821	$2,350
Supplies	438	365
Purchased services	670	608
Depreciation	250	210
Interest	137	92
Other	145	139
Total operating expenses	$4,461	$3,764
Operating income	$ 259	$ 176
Nonoperating income	40	30
Net income for the year	$ 299	$ 206

Included in the definition of current assets are (a) cash available for current operations, (b) temporary investments of such cash, (c) receivables from patients and others that arise from normal and regular operations, (d) inventories of supplies and, (e) short-term prepayments of expenses. Prepaid expenses are not current assets in the sense that they will be converted into cash but that, if not paid in advance, they would require the use of current assets during the next operating cycle. In Figure 14-1, the current assets of Finecare Hospital are shown to be $1,000 at December 31, 1987, and $800 at December 31, 1986.

Current Liabilities

Current liabilities have been defined by the American Institute of Certified Public Accountants as follows:[2]

The term **current liabilities** is used principally to designate obligations whose liquidation is reasonably expected to require the use of existing resources properly classifiable as current assets, or the creation of other current liabilities.

Items typically included in this classification are shown in Figure 14-1. Note that Finecare Hospital's current liabilities are $500 at December 31, 1987, and $320 at the end of 1986.

Definition of Working Capital

Some disagreement exists as to the definition of the term **working capital**. In certain discussions, the term may be used to mean **total current assets**, i.e., it may be said that Finecare Hospital's working capital at December 31, 1987, is $1,000. On the other hand, the term may be used to mean the **difference** between total current assets and total current liabilities, i.e., $500 ($1,000 − $500). The expressions **working capital** (total current assets) and **net working capital** (current assets minus current liabilities) are often employed to distinguish between the two commonly used meanings of the term. Accountants generally use the latter meaning (see Figure 14-2); financial managers, however, sometimes prefer the former meaning (total current assets).

In this book, the term **working capital** is used to refer to the amount of the excess of current assets over current liabilities; the phrase **working capital management** refers to the management of current assets **and** current liabilities, **and** the relationship between them. This is consistent with the meaning given to working capital in the context of the statement of changes in financial position (see Chapter 21).

The Operating Cycle

The ordinary operations of a hospital involve circulation of cash within the current asset classification. Cash is expended for supplies inventories and, as these supplies are used, for employee services and other expenses. In this process, hospital services are provided to patients and these costs are in a sense converted into receivables. The receivables, in turn, are collected and thereby converted into cash. At this point, another cycle begins. An operating cycle, then, may be defined as the average time intervening between the acquisition of supplies and services entering into the production of patient care services and the final cash realization from patients and their sponsors of the charges made for such hospital services. A simplified illustration of the cycle is presented in Figure 14-4.

Figure 14-4.
Any Hospital
The Operating Cycle

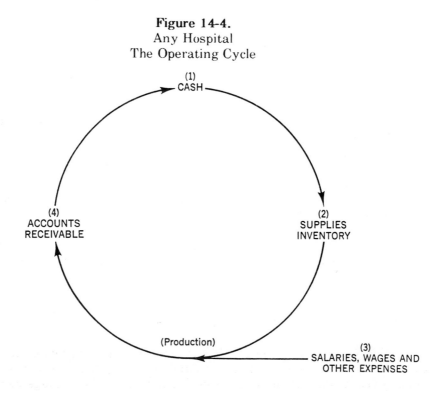

Assume, for example, that a hospital begins operations (with a zero cash balance) on April 1 when a month's supply of inventory is purchased at a cost of $300. These supplies must be paid for on April 10. Payroll and other operating expenses are $2,700 per month, payable 50 percent on April 15 and 50 percent on April 30. Cash requirements for the month of April therefore are $3,000 ($2,700 + $300). If the hospital is to stay in business, $3,000 must be obtained from some source.

A portion of the $3,000 required may be secured from the collection of the amounts charged to patients for services rendered during the month. Assume that the hospital began production of patient care services on April 1, that the average length of stay for a patient is six days, that bills for services are presented to patients on the day of discharge and that 24 days elapse, on the average, between the date of billing and receipt of payment. In other words, billings are $100 per day, or $3,000 for the month (assuming charges are equal to costs). Cash receipts from patients for the month therefore will be $600, consisting of the April 6 billings for six days' services.

As a result, the hospital in this month will receive payments equal to six days' costs but must make payments equal to 30 days' costs. There is an imbalance of $2,400 ($3,000 − $600)! In order to stay in business, therefore, the hospital must secure financing from some source for this $2,400 of costs which cannot be met from cash inflows arising from patient care services. If working capital is viewed as consisting entirely of cash, this hospital has a working capital requirement of $2,400 for the month of April. Unless this minimum amount of working capital is obtained, it will be impossible for the hospital to remain in operation throughout the month. Had the hospital begun the month with $2,400 of working capital (cash), it could have just barely survived the month without additional financing.

Importance of Working Capital Management

The need for a substantial investment in hospital property, plant, and equipment is obvious. Hospital services simply cannot be provided without this investment. Less clearly understood, however, is the equally imperative need for an investment by the hospital in an adequate amount of current resources. Standing alone, the physical plant is not productive of health care services; it is but one of the necessary factors of production. Plant assets become productive only through the catalytic action generated by the addition of a sufficient amount of working capital required for the current financing of the costs of labor, supplies, utilities, and other operating expense items. Since working capital is essential to the continued existence of the hospital, its proper administration is a prime concern of management. Careful attention must be given by the hospital manager to the amount and composition of the investment in current asset items and to the sources from which that investment is financed. If this is not done, the costs of hospital services will be adversely affected and the financial solvency of the hospital may be endangered.

A GENERAL THEORY

Working capital management consists of planning and controlling the amount and composition of current assets and the manner in which these assets are financed. Attention is given in subsequent sections of this chapter to the management of specific components of working capital. First, however, it will be useful to set forth an underlying general theory of working capital management.

The determination of the appropriate amounts of current assets and current liabilities, and therefore the level of working capital, involves a trade-off between risk and the achievement of least-cost operating results. It is certainly reasonable to assume that an investment in current assets generally yields a return (social and monetary) lower than the investment in other hospital assets. It also is safe to assume that short-term financing usually is less expensive than long-term debt in terms of explicit costs and because short-term debts may be paid off in periods when the funds are not needed. These assumptions lead to the conclusion that a hospital should maintain (1) a low proportion of current assets to total assets and (2) a high proportion of current liabilities to total liabilities. Such a strategy would tend to produce a minimum investment in working capital and, presumably, least-cost operations.

On the other hand, the risk factor must be considered. The lower the proportion of current assets to total assets and the higher the proportion of current liabilities to total liabilities, and, in turn, the lower the level of working capital, the greater is the risk of technical insolvency, i.e., the inability to meet currently maturing obligations. The hospital, like any other enterprise, must maintain a reasonable degree of liquidity in order to reduce this risk. The greater the proportion of current assets to total assets and the lower the proportion of current liabilities to total liabilities, the greater the liquidity of the hospital and the lower the risk of technical insolvency.

Under the conditions of uncertainty normally prevailing in hospital operations, an exact synchronization of cash inflows and outflows is not possible. A margin of safety must exist to allow for adverse, unforeseen fluctuations in cash flows. The provision of the necessary margin of safety, however, has a real cost which varies directly with the amount of the safety margin that is maintained. This cost may be viewed as an "opportunity cost," i.e., the return or "profit" foregone on the possible alternative uses of the funds.

The quantity of working capital required is a function of the amounts and timing of cash inflows and outflows during a given time period. This quantity can be managed, i.e., it is subject to management control to a significant degree. The amount of working capital required can be reduced by accelerating cash inflows or by decelerating cash outflows, or both. As noted, however, the greater the amount invested in working capital, the higher the cost that will be incurred by the hospital. Insufficient working capital, on the other hand, exposes the hospital to risk. Hospital managements therefore should seek not to minimize the working capital investment but to **optimize** it. The quantity of working capital should be adequate but not excessive.

The working capital needs of a hospital consist of two components: (1) a relatively stable, permanent working capital requirement and (2) a fluctuating, temporary working capital requirement. A permanent working capital investment is required for the hospital to be able to finance the lowest expected level of operations over a given period of time. When volume of service exceeds this level of operations, a greater investment in current assets is required. The relationship, however, is not linear, i.e., current assets will tend to increase at a decreasing rate. Current liabilities will also tend to increase with volume, thereby financing a portion of the additional current assets. The excess of this increase in current assets over the increase in current liabilities is the hospital's temporary working capital requirement.

Since the minimum working capital requirement is a permanent asset, it ordinarily should be financed through a permanent source of funds, i.e., through retained earnings or contributed equity. It is a generally held principle of finance that permanent or long-term assets should be financed only from permanent or long-term sources of funds. The hospital initially may arrange to finance its permanent working capital needs from the proceeds of bond issues and other long-term debt sources, but it must be recognized that the debt ultimately must be repaid from retained earnings. If not, (1) the hospital will be deprived of its permanent working capital and must close its doors or (2) the hospital must continually refinance its long-term obligations, remain forever in long-term debt, and incur the related high costs of such financing. Except for the possible disadvantages of continued inflation, it is clear that the financing of permanent working capital needs from retained earnings (equity) is fully justifiable for financially pragmatic reasons as well as in terms of opportunity costs to the community.

The temporary working capital needs of the hospital, on the other hand, are eventually self-liquidating over the short run when the period of peak demand for services has passed. These needs arise periodically with increases in volume and are caused by the lag between cash inflows and cash outflows. Until the volume of service subsides and positive cash flows are generated, management must decide how to finance its temporary working capital needs. Assuming again that the rate of return on funds invested in plant assets is higher than either an investment in current assets or the cost of debt, it follows that the opportunity cost of financing these needs through equity is greater than the cost of financing through debt. Therefore, equity financing of temporary working capital requirements is not likely to be desirable. It is not the least-cost alternative available to management.

Management's primary financing choices with respect to temporary working capital needs are (1) short-term debt or (2) long-term debt. If long-term debt is employed, the hospital generally will be paying higher explicit rates for the use of funds and for periods longer than such funds actually are needed for working capital purposes. Temporarily excess funds, of course, may be invested, but such investments are not likely to provide returns equal to the interest costs of long-term debt. Therefore, to minimize financing costs, management should employ short-term debt to finance temporary working capital needs, in excess of what may be satisfied from advances that may be obtained from third-party payers. The particular form this financing should take depends upon the alternative that would result in the least total cost to the hospital. Because of the uncertainty which exists with regard to the timing of cash inflows, however, the maturities of short-term debts should be scheduled so as to provide a margin of safety. This is necessary to avoid default and loss of credit standing with banks and other creditors.

In summary, the general theory of working capital management includes these major points:

1. Working capital management consists of planning and controlling the amount and composition of current assets and the manner in which such assets are financed.
2. Determination of the appropriate quantity of working capital involves a trade-off between risk and achievement of least-cost operational results:

a. The lower the proportion of current assets to total assets and the greater the proportion of current liabilities to total liabilities, the greater the return (social and monetary) on the hospital investment. A strategy based upon this premise tends to lead to a minimum investment in working capital.

b. The greater the proportion of current assets to total assets and the lower the proportion of current liabilities to total liabilities (and the longer the maturity schedule of liabilities), the lower the risk of technical insolvency, all other things held constant. A strategy based upon this premise tends to lead to a maximum investment in working capital.

c. The quantity of working capital required can be managed and will depend upon the risk preferences of management. Management should attempt not to minimize, nor to maximize, the amount of working capital but to **optimize** it.

3.   In financing working capital requirements:

a. Permanent working capital requirements should be financed through retained earnings (equity).

b. Temporary working capital requirements should be financed through short-term credit in whatever form is the least-cost financing alternative.

These broad principles of working capital management will serve as the basis for the following discussion of the management of specific components of hospital working capital.

WORKING CAPITAL RATIOS

A number of ratios are helpful in the analysis and assessment of a hospital's working capital position. Certain of these ratios relate to specific items in the current asset classification and are treated later in this chapter. Others, being of a more general nature, are discussed here. The object of the general analysis is to obtain some insight into the answers to two broad questions of concern to management:

1.   Is the working capital adequate?
2.   Is the working capital effectively employed?

The ratios often utilized as a means of providing a general, overall indication of the answers to these questions are set forth below. Figures used in the computations are drawn from the financial statements of Finecare Hospital (Figures 14-1, 14-2, and 14-3).

Current Ratio

A widely used overall indicator of current financial strength or adequacy of working capital is the **current ratio**, sometimes called the **bankers' ratio**. The current ratio indicates the number of dollars of current assets for each dollar of current liabilities; it shows the number of times the current assets will "pay off" the current debts of the hospital. The computation is shown below:

		December 31	
		1987	1986
1.	Total Current Assets	$1,000	$ 800
2.	Total Current Liabilities	500	320
3.	Current Ratio (1 divided by 2)	2.00	2.50

Thus, Finecare Hospital has $2 of current assets per dollar of current liabilities at December 31, 1987, i.e., its current ratio is 2 to 1. At the end of the previous year, the ratio was higher (2.5 to 1). Generally speaking, it may be said that the hospital was in a stronger overall working capital position last year; its current debt-paying ability has declined somewhat. Although the amount of working capital has increased from $480 to $500, the critically important relationship between current assets and current liabilities is less favorable.

What should a hospital's current ratio be? The popular rule of thumb says that the ratio should be at least 2 to 1, but it is a highly arbitrary and often erroneous notion. There is **no one value** for the current ratio that applies to all hospitals, regardless of type, size, and financial policy. For one hospital, a 1.5 to 1 ratio may be quite acceptable; for another, a 2.5 to 1 ratio may be regarded as somewhat risky. It also is true that for a particular hospital a satisfactory current ratio at the end of one year may not be satisfactory at the end of the next year. In any event, a substantial change in the current ratio from one period to the next should signal the need for an investigation by management to determine its causes, implications, and remedy (if the change is unfavorable).

Quick Ratio

Because the current ratio does not take into account the composition of current assets, the **quick ratio**, sometimes called the **acid test**, also may be computed. It is a more severe test of the current debt-paying ability of the hospital in that it indicates the relationship between the hospital's "quick" or liquid assets and its current debts. The computation is as follows:

		December 31	
		1987	1986
	Cash	$ 180	$ 140
	Temporary Investments	44	99
	Receivables (net)	660	470
1.	Total Quick Assets	$ 884	$ 709
2.	Total Current Liabilities	500	320
3.	Quick Ratio (1 divided by 2)	1.77	2.22

Thus, Finecare Hospital has $1.77 of cash and near-cash assets for every dollar of currently payable obligations at December 31, 1987. Note that inventories and prepaid expenses are excluded from the computation because such assets are not readily convertible into cash.

A modification of the quick ratio is used sometimes. This involves the division of the total of cash and temporary investments by current liabilities. Such a ratio may be helpful in cases where the collection period for receivables is unusually long and where the composition of current liabilities is such that extreme pressure exists for their immediate payment.

Comments made above with respect to the adequacy of the current ratio also apply to the quick ratio. It must be recognized that if a hospital can pay its current debts promptly, take advantage of discount opportunities, and maintain sound credit relationships, then the current and quick ratios, whatever they are, must be adequate. Either ratio can be too high or too low, and a "price" will be paid for either condition.

Current Asset Turnover

The current asset turnover is an overall indicator of how "hard" the management of the hospital "works" the current assets, i.e., the **intensity** of current asset utilization. It is a measure of the average number of times the hospital's current assets were "turned over" in the operating cycle during a given period of time. The computation is shown below:

		December 31	
		1987	1986
1.	Total Operating Revenues	$4,720	$3,940
2.	Total Current Assets	1,000	800
3.	Current Asset Turnover (1 divided by 2)	4.72	4.93

An acceptable, or preferable, alternative is to use total operating **expenses** as the numerator. Another variation of the computation is to divide by working capital to produce a so-called **working capital turnover.** However this may be, a high turnover generally is indicative of the intensity, efficiency, and productivity of the employment of current resources. An extremely high turnover, however, may be indicative of nothing more than an inadequate investment in current resources.

Component Percentages

A general assessment of a hospital's working capital or current financial position should also include an examination of component percentages as reflected in Figures 14-1 and 14-2. As can be seen in Figure 14-1, for example, the hospital's current assets were a greater proportion (12.5%) of total assets at December 31, 1987, than at the end of 1986 (11.4%). Also, in 1987 the proportion of current and noncurrent liabilities to total assets increased substantially, i.e., a higher percentage of the hospital's assets was being financed through debt than at the end of the previous year. And, in Figure 14-2, changes in the relative significance of each component of working capital may be easily perceived. Component percentages bring to light certain relationship and trends that might go largely unnoticed in an examination of dollar amounts alone.

CASH AND TEMPORARY INVESTMENTS

As emphasized in Chapter 10, the proper management of cash requires an effective internal control system sound accounting procedure and the development of cash budgets. The details of these matters are not repeated here.

Quantity of Cash Holdings

The fundamental premise upon which cash management rests is the idea that the holding of assets in the form of cash is nonproductive and, therefore, that perfect cash management consists of maintaining a **zero** cash balance. While a continuous zero cash balance is a theoretically sound ideal, it cannot be achieved in actual practice for a number of valid reasons. Economists generally identify three motives for holding cash balances:

1. **Transactions motive.** There is a measurable need to hold cash in certain amounts at predictable times to meet required payments arising in the ordinary course of business, e.g., a hospital payroll of a known amount must be paid on a determinable date.
2. **Precautionary motive.** There is a need to maintain a cash balance of some amount as a cushion or margin of safety to meet emergency and unexpected contingencies which require cash payments, e.g., a sudden and unanticipated event such as a fire or flood.
3. **Speculative motive.** Finally, cash balances may be held in some arbitrary amount so that the holder may be in a position to take advantage of special profit-making or cost-saving situations which may arise, e.g., a short-lived opportunity to make a cash purchase of a commodity in quantity before its price is expected to rise dramatically.

The more predictable the cash flows of the hospital, the less precautionary cash balances are needed. It should also be noted that not all transactions and precautionary balances need be held in cash. If cash flows are budgeted as they should be, a portion of the hospital's cash resources can be temporarily invested in earning assets.

The critical point to be recognized is that hospitals and all other enterprises hold transactions and precautionary cash balances primarily because of a lack of synchronization between cash inflows and outflows. Influences on the quantity of cash held for transactions and precautionary balances are:

1. Expected net cash flows of the hospital as determined by the cash budget.
2. Possible deviations from expected net cash flows.
3. The maturity structure of the hospital's debts.
4. The hospital's borrowing capacity to meet emergency needs beyond transactions and precautionary balances.

5. The utility preferences of management with respect to the risk of running out of cash.
6. The efficiency of cash management.[3]

Each of these factors must be considered carefully by hospital management in its determination of the quantity of cash holdings by the hospital.

Optimization of Cash Holdings

It must be recognized that a "price" must be paid for the maintenance of a cash balance. If the cash balance is inadequate and shortages are frequent and large, the result will be the loss of purchase discount opportunities, an increase in the costs of short-term borrowing, and the deterioration of credit standing. On the other hand, the holding of excessive cash balances is also costly. The hospital will incur an opportunity cost in terms of the return which would otherwise have been earned had such funds been invested in earning assets. Management therefore must strive to **optimize** hospital cash holdings, i.e., maintain cash balances at levels that are neither insufficient nor excessive.

In attempting to optimize the size of the hospital's cash balances, management should strive to create operating conditions in which a synchronization of cash flows is secured to the degree feasible. The timing of outflows for items such as payrolls and taxes is largely fixed either by contract or custom, and it may not be possible to alter the due dates of such payments to any significant extent. With respect to payments for supplies and purchased services, however, some adjustments in timing may be within the control of management. If so, the deceleration of cash outflows generally is desirable because it (1) gives the hospital the use of cash resources for productive purposes for a longer period of time and (2) increases the ability of management to more closely synchronize cash inflows with outflows. This should be done, however, only if it serves to minimize total costs. The deferral of payments on accounts payable, for example, means foregoing discounts, and this can be extremely expensive. Yet, in certain instances, the least-cost solution may be the substitution of short-term bank loans for accounts payable.

Whereas the objective with respect to cash outflows is to slow them down as much as is economically feasible, the objective in regard to cash inflows is maximum acceleration. The hospital's cash inflows should be accelerated to the fullest extent practicable for the same reasons that pertain to the deceleration of cash outflows. Again, however, the control that can be exercised by the management of a particular hospital is limited. Third-party payers obviously have superior economic power, and no single hospital is able to exert any significant amount of pressure on them to accelerate their reimbursements. Also, the relationship between the financial resources and hospital bills of self-pay patients is such that a limit is placed on what the hospital can do to speed up the collections of such accounts. What can and must be done by every hospital, however, is to minimize the time required for the processing of patients' accounts, third-party billings, and related cash receipts. These are mainly problems of systems design, accounting procedure, and internal control. It is vital that the hospital's revenue system be such that both in-house processing time and revenue losses are reduced to a minimum.

The actual determination of the optimal cash balances is a difficult matter due to the uncertainty of future cash flows and the problems involved in measuring the subjective costs of holding or not holding cash. Yet, as Berman and Weeks point out, it is a problem which must be solved if management is to administer the hospital's cash balances effectively.[4] They also describe how this determination can be made using matrix algebra and the mathematics of probabilities.

In essence, the determination of an optimal cash balance involves a number of subjective judgments concerning alternative cash balance strategies, the dollar value of holding various levels of cash so as to avoid the costs associated with shortages and the opportunity costs of holding cash which might otherwise be invested in earning assets. Given these judgments, the optimal cash balance can be identified as that level of cash holding at which the opportunity cost of holding cash begins to exceed the value of the benefits obtained from such level of cash holding. In other words, the hospital's cash holdings should be kept at that level where a tolerable balance is achieved between the risk of running out of cash and the desire to keep as much cash invested in earning assets as may be possible. Some managements will tackle the problem through a series of mathematical gyrations; others, largely on the basis of experience, will simply develop a "notion" as to what the hospital's cash holdings should be at any given time. While the latter approach often produces satisfactory results, the current trend is toward an increasing use of mathematical tools in the solution of management problems.

Role of Cash Budgeting

Having determined by one process or another the optimal amount of cash to be held, the hospital manager looks to the cash budget for information concerning projected cash flows and cash balances at various future points in time. The cash budgeting procedure allows the manager to anticipate the need for additional cash well in advance of the time it is actually needed. It also may indicate a projected cash balance that is in excess of optimal cash holdings. In either event, the comparison of desired and budgeted cash balances usually points out the necessity for appropriate managerial action. If the budgeted cash balance is below the established optimal level, various corrective measures may be taken. An extreme and long-lived shortage may require revision of the revenue and expense budgets upon which the cash budget is based. If this should not be necessary or feasible, it may be possible to make up the cash deficiency to some extent by adjustments in financial policies and operational procedures (as discussed above) that will accelerate cash inflows and decelerate cash outflows. Or, where the hospital has temporary investments, the manager may plan to sell such securities to acquire the necessary amounts of cash. Consideration may also be given to the desirability of obtaining short-term loans during the periods in which the cash shortages are projected. Whatever the alternatives, cash budgeting gives the hospital manager advance notice of probable cash shortages so that all available remedies can be fully investigated and studied. This lead time tends to produce better decisions and minimization of hospital costs.

On the other hand, the cash budget may predict cash balances in excess of established optimal levels. If so, the problem becomes that of deciding how the cash surplus can be most effectively utilized. This decision, which depends in part upon the amount of the surplus and the length of time it will persist, may be to invest in marketable securities, to increase inventory levels, or to pay certain debts prior to their maturities. However, this may be, cash budgets give the manager time to study the problem long before it arises and to make the best possible arrangements for the most productive investment of cash surpluses. The short-term investment of temporarily excess cash balances in marketable securities often is the most advantageous alternative. U.S. Treasury securities of many kinds are available, and these are almost riskless, being highly marketable and having a wide range of maturities (see Chapter 10). While yields are relatively low, these securities can be readily sold without loss of principal whenever emergency cash needs arise. The varying maturities available also provide a high degree of flexibility which permits a synchronization of investment maturities with projected future cash needs.

Cash and Investment Reports

The fact that most hospitals prepare a daily cash report is good evidence of the great importance assigned to cash flows by management. (An illustration of a daily cash report was provided in Figure 10-7.) This report provides for a day-by-day comparison of actual and budgeted cash receipts, disbursements, and balances. Should the budgeting of cash on a daily basis not be considered feasible, the daily cash report may be prepared as shown in Figure 14-5. Whatever the format, it is important that, in addition to historical cash flow data, the report include a projection of cash flows for an appropriate period into the future (perhaps one month).

Figure 14-5.
(Hospital Name)
Daily Cash Report
(Date)

	Actual		Budget	
	Today	Month to Date	This Month	Next Month
Opening cash balance	$	$	$	$
Cash Receipts:				
Blue Cross	$	$	$	$
Medicare				
Medicaid				
Commercial				
Self-pay				
Other				
Total cash receipts	$	$	$	$
Total cash available	$	$	$	$
Cash Disbursements:				
Payroll	$	$	$	$
Accounts payable				
Mortgage payments				
Equipment purchases				
Other				
Total cash disbursements	$	$	$	$
Closing cash balance	$	$	$	$

In many hospitals, it is also desirable to prepare a monthly report of temporary investments such as the one illustrated in Figure 14-6. The information provided in this report enables the hospital manager to evaluate the productivity and quality of the short-term investment portfolio and to maintain an appropriate allocation of resources between cash balances and temporary investments of surplus cash. Data concerning maturity dates and current market values are helpful in planning future cash inflows.

Figure 14-6.
(Hospital Name)
Monthly Report of Temporary Investments
Month Ended June 30, 19 –

Opening balance of investments, at cost (see last month's
   report for details) $
Additions during current month:
  (Details)
Total $
Disposals during current month:

	Proceeds	Gain (Loss)	Cost	
(Details)	$	$	$	
	$	$		

Closing balance of investments, at cost (detailed in
   schedule below) $

Schedule of Temporary Investments
June 30, 19___

Security	Date of Purchase	Maturity Date	Income Yield	Income to Date	Cost	Market Value
(Details)			% $	$	$	
			% $	$	$	

RECEIVABLES

Accounts receivable is by far the largest single component of a hospital's working capital. In Finecare Hospital's December 31, 1987, balance sheet (illustrated in Figure 14-1), accounts receivable are $660, or 66 percent of total current assets. This sizable investment in patients' accounts, which is typical of most hospitals, arises because of the nature and cost of hospital services and because of the delayed manner in which hospitals are paid for their services by third-party payers. It is not at all unusual for hospitals to have 60, 90, or more days of service charges in accounts receivable, which are uncollected in spite of good credit and collection procedures. Hospitals are in the credit business to a very substantial degree, but not by choice; they literally are forced into extending credit on a large scale because of externally imposed constraints that prohibit operations on a cash-and-carry basis.

The extension of credit and the resultant investment of large amounts of working capital in receivables, of course, is costly. It must be recognized by all parties concerned that the credit-granting hospital, in effect, is lending money. This money has a cost (an opportunity cost) equal to the return (income) that would otherwise have been earned had the funds invested in receivables been invested instead in some earning asset. If funds to finance the investment in receivables must be borrowed, and they often must be, the carrying cost includes the actual cash out-of-pocket cost, i.e., the interest paid on the borrowed funds. The opportunity cost of equity funds invested in receivables, however, is no less real or important. Besides carrying costs, the investment in receivables also gives rise to additional operating costs associated with the necessary credit and collection functions. In addition, thee are **delinquency** costs, i.e., collection agency fees and, ultimately, bad debts.

Since hospitals generally cannot increase their revenues and profits by a liberal extension of credit to customers as do many commercial businesses, credit-granting by hospitals serves only to increase operating costs. Interest sometimes may be charged on delinquent patients' accounts as it often is both necessary and justifiable, but many hospital managers point out that the income thereby generated fails to equal the cost of credit and tends to have an adverse effect on public relations.

In view of these observations, it would seem apparent that the granting of credit and the related investment in receivables by hospitals should be held to a minimum in order to achieve least-cost operating results. Some amount of receivables, of course, is unavoidable, but the size of this investment in credit extended to patients and their sponsors **is** subject to a significant degree of control by hospital managements. This control can be effected through (1) efficient accounting procedures for revenues and receivables, (2) strong internal control systems, and (3) effective credit and collection methods. In these and other areas of control, the emphasis is upon reduction of the length of the accounts receivable cycle (collection period) and protection against the loss of revenues either through bad debts or slipshod accounting practices.[5]

Ratio Analysis

The evaluation of the level of receivables and the effectiveness of receivables management is a continuous process. For this purposes, the computation and reporting of certain ratios may be useful. One widely employed ratio, called the **accounts receivable turnover**, is computed here, using the data for Finecare Hospital provided in Figures 14-1 and 14-3.

		December 31	
		1987	1986
1.	Net Patient Service Revenues	$4,600	$3,840
2.	Patients' Accounts Receivable (net)*	660	470
3.	Accounts Receivable Turnover (1 divided by 2)	7.0	8.2

*Average accounts receivable for the year may be used here rather than the year-end figures.

This ratio indicates the number of times during the year the receivables were "turned over," i.e., collected. A decrease in turnover generally is regarded as an unfavorable sign with respect to the effectiveness of the credit and collection function although several other factors could be involved. The important point to recognize is that the primary value of the ratio lies in the fact that it will reveal a change in the relationship between accounts receivable and the total charges to patients' accounts during a given period. A significant change in this relationship has important implications for receivables management, and an appropriate managerial investigation should be made to determine its cause. Until that investigation is completed, a correct interpretation and management use of the ratio is not possible.

A related ratio used in the analysis of receivables is the **number of days' charges in receivables**, sometimes called **days' revenue in receivables**. This ratio is computed below, using the Finecare Hospital data.

		December 31	
		1987	1986
1.	Days in One Year	365	365
2.	Accounts Receivable Turnover (above)	7.0	8.2
3.	Number of Days' Charges in Accounts Receivable (1 divided by 2)	52.1	44.5

It can be said, for example, that Finecare Hospital has an average of 52.1 days of charges (revenues) uncollected and in accounts receivable at December 31, 1987. At the end of 1986, an average of only 45 days of service remained uncollected. The ratio, in this way, is useful in an assessment of the amount of working capital invested in patients' accounts receivable.

External standards for this ratio are available. National group medians are reported, for example, by the HFMA's Financial Analysis Service and the Hospital Administrative Services Division of the AHA. For instance, assume that it is reported that hospitals of 200-bed size had 67.4 days of revenue in receivables. This indicates that a 200-bed hospital operating at 80 percent capacity with daily revenue of about $300 per inpatient bed might expect to have an investment in accounts receivable approximating $3,200,000 (200 X 80% X $300 X 67.4) = $3,235,200. It must be recognized, however, that the externally developed standards usually represents medians and that factors other than bed size have an effect upon the number of day's charges in receivables for a given hospital.

The number of days' charges uncollected can also be computed by first determining the average revenue per day and then dividing the daily average revenue into accounts receivable. This alternative method is illustrated below:

		December 31	
		1987	1986
1.	Net Patient Service Revenues	$4,600	$3,840
2.	Average Daily Revenue (net revenues divided by 365)	12.6	10.5
3.	Patients Accounts Receivable	660	470
4.	Number of Days' Charges in Accounts Receivable (3 divided by 2)	52.4	44.8

The slight difference in the results obtained under this alternative method of computing is merely the result of rounding the figures.

With respect to both receivables turnover and days' charges uncollected, it must be remembered that the ratios are **averages**. The computed number of days' charges may be 52, for instance, but some of the accounts receivable may well be 90, 200, or even 300 days old. This fact is "hidden" in the average. For this reason and because credit arrangements differ by type of payer, undue reliance should not be placed on general or overall ratios. Instead, using the more detailed information that should be available from a good accounting system, receivable turnovers and days' charges uncollected should be computed **by major categories of payment sources**, i.e., classes of patients and third-party payers. This procedure is far more enlightening and useful for purposes of receivables management than a single overall ratio as computed in the above illustrations. A monthly aging of accounts receivable is also essential to a proper interpretation and use of the receivables ratios.

Other ratios may be developed for use in evaluating receivables. The percentage of the allowance for uncollectibles to gross receivables, for example, is helpful particularly when computed by categories (payment sources) of receivables and compared over time. An increase in this percentage means that the hospital requires a relatively greater working capital investment, which is an undesirable situation calling for managerial attention and correction.

Reports of Receivables

Should the investment in receivables become excessive, the hospital may soon find itself without sufficient cash to pay its currently maturing obligations. A continuous watch therefore must be maintained by management over the level of receivables. This is accomplished in part through monthly reports such as the one illustrated in Figure 14-7. Some of the information summarized in this report is secured from the monthly aging of receivables (see Chapter 11).

Figure 14-7.
(Hospital Name)
Monthly Analysis of Accounts Receivable
(Date)

	Year to Date		Current Month	
	Amount	Percent	Amount	Percent
Accounts receivable, opening balance			$	
Add Gross Charges:				
Blue Cross	$	%	$	%
Medicare/Medicaid				
Other Insurance				
Self-pay				
Other				
Total gross charges	$	100.0%	$	100.0%
Total opening balance and gross charges			$	
Less Noncash Credits:				
Charity care	$	%	$	%
Contractual adjustments				
Bad debt write-offs				
Other				
Total noncash credits	$	100.0%	$	100.0%
Net collectible receivables			$	
Less Cash Collections:				
Blue Cross	$	%	$	%
Medicare/Medicaid				
Other insurance				
Self-pay				
Other				
Total cash collections	$	100.0%	$	100.0%
Accounts Receivable, Closing Balance:				
In hospital				
Blue Cross			$	%
Medicare/Medicaid				
Other insurance				
Self-Pay:				
In hospital over 15 days				
In hospital less than 15 days				
Other				
Total in hospital			$	100.0%
Discharged and outpatient				
Blue Cross			$	%
Medicare/Medicaid				
Other insurance				
Self-pay				
Other				
Total discharged and outpatient			$	100.0%
Accounts receivable, closing balance			$	

Summary

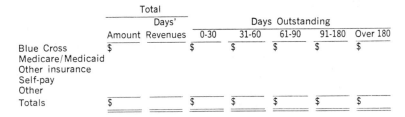

	Amount	Total Days' Revenues	Days Outstanding				
			0-30	31-60	61-90	91-180	Over 180
Blue Cross	$		$	$	$	$	$
Medicare/Medicaid							
Other insurance							
Self-pay							
Other							
Totals	$		$	$	$	$	$

In some instances, the medical staff may be able to assist the hospital in maintaining its accounts receivable and uncollectible accounts at an acceptable level. For this purpose, an additional report of bad debts written off classified by attending physician may be prepared on an annual or quarterly basis.

It is possible to maintain effective credit and collection policies and good public relations at the same time. Good credit and collection policies, as a matter of fact, produce good public relations. Inconsistency in dealing with patients on matters of credit invariably leads to poor public relations. A carefully devised program of credit and collections, placed in writing and understood by all employees involved, must be established. The program should require that the incoming patient make definite arrangements for the payment of his or her account and should set forth those procedures to be followed when such payments are not received according to prearrangements.

If administrative reports indicate laxity and inefficiency in the credit and collection program, management should take immediate corrective measures. A review of existing credit and collection procedures may show that different or additional procedures should be established. Or, it may be discovered that there is insufficient clerical staff to properly carry out existing policies and procedures. Minimization of credit and collection costs should not be the hospital objective, i.e., in many instances it may be possible to decrease total operating costs by increasing credit and collection costs. With increased collection efforts, average collection time and bad debt losses may be so reduced that cost savings exceed the additional costs incurred in such increased efforts. As a general rule, credit and collection expenditures should be extended to a point at which another dollar of expenditure would not produce a dollar of savings, i.e., in the jargon of the economist, the point at which marginal costs and marginal savings are equal.

Early recognition of accounts that eventually may prove uncollectible is an important requirement. The research department of the American Collectors Association, based on a survey conducted in 78 communities, reported the following dollar values of delinquent accounts:

Age of Account:	Value
Current	$1.00
Two months old	.80
Six months old	.67
One year old	.49
Two years old	.27

The Association also reported that an overall recovery of 40 percent occurred during the first 90 days that the accounts were being worked on a collection basis. Also during the first 90 days, 38 percent of the accounts were found to be totally uncollectible and 22 percent of the accounts were deemed doubtful. Approximately 50 percent of the doubtful accounts were uncollectible because of an inability to locate the debtor.

Uncollected accounts should be turned over to a collection agency when the hospital loses effective contact with the debtor. In selecting an agency, the importance of the matter of commissions is often overemphasized. The most important cost consideration is not the percentage rate of commission charged, but the percentage of accounts which are not recovered. An agency charging a 25 percent rate, for example, might actually produce net recoveries in an amount considerably less than an agency whose commission rate is 50 percent. In choosing an agency, the hospital should require that the agency offer prompt and efficient service and have a good reputation, financial stability, bonded and well-trained personnel, forwarding facilities, and affiliation with local and state collectors' organizations.

It is essential that hospital management be kept aware of the progress of collection efforts by outside agencies. For this purpose, a monthly report of the type illustrated in Figure 14-8 may be prepared.

Figure 14-8.
(Hospital Name)
Progress Report on Collections by Agencies
(Date)

Gross amounts of accounts with agency at end of previous month	$
Gross amounts of accounts turned over during the current month	
Total	$
Gross collections on accounts during the current month	
Balance	$
Accounts returned as uncollectible	
Balance with agency at end of the month	$
Collection cost for the month	$
Net cash received by the hospital	$

Financing with Receivables

The accounting aspects of various arrangements by which receivables may be used in financing temporary working capital needs were discussed in Chapter 11. Receivables can be pledged as collateral for a bank loan or they may be discounted with a bank or finance company. In addition, some hospitals have been able to work out direct bank/patient loan arrangements as a means of financing the self-responsible portion of patients' accounts. It may also be noted that patients' accounts can be sold or assigned to financial institutions called **factors**, but this generally is not desirable because of the high costs involved and possible adverse public relations arising from undue harassment of patients by some factoring agencies. In any event, whatever the financing arrangement, cost and public reaction should be management's paramount considerations.

INVENTORIES

The existence of inventories is unavoidable and, as a matter of fact, quite essential to the operation of a hospital. Inventories exist primarily because of the high degree of uncertainty which surrounds the future demand for hospital services, i.e., it is necessary that a margin of safety be provided as assurance that sufficient supplies be available at all times. Given the nature and importance of hospital services, "stockouts" of many types of inventoriable supplies simply cannot be tolerated. Excessive inventories, on the other hand, tend to encourage waste, unnecessarily tie up working capital which might be employed in a more productive manner, increase the hazard of obsolescence and spoilage, and increase the costs of storage and insurance. Yet, only through quantity purchasing can the lowest prices be obtained. The maintenance of excessively **low** levels of inventory will require a high frequency of purchasing, thereby increasing the unit costs of the purchasing, receiving, and handling functions.

Since either insufficient or excessive inventories may have an unfavorable influence on hospital costs and the quality of patient care, hospital management has a responsibility to take steps to avoid both extremes. There is an optimum level of investment for any asset. This has been demonstrated with respect to cash, temporary investments, and receivables. It also is true of the investment in inventories by the hospital. The optimum level of inventories, while highly conceptual, can be reasonably approximated. Management's task is to find and maintain that level of inventory investment. This requires adequate internal control and accounting procedures (see Chapters 8 and 12). This chapter emphasizes the determination of optimum inventory quantity and additional techniques by which management can control the size of the investment in supply inventories. These are important managerial considerations because, while the inventory "asset" may not be substantial in comparison with receivables, supplies expense **is** the single largest nonpayroll cost in most hospitals. If hospital inventories are properly managed, significant cost savings can be effected.

Determination of Optimum Inventory Levels

Optimization of inventory levels begins with accurate estimates of (1) the expected annual usage of supply items, (2) the unit purchase prices, (3) the ordering costs, and (4) the inventory carrying costs. Assume, for example, that the hospital has budgeted the use of 4,380 units of Supply Item A during the coming year, with average daily usage estimated at 12 units (4,380 units/365 days). Also assume the following costs:

1.	Purchase price per unit		$ 2.00
2.	Cost of placing an order (stationery, postage, telephone and clerical costs involved in order preparation, accounting, and paying the invoice)		14.60
3.	**Carrying costs per unit per year:**		
	Storage (space, insurance, taxes, clerical, handling, etc.)	$.08	
	Interest on investment in the inventory (8% x $2.00)	.16	.24

While a precise measurement of these costs generally is impossible, they are susceptible to reasonable approximation which is sufficient for the purposes of this analysis. Minor variations between estimates of the relevant cost factors and "true costs" can be expected to occur, but such variations are unlikely to have any significant effect on the hospital's inventory policy as determined by the following computations.

The two major questions to be answered are (1) how many units of Supply Item A should be ordered at a time and (2) when should such orders be placed so as to maintain the inventory at the optimum level? In other words, determinations must be made of:

1. Economic order quantity (EOQ)
2. Reorder point (ROP)

How much to order? When to order? As shown below, a mathematical solution to these questions is available.

The determination of how much to order at a time (EOQ) may be arrived at by a tabular method or by the use of a formula. Using the tabular method, varying assumptions are made as to order size until the order quantity is found at which total annual costs (ordering and carrying) are minimized. This procedure is illustrated in Figure 14-9.

Figure 14-9.
Annualized Costs of Various Order Sizes

(1) Order Size (Units)	(2) Average Inventory (Units)	(3) Orders Per Year	(4) Annual Carrying Cost	(5) Annual Ordering Cost	(6) Total Annual Cost
4,380	2,190	1	$525.60	$ 14.60	$540.20
2,190	1,095	2	262.80	29.20	292.00
1,460	730	3	175.20	43.80	219.00
1,095	548	4	131.52	58.40	189.92
730	365	6	87.60	87.60	175.20
365	183	12	43.92	175.20	219.12
168	84	26	20.16	379.60	399.76
84	42	52	10.08	759.20	769.28

KEY TO COMPUTATIONS

Column	
(1)	Assumed order sizes
(2)	Column 1 divided by 2
(3)	Annual usage (4,380) divided by column 1
(4)	Column 2 multiplied by 24¢
(5)	Column 3 multiplied by $14.60
(6)	Column 4 plus column 5

As can be seen, total annual costs are minimized at $175.20 when 730 units of Supply Item A are ordered at a time. This is also the order quantity at which annual carrying costs equal annual ordering costs. The same solution is shown in graphic form in Figure 14-10.

Figure 14-10.
Graphic Solution of Economic Order Quantity

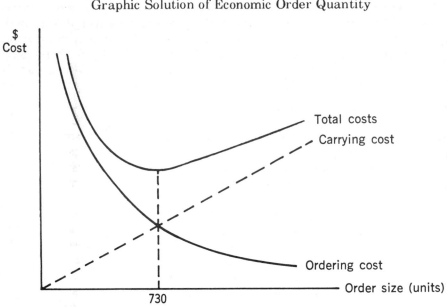

Differential calculus makes it possible, however, to compute the economic order quantity by formula, a variation of which is:

$$EOQ = \sqrt{\frac{2DP}{C}}$$

Where: D = Demand (annual usage in units)
P = Cost of placing an order
C = Annual cost of carrying one unit in inventory

Hence:

$$EOQ = \sqrt{\frac{2 \text{ X } 4{,}389 \text{ X } 14.60}{.24}}$$

$$= \sqrt{\frac{127{,}896}{.24}}$$

$$= \sqrt{532{,}900}$$

$$= \underline{730} \text{ Units}$$

It should be recognized that the optimum order size increases as D (annual usage) or P (ordering cost) get larger or as C (carrying cost) gets smaller.

The second question of when to order (ROP) requires a knowledge of average daily usage and "lead time," i.e., the length of time elapsing between placing an order and receiving delivery of the goods. If, for example, the average daily usage is 12 units and the lead time for Supply Item A is assumed to be 14 days, the reorder point is reached whenever the inventory level falls to 168 units (12 units x 14 days). Thus, either by periodic observation of inventory or by the monitoring of perpetual inventory ledger cards, a determination can be made of the points in time when a new order for 730 additional units should be placed with the supplier.

With respect to many supply items, however, the daily usage is not certain and will fluctuate to some degree. To be sure that stockouts are avoided, it is necessary to maintain a so-called **safety stock**. Department heads generally have some notion, based on past experience and current budgets, of the range of daily demand and of the probabilities that various quantities will be used in excess of average daily demand during a given lead time period. With this in mind, a safety stock quantity is established where the cost of carrying that extra quantity is roughly counterbalanced against the "costs" of a possible stockout. Assume, for example, that maximum daily usage of Supply Item A in all likelihood will be no greater than 15 units. The safety stock, then, could be established as 42 units (excess usage of 3 units per day x 14 days' lead time). This means that the reorder point should be adjusted upward to 210 units (168 + 42) so that a stockout becomes improbable.

In summary, using the EOQ, ROP, and safety stock techniques, the hospital inventory can be maintained at optimum levels. The objective is to minimize the total associated costs of carrying and not carrying inventories. In the example given above, the inventory level of Supply Item A, assuming maximum and minimum probable daily usage, would never fall below zero and would never exceed 772 (730 + 42) units. While the concepts discussed here are useful with regard to all supply items, specific application of the above techniques usually is limited to the more significant components of inventory as determined by the so-called ABC method or some other ranking procedure. As noted in Chapter 12, a cost-benefit analysis is often necessary to determine whether a particular control method is worth what it costs.

Ratio Analysis

Ratio analysis is often helpful to an evaluation of the hospital investment in inventories. There should be, of course, a reasonable relationship between inventories and total current assets. As may be seen in Figure 14-2, for example, Finecare Hospital's December 31, 1987, inventories are 10.2 percent of total current assets, a slight increase over the 9.9 percent position at the end of 1986. Any significant increase in this percentage should be investigated and its causes determined.

In addition, the relationship between inventories and total cost of supplies used should be examined and studied. For this purpose, the **inventory turnover** may be computed and reported to hospital management. The computation is shown below, using the Finecare Hospital data provided earlier in this chapter.

	December 31	
	1987	1986
1. Total Cost of Supplies Used	$ 438	$ 365
2. Inventories*	102	79
3. Inventory Turnover (1 divided by 2)	4.3	4.6

*Average inventory for the year may
be more appropriate.

The fact that the rate of inventory turnover has declined from 4.6 to 4.3 times generally would be interpreted as an unfavorable change. A high or moderately high turnover usually is indicative of a desirable situation, but an extremely high rate of turnover may result from the maintenance of insufficient inventory levels or from waste. On the other hand, a low turnover could be caused by a decrease in service volume, overstocking, and poor purchasing policies. Since turnover rates will naturally vary somewhat for different types of supply items, inventory turnover information is most useful when it is developed by type of inventory and by individual departments or cost centers as illustrated in Figure 14-11. A single overall ratio, computed as above for Finecare Hospital, is not likely to be of much value to hospital management.

Figure 14-11.
(Hospital Name)
Monthly Inventory Report
(Date)

	Current Inventory			Usage	Turnover Rate*	
Cost Center	Dollars	Units	Days' Supply	Last 90 Days	This Month	Year to Date
(Detailed by major categories of supplies)	$					
	$					

*Where the necessary information is available, turnover rates may be determined on the basis of units rather than dollars to avoid distortions caused by price changes.

Another manner in which inventory activity may be measured is the determination of the average **number of days' supply** in inventories. The calculation is as follows, again using the Finecare Hospital data:

	December 31	
	1987	1986
1. Days in One Year	365	365
2. Inventory Turnover	4.3	4.6
3. Number of Days' Supply (1 divided by 2)	84.9	79.3

In other words, Finecare hospital had about 85 days' supply of inventory on hand in its storerooms at December 31, 1987. The interpretation of this ratio would be similar to that provided for inventory turnover. Like turnover data, number of days' supply information must also be developed for each major category of inventory and for each cost center where significant amounts of supplies are used. A material increase **or decrease** in the number of days' supply should always be investigated for cause. It bears repeating that a hospital can be in an understocked as well as an overstocked inventory position, although the latter tends to be more common.

Inventory Reports

Various reports of inventory usage and position may be prepared to assist management in its effort to optimize the hospital investment of working capital in inventories. These reports may compare actual inventory data with maximum and minimum inventory levels established by management policy; they may report differences between book and periodic physical inventory figures; they may provide turnover and number of days' supply data; and they may present comparisons of actual and budgeted inventories. In any event, management should determine the kinds of inventory information it needs, how often it is needed and what reporting format is most appropriate. A sample format is illustrated in Figure 14-11.

CONCLUSION

This concludes the last of a five-chapter sequence concerned with accounting for and managing hospital working capital. As has been discussed, there is for any current asset component of working capital an optimum investment amount. Given that total investment, there is an optimum financing method which results in appropriate relationships among current liabilities, long-term debt, and hospital equity (fund balance). Once these optimum, least-cost investing and financing policies are established, the management task is that of controlling the hospital's activities and affairs so that the objective of those policies are realized to the fullest extent possible. The accounting and reporting methods, internal control measures, and financial management techniques described in the preceding pages are essential to the performance of that task.

CHAPTER 14 FOOTNOTES

1. "Restatement and Revision of Accounting Research Bulletins," Accounting Research Bulletin No. 43 (New York: AICPA, 1953), Chapter 3A, par. 4.

2. Ibid, par. 7.

3. Adapted from James C. Van Horne, *Financial Management and Policy* (Englewood Cliffs, New Jersey: Prentice-Hall, Inc., 1968), pp. 335-336.

4. Howard J. Berman and Lewis E. Weeks, *The Financial Management of Hospitals, 2nd ed.* (Ann Arbor, Michigan: Health Administration Press, School of Public Health, The University of Michigan, 1974), pp. 304-308.

5. These matters are discussed in Chapters 7 and 11. Many excellent articles and textbooks contain a more detailed treatment of the mechanics involved. See, for example, *Managing the Patient Account* (Chicago: Healthcare Financial Management Association, 1970).

excess current asset/liable (handwritten)

QUESTIONS

1. Define the term **working capital.** What, briefly, is meant by the expression **working capital management?** Why is so much importance accorded to the effective management of working capital in hospitals?

2. What is your understanding of the term **operating cycle?** What is the length of an operating cycle in a hospital?

3. What are the basic conclusions of the general theory of working capital management presented in the text of this chapter?

4. State the formula for the computation of (1) the current ratio, (2) the quick ratio, and (3) the current asset turnover. Indicate how each of these ratios may be employed in an evaluation of the hospital's working capital position.

5. Identify three motives for the holding of cash balances. What portion of a hospital's total resources should be held in the form of cash?

6. How can a hospital optimize its cash holdings? What is the role of cash budgeting in this process?

7. State the formula for the computation of (1) the accounts receivable turnover and (2) the number of days' charges in receivables. Indicate how these ratios may be employed in an evaluation of the hospital's investment in receivables.

8. With respect to inventory management, what is your understanding of each of the following terms: (1) stockout, (2) EOQ, (3) reorder point, and (4) safety stock.

9. State the formula for the computation of (1) the inventory turnover and (2) the number of days' supply in inventory. Indicate how these ratios may be employed in an evaluation of the hospital's investment in inventories.

10. What basic information do you think should be included in monthly reports of cash, temporary investments, receivables, and inventories which are prepared for the hospital administrator?

EXERCISES

E1. Rightcare Hospital provides you with the following information relating to patient service revenues and accounts receivable:

	December 31	
	1987	1986
Net patient service revenues	$4,400	$4,320
Patients' accounts receivable (net)	800	720

Required. Compute (1) the accounts receivable turnover and (2) the number of days' charges in receivables. What general interpretation can you make of the computed ratios?

E2. Extracare Hospital provides you with the following information relating to supplies used and in inventory:

$1700|340 = 5$
$365|5 = 73$

	December 31	
	1987	1986
Total cost of supplies used	$1,700	$1,674
Inventory	340	310

Required. Compute (1) the inventory turnover and (2) the number of days' supply in inventory. What general interpretation can you make of the computed ratios?

E3. Overcare Hospital has budgeted the usage of 5,110 units of Supply Item A during the coming year, with average daily usage estimated at 14 units. The following costs are estimated:

$5110/365$

1.	Purchase price per unit	$ 5.00
2.	Cost of placing an order	18.00
3.	Carrying costs per unit per year	.40

The lead time for Supply Item A is 10 days, and the maximum daily usage in all likelihood is 20 units.

Required. Compute (1) the economic order quantity, (2) the reorder point, and (3) the safety stock.

E4. Highcare Hospital's balance sheets provide the following information concerning current assets and liabilities:

	December 31	
	1987	1986
Cash	$ 100	$ 120
Marketable securities	200	140
Receivables (net)	700	660
Inventories	150	170
Prepaid expenses	50	10
Total current assets	$1,200	$1,100
Total current liabilities	$ 520	$ 460

Total operating revenues were $4,560 in 1987 and $4,140 in 1986.

Required. Compute (1) the current ratio, (2) the quick ratio and (3) the current asset turnover. What general interpretations can you make of the computed ratios?

E5. Greatcare Hospital has budgeted the usage of 7,200 units of a certain supply item during the coming year. This item will be purchased at a price of $2.50 per unit. The cost of placing an order is $12.50 and the carrying cost of the inventory is 20 percent. There are no safety stock requirements. $2.50 \times 20\% = .50$

Required. Calculate the economic order quantity and the number of orders needed per year for the acquisition of this supply item.

PROBLEMS

P1. As controller of Memorial Hospital, you have been asked by the administrator to review the buying practices of the purchasing department. You find that the objective of this department has been to keep as small a quantity of each item on hand as possible, thus achieving the highest possible inventory turnover.

After an extensive study, you determine that the average cost of processing an order is $7.50. This figure includes preparation of the requisition, issuance of the purchase order, processing and payment of the invoice, receipt of the merchandise, and so on. You also determine that the average cost of carrying inventory is 6 percent of the value of the inventory on hand.

Required. (1) Explain what is meant by **economic order quantity.** (2) Illustrate the determination of EOQ for the following nonperishable items:

Item A — Annual usage, $20,000
   Price quoted allows a 1/2 percent (.005) discount on purchases of $5,000 or more at one time.

Item B — Annual usage, $600
   Price, net

Item C — Annual usage, $6,000
   Price quoted allows a 1 percent discount on purchases of $5,000 or more at one time.

P2. Your hospital's administrator notices that outstanding accounts receivable has increased 10 days this month compared to the prior month. The number of days receivable this month is 65 days as compared with 55 days the prior month.

Required. What are some of the possible answers or areas that you should investigate before giving a reply to your administrator? Give at least ten possible suggestions.

P3.   You have been engaged to install an accounting system for Kaufman Hospital. Among the inventory-control features the hospital desires as a part of the system are indicators of **how much** to order **when.** The following information is furnished for one item, called a komtronic, which is carried in inventory:

1.   Komtronics are sold by the gross (12 dozen) at a list price of $800 per gross f.o.b., shipper. The hospital receives a 40 percent trade discount off list price on purchases in gross lots.

2.   Freight cost is $20 per gross from the shipping point to the hospital.

3.   The cost of placing an order is $10; the cost of receiving an order is $20. Space storage cost is $12 per year per gross stored.

4.   The hospital uses about 5,000 komtronics during a 259-day year and must purchase a total of 36 gross per year to allow for normal breakage. Minimum and maximum usages are 12 and 28 komtronics per day, respectively.

5.   Normal delivery time to receive an order is 20 working days from the date a purchase request is initiated. A rush order in full gross lots can be received by air freight in five working days at an extra cost of $52 per gross. A stockout (complete exhaustion of the inventory) of komtronics is unacceptable, and the hospital would purchase komtronics locally at list price rather than shut down.

6.   Insurance and taxes are approximately 12 percent of the net delivered cost of average inventory and the hospital expects a return of at least 8 percent on its average investment (ignore return on order and carrying cost for simplicity).

Required. (1) Prepare a schedule computing the total annual cost of komtronics based on uniform order lot sizes of one, two, three, four, five, and six gross. The schedule should show the total annual cost according to each lot size. Indicate the economic order quantity. (2) Prepare a schedule containing the minimum-stock reorder point for komtronics. (3) Prepare a schedule computing the cost of a stockout of komtronics.

PART 4

Long-Term Resources and Obligations

15
Long-Term Investments

The hospital enterprise invests in receivables, inventories, land, buildings, equipment, and other operating assets. But substantial amounts may also be invested in corporate stocks and bonds, government securities of various types, and other assets not directly related to the primary revenue-producing activities of the hospital. These assets appear in balance sheets under the **investments** caption. Short-term or temporary investments were discussed in Chapter 10; the present chapter deals with noncurrent or long-term investments in securities.

NATURE OF LONG-TERM INVESTMENTS

Short-term, or temporary, investments are those which are readily marketable and which management intends to hold only for a brief period, perhaps not longer than one year. The proceeds from their disposition are used to meet current obligations. Investments not meeting these tests are separately classified as long-term, or noncurrent, investments for balance sheet reporting purposes. Accounting procedures for the two categories of investments are similar, but there are some significant differences.

Long-term investments may appear in any fund, although they most often are found as assets of Endowment Funds or Plant Replacement and Expansion Funds. The investments typically consist of corporate stocks and bonds, government bonds, and real estate held for future use or appreciation. Such assets are acquired because of the need for productive long-term employment of endowment and other donor-restricted resources. Sometimes gifts and endowments may be initially received in the form of bonds, stocks, and real estate rather than in cash. The funding of depreciation by action of the hospital governing board may also result in long-term investments which are properly carried in the Unrestricted Fund. In certain instances, the "pooling" of investments may be desirable.

When securities and other noncash assets of a long-term investment nature are acquired by gift or endowment, they are recorded in the appropriate fund at their fair market value when received. This, at times, may require the hospital to obtain an independent appraisal of the donated resources. The cost of bonds and stocks purchased, on the other hand, includes the purchase price, brokerage fees, taxes, and other expenditures necessary to the acquisition. Where investment securities are acquired by exchange, the "cost" of the securities received is the fair market value of the securities given in exchange unless the fair market value of the securities received is more clearly evident. If neither value is determinable, the cost of the securities received is considered to be the book value of the securities given up, and no gain or loss is recognized.

The income from long-term investments may consist of interest, dividends, rentals, royalties, and similar items. In accounting for such income, it is essential that the income be recognized in the appropriate fund and in the proper time period. Gains and losses from dispositions of long-term investments generally are recorded within the fund where such assets were carried. General principles relating to these matters are stated in Chapters 2 and 4; illustrations of the application of these principles are provided in this chapter.

Long-term investments, regardless of the fund of which they are assets, are ordinarily reported at cost (if debt securities), or at the lower of aggregate cost or market (if equity securities). Departures from these valuation bases are not currently acceptable unless there is clear evidence of a material and apparently permanent **decline** in the market value of the investments. Such write-downs are reported as losses of the period in which they are recognized. In no event is it presently appropriate to adjust the carrying value of long-term investments **upward** (above acquisition cost) to reflect higher market values. Certain authorities, however, are challenging this position, calling it inconsistent and saying that "cost" valuation serves no useful managerial purpose. They propose that long-term security investments be carried at current market value, whether higher or lower than acquisition costs. The AICPA, however, has clearly indicated its opposition to this point of view but suggests that market value be disclosed parenthetically or by footnote in hospital financial statements.[1]

The following discussion of accounting procedures with respect to long-term investments assumes, unless otherwise stated, that the investment transactions are those of the hospital's Unrestricted Fund. These procedures generally are the same for the Specific Purpose and Plant Replacement and Expansion Funds. Substantial differences exist, however, in the accounting procedures for investments carried in Endowment Funds. Attention is drawn to these differences at appropriate points.

ACCOUNTING FOR INVESTMENTS IN STOCKS

The investment of hospital resources in corporate stocks involves some degree of risk with regard to price declines, but such investments may offer large rewards in the form of dividends and appreciation in value if intelligently managed. Investments may be made in either preferred or common stocks. All corporations have common stock issues, and some also have preferred stock outstanding. Preferred stock, as the name implies, has certain preferences over common stock. Annual dividends, for example, usually must be paid to a company's preferred stockholders before any dividends may be paid to its common stockholders. Preferred stockholders may also have a preference as to assets in the event of corporate liquidation. On the other hand, annual dividends on preferred stock typically are fixed in amount regardless of the company's profits. The market price of preferred stock therefore is likely to be more stable than that of common stock which may fluctuate widely and provide a greater opportunity for gain through appreciation. Accounting procedures for investments in capital stocks, however, are not much affected by the particular type of stock involved.

Assume the purchase by the hospital's Unrestricted Fund of 500 shares of ABC Company common stock for $25,000 (including brokerage fees, transfer taxes, and other acquisition costs) on January 2, 1987. The Unrestricted Fund entry is:

Investments – Stocks	$ 25,000	
Cash in Bank		$ 25,000

To record purchase of 500 shares of ABC
Company common stock at $50 per share.

The same entry would be made in any other fund. Had this stock (with a market value of $25,000) been donated to the hospital as an endowment, however, the credit would instead be to the Restricted Gifts and Bequests Received account in the Endowment Fund. A similar credit is made for the receipt of stocks that are donor-restricted to the Specific Purpose or Plant Replacement and Expansion Funds. If the stock were received with no donor restrictions whatever, its fair market value should be credited to nonoperating revenues in the Unrestricted Fund of the hospital. In any event, full details concerning the investment should be maintained in well-designed subsidiary ledger records.

A corporation occasionally will "split" its stock, usually in an effort to reduce its per share market price to a level more attractive to investors. For example, assume that the ABC Company subsequently splits its stock on a 2-for-1 basis at a time when the stock is quoted at, say, $80 per share. The hospital then would own 1,000 shares (2 X 500 shares), and the adjusted cost per share becomes $25 ($25,000 X 1,000 shares). The market value of the stock after the split would tend to drop toward $40 from $80 because ABC Company now has twice as many shares of stock outstanding. Even if the market value does not react in precisely this way, however, the hospital does not recognize income as a result of a stock split. The only effects of the split are to increase the number of shares held and reduce the cost per share, although the market value of the holding sometimes may be greater than before the split.

Receipt of Dividends

Hospitals having capital stocks in their investment portfolios will receive cash dividends and sometimes stock dividends. On occasion, corporation may distribute so-called property dividends and liquidating dividends.

There are three important dates with respect to dividends. A typical cash dividend announcement reads somewhat as follows: "On March 1, 1987, the Board of Directors of ABC Company declared a cash dividend of $1.60 per share payable on March 25, 1987, to common stockholders of record at March 10, 1987." March 1 is the **declaration date**, i.e., the date on which the Board of Directors voted approval for the dividend payment. March 10 is the **record date** at which time a determination is made of the names of stockholders entitled to the dividend on the basis of records maintained by ABC Company. All stockholders listed in such records on March 10 will receive the dividend although they may sell their stock prior to March 25, the **payment date**. Similar dates are established for other types of dividends.

Cash Dividends. Assuming that the dividends received on the ABC Company stock are not donor-restricted but available for general operating purposes, the appropriate entries in the Unrestricted Fund are (assuming the stock split previously discussed):

<u>March 1, 1987</u>

Dividends Receivable	$ 1,600	
Dividend Income		$ 1,600

  To record unrestricted dividend income
  receivable on investment in ABC Company
  stock (1,000 shares X $1.60).

<u>March 25, 1987</u>

Cash in Bank	$ 1,600	
Dividends Receivable		$ 1,600

  To record receipt of cash dividends
  on investment in ABC Company stock.

Although theoretically superior, the March 1 entry often is not made in actual practice. Cash dividends may be recorded only when received. So long as the end of a reporting period does not fall between the declaration and payment dates, this practice may be satisfactory.

Similar entries would be made in the Specific Purpose and Plant Replacement and Expansion Funds for cash dividends received on stock investments properly carried as assets in those funds. If the ABC Company stock, however, is an Endowment Fund investment, the dividend would be recorded only in the fund to which the dividend income belongs by reason of donor restrictions, or the absence of any such restrictions. It is inappropriate to record such income initially in the Endowment Fund even though it is subsequently transferred to the proper fund. A memorandum entry of the dividend, however, should be made in the subsidiary ledger records of the Endowment Fund.

To summarize, it is unlikely that investment income would ever be recorded in the Endowment Fund. Depending upon donor restrictions, investment income on Endowment Fund investments is recorded either in the Unrestricted Fund or in one of the other two restricted funds. Gains and losses on the disposition of Endowment Fund investments, however, generally are treated as Endowment Fund gains and losses, but the individual hospital should obtain legal advice on the matter as state laws and interpretations of such laws vary somewhat.

Stock Dividends. In addition to paying cash dividends, corporations frequently distribute stock dividends, i.e., their stockholders are given shares of stock without charge. Assume, for example, that on April 1, 1987, ABC Company's Board of Directors declares a 25% common stock dividend payable April 25, 1987, to common stockholders of record at April 10, 1987. As a result, the hospital would receive 250 (25% X 1,000 shares) additional common shares. Upon receipt of this stock dividend, an appropriate notation of the increased number of shares should be made in the subsidiary ledger records.

No formal entry of any kind, however, is necessary because stock dividends, like stock splits, do **not** give rise to income. This is true regardless of the market value of the shares received. Stock dividends and splits simply increase the number of shares outstanding without any change whatever in the issuing corporation's assets. Subsequently, each stockholder has the same percentage of ownership interest as before. Besides, revenue arises only from sales of products and services, and there is no sales transaction connected with stock dividends or splits. In the above example, the effect of the stock dividend is to reduce the hospital's cost per share of ABC Company stock from $25 ($25,000/1,000 shares) to $20 ($25,000/1,250 shares). When shares of this stock are subsequently sold, the adjusted per share cost of $20 is the basis for determining gain or loss.

Property Dividends. In relatively rare instances, a corporation may distribute certain noncash assets to its stockholders as a property dividend. Should this occur, the hospital should make the same entries as described for cash dividends. The amount of the entry should be the fair market value of the property received. Instead of a debit to cash, however, a debit would be made to an appropriate asset account (inventory, for example).

Liquidating Dividends. A corporation that is going out of business may at times pay liquidating dividends to its stockholders. Such dividends are paid from the corporation's remaining assets, if any, after its creditors have been paid. The dividend will be identified as a liquidating dividend, and the stockholder generally should record the dividend as if it were the proceeds from the sale or redemption of the stock.

Disposition of Stocks

Investments in stocks may be disposed of in response to the need for cash or as a result of management decisions which require changes in the investment portfolio. The legality of such dispositions should be considered in instances where restrictions may have been established by donors as to the disposition of stocks they have donated as endowments to the hospital. This is usually the situation when the hospital holds an endowment consisting of shares of stock in a local, family-owned enterprise.

When stock is sold, the difference between the proceeds of sale (net of any disposition costs) and the cost of the stock (as it may be adjusted on a per share basis for stock dividends and splits) is recorded as a gain or loss of the fund in which the stock was carried as an investment. Assume, for example, that 400 shares of ABC Company stock are sold for $14,000 on September 20, 1987. Assuming brokerage fees of $140, the entry to record the sale is as follows in whatever fund the investment is carried:

Cash in Bank	$ 13,860	
Investments — Stocks		$ 8,000
Gain on Sale of Investments		5,860

To record sale of 400 shares of ABC Company common stock as follows:

Sale price	$14,000	
Less brokerage fees	140	
Net proceeds	13,860	
Less cost of stock (400 shares @ $20)	8,000	
Gain on sale	$ 5,860	

The subsidiary ledger records of the fund, of course, should be properly adjusted for the sale. It should be clear that 850 (1,250 − 400) shares of ABC Company stock remain in the investment portfolio at a cost of $17,000 (850 X $20).

The general rule is that gains and losses on the disposition of investments of restricted funds are **not** recorded in the hospital's Unrestricted Fund. Such gains usually are added back to the principal balance of the restricted fund, and all donor restrictions associated with the principal are considered applicable to the gains. Losses are treated as reductions of the principal balance of the restricted fund involved. Consequently, the Unrestricted Fund income statement generally reflects only those gains and losses resulting from sales of Unrestricted Fund investments, including those on board-designated investments. Such gains and losses must be reported in the Unrestricted Fund income statement.

It is the opinion of some legal authorities, however, that the gains and the losses on dispositions of restricted fund investments should "follow" investment income rather than principal. They argue that, if investment income on the investments of restricted funds is not donor-restricted, gains and losses on the disposition of such investments likewise are unrestricted. Assume, for example, that the dividends on the stock are not donor-restricted but are available for general operating purposes. If the above argument is valid, the sale of ABC Company stock described above might be recorded in the Endowment Fund so as to retain the cost of the stock in the Endowment Fund and transfer the gain to the Unrestricted Fund, as follows:

Endowment Fund

Cash in Bank	$ 13,860	
Investments – Stocks		$ 8,000
Due to Unrestricted Fund		5,860
To record sale of investments.		
Due to Unrestricted Fund	$ 5,860	
Cash in Bank		$ 5,860
To record transfer of gain on sale of		
investments from Endowment Fund.		

Unrestricted Fund

Cash in Bank	$ 5,860	
Gain on Sale of Investments		$ 5,860
To record transfer of gain on sale of		
investments from Endowment Fund.		

Even in this case, there is yet another difference in legal opinion. Some argue that although the above transfer should be made, the transfer itself is **not** Unrestricted Fund income but should be recorded as a direct addition to the Unrestricted Fund Balance. In any event, the matter is controversial and, as yet, generally unresolved.

A problem may also arise with respect to the determination of the cost of shares of stock sold. Consider, for example, the following purchase of capital stock in XYZ Company by a hospital.

Date	Shares	Price Per Share	Brokerage	Cost Per Share	Total
2/1/87	200	$11.00	$200.00	$12.00	$2,400
9/1/87	200	14.50	300.00	16.00	3,200
	400				$5,600

Assume that 100 shares of this stock are sold on December 1, 1987, for $2,000. What is the amount of gain on this sale? This requires a determination of the per share cost of the 100 shares sold. The per share cost may be determined by specific identification if subsidiary ledger records are maintained in a manner that permits the association of costs with stock certificate numbers. Otherwise, the cost per share sold may be determined on a FIFO (first-in, first-out) assumption, i.e., the cost per share sold may be regarded as $12. Or, on an average cost basis, the cost per share is $14 ($5,600/400 shares). If such costs are not determined by specific identification, the hospital should establish an appropriate policy and follow it consistently.

Stock Rights

The hospital having investments in corporate stocks may on occasion receive so-called stock rights. These are certificates issued by corporations to their stockholders entitling them to purchase additional shares of stock in proportion to their holdings and generally at a price lower than the current market value of the stock. This procedure is followed so as to comply with the **pre-emptive rights** of existing stockholders to participate in an issue of additional shares so that their ownership interest in the corporation is not diluted.

To illustrate, assume that RST Company wishes to issue additional shares of capital stock in order to raise funds for expansion purposes. The company therefore issues rights, also called warrants, to its stockholders on April 1 entitling them to purchase one additional share at $38 for each two shares currently held. One right is issued for each shares of stock outstanding. The stock begins to sell ex rights at $46 per share and the rights are quoted at $4 each.

Assume also that General Hospital owns 100 shares of RST Company stock which had been acquired several years ago at a cost of $2,500. Thus, on April 1 the hospital receives 100 rights. These certificates have value because the holder of two rights may purchase a new share of RST Company stock for $38, a price lower than the current market price of $46, i.e., the rights have a theoretical value of $4 each ($46 minus $38, divided by two rights), and it is assumed here that the theoretical value and quoted market value are the same.

Upon receipt of the rights, the hospital owns 100 shares of stock and 100 rights which together are assumed to have cost $2,500. The rights were received because the stock was owned, and the amount originally paid for the stock included payment for any future stock rights. This means that a part of the cost of the stock should be regarded as the "cost" of the rights received, and an allocation therefore is made on the basis of relative market values as follows:

	Market Value	Percent		Allocated Cost
Stock (100 shares)	$4,600	92%	X $2,500 =	$2,500
Rights (100)	400	8	X 2,500 =	200
	$5,000	100%		$2,500

The necessary journal entry is:

```
Investments — Rights                            $ 200
     Investments — Stocks                                  $ 200
  To record receipt of rights to purchase
  RST Company stock.
```

After this allocation, the adjusted cost of the 100 shares of stock is $2,300, or $23 per share. The rights are recorded at a cost of $200 ($2 per right). Note that the receipt of the rights is not income to the hospital although the rights have a market value of $400.

Now, two options are open to the hospital: (1) the rights may be exercised to purchase additional shares of stock, or (2) the rights may be sold. To illustrate both possibilities, assume that the hospital decides to exercise 60 of the rights and to sell the remainder. The entries are:

```
Investments — Stocks                            $ 1,260
     Investments — Rights                                  $  120
     Cash                                                   1,140
  To record exercise of 60 rights for the purchase
  of 30 shares of RST Company stock as follows:
       Cash paid (30 shares @ $38)        $1,140
       Rights exercised (60 @ $2)            120

       Cost of stock acquired             $1,260


Cash                                            $  160
     Investments — Rights                                  $   80
     Gains on Sale of Rights                                   80
  To record sale of 40 rights as follows:
       Proceeds (40 @ $4)                 $ 160
       Cost of rights (40 @ $2)              80

       Gain                               $  80
```

If the 30 shares acquired by exercise of the rights are subsequently sold, their cost would be considered as $1,260, or $42 per share. Should the hospital fail to either exercise or sell the rights before their expiration date, the entire $200 "cost" of the rights should be recognized as a loss on expiration of stock rights. It is important to take careful note of the expiration date of stock rights received in order to avoid such losses.

Equity Method of Accounting

The above discussion of accounting for stock investments assumes the use of the cost method. In other words, investments in stock are recorded and maintained at initial acquisition cost. Cash dividends were recorded as income. This method of accounting applies to most stock investments of healthcare organizations.

In somewhat rare situations, a healthcare entity may own 20% or more of the outstanding voting stock of a corporation. The healthcare entity, in such cases, may be able to exercise significant influence over the operating and financial policies of that corporation. When a situation of this sort exists, APB Opinion No. 18 requires that the investor account for the stock investment by the equity method.[2]   Under the equity method, the investor records (as income) its percentage equity in the investee's reported earnings (net income), and treats cash dividends received as cost recoveries (reductions of the investment account, rather than as dividend income).

To illustrate, assume that a hospital (the investor) purchased 30% of the outstanding voting stock of the Joy Company (the investee) for $30,000 on January 1, 1987. The investee paid $12,000 of cash dividends during 1987, and reported a 1987 net income of $20,000. Entries to be made by the hospital during 1987 are as follows:

Long-Term Investments – Stocks	$ 30,000	
Cash In Bank		$ 30,000
Purchase of 30% of the outstanding		
voting stock of Joy Company.		
Cash In Bank	$ 3,600	
Long-Term Investments – Stocks		$ 3,600
Receipt of dividends on Joy Company		
stock (30% of $12,000)		
Long-Term Investments – Stocks	$ 6,000	
Equity in Investee Earnings		$ 6,000
Equity in 1987 reported earnings of		
Joy Company (30% X $20,000).		

The hospital's December 31, 1987, balance sheet will report this stock investment at $32,400 ($30,000 − $3,600 + $6,000). In other words, the investment is carried at "equity" rather than cost.

This discussion of the equity method is highly simplified. Coverage of the many complications and other aspects of the equity method may be found in standard intermediate accounting textbooks. The interested reader also should refer directly to the provisions of APB Opinion No. 18 for additional information on the subject.

Balance Sheet Valuation

Except for stock investments accounted for the equity method, investments in equity securities should be presented in hospital balance sheets at the lower of aggregate cost or market value. This basis of valuation is required for investor-owned hospitals by FASB Statement No. 12.[3]   The **Hospital Audit Guide** extends this requirement also to not-for-profit hospitals.[4] A marketable equity security is any instrument that represents ownership shares in an enterprise, and for which market prices are readily available.

To illustrate the basic requirements of FASB Statement No. 12 and the **Hospital Audit Guide** as they apply to long-term investments in marketable securities, assume that a hospital holds the following long-term investments in marketable equity securities in its Unrestricted Fund at December 31, 1987:

	Cost	Market Value
Company A stock	$10,000	$11,000
Company B stock	15,000	15,000
Company C stock	20,000	16,000
Totals	$45,000	$42,000

The aggregate cost of this investment portfolio is $45,000; the aggregate market value is $42,000. (Note that the lower of cost or market convention is applied on an aggregate basis; application on an individual stock-by-stock basis is prohibited by FASB Statement No. 12). Because aggregate market value is lower than aggregate cost at the balance sheet date, a valuation allowance is created by the entry shown below:

Net Unrealized Loss on Long-Term Investments
  in Marketable Equity Securities $ 3,000
     Valuation Allowance on Long-Term
      Investments in Marketable Equity
      Securities $ 3,000
Adjustment of portfolio of long-term
investments in marketable equity securities
to lower of aggregate cost or market:
    Aggregate cost $45,000
    Aggregate market   42,000
    Required valuation allowance $ 3,000

The net unrealized loss of $3,000 is not reported in the hospital's 1987 income statement. Instead, it is shown as a deduction in the 1987 statement of changes in the Unrestricted Fund balance. In other words, it is a negative element of the Unrestricted Fund balance at December 31, 1987. The investments are reported in the December 31, 1987, balance sheet as follows:

Noncurrent assets:
  Investments in marketable equity securities,
  at lower of aggregate cost or market value
  (Note X) $42,000

It is important to recognize that these securities continue to be carried in the accounts at acquisition cost; the stocks are not individually written up (or down) to market value. The valuation allowance applies to the portfolio as a whole, and not to the individual stocks in the portfolio.

Now assume that the Company A stock is sold for $11,500 during 1988. The correct entry is given below:

Cash In Bank	$ 11,500	
Long-Term Investments – Stocks		$ 10,000
Gain on Sale of Investments		1,500
Sale of Company A stock:		

Sales proceeds	$11,500
Less cost	10,000
Gain on sale	$ 1,500

Notice that the basis for computing the gain or loss on the sale of stock is acquisition cost rather than the market value of the stock at the end of the previous reporting period.

Transfers of securities from a noncurrent to a current investment portfolio (or vice versa) are accounted for at lower or cost or market. In other words, if market is lower than cost at the transfer date, a loss is recognized in the income statement of the period of transfer. The market value of the stock at the transfer date (if lower than cost) becomes the new cost basis of the stock.

Assume that the long-term investment portfolio at the end of 1988 was as follows (the Company D stock was acquired during 1988):

	Cost	Market Value
Company B stock	$15,000	$16,000
Company C stock	20,000	17,000
Company D stock	25,000	22,000
Totals	$60,000	$55,000

Because the aggregate market is now $5,000 less than aggregate cost, an entry should be made to increase the valuation allowance by $2,000. Had the aggregate market value been $59,000, an entry would be made to reduce the valuation allowance (and the related net unrealized loss account) by $2,000. In other words, the portfolio is adjusted up or down to market value, but not "up" in excess of acquisition cost.

This valuation procedure is applicable only where the decline in market value below cost is deemed to be temporary. If the decline is judged to be other than temporary, the individual securities should be written down, and the amount of the write-down should be recognized as a loss in the income statement of the hospital. The new cost basis should not be adjusted for subsequent recoveries in market value.

When fund accounting is employed by a not-for-profit hospital, the investments of restricted funds in marketable equity securities should be treated as noncurrent investment portfolios. The lower of aggregate cost or market should be applied separately to the portfolios of each restricted fund. Changes in the valuation allowances in the restricted funds should be reported in the respective statements of changes in fund balances. Realized gains and losses on the sale of these investments of restricted funds generally should be charged or credited directly to the fund balance accounts of those funds. Gains and losses arising from investment trading between unrestricted and restricted funds, or between an restricted fund and another restricted fund, should be regarded as realized gains and losses, and should be separately disclosed in the hospital's financial statements.

The following financial statement disclosures should be made with respect to long-term investments in marketable equity securities:

1. As of the date of each balance sheet, the aggregate cost and market values for each separate investment portfolio, with indication of the carrying amount.
2. As of the date of the most recent balance sheet, for each portfolio:
    a. Gross unrealized gains (excess of market value over cost), and
    b. Gross unrealized losses (excess of cost over market value).
3. For each period for which an income statement is presented:
    a. Amount of net realized gain or loss included in nonoperating revenues, and
    b. The basis on which cost was determined in computing realized gains and losses.

The reader is referred to FASB Statement No. 12 and to the **Hospital Audit Guide** for more detailed information concerning the application of the lower of aggregate cost or market principle to long-term investments in marketable equity securities.

ACCOUNTING FOR INVESTMENTS IN BONDS

The larger portion of the hospital investment portfolio is likely to consist of corporate and government bonds. This results from the emphasis usually placed upon safety of principal and stability of income by hospital investment policies. Bond prices tend to fluctuate less spectacularly than do stock prices, and the receipt of interest on bonds is more regular and assured than dividends on stocks.

Both corporate and government bonds are available in varying terms and in different denominations, although bonds of $1,000 face or par value are most common. Interest is quoted at annual percentage rates of face value but generally is paid semiannually on specified dates six months apart. Certain government bonds do not pay interest in this sense but are sold at a discount, i.e., at less than face value. The interest accumulates and is received in the maturity value of the bonds. When all the bonds of a particular issue mature at one time, they are called **term** bonds. **Serial** bonds mature at regular intervals in installments.

Corporate bonds may be **secured** or **unsecured** bonds. Secured bonds involve the pledging of specified corporate assets as security to the bondholders. In many cases, these bonds are described as mortgage bonds or collateral trust bonds. Bonds not protected other than by the general financial strength of the issuer are frequently called **debentures.** Bonds issued by state and local governmental units sometimes are termed **revenue** bonds in that they are secured by specified revenues of the taxing authority.

Certain corporate bonds are **convertible** at the option of the bondholder into the common stock of the issuing corporation. Such bonds may also be callable at a specified price at the option of the corporation. Interest does not accrue after the call date of these bonds.

Bonds may also be classified as **registered** or **coupon** bonds. Registered bonds require that the corporation maintain a current list of bondholders, and periodic interest is received only by bondholders of record on interest payment dates. Coupon, or bearer, bonds are accompanied by coupons which the bondholder must clip and mail to the corporation at appropriate dates so as to receive interest payments.

Acquisition of Bonds

To illustrate accounting procedures for the acquisition of bonds for long-term investment purposes, assume that a hospital purchases 50 of the 12%, 10-year, $1,000 bonds of Indiana Company at 92 on August 1, 1987. The bonds, which have an April 1, 1994, maturity date, pay interest semiannually on April 1 and October 1. Assuming that these bonds are an Unrestricted Fund investment, the entry for the acquisition is:

Investments – Bonds	$ 46,800	
Accrued interest Receivable	2,000	
Cash in Bank		$ 48,800

To record purchase of 50, $1,000 bonds of Indiana company at 92 and accrued interest as follows:

Price of bonds ($50,000 @ 92)	$46,000
Brokerage fees	800
Cost of bonds	46,800
Accrued interest:	
$50,000 x 12% x 4/12 =	2,000
Cash disbursement	$48,800

Observe that the price of bonds is quoted as a percentage of face value and that brokerage fees and related acquisition costs are treated as a part of the cost of the bonds. Note also that since these bonds were purchased between interest payment dates, the hospital must pay the seller the accrued interest since the last interest payment date. This $2,000 will be recovered by the hospital on October 1, 1987, as Indiana Company automatically pays six months' interest on that date regardless of the number of months the bonds have been held. If these bonds had been purchased on an interest payment date (April 1 or October 1), no accrued interest would be involved in the acquisition.

These bonds were acquired at a discount, i.e., at a price less than their face value. This is probably due to the fact that the market rate of interest on similar securities currently was in excess of 12%, the nominal interest rate on the Indiana Company bonds. Since only $46,800 was paid for the bonds, the annual interest of $6,000 (12% of $50,000) provides the hospital with a yield well in excess of 12 percent on the investment.

In instances here the nominal rate of interest is higher than the current market rate of interest, bonds tend to sell at a premium, i.e., at a price that is greater than the face value. Assume, for example, that a hospital purchases 50 of the 15%, 10-year bonds of Carolina Company at 104 on April 1, 1987. These bonds, which have an April 1, 1995, maturity date, pay interest semiannually on April 1 and October 1. The necessary entry is:

Investments – Bonds	$ 52,880	
Cash in Bank		$52,880
To record purchase of 50, $1,000 bonds of		
Carolina Company at 104 as follows:		
Price of bonds ($50,000 @ 104)	$52,000	
Brokerage fees	880	
Cost of Bonds	$52,880	

Because $52,880 was paid for these bonds, the annual interest of $7,500 (15% of $50,000) represents an effective yield of less than 15 percent. The bonds were purchased at a premium of $2,880 ($52,880 − $50,000).

Bond Interest Income – Straight-Line Amortization

Assume the purchase of Indiana Company bonds (described above) on August 1, 1987. At the end of each ensuing month, the hospital should make an adjusting entry to record interest income for the month. Assuming the amortization of bond discount by the **straight-line method**, the entry is:

Accrued Interest Receivable		$ 500	
Investments – Bonds		40	
Interest Income			$ 540
To record accrued interest and amortization of			
bond discount as follows:			
Nominal interest:			
$50,000 x 6% x 1/12		$500	
Discount amortization:			
Maturity value	$50,000		
Cost of bonds	46,800		
Discount	3,200		
Divide by months to			
maturity	80		
Monthly amortization		40	
Monthly interest income		$540	

Note that the difference between the acquisition cost and maturity value of the bonds is taken into income over the 80 months from the acquisition date (August 1, 1987) to the maturity date (April 1, 1994) of the bonds. The credit of $540 to interest income is roughly the effective amount of interest earned monthly on the investment.

The $40 of monthly discount amortization is also added to the carrying value of the investment in Indiana Company bonds. On April 1, 1994, after 80 months, the carrying value of the bonds will be exactly $50,000 ($46,800 plus $40 x 80 months), the maturity value of the bonds. If the bonds are held until the maturity date, the entry at that time is:

Cash in Bank	$ 50,000	
Investments – Bonds		$ 50,000
To record receipt of maturity value of		
Indiana Company bonds.		

Thus, long-term investments in bonds purchased at a discount are carried in the accounts at acquisition cost plus discount amortization to date. It would be incorrect to carry the bonds in the accounts at current market value as discussed earlier in this chapter.

Now consider the investment in Carolina Company bonds described earlier. In this case, the bonds were acquired at a premium rather than at a discount. As a part of the monthly interest accrual, the $2,880 of bond premium is amortized as indicated in the following entry:

Accrued Interest Receivable	$ 625	
Investments – Bonds		$ 30
Interest income		595
To record accrued interest and amortization of		
bond premium as follows:		

Nominal interest:		
$50,000 x 15% x 1/12	$625	
Premium amortization:		
Cost of bonds	$52,880	
Maturity value	50,000	
Premium	2,880	
Divide by months		
to maturity	96	
Monthly amortization		26
Monthly interest income		$595

Note that the difference between the maturity value and the acquisition cost of the bonds is recorded as a reduction of income over the 96 months from the acquisition date (April 1, 1987) to the maturity date (April 1, 1995) of the Carolina Company bonds. The credit of $595 to interest income is roughly the effective monthly yield on the investment.

The $30 of monthly amortization of premium is also deducted from the book value of the investment in the Carolina Company bonds. If the bonds are held until the maturity date, the investment carrying value will be exactly $50,000 ($52,880 minus $30 X 96 months). Thus, long-term investments in bonds purchased at a premium are carried in the accounts at acquisition cost minus amortization of premium to date.

When interest is received on the semiannual interest payment dates (April 1 and October 1), the entry is:

Cash in Bank	$ 3,750	
Accrued Interest Receivable		$ 3,750

    To record receipt of semiannual interest on
investment in Carolina Company bonds (15%
x $50,000 x 1/2).

The receipt of semiannual interest on Indiana Company bonds would be recorded in the same way except that the amount would be $3,000 ($50,000 X 12% X 1/2).

    The procedures discussed above are also applicable to bonds acquired by the hospital as a gift or endowment. In such cases, the cost of the bonds is regarded as their fair market value at the date received.

Bond Interest Income — Effective Yield Method

    The preceding illustrations have assumed the use of the straight-line method for amortization of bond discount or premium. A preferable method of amortization is the effective yield procedure. The objective of this alternative method is to produce a periodic interest income figure that represents a level effective interest rate on the book value of the investment. It results in the "true" amount of interest income for each reporting period.

    Discount Acquisition. Assume that a hospital purchased $20,000 (face value) of 8% bonds on January 1, 1987, at a price to yield 10%. The bonds pay $1,600 interest annually on January 1, and mature on January 1, 1992. The purchase price of the bonds is computed below:

Present value of the maturity amount:	
$20,000 X .6209	$12,418
Present value of the interest receipts:	
$1,600 X 3.7908	6,065
Purchase price	$18,483

In other words, using appropriate present value factors from compound interest tables such as those in Appendix B of this book, a calculation is made of the purchase price that will yield a 10% return to the hospital. The maturity amount of the bonds ($20,000) is multiplied by the present value of $1 to be received in five years, assuming money is worth 10% compounded annually (the appropriate present value factor is .6209). The annual interest to be received ($20,000 X 8% = $1,600) is multiplied by the present value of an ordinary annuity of $1 for five periods at 10% per period (the appropriate present value factor is 3.7908). Thus, to obtain a 10% rate of return, the hospital-investor would pay $12,418 for the maturity amount of the bonds and $6,065 for the five annual $1,600 interest payments. The bonds therefore would be purchased for $18,483, or at a discount of $1,517 ($20,000 − $18,483).

    Figure 15-1 provides an amortization table for this bond investment. The annual effective interest is 10% of the book value of the bonds. Annual discount amortization is the difference between the effective interest and nominal interest. Notice that an increasing amount of interest income is recognized under the effective yield method. Were the straight-line method of amortization used, the annual interest income would be $1,600 of nominal interest plus discount amortization of $303 ($1,517/5 years), or $1,903.

Figure 15-1.
Amortization Table – Bond Investment
Effective Yield Method
Discount Acquisition

Year	Effective Interest*	Nominal Interest	Discount Amortization	Book Value of Bonds
				$18,483
1987	$1,848	$1,600	$ 248	18,731
1988	1,873	1,600	273	19,004
1989	1,900	1,600	300	19,304
1990	1,930	1,600	330	19,634
1991	1,966	1,600	366	20,000
	$9,517	$8,000	$1,517	

*10% of book value of bonds.

The necessary entries at January 1, 1987, December 31, 1987, and January 1, 1988, are given below:

<u>January 1, 1987</u>

Long-Term Investments – Bonds	$ 18,483	
Cash In Bank		$ 18,483
Purchase of bonds.		

<u>December 31, 1987</u>

Accrued Interest Receivable	$ 1,600	
Long-Term Investments – Bonds	248	
Interest Income		$ 1,848
Accrual of interest and amortization		
of bond discount.		

<u>January 1, 1988</u>

Cash In Bank	$ 1,600	
Accrued Interest Receivable		$ 1,600
Receipt of bond interest for 1987.		

Premium Acquisition. A similar procedure is followed when bonds are purchased at a premium and the effective yield method is employed. Assume that the bonds described above were purchased at a price to yield only 6%. The purchase price is computed as shown below:

Maturity amount:
$20,000 X .7473 $14,946
Interest payments:
$1,600 X 4.2124   6,740

Purchase price $21,686

The .7473 factor is the present value of $1 to be received in five years, assuming money
is worth 6% compounded annually. The 4.2124 factor is the present value of an ordinary
annuity of $1 for five periods at 6% per period. In other words, if the bonds are
purchased for $21,686, the rate of return on the investment will be 6%. Figure 15-2
provides the appropriate amortization table.

Figure 15-2.
Amortization Table – Bond Investment
Effective Yield Method
Premium Acquisition

Year	Effective Interest*	Nominal Interest	Premium Amortization	Book Value of Bonds
				$21,686
1987	$1,301	$1,600	$ 299	21,387
1988	1,283	1,600	317	21,070
1989	1,264	1,600	336	20,734
1990	1,244	1,600	356	20,378
1991	1,222	1,600	378	20,000
	$6,314	$8,000	$1,686	

*6% of book value of bonds.

Disposition of Bonds

The entry to be made when bond investments are held to maturity has been
illustrated earlier. Suppose, however, that bonds held as long-term investments are sold
prior to their maturity? Refer to the facts relating to the investment in Indiana Company
bonds and assume that these bonds are sold on November 1, 1989, at 102 and accrued
interest. The necessary entry is:

Cash in Bank		$ 50,680	
Accrued Interest Receivable			$ 500
Investments – Bonds			47,880
Gain on Sale of Investments			2,300

To record sale of Indiana Company bonds at 102
and accrued interest as follows:

Sale price ($50,000 @ 102)	$51,000
Less brokerage fees	820
Net sales price	50,180
Accrued interest:	
$50,000 X 6% X 1/12	500
Cash received	$50,680

Net sales price (above)		$50,180
Less book value of bonds:		
Acquisition cost	$46,800	
Add accumulated discount:		
$40 X 27 months	1,080	
Book value of bonds, 11/1/89	47,880	
Gain on sale	$ 2,300	

Interest for the month of October 1989 is collected from the purchaser. At the date of sale, Indiana Company bonds have been written up in the accounts by monthly amortization of discount for the 27 months since the acquisition date. The difference between this carrying value and the net proceeds of the sale is recorded as the gain on the sale.

Now, refer to the facts relating to Carolina Company bonds and assume that $20,000 face value of these bonds are sold on September 1, 1990, at 98 and accrued interest. The appropriate entry is:

Cash in Bank		$ 20,610	
Loss on Sale of Investments		1,300	
Accrued Interest Receivable			$ 1,250
Investment – Bonds			20,660

To record sale of Carolina Company bonds at
98 and accrued interest as follows:

Book value of bonds:	
Acquisition cost	$52,880
Less premium amortization:	
$30 X 41 months	1,230
Book value of bonds, 9/1/90	51,650
Percentage sold:	
$20,000/$50,000	40%
Book value of bonds sold	$20,660

Sales price of bonds:
    $20,000 @ 98 $19,600
    Less brokerage fees   240

Net sales price   19,360
Loss on sale $ 1,300

Net sales price (above) $19,360
Add accrued interest:
    $20,000 X 15% X 5/12   1,250

Cash proceeds $20,610

Interest and premium amortization, of course, will continue on the remaining $30,000 face value of Carolina Company bonds until they also are sold or reach maturity on April 1, 1995. The monthly interest and premium amortization, however, will be only 60% ($30,000/$50,000) of the amounts illustrated earlier.

In some instances, a hospital may own **convertible bonds** and will elect to exercise the conversion privilege. Assume for example, that a hospital owns $100,000 face value Iowa Corporation convertible bonds having a current book value of $102,000. These bonds, with a market value of $105,000, are converted into 2,000 shares of Iowa Corporation common stock having a current market value of $110,000. The entry for the conversion is indicated below:

Investments – Stocks $105,000
    Investments – Bonds $102,000
    Gain on Conversion of Bonds   3,000
  To record conversion of bonds into 2,000
  shares of Iowa Corporation common stock.

Thus, as stated earlier in this chapter, the "cost" of assets acquired in an exchange generally is considered to be the fair market value of the assets surrendered. In this instance, however, many accountants would record the stock acquired at the book value of the bonds converted, recognizing no gain on the transaction.

Endowment Fund Bond Investments

The preceding discussion of accounting procedures for long-term bond investments of the Unrestricted Fund also applies to the Specific Purpose Fund and the Plant Replacement and Expansion Fund. The investment income of these restricted funds generally should not be recorded as Unrestricted Fund income until it is transferred to the Unrestricted Fund in accordance with donor restrictions. In most instances, such transfers are appropriate only after the Unrestricted Fund has accomplished some activity such as the provision of charity care or the purchase of plant assets. Thus, no particularly difficult problems arise with respect to accounting for bond investments in these funds.

Complications are encountered, however, in attempting to apply the above procedures to bond investments of the Endowment Fund. The reason is that while the income from such investments usually is recorded in another fund, the investments themselves are carried as assets of the Endowment Fund. Special attention therefore must be given to the problems created as a result of this interfund relationship.

To illustrate, refer to the facts provided earlier concerning Indiana Company bonds, but assume that the bonds are Endowment Fund investments. Assume also that the income, including discount amortization, from this investment is not donor-restricted and therefore is to be recorded as Unrestricted Fund income. (Whether or not the discount amortization should be recorded as Unrestricted Fund income is a debatable point.) Any gain or loss on the disposition of the bonds, however, is to be recognized only in the Endowment Fund. (As noted earlier, this also is somewhat controversial.) The entries are:

1. Acquisition of Investments:

Endowment Fund

Investments – Bonds	$ 46,800	
Accrued Interest Receivable	2,000	
Cash in Bank		$48,800
To record purchase of Indiana Company		
bonds at 92 and accrued interest.		

2. Monthly Amortization and Interest Accrual:

Endowment Fund

Accrued Interest Receivable	$ 500	
Investments – Bonds	40	
Due to Unrestricted Fund		$ 540
To record monthly amortization and		
interest accrual.		

Unrestricted Fund

Due from Endowment Fund	$ 540	
Interest Income		$ 540
To record monthly unrestricted investment		
income due from Endowment Fund.		

3. Receipt of Semiannual Interest:

Endowment Fund

Cash	$ 3,000	
Accrued Interest Receivable		$ 3,000
To record receipt of semiannual interest		
on Indiana Company bonds.		

4. Transfer of Semiannual Interest to Unrestricted Fund:

Endowment Fund

Due to Unrestricted Fund	$ 3,240	
Cash in Bank		$ 3,240
To record transfer of semiannual interest		
to Unrestricted Fund ($540 X 6 months).*		

Unrestricted Fund
_____

Cash in Bank	$ 3,240	
Due from Endowment Fund		$ 3,240
To record receipt of transfer for		
unrestricted investment income from		
Endowment Fund.*		

5. Sale of the Investment (11/1/89):

Endowment Fund
_____

Cash in Bank	$ 50,680	
Accrued Interest Receivable		$ 500
Investments – Bonds		47,880
Gain on Sale of Investments		2,300
To record sale of Indiana Company bonds.		
Due to Unrestricted Fund	$ 540	
Cash in Bank		$ 540
To record transfer to Unrestricted Fund		
of interest on Indiana Company bonds for		
previous month.*		

Unrestricted Fund
_____

Cash in Bank	$ 540	
Due from Endowment Fund		$ 540
To record receipt from Endowment Fund of		
interest for October on Indiana Company		
bonds.		

*The initial transfer on October 1, 1987, would be only $1,080 ($540 X 2 months) since the bonds had been held only two months up to that time. Subsequent semiannual transfers would be in the $3,240 amount shown. The previous transfer was on October 1, 1989, for $3,240, the amount of interest income for the prior six months. This final transfer therefore is only $540, interest income for October 1989.

Similar accounting procedures would be employed where income from Endowment Fund investments is donor-restricted to the Specific Purpose Fund or the Plant Replacement and Expansion Fund.

    The reader must be aware that there are other possible procedural alternatives to the entries suggested above. Bond interest, for example, might instead be accrued in the Unrestricted Fund. The receipt of semi-annual interest then would be recorded directly in the Unrestricted Fund, thereby eliminating a certain amount of the "due to" and "due from" procedure. Yet, this alternative leaves the amortization factor unresolved and tends to create other mechanical difficulties not present in the suggested entries.

POOLED INVESTMENTS

Hospitals typically have cash in both unrestricted and restricted funds that can be invested in securities for varying periods of time. The available cash of each fund, of course, may be invested separately, and individual records can be maintained to reflect the investment transactions of each fund. If this is done, there is no question about the amount of investment income, gains, and losses relating to each fund. Consider, for example, the information given in Figure 15-3 in which it is assumed that all investments were purchased at the beginning of 1987 and that no additional purchases or sales occurred during the year. The cash balance in each fund also remained unchanged during 1987.

On an overall basis, the increase in market value and the investment income appears to be quite good. Yet, the reader will note that the investment performance of the individual funds ranges from excellent to poor. The holdings of the Endowment Fund show an extraordinary growth in value and a high return in income. On the other hand, the value of the Specific Purpose Fund investments was cut to almost half and the investment income is rather insignificant. It may also be observed that a total of $18,000 of cash was left uninvested during 1987. The available cash in each fund was perhaps regarded as too little to warrant the purchase of additional securities. But had this cash been in a single fund, it would have made up a total large enough to invest profitably.

Figure 15-3.
Summary of Investments
Year Ended December 31, 1987

	12/31/87		1987
	Cost	Market	Income
Unrestricted Fund:			
Investments	$ 96,000	$120,000	$ 3,600
Uninvested cash	4,000		
Total	$100,000		
Specific Purpose Fund:			
Investments	$ 48,000	25,000	660
Uninvested cash	2,000		
Total	$ 50,000		
Plant Replacement and Expansion Fund:			
Investments	$147,000	165,000	6,500
Uninvested cash	3,000		
Total	$150,000		
Endowment Fund:			
Investments	$191,000	290,000	19,240
Uninvested cash	9,000		
Total	$200,000		
Totals	$500,000	$600,000	$ 30,000

Thus, when investments are made by individual funds, a number of important problems arise: (1) the full effects of a poor, or good, investment decision are confined to a single fund, (2) a relatively large amount of cash goes uninvested, and (3) a considerable amount of bookkeeping is involved in keeping records of specific investments by individual funds. The **pooling** of the investments of all funds into a single "pot" provides a means of solving these problems. Consider, for instance, the results presented in Figure 15-4 in which it is assumed that the investments of the several funds were pooled during 1987.

Figure 15-4.
Summary of Pooled Investments
Year Ended December 31, 1987

	Number of Shares	12/31/87 Cost	12/31/87 Market	1987 Income
Unrestricted Fund	2,000	$100,000	$120,000	$ 6,000
Specific Purpose Fund	1,000	50,000	60,000	3,000
Plant Replacement and Expansion Fund	3,000	150,000	180,000	9,000
Endowment Fund	4,000	200,000	240,000	12,000
Totals	10,000	$500,000	$600,000	$30,000
Per Share		$50.00	$60.00	$3.00

Thus, the investments and cash balances of the four funds were pooled on January 1, 1987, at which time each fund was assigned "shares" on the arbitrary basis of one share for each $50 of assets transferred to the investment pool. Since, for example, the Unrestricted Fund transferred $100,000 of assets to the pool, it received 2,000 shares ($100,000/$50). At December 31, 1987, the market value of the pool is $600,000, or $60 per share ($600,000/10,000 shares). The Unrestricted Fund's interest in the pool therefore is $120,000 ($60 x 2,000 shares). Similarly, the 1987 net income per pool share is $3 ($30,000/10,000 shares), and the Unrestricted Fund's interest is $6,000 ($3 x 2,000 shares).

A comparison of Figures 15-3 and 15-4 indicates the principal advantage of pooling: the spreading of risk, whether good or bad. In Figure 15-3, the Specific Purpose Fund was reduced to almost half, but pooling leaves the fund in fair shape. The superior performance of the securities previously assumed to be Endowment Fund investments is shared by all pool participants on an equitable basis. Thus, pooling provides greater assurance that the integrity of each fund will be maintained by spreading losses and gains over all funds in the pool. Other advantages to be gained from the pooling of investments are:

1.   Broad diversification of investments.
2.   Stable rate of income for all funds.
3.   Elimination of the difficulty of investing small amounts of cash.
4.   Establishment of a single bank account for uninvested cash.
5.   Elimination of the necessity of maintaining separate investment records for each fund.

If there are no stipulations from donors to prevent it, the pooling of investments usually is a highly desirable practice.

Creation of the Investment Pool

In order to effectively illustrate the accounting procedures involved in pooling, assume that an investment pool is created on January 1, 1987, when Fund A contributes $200,000 cash and Fund B contributes securities which cost $200,000 but have a current market value of $300,000. A self-balancing set of accounts is established for the investment pool, and the following entries are made:

Fund A

Investment Pool Shares	$200,000	
Cash in Bank		$200,000
To record purchase of 2,000 shares of $100 par value in investment pool.		

Fund B

Investment Pool Shares	$200,000	
Investments		$200,000
To record contribution of securities which cost $200,000 (market value: $300,000) to investment pool in exchange for 3,000 shares of $100 par value as follows:		

Fund A ($200,000/$100)	2,000
Fund B ($300,000/$100)	3,000
Total shares issued	5,000

Note that noncash contributions are recorded in the pool accounts at **cost**, i.e., in the amount of the participating fund's cost as indicated by its accounts. The participating fund records the pool shares on the same cost basis. At the same time, however, the investment pool distributes its shares in a number determined by the **fair market values** of contributed assets. Subsequent purchases and redemptions by participants are also based upon fair market values. It should be emphasized, however, that fair market values are not recorded in the accounts; the books are maintained on a cost basis adjusted **only** for realized gains and losses.

These observations are in conformity with generally accepted accounting principles as recognized at present. The **Hospital Audit Guide** states: [5]

> Gains and losses on investment trading between unrestricted and restricted funds should be recognized and separately disclosed in the financial statements. Gains or losses resulting from transactions between designated portions of the unrestricted fund should not be recognized.

While the applicability of this statement to transactions between any fund and an investment pool may be uncertain, the **Guide** makes it very clear that hospitals should not give accounting recognition to **unrealized** gains or losses on investments, except for declines in value that result from an other than temporary impairment. Is there a **realized** gain in the above transfer of securities from Fund B to the investment pool? It would appear not.

The matter, of course, would be resolved nicely if the proposal to value securities at fair market value was accepted by the accounting profession. In such case, Fund B would record the transfer at $300,000, already having written the securities up to that fair market value.

Operations of the Investment Pool

Taking certain liberties with account titles and related matters, the assumed investment activities of the pool for the first quarter of 1987 are summarized in the following entries:

<u>Investment Pool</u>

Cash in Bank	$ 8,500	
Investment Income		$ 8,500
To record receipt of investment income net of expenses.		
Cash in Bank	$ 49,500	
Investments		$ 43,000
Gain on Sale of Investments		6,500
To record net gain on sale of investments of pool during first quarter of 1987.		
Investments	$243,000	
Cash in Bank		$ 243,000
To record purchase of additional investments.		

At the end of the quarter, the pool has $15,000 of cash and investments with a "pool cost" of $400,000. Assume, however, that the investments have a current market value of $600,000.

Allocation of Income, Gains, and Losses

The income and gains (net) of the pool for the first quarter now must be allocated to the participating funds. This allocation is determined as indicated below:

	Number of Shares	Market Value	Allocation		
			Income	Net Gain	Total
Fund A	2,000	$240,000	$3,400	$2,600	$ 6,000
Fund B	3,000	360,000	5,100	3,900	9,000
Totals	5,000	$600,000	$8,500	$6,500	$15,000
Per Share		$120,000	$ 1.70	$ 1.30	$ 3.00

The investment income and net gains (or losses) of investment pools generally are allocated on a quarterly basis, or sometimes annually. It could be done on a monthly basis, but that usually is not necessary or worthwhile.

Some indication is given below of the nature of the entries to be made in the accounts of the investment pool and of the participants:

Investment Pool

Distributions to Participants	$ 15,000	
Cash in Bank		$ 15,000
To record transfer of investment income and gain to participants as follows:		
Fund A	$ 6,000	
Fund B	9,000	
Total	$15,000	

Fund A

Cash in Bank	$ 6,000	
Income from Investment Pool		$ 6,000
To record receipt of income from investment pool.		

Fund B

Cash in Bank	$ 9,000	
Income from Investment Pool		$ 9,000
To record receipt of income from investment pool.		

It is assumed here that the distributed income, in accordance with donors' stipulations, is properly recorded as shown. Under certain circumstances, it is possible that the entire income of the pooled investments should be recorded as income of, say, Fund A.

Additional Investments and Withdrawals

The participants in investment pools frequently will make additional investments (purchase additional shares) or will withdraw all or a portion of their investment (redemption of shares). Purchases and redemptions usually are permitted only at the end of a regular reporting period of the pool, e.g., quarterly. It would not be practical to attempt to determine a new market value per share after each purchase or redemption. Or, if purchases and redemptions are allowed at any time, the value of the shares involved may be based upon the share value regularly determined at the end of the next reporting period. It is assumed in this illustration that entry and withdrawal occurs only at the end of a quarter.

At the end of the first quarter of 1987, assume that Fund B increases its participation in the pool by the purchase of 600 additional shares. Fund A, on the other hand, redeems 100 shares. These transactions should be recorded on the basis of the $120 current market value per pool share as computed above. The necessary entries are:

Fund B

Investment Pool Shares*	$ 72,000	
Cash in Bank		$ 72,000
To record purchase of 600 additional pool shares at $120 per share market value.		

Investment Pool

Cash in Bank	$ 72,000	
Fund B Equity		$ 72,000
To record issuance of 600 additional pool shares to Fund B at $120 per share.		

Fund A Equity	$ 10,000	
Premium on Redemption of Shares	2,000	
Cash in Bank		$ 12,000
To record redemption of 100 shares by Fund A as follows:		

Redemption value (100 shares @ $120)	$12,000	
Book value of shares redeemed:		
($200,000/2,000) x 100 shares	<u>10,000</u>	
Premium on redemption	<u>$ 2,000</u>	

Fund A

Cash in Bank	$12,000	
Investment Pool Shares		$ 10,000
Gain on Redemption of pool		2,000
To record redemption of 100 pool shares as follows:		

Redemption proceeds	$12,000	
Cost of shares redeemed:		
($200,000/2,000) x 100 shares	<u>10,000</u>	
Gain on redemption	<u>$ 2,000</u>	

*Fund B now holds 3,600 shares. Should some of these shares be redeemed at a later date, the cost of shares redeemed may be determined by the specific identification method, or on a FIFO or average cost basis.

The Premium on Redemption of Shares account is not closed out at the end of the fiscal year. It is a permanent account reflecting the accumulated gains recorded in the participating funds as a result of redemption transactions with the investment pool. Other than this, the account serves only to maintain the self-balancing feature of the investment pool accounts taken as a group.

Note that Fund A records the redemption in the same manner as a regular sale of stock that has been held as an investment. Under ordinary circumstances, the gain may be regarded as a realized gain subject to the same financial statement treatment as gains recognized in transactions with entities external to the hospital. An extraordinary situation, however, might suggest another treatment if that is necessary in order to reflect the substance of the redemption rather than its form. In other words, redemption transactions must not be artificially arranged merely as a means of manipulating the accounts to create fictional results for whatever purpose.

INTERNAL CONTROLS

Internal controls should be maintained to safeguard the hospital's investments in stocks and bonds, as well as related dividend and interest income, against loss through fraud, error, and mismanagement.

Policies and Authorization

The accumulation of excessive cash balances should be avoided through the prudent investment of such amounts on either a temporary or long-term basis. Some investments may be in the form of bank savings accounts, certificates of deposit, and U.S. Treasury bills or notes; other investments may be corporate stocks and bonds. Responsibility for investment policies rests with the hospital governing board. The board often forms an investment committee to formulate policies, evaluate investments, and decide upon changes in the portfolio. In other cases, management of the investment program may be provided by the trust department of a bank.

In any event, the investment policies of the hospital should be related to its investment requirements. These requirements generally are:

1. High degree of marketability.
2. Protection against loss of principal and income in dollars.
3. Protection against loss of purchasing power.

The need for a high degree of marketability is an important limitation on investment policy mainly with respect to the short-term investment of temporarily excess cash resources. This situation is most likely to be encountered in the current section of the Unrestricted Fund and in the Specific Purpose Fund. At times, some marketability can be sacrificed in the other restricted funds in an effort to obtain greater investment returns in the form of income and principal appreciation.

The need for protection against loss of principal and income in dollars is rather important with respect to the investment portfolio generally. It is least important, however, in connection with investments related to the Endowment Fund. These securities, within limits, usually can be carried through the ups and downs of the market. The need for protection against loss of purchasing power should be the major determinant of investment policies for resources intended for the Plant Replacement and Expansion Fund and for investments of funded depreciation resources. Plant replacements undoubtedly will be made at greatly inflated prices. This is also a critical consideration with respect to the income of the Endowment Fund. A fixed-income security investment of endowment funds is undesirable in periods of rising prices.

In some states, the hospital governing board is required to exercise extraordinary care, and the types of securities in which the hospital may invest are specified in the laws relating to fiduciary responsibilities. Most states, however, require only the degree of care that would be exercised by a "prudent" person in the management of one's own investments in a somewhat conservative manner. In any event, special care must be given to strict compliance with donors' desires and restrictions.

It is important that all purchases and sales of investment securities be authorized by the governing board of the hospital. Should this prove to be inconvenient because of a high volume of investment activity, a nominee partnership arrangement may be advisable. This is particularly imperative with respect to frequent and sizable transactions in investments of a long-term nature. In some cases, however, limited authority for the temporary investment of the hospital's unrestricted funds may be delegated to the administrator, treasurer, or other officer for practical reasons. The hospital controller should determine that the appropriate authorizations are made as investment transactions are recorded.

Safekeeping

Like cash, securities are highly susceptible to misappropriation. Stock and bond certificates therefore should be kept locked in a safe place, preferably in a bank safe-deposit box with entry requiring two hospital officials. In certain instances, a formal bank safekeeping agreement should be established in which a bank is authorized upon proper written notice to accept or release hospital securities in the bank's custody. The advantages of safekeeping agreements are:

1. Securities are safer in a bank than in the hospital's safe.
2. If securities are kept in a safe-deposit vault at a bank, a visit to the bank is necessary each time securities are purchased or sold. This is eliminated by a safekeeping agreement.
3. Securities held in a bank are automatically covered by insurance.
4. Each deposit or withdrawal of securities is evidenced by a copy of the safekeeping receipt in the files of the bank, the investment counselor and the hospital.
5. Once each year, the bank provides a detailed list of securities held for the hospital.

Employees who have access to the accounting records or to cash should not have access to investment securities. Many hospitals using a safekeeping agreement never see stock or bond certificates because they are handled only by a bank.

Investment Records and Reports

Investment record systems vary considerably, but provision generally should be made for one or more control accounts supported by detailed subsidiary ledger records containing all pertinent information concerning individual investments. At a minimum, these records should include (1) a full description of the security, (2) the facts of acquisition, (3) a complete summary of income received, and (4) the facts of disposition. The bookkeeping task is considerably reduced when investments are pooled.

Regular investment reports should be prepared and submitted to the hospital governing board. In most instances, these reports may be made on a quarterly basis in the absence of unusual events. The reports should provide whatever information is necessary to enable the board to fully discharge its responsibilities.

AUDIT OF INVESTMENTS

The objective of the auditor is to ascertain the existence of the investments indicated by the accounting records as being owned by the hospital at the balance sheet date. The auditor also seeks assurance that the investment transactions of the period under review were properly recorded. In preparation for the audit, the hospital accountant should prepare a detailed list of investments classified by funds and by type of investment. The listing should show such information as date acquired, acquisition cost, and location. Since the auditor will want to examine security certificates or otherwise confirm their existence with a safekeeping agent, the hospital accountant must be prepared to make the necessary arrangements. Properly maintained subsidiary investment records will facilitate the auditing process.

CHAPTER 15 FOOTNOTES

1. Subcommittee on Health Care Matters, Hospital Audit Guide (New York: AICPA, 1982), p. 4.

2. "The Equity Method of Accounting for Investments in Common Stock," APB Opinion No. 18 (New York: AICPA, 1971), par. 14.

3. "Accounting for Certain Marketable Securities," Statement of Financial Accounting Standards No. 12 (Stamford, Connecticut: FASB, 1975), par. 8.

4. Subcommittee on Health Care Matters, Hospital Audit Guide (New York: AICPA, 1982), pp. 75-76.

5. Ibid., p. 78.

QUESTIONS

1. When securities and other noncash assets of a long-term investment nature are acquired by a hospital, at what amount are such assets initially recorded in the accounts? If securities are purchased by the hospital, what is included in cost?

2. In what fund should income earned on long-term investments be recorded by the hospital? In what fund should gains and losses on sales of long-term investments be recorded?

3. It has been proposed that long-term security investments be carried in the accounts at current market values, whether higher or lower than acquisition costs. Give the arguments for and against this proposed procedure.

4. What is a **stock split?** What is the effect of a stock split on the long-term investment holdings of the hospital?

5. With respect to corporate dividend distributions, explain what is meant by the declaration date, the record date, and the payment date.

6. Reston Hospital holds an investment in the shares of an American industrial corporation. The hospital receives 100 shares of the corporation's common stock as a dividend at a time when the stock is quoted on the market at $60 per share. Should Reston Hospital record $6,000 of dividend income? Explain fully.

7. A hospital owns 500 shares of stock which were acquired at five different times and at five different per share costs. If the hospital should sell 200 shares of this stock, how would the cost of the 200 shares sold be determined?

8. Briefly describe what is meant by **pooling** of investments. What are the advantages of the procedure?

9. What are the major features of a satisfactory system of internal control over hospital investments in securities?

10. What are the primary investment requirements of a hospital? Should hospitals invest in the common stocks of industrial corporations?

11. Describe the bank safekeeping agreement as a means of internal control over hospital security investments.

12. When investments in bonds are acquired at a discount or a premium, the discount or premium is **amortized.** What is the purpose of such amortization procedures? What is the effect of amortization on reported investment income?

13. If a hospital holds convertible bonds and converts them into shares of capital stock, at what amount should the stock so acquired be recorded in the accounts? Explain.

EXERCISES

E1. Healthy Hospital purchased $600 of the 6% bonds of Indiana Company at 91 on August 1, 1986. Brokerage and other acquisition costs were $10. Interest is payable semiannually on April 1 and October 1. The maturity date of the bonds is April 1, 1990. On January 1, 1987, the bonds are sold at 98 and accrued interest; brokerage costs were $12. The hospital's fiscal year ends December 31 and adjusting entries are made monthly.

Required. Prepare all necessary journal entries relating to the investment in Indiana Company bonds.

E2.   Hartline Hospital purchased $600 of the 8% bonds of Illinois Company at 105 on September 1, 1986. Brokerage costs were $13. Interest is payable semiannually on April 1 and October 1. The maturity date of the bonds is April 1, 1980. On January 1, 1987, the bonds are sold at 103 and accrued interest; brokerage costs were $10. The hospital's fiscal year ends December 31 and adjusting entries are made monthly.

Required. Prepare all necessary journal entries relating to the investment in Illinois Company bonds.

E3.   Hasty Hospital purchased $600 of the 10% bonds of Iowa Company at 112 on January 1, 1987. Brokerage costs were $12. Interest is payable annually on January 1. The maturity date of the bonds is January 1, 1992, but they are callable at 106 beginning July 1, 1989. The hospital's fiscal year ends December 31.

Required. What amount should Hasty Hospital report as investment income in its 1987 income statement?

E4.   Hardy Hospital purchased $400 of the 6% bonds of Ohio Company at 105 on January 1, 1986. Interest is payable annually on January 1. The maturity date of these bonds is January 1, 1991, and they are convertible into Ohio Company common stock ($2 par value) at the rate of 10 shares for each $100 of bonds. On January 1, 1986, the Ohio Company stock was quoted at $10 per share. On January 1, 1988, when the Ohio Company stock was quoted at $15, $100 of the bonds were converted into stock.

Required. Prepare the entry to record the conversion of the bonds into stock.

E5.   Hopeful Hospital purchased $500 of the 6% bonds of Kentucky Company on January 1, 1987, for $720. Received with each $100 of bonds was a stock purchase warrant entitling the holder to purchase 20 shares of the Kentucky Company common stock ($2 par value) at $20 per share. At January 1, 1987, the stock was quoted at $22 per share. On October 1, 1987, when the Kentucky Company stock was quoted at $25 and the warrants at $100, Hopeful Hospital exercised two warrants and sold three warrants.

Required. Prepare the necessary entry at January 1, 1987, and at October 1, 1987.

E6.   Hickey Hospital purchased $500 of the 6% bonds of Idaho Company and 40 shares of Idaho Company common stock at a package price of $950. These securities were quoted separately as follows: bonds, 104; stock, $12.

Required. Prepare the entry to record the purchase of the securities at the package price of $950.

E7. Healy Hospital purchased Carolina Company common stock as shown below:

Date	Shares	Price Per Share	Brokerage	Total Cost
1/1/86	20	$11.00	$20.00	$240.00
1/1/87	20	14.50	30.00	320.00

On October 1, 1987, Healy Hospital sold 10 of these shares at $22 per share less brokerage costs of $40.

Required. Prepare the journal entry to record the sale of the 10 shares.

E8. Happy Hospital owns 50 shares of Georgia Company stock which it had acquired on November 1, 1986, for $1,180. On February 5, 1987, Georgia Company paid a cash dividend of $1.40 per share. On March 10, 1987, when its stock was quoted at $25 per share, Georgia Company distributed an 18% stock dividend. On April 15, 1987, Happy Hospital sold the shares received as a stock dividend for $252.

Required. (1) What is the amount of the hospital's investment income for 1987? (2) What was the amount of gain or loss on the sale of the stock?

E9. Humorous Hospital owns 50 shares of New York Company stock which it acquired on January 1, 1987, for $2,000. On September 23, 1987, when its stock is quoted at $51, New York Company issues rights to its stockholders entitling them to purchase one new share at $42 for each five shares held. On the date that the stock sells ex rights, the market value of a right is $2.50 and the market value of the stock is $47.50 per share. On October 5, 1987, the hospital exercises 60 percent of the rights and sells the remaining rights. The shares acquired by exercise of the rights are sold on November 2, 1987, for $348.

Required. Prepare the necessary entries to record (1) the receipt of the rights, (2) the exercise of the rights, (3) the sale of the rights, and (4) the sale of the stock.

E10. The following multiple-choice items relate to long-term investments in corporate stocks and bonds.

1. On 1/1/87, Schram Hospital purchased at $1,000 (face value) of the 10% bonds of Shively Company at a price to yield 8%. The bonds pay interest annually on 1/1 and mature January 1, 2002. The necessary adjusting entries are made annually on 12/31 under the effective yield method. Schram's 1987 income statement should report bond interest income of

a. $117.12
b. $107.99
c. $ 93.69
d. $ 88.59

2. Refer to the data of Item 1 above, but assume the use of the straight-line amortization method. Schram's 1987 income statement should report bond interest income of

a. $117.12
b. $107.99
c. $ 93.69
d. $ 88.59

3. On 7/1/87, Jenkins Hospital purchased $1,000 (face value) of the 10% bonds of Pardee Company at a price to yield 6%. These bonds pay interest semiannually, 7/1 and 1/1, and mature July 1, 2002. Jenkins makes all adjusting entries semiannually, 6/30 and 12/31 only, using the effective yield method. Jenkins' 1988 income statement should report bond interest income of

a. $109.44
b. $100.00
c. $ 92.14
d. $ 82.77

4. On 1/1/87, Cooper Hospital purchased $800 of the 5% bonds of Capshew Company at a price to yield 10%. The bonds pay interest annually on 1/1 and mature 1/1/97. Cooper makes all adjusting entries annually on 12/31 only, using the effective yield method. The 12/31/88 balance sheet of Cooper should report this investment at

a. $586.56
b. $698.56
c. $705.78
d. $744.92

5. Keener Hospital held the following long-term investments in corporate stocks at 12/31/86 in its Unrestricted Fund:

	Cost	Market
Company A stock	$ 30,000	$ 35,000
Company B stock	50,000	40,000
Company C stock	120,000	115,000

On 6/1/87, the Company B stock was sold for $36,000. Cash dividends of $4,000 were received during 1987. The market values of Company A and Company C stock investments at 12/31/87 were $38,000 and $109,000, respectively. If Keener has a 1987 net income of $100,000 before investment transactions, the net income for the year including investment transactions should be

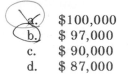

    a. $100,000
    b. $ 97,000
    c. $ 90,000
    d. $ 87,000

6. Cash dividends are usually declared on one date, payable on a subsequent date to stockholders of record on some intermediate date. At which of the following dates has the hospital stockholder realized income from the dividend?

    a.   The date the dividend is declared.
    b.   The date of record.
    c.   The date the dividend check is mailed by the corporation.
    d.   The date the dividend check is received by the hospital.

7. When the interest payment dates of a bond are May 1 and November 1, and the bond is purchased on June 1, the amount of cash paid by the hospital purchaser will be

    a.   Decreased by the accrued interest from June 1 to November 1.
    b.   Decreased by the accrued interest from May 1 to June 1.

    c.   Increased by the accrued interest from June 1 to November 1.
    d.   Increased by the accrued interest from May 1 to June 1.

8. Harper Hospital neglected to amortize the discount on its long-term investments in bonds carried in the Unrestricted Fund. Compare the hospital's net income without this amortization (X) and the hospital's net income with such amortization (Y).

    a.   X greater than Y.
    b.   X equals Y.
    c.   X less than Y.
    d.   Cannot be determined from the information given.

Required. Select the best answer for each of the above multiple-choice items.

PROBLEMS

P1.   Hilltop Hospital completed the following transactions relating to its investment in Hoosier Company common stock ($2 par value):

1.   On January 1, 1987, 25 shares were purchased for $300 (including brokerage).

2.   On April 15, 1987, the Hoosier Company Board of Directors declared a cash dividend of $1 per share payable May 5, 1987, to stockholders of record at April 25, 1987. The dividend was paid.

3.   On September 15, 1987, the Hoosier Company Board of Directors declared a 20% stock dividend to stockholders of record at September 25, 1987. The quoted market price of the stock at various dates was:

9/15	$19
9/25	16
9/30	17
10/5	18

   The stock dividend was distributed on October 5, 1987.

4.   On October 10, 1987, 10 shares of Hoosier stock were sold for $180.

5.   On October 25, 1987, when its stock was quoted at $20, Hoosier Company issued rights to its stockholders entitling them to purchase one new share at $14 for each two shares held. On the date that the stock sold ex rights, the market value of a right was $2 and the market value of the stock was $18.

6.   On November 5, 1987, Hilltop Hospital exercised 10 of the above rights.

7.   On November 10, 1987, Hilltop Hospital sold 10 rights for $16.

8.   On November 20, 1987, Hilltop Hospital sold 5 shares of Hoosier Company stock for $100.

Required. Prepare entries to record all of the above transactions.

P2.   Huber Hospital purchased $100,000 par value XYZ Company bonds at 96 on May 1, 1987. The bonds pay 6% interest per year, payable semiannually on April 1 and October 1. The maturity date of these bonds is April 1, 1996. A brokerage fee and various other acquisition costs totaling $255 were paid. It is management's intention to hold these securities as long-term investments. On January 1, 1988, however, 60 percent of the bonds were sold at 94 and a brokerage fee of $210 was paid.

Required. Assuming that monthly adjustments are made, prepare the entries to record all matters relating to this investment through January 1, 1988.

P3.   Hooper Hospital purchased $100,000 par value ABC Company bonds at 104 on May 1, 1987. The bonds pay 7.5% interest per year, payable semiannually on April 1 and October 1. The maturity date of these bonds is April 1, 1996. Brokerage fees and other acquisition costs were $280. It is management's intent to hold these bonds as long-term investments. On January 1, 1988, however, 40 percent of the bonds are sold at 106 and a brokerage fee of $310 was paid.

        Required. Assuming that monthly adjustments are made, prepare the entries to record all matters relating to this investment through January 1, 1988.

P4.   Huxler Hospital purchases 200 shares of the $10 par value common stock of RST Company on May 15, 1987, for $12,700. A brokerage fee of $60 was paid. On June 1, the Board of Directors of RST Company declared a cash dividend of $2.50 per share, payable June 18 to stockholders of record at June 10. On August 4, the Board of Directors of RST Company declared a 10% stock dividend payable August 30 to stockholders of record at August 15. At August 4, RST Company's stock was selling on the market at $80 per share. On September 19, Huxler Hospital sells 120 shares of RST Company stock for $10,800, with brokerage fees amounting to $140.

        Later, RST Company, wishing to issue additional shares of its stock, distributes stock "rights" to its shareholders entitling them to purchase one new share at $76 for every two shares they currently hold.

        Huxler Hospital received the rights on November 29 when RST Company stock was selling on the market at $94 per share. The rights began to sell in the market at $6 each. On December 6, Huxler Hospital exercised 20 of these rights and sold the remaining rights on December 17 for $560, paying a brokerage fee of $25.

        Required. Prepare entries to record all the above transactions.

P5.   Harper Hospital creates an investment pool on January 1, 1987, when contributions to the investment pool are made as follows:

        1.   Fund A contributes $200,000 cash.

        2.   Fund B contributes $400,000 cash.

        3.   Fund C contributes securities which had cost $120,000 but which have a current market value of $200,000.

        A self-balancing set of accounts is established for the pool which issues "shares" ($50 par value) to the participating funds.

During the first quarter of 1987, the following investment transactions are completed by the investment pool:

1. Purchased investments at a cost of $590,000.

2. Received investment income of $48,000.

3. Sold investments for $96,000. These investments had cost the pool $80,000.

4. Purchased additional investments for $90,000.

The market value of the investments in the pool at March 31, 1987, is $960,000, and a cash distribution is made of the investment income and gains to the participants.

On April 1, 1987, Fund A increases its participation in the pool by the purchase of 1,000 additional shares. Fund B redeems 500 shares.

Required. Prepare entries to be made by the investment pool and by all the participants to record the above activity.

P6.   The investment committee of your hospital board has been told that they have $110,000 to invest. They are also informed that $10,000 of this money will be needed in 12 months for a research project, while the balance will not be needed for about 10 to 15 years when the present building will need to be replaced.

The committee decides to buy $10,000 of U.S. Treasury bonds due in one year, with an interest rate of 6%. Long-term bonds currently are yielding 7.5%. The investment committee also decides to invest the $100,000 in blue-chip stocks. The $100,000 is to be evenly divided over 10 different stocks, covering at least five basic industries, yielding from 3 to 7%.

Required. (1) Explain how the above investments would be classified in the hospital's balance sheet and why they are so classified. (2) Comment on the investment policy of the board, indicating the strong and weak points of the procedure followed.

P7.   The following information concerning investments was taken from the books and records of Martin Hospital at the end of 1987.

Restricted and Endowment Fund principal at January 1, 1987, was $1,084,000, broken down as follows:

Vascular Research Fund	$504,000
Unrestricted Endowments	480,000
Other Endowments	100,000

Unrestricted Fund investment principal at January 1, 1987, amounted to $120,000. All of these funds were pooled investments.

The Vascular Research Fund principal is periodically reduced to cover the research expenses. To accomplish this, $25,000 of investments are cashed and are transferred to a checking account each April 1 and October 1. The Endowment principal must remain intact. On July 1, 1987, $40,000 was added to the Other Endowments investments. During 1987, total investment income on these pooled investments amounted to $60,000.

Required. (1) Calculate the average rate of income earned during the year ended December 31, 1987. (2) How much of the investment income should be transferred to the Unrestricted Fund?

P8.   Following is information relating to Unrestricted Fund noncurrent investments in marketable equity securities for Joycare Hospital.

1.   10/31/86 — Purchased the following corporate stocks:

Company A	$1,000
Company B	2,000
Company C	3,000

2.   12/31/86 — Quoted market value were:

Company A	$1,200
Company B	1,700
Company C	2,500

3.   10/31/87 — Sold Company C stock for $2,200.

4.   11/30/87 — Purchased Company D stock for $4,000.

5.   12/31/87 — Quoted market values were:

Company A	$1,300
Company B	1,800
Company D	3,400

6.   10/31/88 — Sold Company D stock for $4,300.

7.   11/30/88 — Purchased Company E stock for $2,500.

8.   12/31/88 — Quoted market values were:

Company A	$1,200
Company B	1,300
Company E	2,300

9. 11/30/89 — Transferred Company B stock to current investment portfolio when Company B stock had a quoted market value of $1,400.

10. 12/31/89 — Quoted market values were:

Company A $ 900
Company B   1,500
Company E   2,700

Required. Make all necessary entries for the 1986-1989 period for Joycare Hospital.

16
Property, Plant, and Equipment

The balance sheet classification generally labeled **property, plant, and equipment** refers to those assets that have physical substance and a relatively permanent character and are not intended for sale but are held for productive use in the ordinary course of hospital activities. Included in this category of assets are land, buildings, and many different kinds of equipment. Other terms (fixed assets, capital assets, and plant assets) may also be used to describe such properties. The term **plant assets** is employed in the following discussion as a matter of convenience.

This chapter is concerned with the accounting and financial problems and issues associated with the management of the hospital investment in plant assets, including the related subject of depreciation. It is an important topic because a very substantial investment in plant assets exists today in the hospital industry; some sources estimate this investment as more than $100 billion. The individual hospital is likely to have as much as 70 percent of its assets invested in resources of this type. Besides being by far the largest single category of assets in the hospital balance sheet, expenditures for plant assets represent a long-term commitment of resources which can be recovered through operations only over an extended period of years. Usually, the resources used to construct plant assets are obtained through bond issues and other borrowings, and careful consideration must be given to debt repayment requirements. The effects of unwise investments in plant assets are difficult to correct without serious loss and damage to the hospital's ability to meet its obligations, both current and long-term. Sound plant asset investment decisions therefore are critically important. Once these decisions are made and the assets acquired, the effective management of the investment requires detailed plant asset and depreciation records. The first part of this chapter deals with the necessary accounting records; a subsequent section is concerned with capital expenditure budgeting and investment decisions.

ACQUISITION OF PLANT ASSETS

Investments in plant assets should be made only after a careful evaluation of proposed expenditures. These investments should require the approval of the hospital governing board. When such investments are made, the immediate problem is to establish and maintain useful records of the plant assets acquired. This requires an appropriate classification of plant asset accounts and an accurate determination of the cost of such assets. In addition, suitable subsidiary ledger records and effective internal controls are essential.

Classification of Plant Assets

For many years, hospital plant assets and related long-term liabilities were recorded in a self-balancing group of accounts usually referred to as a **Plant Fund.** Depreciation expense, however, was recorded in the **Unrestricted Fund.** This created mechanical bookkeeping problems, but that was not the major objection to the practice. It came to be recognized that plant assets generally are not, in fact, donor-restricted resources. To segregate such assets in an artificial fund, and to report them separately from unrestricted resources, implied legal restrictions which do not ordinarily exist. It was confusing and even misleading to the reader of hospital financial statements. The practice therefore was discarded; it is no longer a generally accepted procedure. Hospital plant assets currently are recorded and reported as resources of the Unrestricted Fund, assuming the absence of unusual donor restrictions that would dictate another treatment. While plant assets may be recorded in board-designated accounts, this should be done within the framework of the hospital's Unrestricted Fund.

Hospital plant assets, with the related accumulated depreciation accounts, traditionally have been classified in the following accounts:

Land
Land Improvements
Buildings
Leasehold Improvements
Fixed Equipment
Major Movable Equipment
Minor Equipment
Construction in Progress

These classifications have proved useful, and it seems likely that they will continue to be used by most hospitals. Subsidiary accounts are employed in a manner appropriate to individual circumstances.

Land. The land account reflects the cost of earth surface owned by the hospital and used in the ordinary course of business. It includes building sites, yards and grounds, offsite sewer and water lines, and parking areas. Land acquired for future expansion, and not presently in use, is reported as a long-term investment of the Unrestricted Fund. Land held for immediate sale is reported as a current asset within the Unrestricted Fund. When land is donated to the hospital, it is recorded as its fair market value at the donation date. Unlike buildings and equipment, land does not deteriorate with use or the passage of time, and it therefore is not subject to depreciation.

Land Improvements. While land itself is not depreciable, depreciation is recorded on land improvements such as onsite water and sewer systems, fencing and walls, sidewalks, shrubbery, and paving of roadways and parking lots. These costs are separately recorded in the accounts to distinguish them from nondepreciable land costs. That land improvements are depreciable assets is a fact sometimes overlooked by healthcare organizations.

Buildings. The control account for buildings should reflect the cost of all buildings owned by the hospital and used in the normal conduct of hospital activity. Included in this account are the hospital building, residences for personnel, garages and storage buildings, and utility structures such as boiler houses. Buildings donated to the hospital for endowment purposes and not used in regular hospital activities are recorded at fair market value at the donation date in the Endowment Fund.

Leasehold Improvements. A leasehold is a contract between a lessor and a lessee. The hospital lessee is granted the right to use certain property owned by the lessor for a specific period of time in return for periodic cash payments. If the lessee makes improvements to the leased property, ownership of the improvements usually reverts to the lessor at the end of the lease term.

A hospital, for example, may construct a building on leased land. The cost of the building is charged to the Leasehold Improvements account. When an existing building is leased, the costs incurred by the hospital to remodel and otherwise make the building suitable for use also are recorded as Leasehold Improvements. The costs of leasehold improvements are depreciated over the term of the lease, or the estimated useful life of the improvements, whichever is shorter. If the lease agreement contains a renewal option and the estimated useful life of improvements is longer than the initial lease term, the cost of the improvements may be depreciated over the initial lease term because the probability of renewal generally cannot be established with reasonable certainty.

Fixed Equipment. The account for fixed equipment is used to record the cost of equipment that is affixed to and is a structural component of the hospital building and not subject to transfer or removal in the ordinary course of activities. Equipment of this type has a relatively long life, but a life shorter than that of the building to which it is affixed. Fixed equipment includes elevators, generators, pumps, boilers, and refrigeration machinery.

Major Movable Equipment. The general characteristics of equipment included in this classification are:

1. A capability of being easily moved as distinguished from fixed equipment.
2. A more or less fixed location in the building although sometimes transferred from one departmental location to another.
3. A unit cost sufficiently large to justify the expense incident to control by means of a subsidiary equipment ledger.
4. A sufficient individuality and size to make feasible control by means of identification tags and numbers.
5. A minimum life of usually three years or more.

Some examples of major movable equipment are desks, charts, beds, automobiles and trucks, computers and accounting machines, sterilizers, operating tables, and x-ray apparatus.

Minor Equipment. This classification includes equipment items having the following characteristics:

1. No fixed location within the hospital and subject to requisition and use by various departments.
2. Relatively small size and unit cost.
3. Large quantity in use and subject to storeroom control.
4. A maximum useful life of three years or less.

Examples of minor equipment are wastebaskets, bedpans, glassware, sheets, basins, buckets, silverware, blankets, ladders, and surgical instruments.

There is some disagreement as to the most appropriate manner of accounting for minor equipment items. It has been suggested that, as a practical matter, only the cost of the original supply of minor equipment should be charged to this asset account. Some accountants argue that this initial cost should not be subject to depreciation, but that all subsequent acquisitions of minor equipment be expensed at the time of purchase. Other accountants believe that the initial cost of minor equipment should be amortized by charges to depreciation expense over a short period, perhaps three years. If this alternative procedure is followed, the Minor Equipment account is eventually eliminated, and all additional purchases of minor equipment items are recorded as expenses of the departments requisitioning and using such equipment. It generally is not feasible to inventory minor equipment.

Construction In Progress. This account should be charged with the costs of constructing new hospital facilities. When the construction project is completed, the accumulated costs are transferred to the appropriate plant asset accounts.

Accumulated Depreciation. A separate accumulated depreciation account is maintained for each major category of depreciable plant assets. The accumulated depreciation accounts reflect the amount of asset cost that has been charged against operations as depreciation expense. In balance sheet reporting, it is permissible to show a single total of accumulated depreciation for all depreciable plant assets.

Determination of Cost

Hospital plant assets that are purchased are recorded at acquisition cost: the cash outlay representing the bargained price for such resources. Frequently, however, plant assets are acquired in ways other than by cash purchase, and special accounting problems arise in the determination of asset cost. In addition, certain incidental outlays relating to the purchase of an asset or to its preparation for use generally should be added to cost. The proper treatment of expenditures incident to the use of plant assets also give rise to difficult cost determination problems.

Capital vs. Revenue Expenditures. Expenditures relating to the acquisition and use of plant assets presumably are made to obtain certain benefits in the form of asset services. A determination must be made as to whether the benefits pertain to the current period only or whether they extend to future periods. In the former case, such expenditures are termed *revenue expenditures*, and they are immediately charged to expense. If, on the other hand, the expenditure provides reasonably measurable benefits beyond the current period, it is referred to as a *capital expenditure* and is initially recorded as an asset. An expenditure that is charged to an asset account is said to be *capitalized*.

It is important that a careful distinction be made in accounting between capital and revenue expenditures. Only in this way will there be an appropriate matching of revenue and expense for the purpose of measuring operating results and financial position. If a capital expenditure is incorrectly recorded as an expense, for instance, the net income of the current period and the assets in the balance sheet at the end of the period will be understated. The same error also results in misstatements in the subsequent period or periods.

In practice, the theoretical distinction between capital and revenue expenditures is not always precisely observed. It may not be possible in some cases to obtain a reasonable estimate of the future benefits, if any, of a current period expenditure. Such expenditures may be charged to expense immediately on grounds of conservatism. In other instances, immaterial property expenditures which may benefit future periods may also be charged to expense as a matter of expediency. Many hospitals have adopted an arbitrary practice of expensing all plant asset expenditures that do not exceed a specified amount, perhaps $500. Application of depreciation procedures to small amounts is not practical. Such a policy for the treatment of acquisition, repair, and improvement expenditures is acceptable, if reasonable and consistently applied. Adherence to such a policy should not result in any material misstatement of net income or assets.

Acquisition for Cash. The cost of a plant asset acquired in a cash purchase is measured by the cash outlay. Includible in cost are the invoice or negotiated price and all incidental outlays for sales taxes, freight charges, installation, and other items related to the acquisition of the asset and its preparation for use. Plant assets should be recorded net of available discounts. Charges arising from a failure to take such discounts should be recorded as a financial expense. When two or more different assets are purchased for a lump sum, that sum should be allocated to the individual assets acquired on the basis of their relative fair values as determined by the best evidence available. Expenditures made to repair or to recondition assets acquired in a secondhand condition should be treated, if material, as a part of the cost of such assets. The cost of purchased land and building includes the negotiated price, realtors' commissions, legal fees, and surveying charges. Any unpaid taxes and other liens on the property assumed by the purchaser are proper additions to cost.

Special problems arise when land is purchased and a building is constructed on the site. Because land is nondepreciable, particular attention must be given to an appropriate identification of land cost as opposed to building cost. The cost of clearing and grading the land is land cost, but excavation costs should be treated as building cost. If a building, not previously owned, must be razed, the cost of tearing down the old building (net of salvage) is land cost. But if the old building was previously owned by the hospital, the cost of razing it is recognized as a part of the loss on retirement of the old building. The cost of temporary buildings erected on the construction site is treated as a cost of the new building. The cost of a constructed building also includes architects' fees, construction permits, insurance, and interest during the construction period.

The amount of interest to be capitalized as part of the cost of a constructed building is determined by the standards provided in FASB Statement No. 34.[1] While interest costs generally are not capitalized as a part of the acquisition cost of plant assets, assets that are constructed or that otherwise require an extended period of time to prepare them for their intended use may qualify for interest capitalization. Capitalization is required only if the effect of capitalization compared to expensing of interest is material.

The amount of interest cost to be capitalized is the actual interest cost incurred that could have been avoided had plant asset expenditures not been made. Avoidable interest usually is calculated by multiplying the weighted-average amount of accumulated expenditures on qualifying assets during the period by a computed weighted-average interest rate. The capitalization period begins with the first expenditures made, and ends when the asset is substantially complete and ready for use.

To illustrate, assume that a hospital begins construction of a small building on January 1, 1987. Actual construction expenditures for 1987 are shown below, along with the computation of average accumulated expenditures, assuming that construction was completed and the building was ready for use on December 31, 1987:

	Expenditures	X	Fraction of Year*	=	Avg. Accum. Expenditures
January 1	$ 80,000		12/12		$ 80,000
March 1	120,000		10/12		100,000
July 1	210,000		6/12		105,000
September 1	240,000		4/12		80,000
December 1	60,000		1/12		5,000
December 31	40,000				
Totals	$750,000				$370,000

*From expenditure date to end of year.

Assume that the hospital issued $300,000 of 10%, 10-year mortgage bonds on January 1, 1987, at face value, with interest payable annually on December 31. These bonds were issued specifically to finance a major portion of the building construction costs. In addition, the hospital had the following other debt outstanding at December 31, 1987:

1. A five-year, 15%, $400,000 note issued on January 1, 1986, with interest payable annually on January 1.
2. A three-year, 12%, $200,000 note issued on July 1, 1986, with interest payable annually on July 1.

The weighted-average interest rate on the debt not specifically incurred to finance construction of the building is computed as shown below:

	Principal	Interest
15% Note	$400,000	$ 60,000
12% Note	200,000	24,000
Totals	$600,000	$ 84,000

$84,000/$600,000 = 14%

The amount of avoidable interest during the 1987 construction period is computed as follows:

	Avg. Accum. Expenditures	Interest Rate	Avoidable Interest
Average accumulated expenditures	$370,000		
Debt specifically related to construction	300,000	10%	$ 30,000
Balance	$ 70,000	14%	9,800
Avoidable interest			$ 39,800

In other words, the actual interest rate on construction-specific borrowings is applied to average accumulated expenditures to the extent of such borrowings. The weighted interest rate on all other debt is then applied to average accumulated expenditures in excess of construction-specific borrowings.

Actual interest costs for 1987 are computed below:

Bonds	$300,000 X 10%	=	$30,000
15% Note	$400,000 X 15%	=	60,000
12% Note	$200,000 X 12%	=	24,000
Total			$114,000

The amount of interest to be capitalized is the actual interest cost ($114,000) or the computed avoidable interest ($39,800), whichever is less. Thus, the amount of capitalizable interest for 1987 is the avoidable interest of $39,800.

The accounting entries for 1987 are summarized below:

Building	$750,000	
Cash In Bank		$750,000
Construction expenditures.		

Building (avoidable interest)	$ 39,800	
Interest Expense ($114,000 − $39,800)	74,200	
Cash In Bank ($300,000 X 10%)		$ 30,000
Accrued Interest Payable		84,000
Interest expense for 1987.		

Had this construction project included the purchase of land as a site for the building, no part of the interest costs incurred should be treated as a land cost. In addition, had any of the bond proceeds been invested temporarily, the interest income is not offset against interest expense in computing the amount of interest to be capitalized.[2]   As a final point, the financial statements for 1987 must disclose the total interest cost for the year, the amount capitalized, and the amount expensed.

Acquisition by Exchange. On occasion, a hospital may acquire plant assets by exchange. For example, a tract of land may be exchanged for another tract of land, or a tract of land may be exchanged for equipment. Cash "boot" also may be given or received in such transactions. In recording such exchanges, what is the "cost" of the asset acquired? What is the gain or loss (if any) to be recognized?

APB Opinion No. 29 specifies that, as a general rule, the cost of a plant asset acquired in an exchange is the fair value of the asset surrendered, or the fair value of the asset received, whichever is more clearly evident.[3]   A gain or loss ordinarily is recognized on the exchange. This general rule, however, is subject to certain modifications.

{a} Dissimilar Assets Exchanged

Assume that a tract of land is exchanged for an item of equipment. The land has a book value of $18,000 and an estimated fair value of $25,000. The entry to record this transaction is indicated below:

Equipment	$25,000	
Land		$18,000
Gain on Exchange		7,000
Exchange of dissimilar plant assets.		

Since the assets exchanged are dissimilar, the exchange represents the culmination of an earnings process. The cost of the equipment acquired is the fair value of the land given in exchange, and a gain is recorded. Had the fair value of the land been only $15,000, the equipment would be recorded at a cost of $15,000 and a loss of $3,000 ($18,000 − $15,000) would be recognized. Thus, the gain or loss is measured by the difference between the fair value and book value of the land. The receipt or payment of cash boot has no effect on the amount of gain or loss recorded. The cost of the plant asset acquired is increased by the cash boot paid, or decreased by the amount of each boot received. If neither the fair value of the asset given up nor the fair value of the asset received is reasonably determinable, the book value of the asset surrendered is the cost of the asset acquired.

{b} Similar Assets Exchanged

Assume that a hospital exchanges Equipment Item A for Equipment Item B. These are similar plant assets; they are similar in type and function. Equipment Item A has a fair value of $25,000 and a book value of $18,000. Because these are similar assets, a culmination of an earnings process has not occurred, and no gain is recognized. The necessary entry is as follows:

Equipment Item B	$18,000	
Accumulated Depreciation	12,000	
Equipment Item A		$30,000
Exchange of similar plant assets.		

On the other hand, assume that the fair value of Equipment Item A was only $15,000. A loss of $3,000 is indicated, and it is recorded as shown below:

Equipment Item B	$15,000	
Accumulated Depreciation	12,000	
Loss on Exchange	3,000	
Equipment Item A		$30,000
Exchange of similar plant assets.		

It is assumed that the fair value of Equipment Item B is $15,000. If the book value of Equipment Item A is recorded as the cost of Equipment Item B, the cost of the acquired equipment would be overstated by $3,000. The acquired asset should not be recorded at a cost greater than its fair value.

To summarize, when similar plant assets are exchanged and no cash boot is received, indicated gains are never recognized, and indicated losses are always recognized. The idea is that, since an exchange of similar assets does not result in the completion of an earnings process, the hospital remains in substantially the same economic position after the exchange as before. There is, then, no justification for recognizing a gain. Losses, however, are recognized in order to obtain a realistic valuation of the asset acquired. The recognition of loss in this situation also is a reflection of the accounting concept of conservatism.

When cash boot is received in an exchange of similar plant assets, a portion of any indicated gain should be recognized. Assume, for example, the exchange of Equipment Item A for $5,000 cash and Equipment Item B. If Equipment Item A has a fair value of $25,000 and a book value of $18,000, the entry to record the exchange would include the recognition of a gain of $1,400, computed as follows:

Fair value of Equipment Item A	$25,000
Fair value of Equipment Item B	18,000
Indicated gain	$ 7,000
Gain to be recognized:	
($5,000/$25,000) X $7,000 =	$ 1,400

Since 20% ($5,000/$25,000) of the total consideration received was in cash, only 20% of the indicated gain is recognized. It is presumed that a portion of Equipment Item A was sold, and that a portion was exchanged. The portion sold had a book value of $3,600 (20% X $18,000), and the selling price was $5,000. Thus, there is a recognized gain of $1,400 ($5,000 − $3,600). The appropriate entry is:

Equipment Item B	$14,400	
Accumulated Depreciation	12,000	
Cash	5,000	
Equipment Item A		$30,000
Gain on Exchange		1,400
Exchange of plant assets.		

The "cost" of Equipment Item B is the portion of the book value of Equipment Item A that was not sold, or $14,400 (80% X $18,000).

When exchanges of plant assets occur, the financial statements for the period should disclose the nature of the exchange transactions, the basis of accounting for the assets involved, and the amount of gain or loss recognized in the reporting period.

Acquisition on Deferred Payment Plans. Plant assets may be acquired under a conditional purchase contract or other deferred payment plan requiring a series of installment payments with interest charged on the unpaid balance of the contract. Such interest charges, whether or not specifically identified by the seller, must be excluded from asset cost and recorded s expense. The excess of total contractual payments over the cash price of the asset is recognized as interest or financing expense.

The fact that legal title to the asset may be retained by the seller until the completion of all payments should be disregarded by the hospital. The transaction is accounted for in terms of its economic substance rather than its legal form. In substance, such transactions represent the acquisition of an asset and the assumption of a liability. When a significant amount of assets is acquired in this manner and substantial future payments are involved, full disclosure of the essential provisions of the purchase agreement should be made in an appropriate note to the hospital's financial statements.

Assume, for example, that equipment is purchased on January 1, 1987, under a contract calling for payments of $5,000 at the end of each year for five years. To record the acquisition as follows would be *incorrect:*

Equipment	$25,000	
Equipment Contract Payable		$25,000
Purchase of major movable equipment on an		
installment purchase contract (5 x $5,000).		

There undoubtedly is an interest element included in the contract although it may not be specified by the seller. As a result, the above entry overstates both the asset and the liability. The cash equivalent price of the equipment should be used as the basis of the entry.

If the cash equivalent price is not known, it may be estimated by assuming an implicit interest rate into the contract. Assuming that an 8% interest rate is reasonable, the cash equivalent price of the equipment may be determined to be $19,963 (the present value of 5 payments of $5,000 each year at 8% per year).[4] Thus, the purchase and the first two annual payments are correctly recorded as shown below (rounded to nearest dollar):

January 1, 1987

Equipment	$19,963	
Equipment Contract Payable		$19,963
Purchase of major movable equipment on		
an installment purchase contract at the		
present value of 5 annual payments of		
$5,000 each, commencing 12/31/87 and		
assuming 3% implicit interest.		

January 31, 1987

Equipment Contract Payable	$3,403	
Interest Expense	1,597	
Cash		$5,000
Payment on contract including 8% interest		
on $19,963 unpaid balance during 1987.		

January 31, 1988

Equipment contract Payable	$3,675	
Interest Expense	1,325	
Cash		$5,000
Payment on contract including 8% interest		
on $16,560 ($19,963 − $3,403) unpaid		
balance during 1988.		

This procedure allows a reasonable estimate of cash equivalent price and provides an accurate measure of the liability as well as the true acquisition cost of the acquired asset.

The leasing of assets in order to conserve working capital and obtain other benefits also is a popular practice in the healthcare industry. Such leases require the payment of periodic rentals and sometimes provide an option for the hospital lessee to buy the leased asset. If the lease contract is in substance an installment purchase, the leased asset and the related lease liability should be recorded by the hospital. This important matter is discussed at length in Chapter 18.

Acquisition by Gift. When plant assets are acquired by gift or donation, there is no cost in the sense of cash outlays directly identifiable with individual assets. Hospitals engage in efforts to obtain such gifts and may make certain expenditures incident to them, but these costs are far less than the value of the assets so obtained. Such costs clearly are unsatisfactory as a measure of asset accountability to donors or as a basis for computing depreciation on donated assets. It would be equally incorrect to assign no value at all to such assets in that they will provide services which should be charged against future operations on some reasonable basis.

If a hospital obtains a plant asset at no cost by gift or donation, the asset should be recorded at its fair value as determined on the basis of the best evidence available. The offsetting credit is made directly to the Unrestricted Fund Balance account, not to revenues. Donated plant assets are considered to be contributions to the hospital's capital. Depreciation of plant assets acquired in this manner should be recorded as if the assets had been purchased. (These same principles, incidentally, apply also to donated assets received by investor-owned hospitals and profit-seeking industrial corporations.) If a gift of plant assets is contingent upon conditions to be met by the hospital, the contingency should be disclosed in a special note to the financial statements. Depreciation should be taken in the usual manner, both before and after title is acquired, so long as it is evident that the hospital intends to comply with the donor's conditions.

Postacquisition Costs. Expenditures of various types relating to plant assets normally are made in periods subsequent to their acquisition. The proper treatment of certain of these expenditures is sometimes difficult to determine, but the general idea is that those expenditures that create additional asset services or more valuable asset services, or extend asset services lives, usually should be capitalized. Major additions, extensions, enlargements, rearrangements, improvements, and renewals generally are so treated. Expenditures that have the effect of merely maintaining plant assets in efficient operating condition and good repair should be expensed immediately. Unusual and extraordinary repairs arising from fire or other casualties not covered by insurance should be treated as losses.

Plant Asset Records and Internal Controls

Hospitals employ many different types of plant assets having widely varying costs, useful service lives, and other characteristics. The maintenance of complete and accurate records of such assets is a substantial but very necessary requirement. Ideally, property records should be kept which provide information for each asset concerning date of acquisition, cost, estimated useful life and salvage value, method and amount of accumulated depreciation, location, and other useful data. Subsidiary ledger records may be maintained manually, but the sheer magnitude of the task generally requires the use of data processing equipment. The subsidiary records support the periodic depreciation charge and balance sheet asset values, provide the basis for insurance coverage and claims, permit the accurate recording of asset retirements and disposals, and assist greatly in securing effective internal controls over the plant asset investment. (Readers may wish to refer to the author's **Introduction to Hospital Accounting** for further discussion of these matters.)

Effective internal control over the hospital investment in plant assets is vital. It begins with an intelligent evaluation and approval of proposed capital expenditures. All expenditures should result only from appropriate budgeting procedures and be subject to approval by the governing board. Once approved, an acquisition should require purchase orders, competitive bids, and receiving reports. Expenditures should be vouchered, with particular care being taken to ensure that expenditures are properly authorized and charged to the appropriate asset accounts in the correct amounts. Plant asset expenditures should be reported regularly to hospital managers and to the governing board. Accountability for individual items of equipment must be established through equipment ledger records that are classified by departments or responsibility centers. This facilitates cost-finding and cost analyses, the taking of physical inventories of plant assets, and regular reconciliations of detailed subsidiary records with general ledger control accounts. Reports of interdepartmental equipment transfers and equipment taken out of service also are essential.

DEPRECIATION OF PLANT ASSETS

Most plant assets employed by a hospital enterprise are depreciable assets. The costs of such assets are apportioned or allocated in some rational and systematic manner to the accounting periods during which the assets are utilized in providing healthcare services. This cost allocation is the income statement deduction referred to as **depreciation expense.** Fifty years ago, the recognition of depreciation as an expense by hospitals was a controversial matter. It was argued by some authorities that depreciation should not be recognized as an expense because most hospital plant assets were acquired through endowments, public subscription, and taxation. This position was rightly refuted, from both a theoretical and a pragmatic standpoint, and neither the desirability nor the propriety of recording depreciation as an expense of hospital operations is seriously challenged today.

An unfortunate amount of confusion, however, persists in this area, and it is important that the nature of depreciation and the methods by which it is determined be clearly understood by all persons with financial decision-making responsibilities in hospitals. Depreciation is a significant element of hospital expense, and misconceptions as to its true character may lead to incorrect judgments concerning operating results and financial position.

Nature of Depreciation

Assume that an item of laboratory equipment is purchased for $60,000 on January 1, 1987. The hospital has acquired a "bundle of asset services" apparently worth $60,000 at the date of acquisition. This equipment will not last forever; its service potential is limited. Each year, as the equipment is used in hospital activities, it expends a portion of its total service capability. After perhaps five years, the bundle of services may be exhausted. The services have been used up or consumed over the five-year period.

Clearly, then, the asset becomes an "expired" cost properly chargeable as an expense against the revenues it directly or indirectly produces during its service life. Recognition of this expense is necessary to obtain a proper matching of revenue and expired costs for the purpose of measuring and reporting periodic net income. Depreciation is as much an expense as the salaries paid to hospital personnel.

The meaning of **depreciation,** as that term is used in accounting and finance, is clearly set forth in the following widely quoted definition:[5]

> The cost of an asset is one of the costs of the services it renders during its useful economic life. Generally accepted accounting principles require that this cost be spread over the expected useful life of the asset in such a way as to allocate it as equitably as possible to the periods during which services are obtained from the use of the asset. This procedure is known as **depreciation accounting,** a system of accounting that aims to distribute the cost or other basic value of tangible capital assets, less salvage (if any), over the estimated useful life of the unit (which may be a group of assets) in a systematic and rational manner. It is a process of allocation, not of valuation.

Thus, the meaning of the word **depreciation** is sharply distinguished from the sense of "fall in value" in which the word is employed in common usage. Annual depreciation expense is not a measurement of loss in market value but is simply an allocation to time periods of the cost of plant assets employed in hospital operations.

It may be helpful to think of the cost of a depreciable plant asset as a prepaid expense. In the example above, the $60,000 disbursed for equipment may be regarded as a prepayment for asset services to be received over a future five-year period. This cost, as the asset services are consumed, must be recognized as expense. The difficulty lies primarily in obtaining a reasonably accurate and systematic measurement of the portion of the total bundle of services that is consumed in operations during any particular year.

Factors in Measuring Depreciation

The measurement of periodic depreciation charges is dependent upon three important factors: (1) depreciable cost, (2) service life, and (3) depreciation method.

Depreciable Cost. The depreciable cost of a plant asset is its acquisition cost minus its estimated salvage value. It is the portion of the asset cost that is charged against revenues during the asset's service life. Problems involved in the determination of acquisition cost were discussed earlier. Typically, acquisition cost is historical cost measured by cash outlay. When plant assets are acquired other than by cash purchase, acquisition cost is the fair value of the asset received or of the asset given up, whichever is more clearly evident. The acquisition cost of donated plant assets is the fair value of the asset at the donation date.

In the depreciation process, each year is charged with the historical acquisition cost of the asset services it consumes. This is done although the current market value of such services may be, and often is, different. (The difference may be attributable to inflation, but price-level and current cost depreciation are not generally accepted procedures at present). Once determined, the recorded acquisition cost of plant assets is continued in the accounts as the basis for subsequent depreciation charges. Subjective adjustments of previously determined plant asset costs are almost never appropriate.

The residual salvage value of a depreciable plant asset is the estimated amount, net of any dismantling or removal costs, for which the asset can be sold when it is retired from use in hospital operations. In some cases, plant assets may be kept in service until they are physically exhausted and the salvage value is an insignificant amount. The hospital may have a policy for certain types of equipment, however, by which the equipment is regularly replaced well before the end of its physical life maximum. In such cases, the salvage value may be established at a relatively high percentage of acquisition cost. There is no simple formula by which salvage value determinations can be made. It is a matter of judgment applied by the individual hospital in consideration of its plant asset retirement policy and experience, expected market conditions for used and scrapped equipment, and other factors. Should dismantling and removal costs be estimated in excess of gross salvage value, the excess should be added to asset acquisition cost in arriving at depreciable cost.

Service Life. Land improvements, buildings, and equipment have a limited service life because of physical and functional factors, and each factor should be taken into account in determining estimated useful service lives. The physical factors include wear and tear resulting from use, and deterioration caused by the elements. Functional or economic factors include inadequacy and obsolescence which result from technological advances, growth in the scale of a hospital's activities, and major changes in methods of delivering healthcare services. Although a plant asset remains in sound condition, its economic service life may be at an end from the standpoint of a particular hospital.

The useful service life of an asset may be expressed in time units (hours or years) and sometimes in output units (miles, pounds, or examinations). In selecting an appropriate basis for measuring service life, consideration should be given to the relative importance of the factors that limit the service life of the asset. Functional factors generally have a greater influence on the service lives of most types of equipment than do physical factors. On the other hand, the physical factors typically are of greater importance with respect to land improvements and buildings. Although the theoretical objective is to select a unit of service measurement basis that is most closely related to the cause of service life expiration, most hospitals express plant asset service lives in time units as a matter of convenience. Even when useful lives are expressed in time units, the adoption of certain depreciation methods tends to result in depreciation charges that reasonably reflect the actual pattern of use in which asset services normally are consumed.

Depreciation Method. Given acquisition cost, estimated salvage value, and estimated service life, a choice is made of the method by which the depreciable cost is allocated to expense over time. The most widely used methods of depreciation are described in the following section of this chapter. Subsequently, consideration is given to the choice of depreciation method by hospital management.

Methods of Depreciation

A number of methods for determining periodic depreciation charges are generally accepted in accounting for the hospital investment in plant assets. To illustrate these methods, the following data are assumed with respect to an item of new equipment purchased on January 1, 1987:

Acquisition cost	$60,000
Less estimated salvage value (20%)	12,000
Depreciable cost	$48,000

This $48,000 of depreciable cost may be allocated as depreciation expense over the assumed five-year service life by any of the several methods described below. Whatever the method may be, (1) it should be systematic and rational, and (2) it should result in an appropriate matching of revenue and expense.

Straight-Line. The straight-line (abbreviated as SL) method of depreciation is a widely used procedure under which an equal amount of depreciation is assigned to each year of service life. The formula is:

$$\frac{\text{Cost} - \text{Salvage Value}}{\text{Estimated Useful Life}} = \text{Annual Depreciation Expense}$$

Application of the formula to the data assumed above results in annual depreciation expense of $9,600, as follows:

$$\frac{\$60,000 - \$12,000}{5} = \$9,600$$

Thus, each year of the 1987-1991 period is charged with $9,600 of depreciation expense for this item of equipment. As shown in Figure 16-1, a graphic presentation of these annual charges produces a straight line. This is the origin of the expression **straight-line depreciation.**

Figure 16-1.
Straight-Line Depreciation
Graphic Presentation

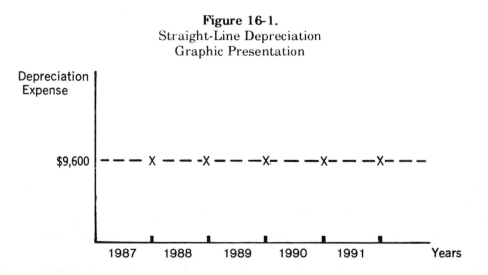

Because monthly financial statements should reflect all expenses, including depreciation, the following adjusting entry is required at the end of each monthly reporting period:

Depreciation Expense	$800	
Accumulated Depreciation		$800

Monthly straight-line depreciation on item of major movable equipment (1/12 X $9,600).

The entry is posted to the general ledger accounts. No postings, however, are ordinarily made to the subsidiary ledger at this time; depreciation is generally recorded in the subsidiary plant assets ledger only on an annual basis.

A summary of the results produced by the straight-line method of depreciation is given in Figure 16-2. The popularity of the method is attributable to its simplicity. It requires a minimum of mathematical exercise, and its effect on expense and asset book values is easily understood. Although these considerations are important, they should hardly be decisive factors in the choice of a depreciation method.

Figure 16-2.
Straight-Line Depreciation
Summary of Results

		December 31		
Year	Depreciation Expense	Acquisition Cost	Accumulated Depreciation	Undepreciated Cost*
1987	$ 9,600	$60,000	$ 9,600	$50,400
1988	9,600	60,000	19,200	40,800
1989	9,600	60,000	28,800	31,200
1990	9,600	60,000	38,400	21,600
1991	9,600	60,000	48,000	12,000†
	$48,000			

*Book value.
†Salvage value.

Sum-of-Years'-Digits. The sum-of-years'-digits (abbreviated as SYD) method of depreciation results in a declining annual amount of depreciation expense. This is an accelerated depreciation method in that it provides for the depreciation of depreciable assets at a more rapid pace than does the SL method. Observe the computational procedure illustrated in Figure 16-3.

The sum of the year's digits is 15. (Had the asset an eight-year useful life, the sum would be 36.) In 1987, the first year of the asset's life, the depreciation charge is calculated by the application of a multiplier fraction, the numerator of which is the remaining life from the beginning of the year and the denominator of which is the sum of the life digits. A similar procedure is followed in subsequent years with the results shown in Figure 16-4.

Figure 16-3.
Sum-of-Years'-Digits Depreciation
Computational Procedure

Year	Remaining Life*	Fraction ×	Depreciable Cost	=	Depreciation Expense
1987	5	5/15	$48,000		$16,000
1988	4	4/15	48,000		12,800
1989	3	3/15	48,000		9,600
1990	2	2/15	48,000		6,400
1991	1	1/15	48,000		3,200
	15	15/15			$48,000

*From January 1 of each year.

Figure 16-4.
Sum-of-Years'-Digits Depreciation
Summary of Results

			December 31	
Year	Depreciation Expense	Acquisition Cost	Accumulated Depreciation	Undepreciated Cost*
1987	$16,000	$60,000	$16,000	$44,000
1988	12,800	60,000	28,800	31,200
1989	9,600	60,000	38,400	21,600
1990	6,400	60,000	44,800	15,200
1991	3,200	60,000	48,000	12,000†
	$48,000			

*Book value.
†Salvage value.

The computation of SYD depreciation can be bothersome where assets are not acquired at the beginning of a fiscal year. Suppose, for instance, that the above equipment were acquired on April 1, 1987. Depreciation expense for 1987 and 1988 would be determined as follows:

1987
$16,000 X 3/4 = $12,000

1988
$16,000 X 1/4 = $4,000
$12,800 X 3/4 =   9,600

Total $13,600

A similar procedure is applied in subsequent years. This computational difficulty can be easily avoided by adopting a policy of recording a full year's depreciation in the year of acquisition regardless of the actual month of acquisition. If the assets are disposed of prior to scheduled retirement, no depreciation is taken in the year of disposal. When a consistently followed policy of this kind is employed, it should be acceptable to independent auditors and third-party payers.

Declining-Balance. Under the declining-balance method (abbreviated as DB), a constant rate of depreciation is applied to a declining base (the undepreciated cost of the asset **not** reduced by salvage value). The rate may be derived from a mathematical formula, or from specially constructed depreciation tables, but it usually is determined as a percentage of the straight-line rate, e.g., 150 or 200 percent of the straight-line rate. If, for example, a depreciable asset has a five-year useful life, the straight-line rate of depreciation is 20 percent per year. The 150 percent declining-balance rate on that asset is 30 percent (150% X 20%); the 200 percent declining-balance rate is 40 percent. Assuming the former rate, depreciation expense would be determined as indicated in Figure 16-5.

Figure 16-5.
150 Percent Declining-Balance Depreciation
Computational Procedure

December 31

Year	Acquisition Cost	− Prior Years' Depreciation =	Depreciation Base	X Rate =	Depreciation Expense
1987	$60,000	(none)	$60,000	30%	$18,000
1988	60,000	$18,000	42,000	30%	12,600
1989	60,000	30,600	29,400	30%	8,820
1990	60,000	39,420	20,580	30%	6,174
1991	60,000	45,594			2,406*
					$48,000

*Remaining depreciable cost ($48,000 − $45,594).

Observe that salvage value is not considered in the declining-balance method until the last year of useful life. At that time, depreciation is taken in an amount to adjust the five-year total to equal acquisition cost less salvage value ($48,000). No method of depreciation should reduce the book value of an asset below salvage value. Under the declining-balance method, the estimate of salvage value need not be made until late in the life of the asset when the estimate is likely to be more accurate.

The results produced by the 150 percent declining-balance method are presented in Figure 16-6. Note that these results, while similar to SYD depreciation, reflect a greater acceleration of expense recognition. Had the 200 percent (or double) DB method been used, the results would have been even more accelerated.

Productivity. The depreciation methods described above determine cost allocations on the basis of the passage of time. It may be feasible, however, to compute depreciation charges in terms of asset productivity as measured by hours of service provided or units of "product" produced. The use of this method requires (1) an estimate of asset lifetime performance in hours or units of service and (2) the keeping of records of actual performance in those terms. Such estimates may be difficult, and the accumulation of the necessary records of output hours or units may not be justifiable if such records serve no other useful purpose. On the other hand, the productivity method does produce depreciation charges that vary directly and proportionately with the level of asset use, thereby tending to result in a particularly appropriate matching of revenue and expense. Thus, the productivity method has considerable theoretical merit when the useful life of an asset is affected primarily by the intensity of use.

Figure 16-6.
150 Percent Declining-Balance Depreciation
Summary of Results
December 31

Year	Depreciation Expense	Acquisition Cost	Accumulated Depreciation	Undepreciated Cost*
1987	$18,000	$60,000	$18,000	$42,000
1988	12,600	60,000	30,600	29,400
1989	8,820	60,000	39,420	20,580
1990	6,174	60,000	45,594	14,406
1991	2,406	60,000	48,000	12,000†
	$48,000			

*Book value.
†Salvage value.

Assume that the equipment has a service life estimated at 80,000 units of service. (These units may be number of hours, number of tests, number of x-ray films, etc.) Depreciation per unit of service is 60 cents ($48,000/80,000). With assumed data as to actual units of service provided annually, the results produced by the productivity method of depreciation are in Figure 16-7.

Figure 16-7.
Productivity Depreciation Method
Summary of Results

				December 31		
Year	Units of Service ×	Rate =	Depreciation Expense	Acquisition Cost	Accumulated Depreciation	Undepreciated Cost*
1987	10,000	60¢	$ 6,000	$60,000	$ 6,000	$54,000
1988	30,000	60¢	18,000	60,000	24,000	36,000
1989	20,000	60¢	12,000	60,000	36,000	24,000
1990	15,000	60¢	9,000	60,000	45,000	15,000
1991	5,000	60¢	3,000	60,000	48,000	12,000†
	80,000		$48,000			

*Book value.
†Salvage value.

Group and Composite Rates. All the depreciation methods discussed above assumed unit depreciation, i.e., the methods were applied to individual items of property as separate units. Because this procedure involves considerable clerical work, hospitals may find it advantageous to associate depreciation with groups of assets and compute depreciation on the collective cost of each group rather than for each particular asset item. This procedure leads to group and composite depreciation methods in which a single depreciation rate is applied to the total cost of all assets in a particular group.

Under the **group depreciation** procedure, a number of similar plant assets are depreciated as a single unit. To illustrate, assume that 10 smaller items of equipment having an average useful life of five years are acquired at a total cost of $50,000 on January 1, 1987. Assume also that three items of this equipment are retired from service on December 31, 1990, four on December 31, 1991, and the remaining three on December 31, 1992. As the average life of this asset group is five years, the annual straight-line depreciation charge is 20 percent of the group cost of those assets in service during each year. A summary of the results of this procedure is given in Figure 16-8.

Figure 16-8.
Group Depreciation Method
Summary of Results

December 31	Depreciation Expense	Cost of Asset Group			Accumulated Depreciation			Book Value
		Dr.	Cr.	Balance	Dr.	Cr.	Balance	
		$50,000		$50,000				$50,000
1987	$10,000			50,000		$10,000	$10,000	40,000
1988	10,000			50,000		10,000	20,000	30,000
1989	10,000			50,000		10,000	30,000	20,000
1990	10,000		$15,000	35,000	$15,000	10,000	25,000	10,000
1991	7,000		20,000	15,000	20,000	7,000	12,000	8,000
1992	3,000		15,000	. . .	15,000	3,000	. . .	. . .
	$50,000	$50,000	$50,000		$50,000	$50,000		

No gain or loss is recognized on the early retirements or other disposal of assets from the group. The entry for retirement of the three units on December 31, 1990, assuming a zero actual salvage value, is a debit to Accumulated Depreciation and a credit to Equipment for $15,000, i.e., the acquisition cost of the assets retired. Had these assets an actual salvage value of $4,000, the retirement entry would be:

Cash	$ 4,000	
Accumulated Depreciation	11,000	
Equipment		$15,000
Retirement of three units of equipment		
with a $4,000 salvage value.		

Thus, the accumulated depreciation account is debited for the cost of assets retired minus any proceeds from salvage. Recognition of gains and losses, if any, is postponed until the last asset item in the group is retired. Depreciation continues to be taken on the cost of assets remaining in service until total cost has been assigned to expense.

The schedule presented in Figure 16-8 assumes that the estimated useful life of the asset group is nicely configured by actual experience. This is unlikely to prevail in practice. So, assume that three asset units are retired on December 31, 1990, and that the remaining seven units are all retired on December 31, 1991. The necessary entries are as follows, assuming no salvage value:

<u>December 31, 1990</u>

Accumulated Depreciation	$15,000	
Equipment		$15,000
Retirement of three units of equipment		
with no salvage value.		

<u>December 31, 1991</u>

Loss on Retirement of Equipment	$ 3,000	
Accumulated Depreciation	32,000	
Equipment		$35,000
Retirement of seven units of		
equipment with no salvage value.		

The above loss, of course, is the undepreciated cost of the equipment retired prematurely. On the other hand, should some of the 10 units remain in service after 1992 when the total group cost has been expensed, no further depreciation expense is recognized.

Under the **composite depreciation** procedure, a number of **dissimilar** assets may be depreciated as a single unit. To illustrate, assume that five different items of equipment are acquired on January 1, 1987, with acquisition costs, salvage values, and useful lives as indicated in Figure 16-9. These are major movable equipment items employed in a newly created department of a hospital.

Figure 16-9.
Composite Depreciation Method
Computational Procedure

Asset	Acquisition Cost	Salvage Value	Depreciable Cost	Useful Life (Years)	Annual Depreciation
A	$ 2,000	$ 500	$ 1,500	5	$ 300
B	2,800	700	2,100	6	350
C	5,000	1,000	4,000	8	500
D	3,500	500	3,000	12	250
E	1,700	300	1,400	14	100
	$15,000	$ 3,000	$12,000		$1,500

The composite rate of depreciation for these departmental assets is 10 percent ($1,500/$15,000); the composite life of the assets is eight years ($12,000/$1,500). Depreciation is recorded annually at 10 percent of the total acquisition cost of the assets so that accumulated depreciation amounts to $12,000 in eight years. When an asset is retired, the acquisition cost is eliminated from the asset account, and accumulated depreciation is debited for the difference between that cost and the salvage proceeds, if any. As with the group depreciation procedure, no gain or loss is recognized when the individual assets are retired. The composite rate method presumes that retired assets are replaced with assets having similar costs and useful lives. If not, the composite depreciation rate must be recomputed.

Group and composite depreciation methods obviously provide simplicity, convenience, and other substantial advantages. If properly applied, these methods produce satisfactory results.

Changes in Depreciation Rates or Methods

The development of depreciation schedules involves certain assumptions, estimates, and choices which subsequently may be found to be incorrect or unwise. Material judgmental errors in previously established useful service lives or salvage values, for example, may become apparent before plant assets are fully depreciated. Or, after adoption of a particular depreciation method, circumstances may make the continued use of that method inappropriate, suggesting the desirability of switching to another method.

For illustrative purposes, assume the purchase for $60,000 of an item of equipment on January 1, 1987. This equipment, which has an estimated useful life of five years and a $12,000 salvage value, is to be depreciated on a straight-line basis. At January 1, 1990, therefore, the relevant general ledger balances would be as follows:

Equipment	$60,000
Accumulated Depreciation (3 years x $9,600)	28,800

Assume that it becomes evident at this time that the useful service life of the asset should have been established originally at seven years rather than five. That is, at January 1, 1990, the asset has four years of remaining life. Also assume that it is determined that the salvage value should be reduced to $7,200. What, if anything, should be done?

The accepted procedure is to revise the depreciation plan so as to allocate the remaining depreciable cost over the remaining currently determined useful service life. Although the $9,600 annual depreciation charge during the 1987-89 period has proved to be incorrect, no adjustment or restatement should be made of previously recorded depreciation. The computation of revised future depreciation charges is as follows:

Acquisition Cost	$60,000
Less Accumulated Depreciation	28,800
Undepreciated Cost, 1/1/90	31,200
Less Revised Salvage Value	7,200
Depreciable Cost, 1/1/90	24,000
Divide by Remaining Useful Service Life	4
Revised Annual Depreciation Expense	$ 6,000

The procedure described here is prescribed by the AICPA in an opinion of its Accounting Principles Board.[6] Adjustments for the effect of a change in accounting estimates should be considered prospective in nature and not prior period adjustments. Even when fully depreciated assets are continued in service, no correction or adjustment should be made for depreciation assigned to prior periods.

To illustrate another possibility giving rise to a revision of depreciation charges, assume the purchase of an item of equipment for $60,000 on January 1, 1987. The equipment, with an estimated useful service life of five years and a salvage value of $12,000, is to be depreciated on a straight-line basis. On January 1, 1990, a $8,800 capital expenditure is made on this equipment. If this expenditure does not prolong the equipment's useful life, the entry for the expenditure is:

Equipment	$ 8,800	
Cash		$ 8,800
Capital expenditure that does not alter		
the useful life of the equipment.		

The revised depreciation charge for 1990 and 1991 is $14,000, i.e., ($9,600 plus $8,800) divided by two years.

Assume, however, that the above expenditure extends the remaining service life of the equipment to four years. The entry for the expenditure is:

Accumulated Depreciation	$ 8,800	
Cash		$ 8,800
Capital expenditure that extends the		
remaining service life of the equipment		
to four years.		

Subsequent annual depreciation charges should be revised to $7,000, as follows:

Acquisition Cost	$60,000
Less Accumulated Depreciation	28,800
Undepreciated Cost, 1/1/90	31,200
Less Salvage Value	12,000
Balance	19,200
Add Capital Expenditure	8,800
Revised Depreciation Base	28,000
Divide by Extended Remaining Life	4
Revised Annual Depreciation Expense	$ 7,000

Expenditures of this type often require a revision of the estimate of salvage value. This consideration, however, is excluded from the above illustration.

Yet another possibility is that the $8,800 expenditure represents the replacement of a worn-out part of the equipment. Assume that it is estimated that the replaced part is 10 percent of the original asset cost, but that the replaced part has no salvage value. Assume also that the replacement of the part does not affect the remaining service life of the asset. The correct entries are:

Accumulated Depreciation	$ 2,880	
Loss on Replacement of Equipment Part	3,120	
Equipment		$ 6,000

Loss on replacement of equipment part
as follows:

Cost (10% X $60,000)	$6,000	
Accumulated depreciation:		
(10% X $28,800)	2,880	
Loss	$3,120	

Equipment	$ 8,800	
Cash		$ 8,800

Cost of replacement part for equipment.

Subsequent annual depreciation charges for 1990 and 1991 are determined as follows:

Original Asset ($9,600 X 90%)	$ 8,640
Replacement Part ($8,800/2)	4,400
Revised Annual Depreciation Expense	$13,040

Should replacement of the worn-out part extend the asset service life or affect the asset's salvage value, the procedure would be modified to conform to the adjustments described in the earlier illustrations.

As to changes in depreciation **method**, two initial points should be made. First, careful consideration should be given to the short-run and long-range implications of the original choice of depreciation method so that subsequent changes in depreciation method generally are not necessary. This is not to say that there is virtue in being consistently wrong or that the principle of consistency precludes a desirable change in accounting method. But it is true that changes in depreciation methods are not always met with approval. Certainly, an indiscriminate changing of methods without good business reasons cannot be condoned. The second point to be made is that when changes in depreciation methods **are** made, the effects of such changes on the reported expenses and net income must be fully disclosed in the hospital financial statements. Users of financial data have a right to know the accounting methods by which such data were determined.

Perhaps the most likely change in depreciation method is one in which an accelerated depreciation method is discontinued in favor of the straight-line method. To illustrate, assume the acquisition on January 1, 1987, of depreciable plant assets with a depreciation base of $550,000 and an estimated useful service life of 10 years. If SYD depreciation is taken for the first five years of the assets' life, the results are:

		Depreciation Expense
1987	$550,000 X 10/55	$100,000
1988	$550,000 X 9/55	90,000
1989	$550,000 X 8/55	80,000
1990	$550,000 X 7/55	70,000
1991	$550,000 X 6/55	60,000
Accumulated depreciation, 1/1/92		$400,000

If a change to the straight-line method is made in 1992, the cumulative effect of the change in accounting principle on previously reported income must be determined. Had straight-line depreciation procedures been followed in the five years prior to 1992, depreciation expense would have been $275,000 ($55,000 X 5 years). The retroactive and cumulative effect of the change in method, then, is $125,000 ($400,000 - $275,000).

In accounting for the change in depreciation method as prescribed in APB Opinion No. 20, the following entry is required in 1992:

Accumulated Depreciation	$125,000	
Cumulative Effect of Change in Accounting Principle		$125,000
Cumulative effect of change in method of depreciation, retroactively applied to prior periods involved.		

The cumulative effect should be reported in the 1992 income statement as a special item includible in the determination of the net income for the year.[7] Full disclosure, by footnote or otherwise, also must be made of the justification for the change. The previously issued financial statements for the 1987-91 period are not adjusted or revised in any manner. Depreciation expense for the year of change (1992) and each subsequent year should be reported on a straight-line basis, i.e., $55,000 annually.

Funding of Depreciation

The "funding" of depreciation is practiced by many hospitals. Although the concept is not a difficult one, it often is misunderstood. The funding of depreciation refers to the process by which cash resources are set aside periodically and accumulated for the purpose of financing the renewal or replacement of plant assets. Since depreciation is an operating expense, it should be taken into account in rate-making. Hospital revenues therefore include an element representing the cost of plant asset services consumed during the period. That portion of periodic revenue is often set aside for the future replacement of consumed asset services so that management may be enabled to meet its obligation to preserve and maintain the hospital capital investment. Monies set aside in this way should, of course, be invested in accordance with sound policies and objectives.

The funding of depreciation is a desirable practice that should be observed to the maximum extent allowed by available resources and consistent with the hospital's primary objective, i.e., the current provision of quality patient care. If, because of inadequate revenues, a conflict arises between the objectives of funding depreciation and of meeting current financial obligations associated with quality patient care, the latter necessarily must be given priority. But it must be understood that the inability to fund depreciation adequately is clearly indicative of the under-financing of hospital operations. A long-run continuation of such situations has serious implications and will eventually lead to an impairment of the hospital's ability to meet the community's healthcare requirements.

To illustrate the accounting procedure for the funding of depreciation, assume that a hospital's depreciation expense for a particular year is $120,000:

Depreciation Expense	$120,000	
Accumulated Depreciation		$120,000
Depreciation expense for the year.		

This entry, in itself, provides no resources. Only through the operation of the mechanisms of adequate rate structures and third-party reimbursement formulas will $120,000 of "funds" be generated. It is a popular misconception that the Accumulated Depreciation account (sometimes unwisely called **reserve for depreciation**) somehow contains money!

In those instances where the funding of depreciation is a voluntary action prescribed by the hospital governing board, the appropriate annual entry in the accounting records, assuming 100 percent funding, is:

Board-Designated Assets — Cash	$120,000	
Cash In Bank		$120,000
Funding (100%) of depreciation		
expense for the year.		

Thus, $120,000 is transferred from the hospital's general checking account and set aside in a special account established **within** the Unrestricted Fund. Although earmarked for a specific purpose, the actual future use of this money remains entirely in the board's control. It would be most **improper** to transfer these resources to the Plant Replacement and Expansion Fund, and to report them as if they were donor-restricted.

If the hospital receives resources that **are** donor-restricted to the funding of depreciation or to plant asset replacement, such resources should always be regarded as restricted fund assets.

Assume, however, that the hospital receives a $45,000 reimbursement for depreciation from a third-party payer under a contract that restricts the use of such reimbursement to plant asset acquisitions. In earlier years, these resources were transferred to the Plant Replacement and Expansion Fund where they were reported as restricted resources. The AICPA Subcommittee on Health Care Matters, however, has recently concluded that this practice is not correct. Statement of Position (SOP) 85-1 states that:[8]

> Assets whose use is limited in substance under terms of debt indentures, trust agreements, third-party reimbursement agreements, or other similar arrangements should be reported in the [Unrestricted Fund] section of the balance sheet as assets whose use is limited.

The Subcommittee argues that such agreements are normal and recurring hospital activities necessary for carrying out the general and unrestricted operating objectives, and are entered into at the discretion of the governing board. To comply with SOP 85-1, the following entry is necessary:

Unrestricted Fund

Noncurrent Limited-Use Assets	$ 45,000	
Cash In Bank		$ 45,000
To record assets whose use is limited by		
contract with third-party payers.		

These resources are invested until such time as plant assets are acquired. Income earned on such investments is reported as nonoperating revenues in the income statement of the Unrestricted Fund.

It is important to note that neither the economic reality of depreciation nor its proper amount is dependent in any way upon whether or not depreciation is funded or upon the amount that may be funded. The objective of depreciation accounting is to allocate historical costs; the objective of funding depreciation is to accumulate resources to finance the replacement of plant assets. The degree to which the latter objective is achieved has no bearing whatever on the former. It is unfortunate that some credence has been given to the denial of depreciation as a valid operating expense unless it is funded.

Choice of Depreciation Method.

As indicated earlier, a number of different generally accepted depreciation methods are available to hospitals. While each method produces the same total amount of depreciation expense in the long-run, the amount assigned to individual years varies widely. Which method should hospitals use?

From a theoretical point of view, an enterprise should adopt the depreciation method that most accurately measures the consumption of asset services so as to obtain an appropriate matching of revenues and expenses for the purpose of net income determinations. The resulting balance sheet asset valuation is of secondary consideration. An evaluation of a depreciation method should be centered on its impact on operating results. Even where agreement is found on this point, theoretical support abounds for all the generally accepted depreciation methods.

Today's hospital manager is likely to be a pragmatist of the first order. Theoretical considerations are not at all unimportant, but the choice of depreciation method tends to be made on the basis of practical concerns. These concerns are the simplicity of the method and its effect on hospital cash flows. The reader will agree that the straight-line depreciation method has the advantage of simplicity. Its mathematics are simple; it requires the least clerical effort; it is easily understood. When applied on a group or on a composite basis, the straight-line method minimizes accounting complications.

A far more important practical consideration in the choice of depreciation method, however, is the effect of depreciation method on cash flows. To the extent that a hospital obtains third-party reimbursement on the basis of its costs (or on the basis of service rates established on the basis of the hospital's costs), the use of accelerated depreciation methods tend to produce larger reimbursements than would be the case under straight-line depreciation, at least during the early years of depreciable asset lives.

The reader, however, is cautioned to observe that smaller cash flows may be realized in the later years of plant asset life when annual depreciation under an accelerated method is less than under the SL method. It may be said that a bird in hand is worth two in the bush and let the future take care of itself, but these short-sighted views can lead to serious long-run difficulties. The adoption of an accelerated depreciation method in an effort to improve current cash flows must be recognized plainly as a mortgage on the future. Whether such borrowing from the future is wise will depend upon many factors other than the urgencies of the moment. These factors include the use of the borrowed cash flow, the estimated trend of inflation, the impact of depreciation method on rate structure, the probable expansion in plant asset investment and anticipated changes in reimbursement contracts.

DISPOSAL OF PLANT ASSETS

It is important that an accurate accounting be made of disposals of plant assets through normal retirement, sale, and involuntary conversion. Each of these possibilities is examined here briefly. To illustrate, assume the January 1, 1987, purchase of a plant asset for $60,000. The asset has an estimated useful life of five years and a salvage value of $12,000. It is depreciated by the straight-line method.

Normal Retirement

If the asset's useful service life ends on December 31, 1991, as estimated and its expected salvage value is realized, the appropriate accounting entry is:

Cash	$ 12,000	
Accumulated Depreciation	48,000	
Equipment		$ 60,000
Normal retirement of item of		
major movable equipment.		

Should the actual salvage value prove to be more or less than $12,000, the entry would include the recognition of a gain or loss on retirement of plant assets. In cases where fully depreciated assets remain in service, no further depreciation is taken and no adjustment is made of previously recorded depreciation. The cost of such assets, and the related accumulated depreciation, remains on the books until the assets are eventually retired from service.

Sale of Plant Assets

A plant asset may be sold prior to the end of its scheduled useful service life for reasons not anticipated when it was acquired. Assume, for example, that the above equipment is sold for $30,000 on April 1, 1989:

Cash		$ 30,000	
Accumulated Depreciation		21,600	
Loss on Sale of Plant Assets		8,400	
Equipment			$ 60,000

Sale of item of equipment as follows:

Acquisition cost		$60,000	
Accumulated depreciation:			
1987	$9,600		
1988	9,600		
1989 ($9,600 x 1/4)	2,400	21,600	
Book value		38,400	
Less sale proceeds		30,000	
Loss		$ 8,400	

It is interesting to observe that had SYD depreciation been taken on this equipment, the sale transaction would have produced a gain of $1,200:

Sale proceeds			$ 30,000
Acquisition cost		$60,000	
Accumulated depreciation:*			
1987	$16,000		
1988	12,800		
1989 ($9,600 X 1/4)	2,400	31,200	
Book value			28,800
Gain on sale			$ 1,200

*See Figure 16-3.

Yet another factor that may have some important implications in regard to the choice of depreciation method is seen in the above example. Accelerated depreciation tends to minimize or eliminate the recognition of loss on premature retirements of plant assets.

Involuntary Conversion

Involuntary conversion refers to the loss of a plant asset due to fire, flood, earthquake, or other casualty. Such losses typically are covered by appropriate insurance. Assume, for example, that an outlying structure on the hospital premises was 60 percent destroyed by fire on April 1, 1987. This building was constructed on January 1, 1983, at a cost of $150,000. It was being depreciated on a straight-line basis, assuming a salvage value of $30,000 and a useful life of 20 years. At the date of the fire, the fire insurance coverage was:

Insurance Company	Policy Face	Coinsurance Required
A	$40,000	90%
B	60,000	75

The insurance companies and the hospital reach an agreement that the insurable value of the building at the date of the fire was $125,000. The amount of the economic loss, then, was $75,000 (60% of $125,000). What, in these circumstances, would be the amount of insurance recovery?

Each insurance company ordinarily will pay the lesser of four figures: (1) policy face, (2) amount of loss, (3) contribution limitation, or (4) coinsurance limitation. The first two of these amounts are indicated above.

The contribution limitation is derived from the contribution or pro rata liability clause which is a standard feature of fire insurance policies. This clause reads somewhat as follows:

This insurance company shall not be liable for a greater proportion of any loss than the amount hereby insured shall bear to the whole insurance covering the property against the peril involved, whether collectible or not.

The effect of this clause is to prevent the insured from collecting more than the amount of loss when a single property is covered by two or more insurance companies. In the illustration provided, insurance Company A's share of the loss is limited to $40,000/$100,000 of $75,000, or $30,000. Similarly, Company B's contribution to the suffered loss is limited to $60,000/$100,000 of $75,000, or $45,000.

Many fire insurance policies also contain a coinsurance clause which often reads as follows:

The insured shall at all times maintain contributing insurance on the property covered by this policy to the extent of at least _% of the actual cash value at the time of loss, and that, failing to do so, the insured shall to the extent of such deficit bear a proportion of such loss.

The effect of this clause is to discourage gambling by insureds who might otherwise greatly underinsure their properties. This clause also makes it possible to establish more equitable fire insurance rates. With the coinsurance clause, the insurance company's liability is limited to an amount determined by application of the following formula:

$$\frac{\text{Policy Face}}{\text{Insurance Required}} \; X \;\; \text{Loss} = \text{Coinsurance Limitation}$$

The amount of "insurance required" is determined by multiplying the coinsurance percentage (stated in the policy) by the insurable value of the property at the date of the fire.

The coinsurance limitation for insurance Company A is $26,667; Company B will pay not more than $48,000. The computation of these amounts is:

Company A:

$$\frac{\$40,000}{90\% \text{ X } \$125,000} \quad \text{X} \quad \$75,000 = \underline{\$26,667}$$

Company B:

$$\frac{\$60,000}{75\% \text{ X } \$125,000} \quad \text{X} \quad \$75,000 = \underline{\$48,000}$$

Company A, in this example, will pay the $26,667 coinsurance clause amount because it is smaller than the policy face ($40,000), the loss ($75,000), or the contribution limitation ($30,000). Using the same reasoning, it can be seen that the recovery from Company B is limited to $48,000, as determined by the contribution clause. The total insurance recovery by the hospital therefore is $74,667.

In accounting for the fire and related insurance recovery, the following entry would be appropriate:

Cash	$ 74,667	
Accumulated Depreciation	15,300	
Loss Arising from Fire	33	
Buildings		$ 90,000
To record building fire and related insurance		
recovery as follows:		
Building cost	$150,000	
Accumulated depreciation:		
1983 ($150,000 − $30,000)/20	6,000	
1984	6,000	
1985	6,000	
1986	6,000	
1987 ($6,000 x 1/4)	1,500	
Total	25,500	
Book value of building	124,500	
Portion lost in fire	60%	
Book value of building destroyed	74,700	
Less insurance recovery	74,667	
Loss	$ 33	

It should be noted that the actual economic loss resulting from this fire is a bit larger than the "accounting" loss recorded above. The value of the portion of the building destroyed was $75,000, but the insurance recovery was $74,667. In real terms, then, the loss was $333. The "accounting" loss is measured in terms of historical cost.

If, due to inflation, the insurable or fair market value of the building had been, say, $200,000, the hospital's economic loss would have been substantial. The assumed insurance coverage, in such case, would have been grossly inadequate. Hospitals are in no way immune to casualty losses of this type, and insurance coverages should be reviewed annually for completeness and adequacy if uninsured losses are to be avoided. Detailed plant asset records are useful for this and other insurance purposes, but it should be recognized that the accounting records reflect historical costs rather than insurable values. The reader having a deeper interest in these matters should refer to the AHA's **Manual on Insurance for Hospitals and Related Health Care Facilities** and to leading insurance textbooks.

CAPITAL EXPENDITURE BUDGETING

The general features of capital expenditure budgeting were presented in Chapter 6. In this section, a single aspect of capital expenditure budgeting—the evaluation of capital expenditure proposals—is considered briefly and in an introductory fashion as an in-depth treatment of the subject is beyond the scope of this book.

Unwise plant asset expenditures are particularly serious because of the long-term nature and magnitude of such commitments. There are few management decisions that affect the long-range operating results and financial position of the hospital as do those relating to capital expenditures. In addition, such spending opportunities far exceed available funds, and choices usually must even be made between clearly desirable expenditure proposals. The primary purpose of capital expenditure evaluation, then, is not to prevent or restrict needed investments but to assign priorities to alternatives and select the most desirable proposals consistent with the hospital's objectives and the available resources.

A number of different techniques and bases for evaluating proposed capital expenditures is available. Those discussed here are based on economics and involve a consideration of factors that may be reasonably quantified. While capital spending proposals should not be approved in chronological or alphabetical order as funds become available or in terms of the relative persuasive powers of department heads, the approval decision should not be entirely reduced to a mathematical formula. The hospital manager's judgment and other qualitative factors should play an important role in the evaluation process.

Three evaluation techniques of a mathematical nature are described here. They are (1) the payback method, (2) the return on investment method, and (3) the net present value method. A more sophisticated technique, the discounted cash flow or yield method, is often preferred by academic theorists but it is not included in this discussion.[9]

As a basis for illustration, assume a departmental proposal to expend $65,000 for an item of equipment having a salvage value of $12,000 and a useful life of five years. This equipment would replace an item of equipment with a present trade-in value of $5,000. In other words, the initial investment outlay would be only $60,000 ($65,000 − $5,000), the net cash cost of the new equipment. It also is estimated that the new equipment will produce annual net cash inflows as follows:

Year	Net Cash Inflows
1	$20,000
2	30,000
3	20,000
4	15,000
5	5,000*
	$90,000

*In addition, the $12,000 salvage value would be realized
at the end of the fifth year.

The net cash inflow is determined as the net positive change (increase) in the cash balance of the hospital, assuming that the proposed expenditure is made. It involves a consideration of cash income generated by the equipment, savings in operating costs (labor, supplies, and maintenance), and any other relevant factors affecting annual cash flow.

Payback Method

The payback method permits a rough evaluation of a proposed expenditure for new equipment in terms of the length of time required for the equipment to pay for itself, i.e., produce net cash inflow equal to the initial investment outlay. The computation is illustrated in Figure 16-10. In this case, it would appear that the equipment in question would pay for itself in about 2.5 years. Should an alternative exist under which the required investment outlay would be recovered in a shorter time period, the alternative might be preferable. Capital expenditure proposals can be ranked, at least tentatively, in this way. The major fault of the method is its failure to consider the time value of money. Yet, it is a widely used decision model, and one must agree that it is a definite improvement over the criterion of urgency or postponement.

Figure 16-10.
Evaluation of Capital Expenditures
Payback Method

Year	Net Cash Inflow Total	Net Cash Inflow Required	Payback Years
1	$20,000	$20,000	1.0
2	30,000	30,000	1.0
3	20,000	10,000	0.5
Investment Outlay		$60,000	
Payback Period			2.5 years

Return on Investment Method

There are different concepts of return on investment, and variation are found in the manner in which it is computed. The computation assumed here is shown in Figure 16-11. Alternate investment opportunities having a return of greater than 21 percent might be favored. Like the payback method, however, this procedure also ignores the time value of money. But it does provide a rough-and-ready measurement of "profitability."

Figure 16-11.
Evaluation of Capital Expenditures
Return on Investment Method

Average Annual Net Cash Flow ($90,000/5 years)	$18,000
Less Annual Depreciation ($53,000/5 years)	10,600
Average Annual Net Cash Flow, Less Depreciation	$ 7,400
Initial Investment Outlay	$60,000
Add Salvage Value	12,000
Total	$72,000
Average Investment ($72,000/2)	$36,000

Average Return on Investment ($7,400/$36,000) = 21% (approx.)

Net Present Value Method

This method takes into account the time value of money, i.e., a dollar received in a future year is not the equivalent of a dollar received today. The use of money has a value which, in this illustration, is assumed to be 10 percent. In Figure 16-12, the annual cash flows are converted to present values by application of factors from Table 2 in Appendix B of this book, assuming a 10 percent "cost of capital." As indicated, the investment proposal has a positive net present value. The present value of cash inflows exceeds the present value of cash outflows by $18,800, indicating that the true rate of return is greater than 10 percent. Capital expenditures having the greatest net present values generally would be regarded with favor.

The extensive use of computers by hospitals makes feasible the refinement of capital expenditure analysis to a degree of sophistication far beyond this greatly simplified discussion. Hospital accountants must be proficient in the use of models and simulation in this area so that they may assist management in the application of advanced techniques to the solution of complex problems.

Figure 16-12.
Evaluation of Capital Expenditures
Net Present Value Method

Year	Cash Inflow (Outflow)	Present Value of $1 @ 10%	Net Present Value of Cash Flow
0	$ (60,000)	1.0000	$ (60,000)
1	20,000	.9091	18,182
2	30,000	.8264	24,792
3	20,000	.7513	15,026
4	15,000	.6830	10,245
5	17,000*	.6209	10,555
Net Present Value			$ 18,800

*Including $12,000 salvage value.

CHAPTER 16 FOOTNOTES

1. **"Capitalization of Interest Costs,"** Statement of Financial Accounting Standards No. 34 (Stamford, Connecticut: FASB, 1979).

2. **"Offsetting Interest to Be Capitalized with Interest Income,"** Technical Bulletin No. 81-5 (Stamford, Connecticut: FASB, 1981).

3. **"Accounting for Nonmonetary Transactions,"** APB Opinion No. 29 (New York: AICPA, 1973).

4. A discussion of compound interest and present value concepts is provided in the Appendix to this book.

5. **"Accounting Standards — Current Text"** (New York: McGraw-Hill, 1985), Section D40, par. 101.

6. **"Accounting Changes,"** APB Opinion No. 20 (New York: AICPA, 1971), par. 31.

7. Ibid., par. 18.

8. **"Financial Reporting By Not-for-Profit Health Care Entities for Tax-Exempt Debt and Certain Funds Whose Use Is Limited,"** Statement of Position 85-1 (New York: AICPA, 1985), p. 12.

9. Suver and Newman, **"Management Accounting for Health Care Organizations"** (Chicago: HFMA, 1981), Ch. 10.

QUESTIONS

1. List five items of expenditure which should be included in the cost of a purchased item of depreciable equipment.
2. Distinguish between capital expenditures and revenue expenditures.
3. Define the term **depreciation** as it is used in accounting.
4. Two elements affecting the computation of depreciation on plant assets are useful life and salvage value. How are useful lives and salvage values of plant assets determined?
5. Defend the position that depreciation should be included in costs for third-party cost reimbursement purposes even if not funded.
6. Under a coinsurance policy covering plant assets against fire losses, why is it important to insure at replacement or sound values?
7. Assume that your hospital's entire plant and equipment have become fully depreciated. An appraisal is made by a professional team of independent appraisers and it is found that the assets have a present value of $750,000. Justify the inclusion of depreciation, on the appraised valuation, in subsequent statements of reimbursable cost.
8. Your hospital is contemplating air-conditioning the hospital building. The choice of methods lies only with window and package units or a complete central system. The hospital building, housing all hospital facilities, is 20 years old and five stories high, with basement. It is estimated that this building can be used for another 20 years as a hospital with no major structural changes. List the points you, as controller, would consider in preparing a cost comparison of the two systems which would be comprehensive enough in scope to provide management with a sound basis for a decision.
9. As the accountant for a newly built hospital, you are faced with the problem of establishing estimated useful lives for hospital properties and equipment. How would you determine the estimated useful lives? In addition, you are faced with the problem of determining the method of depreciation to be used for each classification of plant assets. Describe the various possible methods of depreciation, giving the advantages and disadvantages of each method.
10. What is meant by "funding" depreciation? What are the arguments for and against funding depreciation by hospitals?
11. List the major categories into which hospital plant assets usually are classified and recorded in the accounts. Describe the major characteristics of the types of assets in each classification.
12. Explain what is meant by the coinsurance clause in a fire insurance policy.
13. What procedure should be followed in the accounts if it is determined that depreciation has been incorrectly estimated in prior years?
14. Hartman Hospital has a number of items of equipment that, while fully depreciated, are still being used in hospital operations. How would you suggest that these items be carried in the accounts?
15. In what ways, if any, do accelerated methods of depreciation increase the flow of cash in a hospital?
16. Hospitals sometimes receive plant assets by donation. Present the accounting justification for recording such property at fair market value and subsequently recording depreciation based upon such value.

17.   The administrator of your hospital has asked you to prepare a rationale, directed
       to the hospital board of trustees, to support a request for an appraisal of plant
       and equipment assets by an independent appraisal firm. You presently use
       depreciation lapse schedules for your depreciation calculation and have no
       equipment ledger or property inventory reports. Prepare the rationale and outline
       the benefits over your present system.

18.   What amount of interest should be capitalized during the construction of a new
       hospital building. What interest rates should be used? What treatment should be
       given to interest revenue from temporarily invested excess funds borrowed to
       finance the construction?

EXERCISES

E1.   The XYZ Hospital purchased an x-ray machine on October 1, 1987, at a cost of
       $20,000. In addition, the hospital paid $200 for freight and $800 for the
       construction of a concrete base and for making the proper electrical connections.
       The estimated useful life of the machine is six years with no salvage value. The
       hospital's fiscal year ends September 30.

Required.

   1.   Prepare a schedule showing annual depreciation expense under:

        (a)   The straight-line method
        (b)   The sum-of-years'-digits method
        (c)   The fixed percentage on declining-balance method, assuming a 40
              percent depreciation rate

   2.   Prepare journal entries to record:

        (a)   The purchase of the machine
        (b)   Depreciation expense (straight-line method) for the first year
        (c)   The write-off of the fully depreciated asset after six years
        (d)   The funding of depreciation at the end of the first year

E2.   Your hospital acquires a new asset for $10,000. It has a useful life of 10 years
       and a negligible salvage value.

       Required. Prepare a schedule showing depreciation for the first three years using
       (1) the straight-line depreciation method, (2) the double-declining-balance method
       and (3) the sum-of-the-years'-digits method. Comment briefly on the advantages
       and disadvantages of accelerated depreciation.

E3.   Following are data relating to three assumed cases involving the loss of plant assets by fire:

	Book Value	Insurable Value	Loss	Company	Amount	Coinsurance Clause
				Insurance Coverage		
(1)	$300,000	$1,200,000	100%	X	$1,000,000	80%
(2)	300,000	1,200,000	75	Y	1,000,000	80
(3)	100,000	400,000	50	A	50,000	80
				B	50,000	90
				C	60,000	None

Required. Determine the insurance proceeds from each insurance company.

E4.   Oberhausen Hospital purchased a new item of equipment for $800 on January 1, 1985. The equipment has an estimated salvage value of $80 and an estimated useful life of eight years. This equipment, which was depreciated by the straight-line method, is sold for $535 on September 1, 1987.

Required. Compute the amount of the gain or loss on the sale of the equipment.

E5.   O'Bryan Hospital purchased a new item of equipment for $800 on April 1, 1986. The equipment, which has an estimated salvage value of $80 and an estimated useful life of eight years, is depreciated by the sum-of-the-years'-digits method.

Required. What is the amount of depreciation expense for 1987?

E6.   Ogden Hospital purchased a new item of equipment for $800 on January 1, 1986. The equipment, which has an estimated salvage value of $80 and an estimated useful life of 10 years, is depreciated by the double-declining-balance method.

Required. What is the amount of depreciation expense for 1987?

E7.   Stacey Hospital purchased a new item of equipment for $800 on January 1, 1985. The equipment has an estimated salvage value of $80 and an estimated useful life of eight years. This equipment, which was depreciated by the straight-line method, was traded January 1, 1988, for a new item of equipment having a list price of $900. Cash "boot" of $420 was paid to effect the trade.

Required. Prepare the entry to record the trade.

E8. Simmons Hospital constructed an outlying storage building for $900 on January 1, 1978. The building, which had an estimated salvage value of $100 and an estimated useful life of 20 years, was being depreciated on a straight-line basis. On October 1, 1987, the building was 60 percent destroyed by fire. At the time of the fire, the building had an insurable value of $600 and was insured against fire as follows:

540

    Company A, $390 (90% coinsurance required)
    Company B, $130 (75% coinsurance required)

Both policies contained the standard contribution clause.

Required. Compute the gain or loss arising from the fire.

E9. Expando Hospital acquired the following depreciable assets on January 1, 1987:

Asset	Cost	Salvage Value	Estimated Life*
A	$ 8,800	$ 800	8
B	17,000	2,000	5
C	25,000	5,000	10

    *Years

Required. Compute the amount of depreciation expense for 1987 and 1988, assuming that:

  1. The assets will be depreciated as follows:

Asset	Method
A	SL
B	SYD
C	DDB

  2. The assets will be depreciated on a complete basis using the straight-line method.

E10. Client Hospital purchased a new item of equipment for $60,000 on January 1, 1986. This equipment had a salvage value of $6,000 and an estimated useful life of five years. It has been depreciated on a straight-line basis.

Shortly after the accounts had been closed for 1987, it was decided that the equipment had four years of useful life left and a revised salvage value of $5,000.

no Entry - but new deprec

Required. Prepare whatever journal entry is necessary at January 1, 1987, and explain the reason for the procedure you recommend.

E11.   Clarity Hospital purchased an item of equipment for $50,000 on January 1, 1986. This equipment has a salvage value of $5,000 and an estimated useful life of five years. It was to have been depreciated on a SYD basis.

Shortly before the accounts are closed for the 1987 fiscal year, it is discovered that the equipment was inadvertently omitted from the hospital's depreciation schedules and that no depreciation has ever been recorded on it.

Required. Prepare the necessary journal entry at December 31, 1987.

E12.   Maryville Hospital owns a building which it acquired at a cost of $300,000 on January 1, 1982. The building has a $25,000 salvage value and an estimated useful life of 10 years; it has been depreciated on a SYD basis for the last four years. Now, beginning January 1, 1987, the accelerated depreciation method is to be discontinued in favor of the straight-line method.

Required. Calculate the amount of depreciation expense to be taken in 1987 and in ensuing years on the building.

E13.   Cabot Hospital began operations on January 1, 1986, with plant assets having a depreciable cost of $1,100,000 and an estimated useful life of 10 years. All the hospital's expenses are 100 percent reimbursed. The hospital will use straight-line depreciation for financial reporting purposes but elects the SYD method for reimbursement purposes.

Required. (1) Calculate the amount of reimbursement for depreciation for 1986 and 1987. (2) What amount should be shown as "deferred income" in the hospital's December 31, 1987, balance sheet?

E14.   Hillside Hospital acquired its building 15 years ago at a cost of $800. It has been depreciated by the straight-line method on the basis of a 40-year life, with no salvage value expected. A professional engineering firm provides the following data with respect to a current appraisal of the building:

Reproduction cost	$1,000
Depreciation to date	333
Sound value	$ 667
Remaining life	30 years

Required. Prepare entries to (1) record the appraisal and (2) record depreciation expense for the sixteenth year.

E15.　The budget committee of Hallmark Hospital is considering a departmental proposal to expend $100,000 for an item of equipment having a salvage value of $20,000 and a useful life of five years. It is estimated that the equipment will produce annual net cash inflows as follows:

Year	
1	$ 25,000
2	40,000
3	35,000
4	20,000
5	10,000
	$130,000

The time value of money is 10 percent.

Required. Compute (1) the payback period, (2) the average return on investment, and (3) the net present value of cash flows. How would the results of these computations be used in evaluating the desirability of the proposed capital expenditure?

E16.　Kovener Hospital began construction on a new building on 1/1/87 and completed the construction on 12/31/87. Additional information:

1.　Average accumulated expenditures for construction of the new building, $400,000.

2.　Interest cost incurred on specific borrowings related to construction of the building, $48,000 ($300,000 X 16%).

3.　Interest cost incurred on other borrowings:

$200,000 X 12%	$24,000
$100,000 X 15%	15,000
	$39,000

4.　Interest earned on temporary investment of funds obtained from specific borrowings noted above, $10,000.

Required. What amount of interest should be capitalized in 1987?

E17. The following multiple-choice items relate to accounting for plant assets.

1. Bolinger Hospital purchased a new item of equipment for $800 on 1/1/84. The equipment has an estimated salvage value of $80 and an estimated useful life of 8 years. The equipment, which was depreciated by the straight-line method, was traded on 1/1/87 for a similar item of equipment. Cash "boot" of $420 was paid to effect the trade. The old equipment had a fair value of $400; the new equipment had a fair value of $900. The cost of the new equipment is

   a. $820
   b. $900
   c. $930
   d. $950

2. Herr Hospital has a fiscal year ending April 30. On May 1, 1987, Herr borrowed $10,000,000 at 15% to finance construction of a new building. Repayments of the loan are to commence the month following completion of the building. During the year ended April 30, 1988, expenditures for the partially completed building totaled $6,000,000. These expenditures were incurred evenly throughout the year. Interest earned on the unexpended portion of the loan amounted to $400,000 for the year. How much should be reported as capitalized interest in Herr's financial statements at April 30, 1988?

   a. $--0--
   b. $50,000
   c. $450,000
   d. $1,100,000

3. In October, 1987, Ewing Hospital exchanged an old item of equipment, which had cost $120,000 and was 50% depreciated, for a dissimilar used item of equipment and paid a cash difference of $16,000. The market value of the old equipment was determined to be $70,000. For the year ended 12/31/87, what amount of gain or loss should Ewing recognize on this exchange?

   a. $--0--
   b. $6,000 loss.
   c. $10,000 loss.
   d. $10,000 gain.

4. Lara Hospital traded its old computer for a new model. The following information is pertinent to this transaction:

Cost of old computer	$60,000
Accumulated depreciation on the old computer	20,000
Fair value of old computer	30,000
List price of new computer	80,000
Trade-in allowance for the old computer	45,000

How much loss should Lara immediately recognize on this trade?

a. $--0--
b. $5,000
c. $10,000
d. $15,000

5. On February 1, 1987, Tilden Hospital purchased a tract of land as a site for a new hospital building for $250,000. An existing building on the property was razed and construction was begun on the new hospital building in March, 1987. Additional data:

Cost of razing old building, $30,000.
Proceeds from sale of salvaged materials, $3,000.
Title insurance and legal fees to purchase land, $15,000.
Architect's fees, $60,000.
New building construction cost, $1,500,000.

The capitalized cost of the completed building should be

a. $1,560,000
b. $1,575,000
c. $1,587,000
d. $1,590,000

6. A donated plant asset for which the fair value has been determined, and for which incidental costs were incurred in acceptance of the asset, should be recorded at an amount equal to its

a. Incidental costs incurred.
b. Fair value and incidental costs incurred.
c. Book value on books of donor and incidental costs incurred.
d. Book value on books of donor.

7. In an arm's-length transaction, Hospital A and Hospital B exchanged nonmonetary assets with no monetary consideration involved. The exchange did culminate an earnings process for both hospitals, and the fair value of the nonmonetary assets were both clearly evident. The accounting for the exchange should be based on the

a. Fair value of the asset surrendered.
b. Fair value of the asset received.
c. Book value of the asset surrendered.
d. Book value of the asset received.

8. Plant assets may properly include

a. Deposits on equipment not yet received.
b. Idle equipment awaiting sale.
c. Property held for investment purposes.
d. Land held for possible use as a future building site.

Required. Select the best answer for each of the above multiple-choice items.

PROBLEMS

P1. As a hospital controller, you have been asked to prepare certain information relating to a comparison of the following three methods of computing depreciation:

1. Straight-line

2. Sum-of-the-years'-digits

3. Double-declining-balance

Required. Assuming the following information, prepare a summary of property and accumulated depreciation, showing beginning balances, additions and retirements, and ending balances for the years 1986 and 1987 based on the above three methods. For the purpose of recording depreciation, take one-half year in the year of acquisition and a full year in the year of retirement.

| | | | Retirements | |
| | | | --- | --- |
Year	Property Acquired	Useful Life (Years)	Year Acquired	Cost
1986	$ 50,000	10		
1987	20,000	10	1986	$7,000

Disregard any salvage value for depreciation purposes.

P2.   Hilltop Hospital is a progressive 220-bed hospital having been in operation for 20
        years as of June 30, 1987. Certain of its account balances are shown below:

Building (40-year life)	$1,000,000
Accumulated depreciation of building	500,000
Plumbing & electric system (20-year life)	500,000
Accumulated depreciation on plumbing and electric system	500,000

Depreciation has been recorded on a straight-line basis with no salvage value
expected. The hospital has decided to extend the useful life of the building to 50
years and the plumbing and electric system to 25 years.

Required. (1) Prepare the necessary entries at July 1, 1987, to reflect the
changes in asset lives. (2) Prepare the entry to record depreciation expense for
the year ending June 30, 1988.

P3.   Community Hospital opened on January 1, 1981 and experienced a fire on January
        1, 1988 that totally destroyed the nursing home and equipment. The acquisition
        cost of the nursing home building and equipment was $200,000 and $50,000
        respectively. The total acquisition cost of all hospital buildings and equipment
        including the nursing home is $2,400,000 of which $1,700,000 is in buildings and
        the remainder in equipment. The expected life of all buildings is 50 years and of
        equipment 20 years. The insurance policy held by the hospital is the standard
        fire and extended coverage policy, carrying blanket coverage and including an 80
        percent coinsurance clause. The amount of insurance carried is for $1,500,000.
        The hospital schedule of unexpired insurance shows the policy premium with an
        unexpired balance of $1,800.

Required. (1) Compute the amount owed to the hospital by the insurance
company. (2) Prepare entries to record all matters associated with the fire.

P4.   Having been appointed controller of Paragon Hospital, you find it necessary to
        make certain adjustments in the accounts for the year ended December 31, 1987.

Fixed equipment and movable equipment have been carried in one account titled
"equipment". On December 31, 1986, the balance of the account was $694,250 of
which $620,150 is the cost of the fixed equipment and $74,100 is the cost of the
major movable equipment. These assets were purchased March 15, 1986. By using
the composite method of depreciation for 1986, depreciation of $69,425 was
recorded; depreciation of $72,837 was taken in 1987.

It is now decided to adjust the accounts so as to provide accumulated
depreciation at the rate of 5 percent per annum for fixed equipment and 10
percent per annum for major movable equipment. It is also decided to separate
the asset and accumulated depreciation accounts on the books, and that only
one-half year's depreciation is to be claimed on assets in the year of acquisition.

During 1987, the following asset additions were made:

Fixed Equipment

March 15	$ 38,750
October 1	75,125

Major Movable Equipment

August 1	19,750
November 15	14,375

At December 31, 1987, the balances shown on the books were:

Equipment	$842,250
Accumulated depreciation	142,262

Required. Assuming that the books have already been closed for 1987, prepare the necessary entries at January 1, 1988.

17
Long-Term Debt: Bonds Payable

Every hospital management is faced at one time or another with the need to procure long-term financing. Historically, the sources of capital funds for most hospitals have been:

1. **External financing:**
   a. Nondebt.
      (1) Individual philanthropy.
      (2) Community subscription to fund raising campaigns.
      (3) Government grants.
   b. Debt (mortgages and bonds).

2. **Internal financing:**
   a. Funding of depreciation.
   b. Production and retention of an excess of operating revenues over operating revenues.
   c. Investment income.
   d. Value appreciation of investments.

Yesterday's hospital was almost totally dependent upon individual philanthropy. A later era was marked by heavy reliance upon the participation of the entire community in fund raising campaigns. More recently, various government programs have been the source of much of the long-term funds required by hospitals.

Philanthropy and public subscription are no longer major sources of funds. Contributed funds probably account for less than 20 percent of the annual capital investments by nonprofit hospitals today. Government assistance appears to be shifting from direct to indirect support through interest subsidies and the guarantee of hospital borrowing in the private capital markets. The voluntary, not-for-profit hospital is in a particularly difficult position in that it does not have direct access to public funds as do state and municipal hospitals. Its not-for-profit status also precludes entry into the equity markets in the manner of investor-owned hospitals and other profit-seeking enterprises.

Thus, the procurement of any substantial portion of the long-term funds required by most hospitals directly from nondebt, external sources is unlikely in the foreseeable future. The major sources of long-term funds must continue to be debt and internal financing. Under current third-party reimbursement conditions, however, it has become more difficult to generate sufficient cash flow from operations to meet debt service charges, provide needed working capital, and finance noncurrent asset growth. Only those hospitals that are successful in controlling costs at levels below the payments received from third-party payers are likely to survive.

It seems clear that the majority of hospitals can no longer expect to tap traditional sources for new long-term funds in any significant way. Their only recourse is to borrow and then to repay with internally generated cash. The rapid increase in debt financing by hospitals provides sufficient documentation on the matter. This practice, encouraged by legislation which enables hospitals to issue tax-exempt revenue bonds, naturally places a premium on superior financial management and its accounting prerequisites. Particular attention therefore is given in this chapter to some of the more important financial management accounting considerations related to bond issues. A discussion of accounting procedures with respect to long-term leases, pension plans, and other noncurrent liabilities is deferred to Chapter 18.

NATURE OF LONG-TERM LIABILITIES

In addition to the current liabilities described in Chapter 13, a hospital will have economic obligations that will not be discharged with resources that presently are classified in the balance sheet as current assets. These obligations are variously referred to as **long-term, noncurrent,** or **fixed** liabilities. Such liabilities typically are in the form of mortgages and bonds payable but also include notes, long-term contract obligations and leases, employee pension and retirement plan obligations, and certain deferred revenues. These obligations typically are included in the hospital's Unrestricted Fund but, in somewhat unusual cases, a long-term liability may properly appear in a restricted fund. A long-term liability ordinarily is based upon a written contract such as a mortgage, lease, or bond indenture, whereas current liabilities generally arise from informal contractual arrangements. A proper distinction between current and noncurrent obligations is of considerable importance in evaluating the financial position of a hospital as well as in managing its financial affairs.

CHARACTERISTICS OF BONDS

The power of a hospital corporation to issue bonds arises in the laws of the State of incorporation and is exercised by authorization of the governing board. In the case of State and municipal hospitals, bonded indebtedness also may require the approval of a majority of the citizenry.

The interest on bonds issued by hospitals may or may not be taxable to the bondholder-investor. Hospitals generally prefer to issue tax-exempt debt because such debt usually provides a higher ratio of project financing, longer maturities, and lower interest costs than would be the case with taxable bond issues. In fact, about three-fourths of the long-term debt issued by hospitals has been tax-exempt bonds.

Because most hospitals are legally prohibited from issuing tax-exempt debt directly, hospitals have established separate entities referred to as "financing authorities." The financing authority issues the tax-exempt bonds, and then loans the proceeds to the hospital. This creates some rather interesting accounting and reporting problems which will be discussed at a later point in this chapter.

Bonds ordinarily are issued in $1,000 denominations (referred to as face, par, or maturity value), although so-called "baby" bonds of $500 or $100 are increasingly encountered. The terms of a bond issue are spelled out in a contract known as a **bond** indenture. It details the rights and obligations of the hospital (or financing authority) and the bondholders, names the bank or other entity that is to act as trustee to protect the rights and enforce the obligations of both parties, and describes the bonds as to security, interest rate, maturity date, and other matters. While bonds may be sold directly to the general public, they more often are underwritten by investment bankers or a syndicate on either a purchase or commission basis. In the case of bonds that are publicly distributed, registration may be required under various state laws. Bonds of not-for-profit hospitals, however, are exempt from registration with the Securities and Exchange Commission. Private, or direct, placement of bonds with institutional investors such as insurance companies and savings banks has also been effected with good results.

As indicated in Chapter 15, bonds may be classified into different types. **Registered bonds** are bonds on which interest is paid only to bondholders of record, i.e., those whose holdings are recorded by the issuing hospital or its registrar agent. Interest on **coupon bonds** is paid to all bondholders who present the periodic interest coupons which accompany the bond certificates. **Serial bonds** mature in installments over a period of years, while a **term bond** issue matures on a single fixed maturity date. Some bonds, at the option of the hospital, may be **callable** at specified times upon payment of a "call price" that usually is excess of the maturity value.

In addition, bonds may be secured or unsecured. **Secured bonds**, often known as **mortgage bonds**, involve the pledging of specific plant assets under liens as security to bondholders. Hospital bond issues may also be secured in the sense that payment of principal and/or interest may be **guaranteed** by a governmental authority or some other parent organization. The security for a hospital bond issue may also arise from the accumulation of a bond "sinking fund" as might be required by certain bond indentures. This basically is a matter of setting aside resources periodically for the eventual retirement of the bond issue. In many cases, hospitals issue **revenue bonds**, i.e., interest on the bonds is paid from specified revenue sources. Finally, hospitals may issue general obligation bonds that are secured only by the hospital's fiscal history and general financial strength. Unsecured bonds of this type are termed **debentures**.

The decision to issue bonds is a critical matter. All relevant factors must be carefully considered and evaluated. It should be clearly evident that the bond issue is the most desirable means of obtaining the necessary long-term funds at reasonable cost and on acceptable terms. There must be assurance that the debt burden (periodic interest charges and principal retirement) will not lead to serious financial embarrassment and endanger the hospital's ability to meet its social obligations to the community. In most cases, the assistance of reputable professional firms specializing in feasibility studies for hospital financing should be secured.

ISSUANCE OF BONDS

When the hospital corporation issues bonds, it contracts to pay (1) the face value of the bonds at a specified maturity date and (2) interest, expressed as a percentage of face value, at periodic intervals, usually each six months. This **nominal**, or **coupon**, interest rate is predetermined on the basis of expectations concerning the rate of interest investors will demand at the time the bonds are actually issued. The market rate of interest varies according to the degree of credit risk, the term of the loan, the supply of and demand for money, and the taxability of the bond interest to investors, among other factors. If the nominal interest rate should equal the market rate, the hospital's bonds generally will sell at face value. There frequently is a difference, however, between the nominal and market rates of interest. Bonds will sell at a premium (a price greater than face value) if the nominal interest rate is higher than the market rate; they will sell at a discount (a price lower than face value) if they pay less than the market rate. Thus, differences between the contractual and market rates of interest are reflected in the prices investors are willing to pay for the bonds, thus eliminating the need to amend the bond contract.

Assume, for example, that a hospital decides to issue $600,000 of 10-year, 8% bonds. (Bond issues generally are of considerably larger amounts, but smaller amounts are employed here for ease of illustration.) In other words, the hospital promises to pay $600,000 at a date 10 years into the future and $24,000 ($600,000 X 8% X 6/12) every six months for the next 10 years. Figure 17-1 indicates the probable price at which these bonds might be sold if the market rate of interest is assumed to be 6%, 8%, or 10%. The calculations are based upon compound interest and present value concepts which may not be entirely understood. The reader may wish to read Appendix B to this book before continuing with the materials of this chapter.

Figure 17-1.
Calculations of Bond Issue Prices

	Price to Yield		
	6%	8%	10%
Present value of $600,000 maturity payment in 10 years, assuming:			
6% yield ($600,000 X .5537)	$332,220		
8% yield ($600,000 X .4564)		$273,840	
10% yield ($600,000 X .3769)			$226,140
Present value of $24,000 interest payments due every six months for 10 years, assuming:			
6% yield ($24,000 X 14.8775)	357,060		
8% yield ($24,000 X 13.5903)		326,160	
10% yield ($24,000 X 12.4622)			299,093
Proceeds of bond issue	689,280	600,000	525,233
Face value of bonds	600,000	600,000	600,000
Bond premium (discount)	$ 89,280	$ -0-	$(74,767)

Thus, if the purchasers of these bonds require a yield of only 6%, they will price the bonds at $689,280. Purchasers who demand a 10% return on their investments, however, would be willing to pay only $525,233 for the bonds. Assuming the bonds are of $1,000 denomination, the prices would be $875.39 and $1,148.80, or about 87.5% and

114.9% of face value, respectively. If investors are willing to accept an 8% return, the bonds will sell at 100, or at $1,000 each. Bond prices typically are quoted as a percentage of face value.

Issue at Discount

Where the nominal and market rates of interest are identical, a bond issue may be sold at face value. It is likely, however, that a premium or discount will be involved. To illustrate the accounting procedure for bonds issued at a discount, assume that a hospital issues $600,000 of 8%, 10-year bonds at 87.5 on April 1, 1987. These bonds pay interest semiannually on April 1 and October 1, and mature on April 1, 1997. Assume also that bond issue costs amount to $18,000. Issue costs include sales commissions, legal and accounting fees, registration and filing fees, engraving and printing expenses, and other related costs.

Assuming that all the bonds are issued on April 1, 1987, the following Unrestricted Fund entries would be made:

Cash In Bank	$525,000	
Unamortized Bond Discount	75,000	
Bonds Payable		$600,000

To record issue of $600,000 of 8%, 10-year bonds at 87.5 as follows:

Face value	$600,000
Price of bonds ($600,000 @ 87.5)	525,000
Discount	$ 75,000

Unamortized Bond Issue Costs	$ 18,000	
Cash In Bank		$ 18,000

To record issue costs associated with 8%, $600,000 bond issue.

In some instances, bond issue costs are combined with bond discount in a single account. It is the usual practice, however, to record the issue costs and the discount in separate accounts as shown above. Bond issue costs generally are treated as deferred charges and reported among the noncurrent assets in the hospital's balance sheet. It is never proper to treat bond discount as an asset; bond discount should be shown in the balance sheet as a deduction from the face value of the bonds payable in the manner illustrated later.

The entire bond issue may not always be disposed of on a single date. In such cases, sales are recorded as made but, once the entire issue is sold, an average issue price usually is computed for subsequent accounting purposes involving the amortization of discount and issue costs in the manner described subsequently.

When bonds are issued or sold between interest payment dates, the seller collects accrued interest from the purchaser as a part of the transaction. If the above bonds were issued on June 1, 1987, for example, the hospital would collect two months' accrued interest, or $8,000 ($600,000 X 8% X 2/12), from the purchasers. The above entry would be modified as follows:

Cash In Bank	$ 8,000	
Accrued Bond Interest Payable		$ 8,000
To record collection of accrued interest on		
bonds at date of issue.		

This procedure enables the hospital to pay a full six-months' interest to each bondholder at every semiannual interest payment date regardless of the length of time individual bondholders may have held their bonds. It would be impractical for the issuer of bonds to compute the amount of interest actually due to each individual bondholder at each interest payment date. Accrued interest settlements are made between sellers and buyers of bonds at the trading date. This matter also was discussed in Chapter 15.

    Were a balance sheet prepared immediately after the above bond issue, it would present the bonds as a long-term liability of the Unrestricted Fund in the following manner:

8% Bonds Payable, Due 1997	$600,000	
Less Unamortized Bond Discount	75,000	$525,000

The unamortized bond issue costs usually are included among the assets of the Unrestricted Fund in a "deferred charges" or "other noncurrent assets" category. Only the unamortized bond discount would be shown in the contra-liability position above. It is never correct to classify the bond discount as an asset.

Issue at Premium

    When the nominal interest rate is higher than the market rate of interest, the bonds ordinarily will be issued at a premium. Assume, for example, that the hospital issues $600,000 of 8%, 10-year bonds for $689,280 on April 1, 1987. These bonds pay interest semiannually on April 1 and October 1, and mature on April 1, 1997. Issue costs are $9,600. The issue of the bonds would be recorded in the Unrestricted Fund as follows:

Cash In Bank	$689,280	
Unamortized Bond Premium		$ 89,280
Bonds Payable		600,000
To record issue of $600,000 of 8%, 10-year		
bonds.		
Unamortized Bond Issue Costs	$ 9,600	
Cash In Bank		$ 9,600
To record bond issue costs.		

The bond premium ($89,280) and the issue costs ($9,600) usually are recorded in separate accounts as shown above, but sometimes these two items are combined into a net premium account.

If a balance sheet is prepared immediately after the above bond issue, it would present the bonds as a long-term liability of the Unrestricted Fund in the following manner:

8% Bonds Payable, Due 1997	$600,000	
Add Unamortized Bond Premium	89,280	$689,280

The unamortized bond issue costs ($9,600) usually is reported among the noncurrent assets of the Unrestricted Fund in a "deferred charges" classification. As indicated later, the bond issue costs are amortized and reported as expense over the term of the bonds.

BOND INTEREST AND STRAIGHT-LINE AMORTIZATION

The amount of periodic bond interest expense is affected by amortization of the discount or premium recorded at the time the bonds are issued. Amortization of bond discount is regarded as an addition to bond interest expense; the amortization of bond premium is treated as a reduction of interest expense. In practice, bond discount and premium usually are amortized (allocated) evenly throughout the life of the bond issue by the straight-line, or average, method. Theoretically, however, the "interest" or effective yield method is superior. Both methods are illustrated here.

Interest and Discount

Refer to the illustration above in which the proceeds of a $600,000 bond issue amounted to only $525,000. The $75,000 of bond discount is amortized by charges to interest expense over the 120-month term of the bond issue. (The process is similar to depreciation of plant assets.) The idea is that because the hospital received $525,000 but must repay $600,000, the $75,000 difference represents a cost that is properly allocable to the 10-year period presumed to benefit from the resources provided by the bond issue. It is a matter of cost allocation and of matching costs against revenues on a periodic basis. The straight-line procedure produces a rough approximation of the effective interest expense for each year.

The bonds were issued on April 1, 1987. At the end of April and at the end of each subsequent month of the 120-month period during which the bonds are scheduled to be outstanding, the following Unrestricted Fund entries are made:

Bond Interest Expense	$ 4,625	
Unamortized Bond Discount		$ 625
Accrued Bond Interest Payable		4,000
To record monthly amortization of bond		
discount and accrue monthly interest:		
Nominal interest:		
$600,000 X 8% X 1/12	$4,000	
Discount amortization:		
$75,000/120 months	625	
Monthly interest expense	$4,625	

| Amortization of Bond Issue Costs | $ 150 | |
| Unamortized Bond Issue Costs | | $ 150 |

To record monthly amortization of bond
issue costs ($18,000/120 = $150).

It should be clear that the entire $75,000 of discount will have been charged to expense, and that the Unamortized Bond Discount account decreases by $625 monthly, until the April 1, 1997, maturity date of the bonds. To reduce the clerical effort, the hospital may adopt a policy of amortizing discount and issue costs only at the end of each fiscal year.

Interest and Premium

Refer to the above illustration in which a bond issue of $600,000 produced proceeds of $689,280. The $89,280 premium is amortized by credits to interest expense over the 120-month life of the bond issue. Since the hospital received $689,280 but must repay only $600,000, the $89,280 may be regarded as a "gain" to be recognized on a pro rata basis during the 10-year period presumed to benefit from the resources provided by the bond issue. It is recognized as a reduction of the periodic charge to bond interest expense. This results in an approximation of the effective amount of interest expense.

The bonds were issued on April 1, 1987. At the end of April and at the end of each subsequent month, the following Unrestricted Fund entries are made:

Bond Interest Expense		$ 3,256	
Unamortized Bond Premium		744	
Accrued Bond Interest Payable			$ 4,000

To record monthly amortization of bond
premium and accrue monthly interest:

Nominal interest:		
$600,000 X 8% X 1/12	$4,000	
Premium amortization:		
$89,2800/120 months	744	
Monthly interest expense	$3,256	

| Amortization of Bond Issue Costs | $ 80 | |
| Unamortized Bond Issue Costs | | $ 80 |

To record amortization of bond
issue costs ($9,600/120 = $80).

Thus, the Unamortized Bond Premium account is reduced by $744 per month until it is fully amortized by April 1, 1997, the maturity date of the bonds. A hospital, of course, may adopt a policy of amortizing bond premium and issue costs only at the end of each fiscal year in order to minimize clerical effort.

Semiannual Interest Payment

For both bond issues described above, the semiannual interest payment is $24,000 ($600,000 X 8% X 6/12). Each April 1 and October 1 interest payment date therefore requires this entry in the Unrestricted Fund:

Accrued Bond Interest Payable	$ 24,000	
Cash In Bank		$ 24,000
To record payment of semiannual interest.		

In the case of coupon bonds, the hospital or its agent writes interest checks to those bondholders who present interest coupons on the interest payment dates. If the bonds are registered as to interest, subsidiary ledger records must be maintained to identify the bondholders entitled to interest payments.

BOND INTEREST AND EFFECTIVE-YIELD AMORTIZATION

Again assume that a hospital issues $600,000 of 8%, 10-year bonds on April 1, 1987. The bonds pay interest semiannually on April 1 and October 1, and mature on April 1, 1997. Disregard issue costs.

Interest and Discount

If the bonds are issued to yield 10%, the proceeds of the issue will be $525,233, as indicated in Figure 17-1. A partial amortization table, assuming the effective-yield method, is presented in Figure 17-2. Note that the effective ("true") interest expense for the six months ended October 1, 1987, is $26,262 (5% of $525,233). Interest expense for the second six-month period is $26,375 (5% of $527,495). In other words, the bonds were issued at a price that results in a 10% annual interest rate, or 5% semiannually. Discount amortization is the difference between the effective and nominal interest for each six-month period. Observe that interest expense, amortization of bond discount, and the book value of the bonds increases each period over the 10-year term. At the maturity date, the bonds will have a book value of exactly $600,000.

Interest and Premium.

If the bonds are issued to yield only 6%, the proceeds of the issue will be $689,280, as indicated in Figure 17-1. A partial amortization table, assuming the effective-yield method, is provided in Figure 17-3. The bond interest expense for the first six-month period is $20,678 (3% of $689,280); interest expense for the second period is $20,579 (3% of $685,958). Note that the amount of interest expense declines, and the amount of premium amortization increases, over the 10-year term of the bonds. The book value of the bonds is gradually reduced to exactly $600,000 at the maturity date.

Figure 17-2.
Amortization Schedule
Bonds Issued at A Discount

Date	Effective Interest*	Nominal Interest	Discount Amortization	Book Value of Bonds
				$525,233
10/1/87	$ 26,262	$ 24,000	$ 2,262	527,495
4/1/88	26,375	24,000	2,375	529,870
10/1/88	26,494	24,000	2,494	532,364
4/1/89	26,618	24,000	2,618	534,982
	/	/	/	/
	/	/	/	/
	/	/	/	/
	/	/	/	/
	$554,767	$480,000	$74,767	

*5% of book value of bonds during preceding six months.

Figure 17-3.
Amortization Schedule
Bonds Issued at A Premium

Date	Effective Interest*	Nominal Interest	Discount Amortization	Book Value of Bonds
				$689,280
10/1/87	$ 20,678	$ 24,000	$ 3,322	685,958
4/1/88	20,579	24,000	3,421	682,537
10/1/88	20,476	24,000	3,524	679,013
4/1/89	20,370	24,000	3,630	675,383
	/	/	/	/
	/	/	/	/
	/	/	/	/
	/	/	/	/
	$390,720	$480,000	$89,280	

*3% of book value of bonds during preceding six months.

RETIREMENT OF BONDS

This discussion of the retirement of bonds requires an examination of a number of matters. Term bonds may be retired normally at the specified maturity date, but they may be reacquired prior to maturity. In some cases, this is accomplished through a sinking fund. In other instances, a hospital may "refund" an entire outstanding bond issue. Finally, consideration also is given to serial bonds that are redeemed regularly in accordance with an established schedule.

Term Bonds Retired at Maturity

In each of the above illustrations, the 10-year term bonds have an April 1, 1997, maturity date. The entry to be made at that time when the bonds are retired is as follows:

Bonds Payable	$600,000	
Cash in Bank		$600,000
To record retirement of $500,000 bond issue at scheduled maturity date.		

Due to the amortization process, the discount (or premium) and issue costs initially recorded at the time of issue have been eliminated from the accounts so that the retirement requires only this simple entry. As can be seen below, the matter is more involved when bonds are reacquired prior to scheduled maturity.

Term Bonds Reacquired Prior to Maturity

A hospital may reacquire its own bonds in the market prior to maturity when prices or other factors would make such action desirable. To illustrate, refer to the earlier example in which a $600,000 bond issue was sold at a discount on April 1, 1987. Assume that the hospital reacquires $120,000 of these bonds at 82 and accrued interest on August 1, 1990, with brokerage and other reacquisition costs of $450 being paid. At the reacquisition date, the relevant accounts on the hospital's books would have the following balances:

Accrued Bond Interest Payable ($4,000 X 4 months)	$ 16,000 Cr.
Bonds Payable	600,000 Cr.
Unamortized Bond Discount:	
($75,000) − ($625 X 40 months)	50,000 Dr.
Unamortized Bond Issue Costs:	
($18,000) − ($150 X 40 months)	12,000 Dr.

The entry to record the reacquisition requires the recognition of a gain (loss) of the difference between the amount paid for the bonds and their book value. Assuming discount amortization by the straight-line method, the Unrestricted Fund entry is:

Bonds Payable	$120,000	
Accrued Bond Interest Payable	3,200	
Unamortized Bond Discount		$ 10,000
Unamortized Bond Issue Costs		2,400
Cash In Bank		101,150
Gain on Reacquisition of Bonds		9,650

To record reacquisition of 20% of bond issue
in open market as follows:

Bonds payable (20% X $600,000)	$120,000	
Unamortized bond discount and		
issue costs:		
($50,000 + $12,000) X 20%	12,400	
Book value of bonds reacquired	107,600	
Reacquisition price:		
$120,000 @ 82	$98,400	
Less brokerage cost	450	97,950
Gain on reacquisition	$ 9,650	
Reacquisition price (above)	$ 97,950	
Add accrued interest:		
$120,000 X 8% X 4/12	3,200	
Cash disbursed	$101,150	

This entry assumes that the reacquired bonds are retired. If these bonds are to be held for possible future reissue, however, the above debit to Bonds Payable would instead be made to Treasury Bonds. Should Treasury Bonds be reissued at a later date, the accounting procedure is similar to that for the original issue of bonds at a premium or discount, depending upon the reissue price.

After the reacquisition of $120,000 of bonds, accounting continues as before and until maturity with respect to the remaining $480,000 of bonds. The monthly amount of interest expense, however, would be adjusted to $3,600, or 80 percent of the previously determined figure of $4,675. Similarly, the monthly amortization of bond issue costs would be 80 percent of $625, or $500.

Redemption of Callable Bonds

The bond indenture may permit the hospital to call all or a portion of its bond issue within a specified time period. It is a feature of bond issues that favors the issuer. In other words, the hospital may be able to terminate the bond issue and eliminate future interest charges. It may also permit the hospital to take advantage of a decline in market rates of interest by retiring an expensive bond issue with the proceeds of a new and less expensive issue.

In any event, the bond indenture for callable bonds typically requires the payment of a premium to bondholders if their bonds are called. Refer to the facts of the $600,000 bond issue at a discount, and assume that $120,000 of these bonds are called on April 1, 1990, at 101. At this call date, the relevant accounts have the following balances:

Bonds Payable	$600,000 Cr.
Unamortized Bond Discount:	
($75,000) − ($625 X 36 months)	52,500 Dr.
Unamortized Bond Issue Costs:	
($18,000) − ($150 X 36 months)	12,600 Dr.

Assuming discount amortization by the straight-line method, the following Unrestricted Fund entry is required:

Bonds Payable	$120,000	
Loss on Redemption of Bonds	25,020	
Unamortized Bond Discount		$ 10,500
Unamortized Bond Issue Costs		2,520
Cash In Bank		132,000

To record call of $120,000 of bonds at 101 as follows:

Call price ($120,000 @ 101)	$132,000	
Face value	120,000	
Less unamortized bond discount and issue costs:		
($52,500 + $12,600) X 20%	13,020	
Book value of bonds called	106,980	
Loss on redemption of bonds	$ 25,020	

The future interest charges of $67,200 ($800 X 84 months) saved on the bonds called more than compensates for the redemption loss.

Retirement by Sinking Funds

A bond sinking fund may be established by the voluntary action of hospital management or it may be created as a result of a legal requirement in the bond indenture. The purpose of such a fund is to accumulate resources for the eventual retirement of a bond issue. In most cases, the hospital is required to make periodic payments to a trustee during the term of the bond issue. The fund is administered by the trustee under the provisions of a trust indenture. In most cases, the fund is carried as a long-term investment among the assets of the hospital's Unrestricted Fund. Interest earned on the investments of the fund is recorded as nonoperating income.

Assume, for example, that a bond indenture dated January 1, 1987, requires a hospital to accumulate $500,000 in a sinking fund by January 1, 1998, through a series of 10 equal annual deposits, starting January 1, 1988. If the sinking fund investments are expected to earn 8% compounded annually, the annual deposit required would be $34,515. The required annual deposit is determined by dividing $500,000 by 14.4866 (the amount of an ordinary annuity of $1 for 10 periods at 8% per period). A schedule showing the sinking fund accumulation is provided in Figure 17-4.

Table (3) Rf 706

Figure 17-4.
Bond Sinking Fund Accumulation Schedule

	Additions to Fund			
Year	Deposits	Earnings*	Total	Balance
1987	$ 34,515	$ 2,761	$ 37,276	$ 37,276
1988	34,515	5,743	40,258	77,534
1989	34,515	8,964	43,479	121,013
1990	34,515	12,442	46,957	167,970
	/	/	/	/
	/	/	/	/
	/	/	/	/
	/	/	/	/
	$345,150	$254,850	$500,000	

*8% earnings assumed.

The 1987 earnings of the fund are $2,761 (8% of $34,515). In 1988, the earnings are $5,743, or 8% of $71,791 ($37,276 + $34,515). By January 1, 1997, a total of $500,000 will have been accumulated. The record to be made in the Unrestricted Fund for the annual deposits and earnings is indicated by the following illustrative entries for 1988 and 1989.

January 1, 1988

Bond Sinking Fund	$ 34,515	
Cash In Bank		$ 34,515
To record annual deposit with trustee		
of bond sinking fund.		

December 31, 1988

Bond Sinking Fund	$ 2,761	
Bond Sinking Fund Income		$ 2,761
To record earnings of bond sinking fund for 1988.		

January 1, 1989

Bond Sinking Fund	$ 34,515	
Cash In Bank		$ 34,515
To record annual deposit with trustee		
of bond sinking fund.		

December 31, 1989
_____

Bond Sinking Fund	$ 5,823	
Cash In Bank		$ 5,823
To record earnings of bond sinking		
fund for 1989.		

Should sinking fund earnings be greater or less than 8%, however, the annual deposits must be adjusted in amount so that the fund is accumulated in accordance with scheduled requirements.

When bonds are retired out of the resources of the sinking fund, the entries are the same as illustrated previously except that a credit is made to the Bond Sinking Fund asset account rather than to Cash in Bank.

Refunding a Bond Issue

When a hospital has a bond issue outstanding and a substantial decline occurs in interest rates in the money markets, it may be advantageous for the hospital to sell a new bond issue at the lower interest rate, using the proceeds to retire the outstanding issue carrying the higher interest rate. The procedure is referred to as **refunding** or **refinancing** a bond issue.

To illustrate, assume that a hospital has an 8%, $500,000 bond issue outstanding that is exactly 20 years away from maturity. The relevant account balances at this time are as follows:

8% Bonds Payable	$500,000
Unamortized Bond Discount and Issue Costs	4,000

These bonds are callable at 103. Also assume that the hospital is in a situation which would enable it to sell a new bond issue with a 6% coupon rate. This new issue should sell approximately at face value because the coupon rate is equal to the market rate of interest. After a thorough analysis and evaluation, a decision is made to refund the old issue with a new, 6% bond issue. The new issue is sold and recorded in the manner previously described, providing the hospital with $500,000 that can be used to retire the outstanding 8% bonds.

The entry to be made in the hospital's Unrestricted Fund to record the retirement of the 8% bond issue is as follows:

8% Bonds Payable	$500,000	
Loss on Bond Refunding	19,000	
Unamortized Bond Discount and Issue Costs		$ 4,000
Cash In Bank		515,000
To record retirement of 8% bond issue at 103		
with the proceeds of new 6% bond issue:		
Call price of 8% bonds:		
$500,000 X 103	$515,000	

Face value of 8% bonds	500,000	
Less unamortized bond discount and issue costs	4,000	
Book value of 8% bonds	496,000	
Loss on bond refunding	$ 19,000	

The $19,000 loss, of course, consists of the $15,000 call premium and the $4,000 of unamortized bond discount and issue costs on the 8% bonds retired, and is reported in the hospital's income statement as an extraordinary loss in the manner prescribed by FASB Statement of Financial Accounting Standards No. 4.[1]

The decision to refund a bond issue should be made only after a careful consideration of all relevant factors. A substantial decline in interest rates is not in itself a sufficient basis for the decision. A present value analysis should be made of the costs of refunding in comparison with the cash flow effects of interest savings in the future. Consideration also must be given to probable future interest rates. It may be that refunding at some later date could be even more advantageous. Other factors, many of which cannot be quantified, must also be taken into account.

SERIAL BONDS

The illustrations to this point have assumed that the bonds in question were term bonds, i.e., all bonds in the issue had a fixed single maturity date. Serial bonds, however, mature in periodic installments. Hospitals may find serial bond issues to be a means of adjusting debt repayment requirements to the pattern of its cash flows. Also, if short-term interest rates are substantially lower than long-term rates, a serial bond issue may prove less costly to the hospital than a term bond issue of identical face value. In other words, the average price obtained for the serial bonds may be greater than the price for which term bonds can be sold.

Due to the fact that serial bonds are retired in periodic installments, a special procedure is employed in accounting for them. To facilitate the illustration, assume a simplified case in which a hospital issues $500,000 of 6% serial bonds on January 1, 1987, for $485,000 (net of issue costs). The bonds mature at the rate of $100,000 annually, starting January 1, 1988. Figure 17-5 provides a summary of annual amortization and bond interest expense as computed by the "bonds outstanding" method. This method generally is used for serial bonds rather than the straight-line or the effective-yield methods described earlier in this chapter.

Figure 17.5
Summary of Amortization and Interest
Bonds Outstanding

Year	Bonds Outstanding	Fraction ×	Bond Discount =	Discount Amortization +	6% Nominal Interest =	Interest Expense
1987	$ 500,000	5/15	$15,000	$ 5,000	$ 30,000	$ 35,000
1988	400,000	4/15	15,000	4,000	24,000	28,000
1989	300,000	3/15	15,000	3,000	18,000	21,000
1990	200,000	2/15	15,000	2,000	12,000	14,000
1991	100,000	1/15	15,000	1,000	6,000	7,000
	$1,500,000			$15,000	$ 90,000	$105,000

Assuming that interest on these serial bonds is paid annually on January 1 and that $100,000 of the bonds are retired as scheduled on January 1, 1988, the accounting would proceed as follows:

January 1, 1987

Cash in Bank	$485,000	
Unamortized Bond Discount	15,000	
Bonds Payable		$500,000
To record issue of $500,000 of 6% serial		
bonds on January 1, 1987		

December 31, 1987

Bond Interest Expense	$ 35,000	
Unamortized Bond Discount		$ 5,000
Accrued Bond Interest Payable		30,000
To record discount amortization and		
interest accrual at December 31, 1987.		

January 1, 1988

Accrued Bond Interest Payable	$ 30,000	
Cash in Bank		$ 30,000
To record payment of 1987 bond interest.		
Bonds Payable	$100,000	
Cash in Bank		$100,000
To record retirement of $100,000 of serial		
bonds on January 1, 1988.		

Should serial bonds be retired prior to scheduled dates or in amounts other than those originally scheduled, the discount amortization schedule would have to be revised accordingly.

BONDS ISSUED THROUGH A FINANCING AUTHORITY

Most hospitals are legally prohibited from issuing tax-exempt bonds directly. To issue such bonds, a hospital may create a separate entity known as a **financing authority**. The authority issues tax-exempt debt for the benefit of the hospital. After the bonds are issued, the authority loans the proceeds to the hospital for acquisition of plant assets or other appropriate uses. If the proceeds are used for construction, the proceeds usually will be invested until needed to pay project costs. How should the debt proceeds, the debt obligation, interest expense, and investment income be reported in the hospital's financial statements?

The AICPA Subcommittee on Health Care Matters has concluded in its Statement of Position (SOP) 85-1 that not-for-profit hospitals should report as Unrestricted Fund liabilities the obligations issued for their benefit and for repayment of which they are responsible, whether or not the debt covenant contains any spending restrictions.[2] The resources obtained from the debt issue also should be reported in the Unrestricted Fund as assets whose use is limited. Interest expense on the debt and income from the investment of the debt proceeds should be reported separately as operating expense and operating revenue, respectively. An acceptable alternative is to net the interest expense and investment income, reporting the result as either operating expense or operating revenue, whichever is appropriate. Parenthetical disclosure should be made, however, of the offsetting amount. Several illustrations of these reporting requirements appear in SOP 85-1.

CHAPTER 17 FOOTNOTES

1. **"Reporting Gains and Losses from Extinguishment of Debt,"** Statement of Financial Accounting Standards No. 4 (Stamford, Connecticut: FASB, 1975), par. 8. Also, see "Extinguishment of Debt Made to Satisfy Sinking-Fund Requirements," Statement of Financial Accounting Standards No. 64 (Stamford, Connecticut: FASB, 1982), par. 4.

2. Subcommittee on Health Care Matters, **"Financial Reporting By Not-for-Profit Health Care Entities for Tax-Exempt Debt and Certain Funds Whose Use Is Limited,"** Statement of Position 85-1 (New York: AICPA, 1985), pp. 11-12.

QUESTIONS

1.   Historically, from what sources have hospitals been able to meet their needs for long-term capital funds? Are all these sources still available to hospitals to a significant degree?

2.   Briefly identify each of the following terms:
        1. "Baby" bonds -
        2. Bond indenture -
        3. Registered bonds -
        4. Coupon bonds -
        5. Serial bonds -
        6. Guaranteed bonds -
        7. Revenue bonds -
        8. Debentures -
        9. Mortgage bonds -

3.   What is meant by "refunding" a bond issue? For what reasons are bond issues referred?

4.   Briefly describe the operation of a bond sinking fund. How is a bond sinking fund reported in a hospital's balance sheet?

5.   How should (1) unamortized bond discount, (2) unamortized bond premium, and (3) unamortized bond issue costs be presented in the hospital's balance sheet?

6.   Outline the considerations involved in carrying out a fund raising campaign for the purpose of acquiring funds for the addition of a new wing to a hospital building.

7.   Below is a list of methods for raising funds for long-term capital financing by private businesses and hospitals. Indicate those methods which you believe are applicable to not-for-profit voluntary hospitals. If applicable, give a brief description of the advantages and disadvantages of each.
        1. Issuance of preferred or common stock
        2. Retained earnings
        3. Notes secured by mortgages
        4. Donations
        5. Liquidation of Endowment Funds
        6. Trading on the equity
        7. Issuance of bonds
        8. Sale of fixed assets

8.   On January 1, 1987, a hospital issued serial bonds with a total face value of $1,000,000. These bonds mature annually in $200,000 amounts beginning January 1, 1988. Indicate how these bonds should be presented in the hospital's balance sheet at December 31, 1987.

9.   A hospital bond issue, dated April 1, 1987, is actually issued for cash on June 1, 1987. The purchasers of these bonds will pay the hospital for two months of accrued interest. Why?

10.   Distinguish between the nominal (or coupon) rate of interest and the effective rate of interest with respect to a hospital bond issue.

11.   For what reasons might a hospital bond issue sell at a price that is higher or lower than face value?

12.   If a hospital bond issue is sold at a discount, will the monthly charge to bond interest expense be greater or less than the nominal amount of interest per month? Explain.

13.   A hospital bond issue is sold at a premium on January 1, 1987. Interest on the bonds is payable annually on December 31. Will the annual interest expense recorded on the hospital's books be greater or less than the amount of annual interest actually paid to the bondholders? Explain.

14.   If the market rate of interest is higher than the nominal or coupon rate of interest specified in a hospital bond issue, will the hospital's bonds sell at a price that is higher or lower than face value? Explain.

EXERCISES

E1.   A hospital issues $1,000 of five-year, 6% bonds at 100 and accrued interest on August 1, 1987. Issue costs were $56. Interest is payable semiannually, on April 1 and October 1. The maturity date of the bonds is April 1, 1992. On February 1, 1988, $200 of these bonds are reacquired at 98 and accrued interest.

Required. Prepare entries to record all transactions through February 1, 1988. State how all matters should be presented in the hospital's financial statements for 1987.

E2.   A hospital issues $1,000 of five-year, 4.8% bonds at 94.2 and accrued interest on June 1, 1987. Interest is payable semiannually, April 1 and October 1. The maturity date of these bonds is April 1, 1992. On December 1, 1987, $250 of the bonds are reacquired at 92 and accrued interest.

Required. Compute the gain or loss on reacquisition of the bonds on December 1, 1987.

E3.   A hospital issues $1,000 of five-year, 9.6% bonds at 111 and accrued interest on September 1, 1987. Interest is payable semiannually, April 1 and October 1. The maturity date of the bonds is April 1, 1992. On February 1, 1988, $250 of these bonds are reacquired at 108 and accrued interest.

Required. Compute the gain or loss on reacquisition of the bonds on February 1, 1988.

E4.   On January 1, 1987, a hospital issues $500 of 4%, five-year serial bonds at 94. The bonds mature at the rate of $100 annually, beginning January 1, 1988. Interest is payable annually on January 1.

Required. Prepare a schedule showing amortization of bond discount and bond interest expense for the 1987-91 period.

E5.   A hospital issued $500 of 10-year, 8% bonds at 96 on January 1, 1987. Interest is payable annually on January 1. The maturity date of these bonds, callable at 105 and accrued interest, is January 1, 1997.

On January 1, 1989, the hospital issues $525 of 10-year, 6% bonds at face value and uses the proceeds to call the outstanding 8% bond issue.

Required. Prepare the entry to record the refunding of the 8% bond issue.

E6.   A hospital issues $500 of five-year bonds on January 1, 1987. The provisions of the indenture require a sinking fund, accumulated to $500 by January 1, 1992. Five equal annual contributions of $92.31 are to be made, beginning January 1, 1988. It is estimated that the fund will earn 4% compounded annually.

Required. Prepare a bond sinking fund accumulation schedule for the 1988-92 period.

E7.   On 1/1/87, Indiana Hospital issued $750 (face value) of 8%, 5-year bonds at a price to yield 6%. These bonds pay interest annually on 1/1, and mature 1/1/92. Adjusting entries are made annually on 12/31 only.

Required. Assuming the use of the effective yield method of amortization, prepare all necessary entries for 1987 and 1988.

E8.   On 1/1/87, Ruth Hospital issued $750 (face value) of 8%, 5-year bonds at a price to yield 10%. These bonds pay interest annually on 1/1, and mature 1/1/92. Adjusting entries are made annually on 12/31 only.

Required. Assuming the use of the effective yield method of amortization, prepare all necessary entries for 1987 and 1988.

E9.   Saxton Hospital issued $600 of 10%, 5-year bonds on 1/1/87 at a price to yield 8%. The bonds pay interest semiannually, 6/30 and 12/31, and mature 1/1/92.

Required. Assuming the use of the effective yield method of amortization, prepare all necessary entries for 1987 and 1988.

E10. The long-term debt section of Cockerham Hospital's Unrestricted Fund balance sheet at 12/31/87 included 6% bonds payable of $100,000 less unamortized bond discount of $5,000. Further examination revealed that these bonds were issued to yield 8%. The amortization of the bond discount was recorded using the effective yield method. Interest was paid on 1/1 and 7/1 of each year. On 7/1/88, Cockerham retired the bonds at 102 before their maturity.

Required. What loss should Cockerham record on the retirement of the bonds on 7/1/88? Explain how this loss should be reported in Cockerham's income statement.

E11. The following multiple-choice items relate to accounting for bonds payable.

1. If bonds are issued initially at a discount and the straight-line method of amortization is used for the discount, interest expense in the earlier years will be

    a. Greater than if the effective yield method were used.
    b. The same as if the effective yield method were used.
    c. Less than if the effective yield method were used.
    d. Less than the amount of the interest payments.

2. Unamortized debt discount should be reported on the hospital's balance sheet as a

    a. Direct deduction from the face amount of the debt.
    b. Direct deduction from the present value of the debt.
    c. Deferred charge (asset).
    d. Part of the issue costs.

3. Cole Hospital retired an issue of bonds before its maturity date through a direct exchange of securities. The best value for Cole to assign to the new issue of debt is the

    a. Maturity value of the new issue.
    b. Net carrying amount of the old issue.
    c. Present value of the new issue.
    d. Maturity value of the old issue.

4. A hospital issued bonds with a maturity amount of $200,000 and a maturity ten years from the date of issue. If the bonds were issued at a premium, this indicates that

    a. The yield (effective or market) rate of interest exceeded the nominal (coupon) rate.
    b. The nominal rate of interest exceeded the yield rate.
    c. The yield and nominal rates were identical.
    d. No necessary relationship exists between the two rates.

5. When debt is extinguished before its maturity date through a refunding transaction, any difference between the reacquisition price of outstanding debt and its net carrying amount per books should be

    a. Amortized over the remaining original life of the extinguished issue.
    b. Amortized over the life of the new issue.
    c. Recognized currently in income as a loss or gain.
    d. Treated as a prior period adjustment.

6. The presence of unamortized debt premium indicates that at the time of issuance the underlying obligation

    a. Carried interest at the prevailing market rate.
    b. Carried interest below the prevailing market rate.
    c. Carried interest above the prevailing market rate.
    d. Was noninterest-bearing.

7. What is the preferred method of handling unamortized discount, issue cost, and redemption premium on bonds refunded?

    a. Expense them in the period the bonds are refunded.
    b. Amortize them over the life of the new issue.
    c. Amortize them over the remaining life of the issue retired.
    d. Amortize them over the remaining life of the issue retired or the life of the new issue, whichever is shorter.

8. For bonds payable with a term of 20 years, originally issued at a discount and outstanding for 10 years, the theoretically preferred presentation in the hospital's balance sheet is the

    a. Amount expected to be paid to the bondholders at bond maturity date less the present value of interest to be paid in future periods.
    b. Face amount of the bonds less the discount at the date of issue.
    c. Bond maturity value less the unamortized discount when the effective yield method of amortization is used.
    d. Face amount of the bonds.

Required. Select the best answer for each of the above multiple-choice items.

E12. The following multiple-choice items relate to accounting for bonds payable.

1. Which of the following types of debt extinguishments do not result in the classification of a gain or loss as an extraordinary item?

    a. Early extinguishment of term bonds at a discount.
    b. Sinking fund purchases of outstanding bonds.
    c. Refunding existing debt with a new bond issue.
    d. Retirement of debt maturing serially.

2. Kappa Hospital neglected to amortize the premium on its bonds payable. Compare the hospital's net income without this amortization (X) and the hospital's net income with such amortization (Y).

    a. X greater than Y.
    b. X equals Y.
    c. X less than Y.
    d. Cannot be determined from the information given.

3. When bonds are issued at a discount, amortization of the discount has the effect of

    a. Increasing bond interest expense and increasing the balance sheet valuation of the bonds.
    b. Decreasing bond interest expense and decreasing the balance sheet valuation of the bonds.
    c. Decreasing bond interest expense and increasing the balance sheet valuation of the bonds.
    d. Increasing bond interest expense and decreasing the balance sheet valuation of the bonds.

4. Bond issue costs should be

    a. Reported in the balance sheet as deferred charges (assets).
    b. Added to unamortized bond discount or netted against unamortized bond premium in the balance sheet.
    c. Reported as bond interest expense in the income statement.
    d. Reported as a direct deduction from bonds payable.

5. When the issuer of bonds exercises the call provision to retire the bonds, the excess of cash paid over the carrying amount of the bonds should be recognized separately as a (an)

    a. Extraordinary loss.
    b. Extraordinary gain.
    c. Other operating income.
    d. Nonoperating income.

6. Should the following bond issue costs be expensed as incurred?

	Legal Fees	Underwriting Costs
a.	No	No
b.	No	Yes
c.	Yes	No
d.	Yes	Yes

7. When the interest payment dates of a bond are May 1 and November 1, and a bond issue is sold on June 1, the amount of cash that is received by the issuer will be

    a. Increased by accrued interest from June 1 to November 1.
    b. Increased by accrued interest from May 1 to June 1.
    c. Decreased by accrued interest from June 1 to November 1.
    d. Decreased by accrued interest from May 1 to June 1.

8. The generally accepted method of accounting for gains or losses from the early extinguishment of debt is based on the assumption that any gain or loss on the transaction reflects

       a. An adjustment to the cost basis of the asset obtained by the debt issue.

       b. An amount that should be considered a cash adjustment to the cost of any other debt obtained over the remaining life of the old debt.

       c. An amount received or paid to obtain a new debt instrument and, as such, should be amortized over the life of the new debt.

       d. A change in the market rate of interest which should be recognized in the period of extinguishment.

E13.   On January 1, 1987, Hopewell Hospital sold its 8% bonds that had a face value of $1,000,000. Interest is payable annually on December 31, and the bonds mature on January 1, 1997. The bonds are sold to yield a rate of 10%.

      Required. Prepare a schedule to compute the total amount received from the issue of the bonds.

E14.   On December 1, 1987, Cone Hospital issued its 7%, $2,000,000 face value bonds for $2,200,000, plus accrued interest. Interest is payable semiannually, May 1 and November 1. On December 31, 1989, the book value of the bonds, inclusive of the unamortized premium, was $2,100,000. On July 1, 1990, Cone reacquired the bonds at 98, plus accrued interest. Cone appropriately uses the straight-line method of amortization.

      Required. Prepare a schedule to compute the gain or loss on this early extinguishment of debt.

18
Long-Term Debt: Leases and Pension Plans

Accounting procedures for long-term debt in the form of bonds payable were discussed and illustrated in the preceding chapter. This chapter deals with two other types of long-term debt: leases and pension plans. Most hospitals have employee pension plans, and many hospitals lease equipment and other kinds of plant assets. At this writing, however, many of the problems of accounting for leases and pension plans are largely unresolved, and the FASB is currently in the process of issuing new requirements related to pension plan accounting. The discussion in this chapter therefore is somewhat general in nature and is limited to the basic principles involved in accounting for leases. The discussion of accounting for pension plans is based on APB Opinion 8 and FASB Statement 36 which probably will be superceded by the issuance of new FASB requirements by the time this book is published.

ACCOUNTING FOR LEASES

A lease may be defined as a contract under which the owner of real or personal property (the **lessor**) conveys to another party (the **lessee**) the right to use the property for a specified period of time in return for periodic cash payments. Lease provisions vary greatly. The lease term may range from a few months to many years. Lease payments may be fixed or variable in amount. Maintenance, taxes, and insurance (**executory costs**) on the leased property may be paid by the lessee or by the lessor. The lease contract may be cancelable or noncancelable. It may contain restrictions that limit the lessee's ability to incur additional debt. The lease contract may provide for passage of title to the lessee at the end of the lease term. It may give the lessee the right of renewal, or it may provide a bargain purchase option.

Leasing often is an attractive alternative to ownership. By allowing 100 percent financing, leasing arrangements conserve the lessee's working capital. Leasing provides greater flexibility to the hospital lessee in making equipment changes in response to technological advances, thereby reducing the risks of obsolescence. Lease contracts may contain less restrictive provisions than are found in other debt agreements. Under some types of leases, the lessee is not required to record either the leased asset or the lease obligation and, as a result, certain financial ratios are not affected by leasing.

The claimed advantages of leasing, however, may or may not be realized by a particular lessee. It depends on many factors including, among other things, the nature and intended use of the leased asset, the lease term, the financial position of the lessee, and the pace of technological change. The leasing of property is not without disadvantages, and the decision to lease should be made only after a thorough analysis of all relevant factors.

Lessee Accounting

The accounting procedures to be followed by a hospital lessee depend upon the type of lease involved. From the lessee's viewpoint, leases are of two types: (1) operating leases and (2) capital leases. If the lease is in substance an installment purchase of property, the lessee must account for the lease as a capital lease, i.e., the lease payments must be capitalized at their present value, and lessee records both an asset and a liability. If the lease is not tantamount to a purchase transaction, the lessee accounts for the lease as an operating lease, i.e., a rental agreement.

If at its inception the lease meets any one or more of the following four criteria, the lessee must classify and account for the lease as a **capital lease:**[1]

1.   The lease transfers ownership of the property to the lessee by the end of the lease term.

2.   The lease contains a bargain purchase option, i.e., the lessee has the right to purchase the property at a price significantly lower than its expected fair value at the date the option becomes exercisable.

3.   The lease term is equal to 75 percent or more of the estimated economic life of the leased property (this criterion does not apply to a lease that begins with the last 25 percent of the total economic life of the property, including earlier years of use).

5.   The present value of the minimum lease payments, excluding executory costs, equals or exceeds 90 percent of the fair value of the leased property (this criterion does not apply to a lease that begins with the last 25 percent of the total economic life of the property, including earlier years of use).

If a lease does not meet any of the above criteria, the lessee must classify and account for the lease as an **operating lease.**

Operating Leases. As a basis for illustration, assume that Broughton Hospital leases an item of equipment on January 1, 1987, under a five-year lease requiring annual lease payments of $12,000, commencing January 1, 1987. Also assume that the lease does not meet any of the four criteria for capitalization, and therefore is to be accounted for as an operating lease by the hospital. The necessary entry at January 1, 1987, and at each succeeding lease payment date, is given below:

Rent Expense $12,000
    Cash in Bank $12,000
  To record payment of rent under an
  operating lease.

Note that the leased equipment is not recorded as an asset of the hospital, nor is the legal obligation to make lease payments in the future recorded as a liability.

For external financial reporting purposes, the hospital lessee is required to make the following footnote disclosures:[2]

1. For operating leases having initial or remaining noncancelable lease terms in excess of one year:
    a. Future minimum rental payments required as of the date of the latest balance sheet presented, in the aggregate and for each of the five succeeding fiscal years.
    b. The total of minimum rentals to be received in the future under noncancelable subleases as of the date of the latest balance sheet presented.

2. For all operating leases, rental expense for each period for which an income statement is presented, with separate amounts for minimum rentals, contingent rentals, and sublease rentals.

3. A general description of the lessee's leasing arrangements, including but not limited to:
    a. The basis on which contingent rental payments are determined.
    b. The existence and terms of renewal or purchase options and escalation clauses.
    c. Restrictions imposed by lease agreements, such as those concerning dividends, additional debt, and further leasing.

Capital Leases. On January 1, 1987, a hospital leased equipment under a five-year lease requiring annual lease payments of $12,000, commencing January 1, 1987. The equipment has an economic life of 5 years but no expected residual (salvage) value, and is depreciable by the straight-line method. The hospital's incremental borrowing rate is 10 percent.

Assuming this lease is properly classified as a capital lease, the hospital should treat the lease as an installment purchase of the equipment. A capital lease is recorded as an asset and a liability at the lower of (1) the present value of the minimum lease payments, excluding executory costs, during the lease term or (2) the fair market value of the leased asset at the inception of the lease. The term **minimum lease payments** is defined as the total of:

1. The minimum rental payments required during the lease term.
2. The amount of any bargain purchase option, or if there is no such option:
    a. The amount of any lessee-guaranteed residual value.
    b. The amount payable, if any, for failure to renew the lease.

It is assumed here that there is no lessee-guaranteed residual value and no penalty for failure to renew the lease. It is also assumed that the present value of the minimum lease payments and the fair market value of the leased asset are approximately equal.

In computing the present value of the minimum lease payments, the hospital ordinarily will use its incremental borrowing rate. This is the interest rate that, at the inception of the lease, the hospital would have incurred to borrow the money necessary to buy the leased asset on a secured loan with repayment terms similar to the payment schedule required by the lease. However, if the hospital knows the interest rate used by the lessor (the interest rate implicit in the lease), and if that rate is lower than the hospital's incremental borrowing rate, the hospital must use the implicit rate. It is assumed here that the hospital does not know the implicit rate.

In this illustration, the present value of the minimum lease payments is $50,039 ($12,000 X 3.7908 X 1.10). In other words, the $12,000 annual payment is multiplied by the present value of an ordinary annuity of $1 for five periods at 10 percent per period, or 3.7908 (see Appendix B to this book). Because the first payment is due immediately, however, the periodic lease payments do not represent an ordinary annuity, but an **annuity due.** To convert the present value factor for an ordinary annuity to the present value factor for an annuity due, the present value factor for an ordinary annuity must be multiplied by one plus the interest rate (in this case, 1.00 plus .10, or 1.10).

Figure 18-1 provides a lease amortization schedule. Note that the first lease payment does not include interest, but is applied totally to the reduction of the principal amount of the lease obligation. In other words, the lease obligation outstanding during 1987 is $38,039. The $12,000 lease payment on January 1, 1988, includes interest of $3,804 (10% of $38,039) which should be treated as 1987 interest expense. The $8,196 remainder of the January 1, 1988, payment reduces the lease obligation to $29,843. This process continues over the lease term. In the January 1, 1989, payment, for example, there is interest of $2,984 (10% of $29,843).

Figure 18-1.
Lease Amortization Schedule
(Annuity Due)

| | Lease Payments | | | Lease |
Date	Total	Interest	Principal	Liability
				$50,039
1/1/87	$12,000		$12,000	38,039
1/1/88	12,000	$ 3,804	8,196	29,843
1/1/89	12,000	2,984	9,016	20,827
1/1/90	12,000	2,083	9,917	10,910
1/1/91	12,000	1,090	10,910	-0-
	$60,000	$ 9,961	$50,039	

Had the terms of the lease called for $12,000 annual payments with the first payment due on December 31, 1987, the present value of the minimum lease payments would have been $45,490 ($12,000 X 3.7908) because the periodic payments represent an ordinary annuity. The related amortization schedule is provided in Figure 18-2. Note that each of the five payments include interest at 10 percent on the lease obligation outstanding during each year.

Figure 18-2.
Lease Amortization Schedule
(Ordinary Annuity)

Date	Lease Payments Total	Lease Payments Interest	Lease Payments Principal	Lease Liability
				$45,490
12/31/87	$12,000	$ 4,549	$ 7,451	38,039
12/31/88	12,000	3,804	8,196	29,843
12/31/89	12,000	2,984	9,016	20,827
12/31/90	12,000	2,083	9,917	10,910
12/31/91	12,000	1,090	10,910	-0-
	$60,000	$14,510	$45,490	

Assuming the first lease payment is due at the inception of the lease on January 1, 1987, the hospital lessee's entries for 1987 and 1988 would be as follows:

January 1, 1987

Leased Equipment	$50,039	
Obligation Under Capital Leases		$50,039
To record signing of capital lease and the capitalization of the lease payments.		

Obligations Under Capital Leases	$12,000	
Cash in Bank		$12,000
To record first annual lease payment.		

December 31, 1987

Interest Expense	$ 3,804	
Accrued Interest Payable		$ 3,804
To accrue interest on lease obligation outstanding during 1987.		

Depreciation Expense	$10,008	
Accumulated Depreciation		$10,008
To record depreciation on leased equipment ($50,039/5).		

January 1, 1988

Accrued Interest Payable	$ 3,804	
Obligation Under Capital Leases	8,196	
Cash in Bank		$12,000
To record second annual lease payment.		

December 31, 1988

Interest Expense	$ 2,984	
Accrued Interest Payable		$ 2,984
To accrued interest on lease obligation		
outstanding during 1988.		
Depreciation Expense	$10,008	
Accumulated Depreciation		$10,008
To record depreciation on leased equipment.		

How would depreciation be recorded in this illustration if the estimated useful life of the equipment had been, say, six years? The equipment would be depreciated over its six-year life if the lease contained a bargain purchase option or provided for passage of title to the lessee at the end of the lease term. Otherwise, the leased equipment should be depreciated over the lease term (as was done above).

Executory costs (insurance, taxes, and maintenance) usually are paid by the lessee in capital lease arrangements. In such cases, the hospital lessee records such costs as expenses in the period incurred.

In addition to a general description of the lessee's leasing arrangements (as described earlier for operating leases), the following financial statement disclosures are required for capital leases:[3]

1. The gross amount of assets recorded under capital leases as of the date of each balance sheet presented by major classes according to nature or function.
2. Future minimum lease payments as of the date of the latest balance sheet presented, in the aggregate and for each of the five succeeding fiscal years, with separate deductions from the total for the amount representing executory costs, including any profit thereon, included in the minimum lease payments and for the amount of the imputed interest necessary to reduce the net minimum lease payments to present value.
3. The total of minimum sublease rentals to be received in the future under noncancelable subleases as of the date of the latest balance sheet presented.
4. Total contingent rentals actually incurred for each period for which an income statement is presented.
5. Assets recorded under capital leases and the accumulated depreciation thereon should be separately identified in the lessee's balance sheet or in footnotes thereto. Likewise, the related obligations shall be separately identified in the balance sheet as obligations under capital leases and shall be subject to the same considerations as other obligations in classifying them with current and noncurrent liabilities in classified balance sheets. The amount of depreciation on capitalized leased assets should be separately disclosed.

Lessor Accounting

If at its inception a lease meets one or more of the following Group A criteria and **both** of the Group B criteria, the hospital lessor must classify and account for the lease either as a **direct-financing lease** or as a **sales-type lease.**[4]

Group A

1. The lease transfers ownership of the property to the lessee by the end of the lease term.
2. The lease contains a bargain purchase option.
3. The lease term is equal to 75 percent or more of the estimated economic life of the leased property.
4. The present value of the minimum lease payments (excluding executory costs) equals or exceeds 90 percent of the fair value of the leased property.

Group B

1. The collectibility of the lease payments is reasonably predictable.
2. No important uncertainties exist as to the amount of unreimbursable costs yet to be incurred by the lessor.

Otherwise, the hospital lessor is required to classify and account for the lease as an **operating lease**. Thus, from the viewpoint of the lessor, there are three types of leases: (1) operating leases, (2) direct-financing leases, and (3) sales-type leases.

Operating Leases

On January 1, 1987, Midcity Hospital leased equipment to Troymaw Clinic under a five-year lease requiring annual payments of $12,000, commencing January 1, 1987. The new equipment, which cost $100,000, has an estimated economic life of 20 years but no expected salvage value, and is depreciable by the straight-line method. Midcity Hospital incurred $3,000 of initial direct costs (the costs of negotiating and consummating the lease, e.g., credit investigations, commissions, and legal fees). Executory costs for 1987 amounted to $1,300, and were paid by Midcity Hospital.

Assuming that the lease is properly classified as an operating lease, the necessary 1987 entries for Midcity Hospital are as follows:

January 1, 1987

Deferred Leasing Costs	$ 3,000	
Cash in Bank		$ 3,000
To record payment of initial direct costs.		

Cash in Bank	$12,000	
Rental Income		$12,000
To record receipt of first annual lease payment.		

December 31, 1987

Depreciation Expense	$ 5,000	
Accumulated Depreciation		$ 5,000
To record depreciation on leased equipment for 1987 ($100,000/20).		

Amortization of Leasing Costs (Expense) $ 600
    Deferred Leasing Costs $ 600
    To record amortization of leasing costs
for 1987 ($3,000/5).

Taxes, Insurance, and Maintenance Expense $ 1,300
    Cash in Bank $ 1,300
    To record 1987 executory costs on leased
equipment.

Note that, under an operating lease, the lessor continues to carry the leased property on its books as a depreciable asset. Because the leasing costs relate to the lease, they are amortized over the term of the lease in proportion to the recognition of rental income so as to obtain a proper matching of revenue and expense.

Supplementary disclosures required of the lessor in connection with operating leases include:[5]

1. The cost and carrying amount, if different, of property on lease or held for leasing by major classes of property according to nature or function, and the amount of accumulated depreciation in total as of the date of the latest balance sheet presented.
2. Minimum future rentals on noncancelable leases as of the date of the latest balance sheet presented, in the aggregate and for each of the five succeeding fiscal years.
3. Total contingent rentals included in income for each period for which an income statement is presented.
4. A general description of the lessor's leasing arrangements.

Direct-Financing Leases

On January 1, 1987, Hartsburg Hospital leased equipment to Carewell Health Center under a five-year lease requiring annual payments of $12,000, commencing January 1, 1987, to provide Hartsburg a 10 percent return. The equipment, which has a book value of $50,039 and an approximately equal fair value, has an estimated economic life of five years but no expected salvage value. Executory costs are to be paid by the lessee.

As indicated earlier in Figure 18-1, the present value of the lease payments is $50,039. The total interest income to the lessor over the term of the lease is $9,961 ($60,000 − $50,039). Entries to be made by Hartsburg Hospital during 1987 are as follows:

January 1, 1987

Lease Payments Receivable $60,000
    Unearned Interest Income $ 9,961
    Equipment   50,039
    To record direct-financing lease of
equipment to Carewell Health Center.

Cash in Bank	$12,000	
Lease Payments Receivable		$12,000
To record receipt of first annual lease payment.		

<u>December 31, 1987</u>

Unearned Interest Income	$ 3,804	
Interest Income		$ 3,804
To record 1987 interest income earned on direct-financing lease (see Figure 18-1).		

Observe that the hospital records the gross amount of lease payments (5 X $12,000) as a receivable. Unearned interest income is reported in the balance sheet as a contra-receivable. The supplementary disclosures required of the lessor are itemized in the next section of this chapter.

Sales-Type Leases

Assume the facts given above for a direct-financing lease, except that the leased equipment has a fair value of $50,039 but a book value of only $35,039. The necessary 1987 entries by the hospital lessor are as follows:

<u>January 1, 1987</u>

Lease Payments Receivable	$60,000	
Cost of Equipment Sold	35,039	
Unearned Interest Income		$ 9,961
Equipment		35,039
Sales		50,039
To record sales-type lease of equipment to Carewell Health Center.		

Cash in Bank	$12,000	
Lease Payments Receivable		$12,000
To record receipt of first annual lease payment.		

<u>December 31, 1987</u>

Unearned Interest Income	$ 3,804	
Interest Income		$ 3,804
To record 1987 interest income earned under a sales-type lease (see Figure 18-1).		

Notice the distinction between a direct-financing lease and a sales-type lease: a sales-type lease results in a gain (profit), but a direct-financing lease does not. The gain, under a sales-type lease, is the excess of the leased property's fair value over its book value. In this illustration, the fair value is $50,039 (the present value of the lease payments) and the book value is $35,039. The difference of $15,000 ($50,039 − $35,039) is a gain or profit to be fully recognized in the year the lease is consummated.

The supplementary disclosures required of the hospital lessor under sales-type and direct-financing leases are as follows:[6]

1. The components of the net investment in the leases as of the date of each balance sheet presented:
    a. Future minimum lease payments to be received, with separate deductions for:
        (1) Amounts representing executory costs, including any profit thereon, included in the minimum lease payments, and
        (2) The accumulated allowance for uncollectible minimum lease payments receivable.
    b. The unguaranteed residual values accruing to the benefit of the lessor.
2. Future minimum lease payments to be received for each of the five succeeding fiscal years as of the date of the latest balance sheet presented.
3. The amount of unearned revenue included in income to offset initial direct costs charged against income for each period for which an income statement is presented. (In a sales-type lease, the lessor expenses all initial direct costs in the year in which they are incurred.)
4. Total contingent rentals included in income for each period for which an income statement is presented.
5. A general description of the lessor's leasing arrangements.

Sale-and-Leaseback Arrangements

On January 1, 1987, Vera Hospital sold certain equipment which had a book value of $39,490 to Bryce Medical Center for $45,490, and immediately leased the equipment back under a five-year lease requiring annual payments of $12,000, commencing December 31, 1987, to provide a 10 percent return to Vera Hospital. The equipment has an estimated useful life of six years but no expected residual value, and is depreciable by the straight-line method. The lease contains a bargain purchase option. The present value of the periodic lease payments is $45,490 ($12,000 X 3.7908). The lease amortization schedule is provided in Figure 18-3.

Figure 18-3.
Lease Amortization Schedule
(Sale-and-Leaseback)

Date	Lease Payments Total	Interest	Principal	Lease Liability
				$45,490
12/31/87	$12,000	$ 4,549	$ 7,451	38,039
12/31/88	12,000	3,804	8,196	29,843
12/31/89	12,000	2,984	9,016	20,827
12/31/90	12,000	2,083	9,917	10,910
12/31/91	12,000	1,090	10,910	-0-
	$60,000	$14,510	$45,490	

The necessary 1987 entries by Bryce Medical Center (lessor) are given below (a direct-financing lease):

January 1, 1987

Equipment	$45,490	
Cash in Bank		$45,490
To record purchase of equipment from Vera Hospital.		

Lease Payments Receivable	$60,000	
Unearned Interest Income		$14,510
Equipment		45,490
To record direct-financing lease of equipment to Vera Hospital.		

December 31, 1987

Cash in Bank	$12,000	
Lease Payments Receivable		$12,000
To record receipt of first annual lease payment from Vera Hospital.		

Unearned Interest Income	$ 4,549	
Interest Income		$ 4,549
To record 1987 interest income on Vera Hospital lease (10% of $45,490). See Figure 18-3.		

The necessary 1987 entries for Vera Hospital with respect to this sale-and-leaseback are as follows:

January 1, 1987

Cash in Bank	$45,490	
Equipment		$39,490
Deferred Profit		6,000
To record sale of equipment to Bryce Medical Center under a sale-leaseback arrangement.		

Leased Equipment	$45,490	
Obligation Under Capital Lease		$45,490
To record capital lease of equipment.		

December 31, 1987

Interest Expense	$ 4,549	
Obligation Under Capital Leases	7,451	
Cash in Bank		$12,000
To record lease payment for 1987 (see Figure 18-3).		
Depreciation Expense	$ 7,582	
Accumulated Depreciation		$ 7,582
To record 1987 depreciation expense on leased equipment ($45,490/6).		
Deferred Profit	$ 1,000	
Depreciation Expense		$ 1,000
To record amortization of profit on sale- and-leaseback ($6,000/6).		

Notice that Vera Hospital is depreciating the leased equipment over six years (its estimated useful life) rather than over the five-year term of the lease. As noted earlier, this practice is followed when the lease contains a bargain purchase option or provides for passage of title to the lessee by the end of the lease term. Because depreciation is taken over a six-year period, the deferred profit also is amortized over six years as a credit adjustment to depreciation expense.

ACCOUNTING FOR PENSION PLANS

A pension plan is an arrangement under which a hospital undertakes to provide its employees with retirement benefits. Under a defined-benefit plan the retirement benefits can be determined or estimated in advance. A defined-contribution plan, on the other hand, is a plan under which the hospital agrees to make stipulated periodic contributions to a pension fund, with retirement benefits depending upon the investment earnings of the assets in the fund. Pension plans generally are funded, i.e., the hospital makes periodic payments to an independent funding agency that is responsible for managing the pension fund assets and paying benefits to employees during their retirement years. Some plans are contributory (employees pay a part of the pension plan costs through payroll withholdings); other plans are noncontributory (the hospital pays all of the pension plan costs).

To illustrate the concepts and procedures involved in accounting and reporting for pension plans, assume that a hospital establishes a pension plan for its employees on January 1, 1987. A professional actuary, using acceptable actuarial cost methods, determines the following:

Past service cost at January 1, 1987	$500,000
Normal cost for 1987	60,000

The term **past service cost** means the cost of future retirement benefits earned by employees prior to the inception of the pension plan. It is customary, when a pension plan is established, to give current employees credit for their previous services to the hospital. **Normal cost**, on the other hand, is the cost of future retirement benefits that employees earn in a given year subsequent to the inception of the pension plan. The normal cost will vary from year to year, depending on the number of employees and changes in actuarial assumptions.

Assume also that the hospital has agreed to fund (pay) the normal cost annually as incurred and to fund the past service cost over a period of 20 years by equal annual payments to a funding agency (an insurance company or other financial institution), beginning December 31, 1987. If the actuary specifies an interest rate of 5 percent, the annual funding of the past service cost can be determined by dividing the past service cost by the present value of an ordinary annuity of $1 for 20 periods at 5 percent interest per period (see Appendix B to this book). In this case, the annual funding of the past service cost would be $40,121 ($500,000/12.4622).

APB Opinion No. 8 requires that all pension plan costs (both past service cost and normal cost) be charged against income subsequent to the adoption of the pension plan by an accrual basis accounting method that results in an annual provision for pension plan cost that falls between a specified minimum and maximum. The minimum and maximum limits are as follows:[1]

1. **Minimum.** The annual provision for pension cost should not be less than the total of the following:
    a. Normal cost.
    b. Interest on any unfunded prior service cost.
    c. A provision for vested benefits, if required. Vested benefits are earned pension benefits that are not contingent upon the employee continuing in the service of the hospital.
2. **Maximum.** The annual provision for pension cost should not be greater than the total of the following:
    a. Normal cost.
    b. Ten percent of the past service cost.
    c. Ten percent of the amounts of any increases or decreases in prior service costs arising from plan amendments.
    d. Interest on the difference between amounts expensed and amounts funded, i.e., interest on expensed but unpaid prior service cost.

At any date subsequent to the inception of a pension plan, the term **prior service cost** refers to the total of past service cost and normal cost for all years since inception of the plan.

The hospital may elect to amortize (expense) the past service cost over any reasonable period of time, but not less than ten years. Should the hospital elect to amortize the past service cost over 15 years, the annual charge to expense for that cost can be determined by dividing the past service cost by the present value of an ordinary annuity of $1 for 15 periods at 5 percent per period (see Appendix B to this book). In this case, the annual amortization of past service cost is $48,171 ($500,000/10.3797).

Assuming that the hospital will amortize the past service cost over 15 years, fund the past service cost over 20 years, and fund the normal cost in the year it is incurred, the required entry at December 31, 1987, is as shown below:

Pension Plan Expense − Normal Cost	$ 60,000	
Pension Plan Expense − Past Service Cost	48,171	
Liability for Unfunded Pension Expense		$ 8,050
Cash in Bank		100,121
To record 1987 pension plan expense and		
funding of pension plan costs.		

Thus, when pension plan costs are amortized over a period shorter than the funding period, a liability arises. This liability will increase each year for 15 years. Starting in the sixteenth year, the hospital will be funding a greater amount than it is expensing, and the liability account will be decreased. At the end of the twentieth year, the liability will be totally eliminated.

The hospital might have elected to fund the past service cost over 10 years and amortize it over 15 years. In this case, the amortization period is longer than the funding period, and an asset (deferred pension plan expense) would result. This asset would increase for ten years. After ten years, because the hospital then would be expensing more cost than it is funding, the asset would begin to decrease (and would be totally eliminated by the end of the fifteenth year.)

As noted earlier, the pension plan expense for the year must fall between the minimum and maximum limits established by APB Opinion No. 8. In this illustration, the minimum and maximum amounts are as follows:

Minimum

Normal cost	$ 60,000
Interest on unfunded prior service cost	
($500,000 X 5%)	25,000
Provision for vested benefits	-0-
Total	$ 85,000

Maximum

Normal cost	$ 60,000
10% of past service cost (10% X $500,000)	50,000
10% of cost of plan amendments	-0-
Interest on expensed but unfunded prior	
service costs	-0-
Total	$110,000

Thus, the total pension plan expense of $108,171 charged against 1987 income falls within the limits specified by APB Opinion No. 8.

Assuming a normal cost of $65,000 for 1988, the required entry at December 31, 1988, is as follows:

Pension Plan Expense — Normal Cost	$ 65,000	
Pension Plan Expense — Past Service Cost	48,574	
Liability for Unfunded Pension Expense		$ 8,453
Cash in Bank		105,121
To record 1988 pension plan expense and		
funding of pension plan costs.		

The amount charged to expense for past service cost, assuming no changes in the factors entering into the determination of past service cost, is the scheduled amount of $48,171 plus $403 of interest on the expensed but unfunded costs in 1987, i.e., 5% of $8,050 = $403. To put it another way, the recorded pension expense for 1987 was $108,171 but only $100,121 was paid in 1987; the pension fund was underpaid by $8,050. Because the $8,050 was not available for investment by the pension fund, the hospital must record the "lost" interest of $403 as an expense and increase its liability to the pension fund by the same amount.

FASB Statement of Financial Accounting Standards No. 36 requires the following disclosures relative to pension plans in the financial statements or in accompanying footnotes:[8]

1. A statement that pension plans exist, identifying or describing the employee groups covered.
2. A statement of the hospital's accounting and funding policies.
3. The provision for pension plan expense for the period.
4. The nature and effect of significant matters affecting comparability for all periods presented, such as changes in accounting methods, changes in circumstances, or adoption or amendment of a plan.
5. For defined benefit plans:
    a. The actuarial present value of vested accumulated plan benefits.
    b. The actuarial present value of nonvested accumulated plan benefits.
    c. The plan's net assets available for benefits.
    d. The assumed rates of return used in determining the actuarial present values of vested and nonvested accumulated plan benefits.
    e. The date as of which the benefit information was determined.

If the information in Item 5 is not available, the hospital must disclose the excess, if any, of the actuarially computed value of vested benefits over the total of the pension fund assets and any balance sheet pension accruals, less any pension prepayments or deferred charges. Figure 18-4 illustrates how the financial statements of a hospital might make these disclosures in an accompanying footnote.

Figure 18-4.
Pension Plan Disclosures

Note X. The hospital has several pension plans covering substantially all of its employees. The total pension expense for 19X2 and 19X1 was $xx,xxx and $xx,xxx, respectively, which includes, as to certain defined benefit plans, amortization of past service cost over (number specified) years. The hospital makes annual contributions to the plans equal to the amounts accrued for pension expense. A change during 19X2 in the actuarial cost method used in computing pension cost had the effect of reducing net income for the year by approximately $xx,xxx. A comparison of accumulated plan benefits and plan net assets for the hospital's defined benefit pension plans is presented here:

	January 1, 19X2	January 1, 19X1
Actuarial Present Value of Accumulated Plan Benefits:		
Vested	$x,xxx	$x,xxx
Nonvested	x,xxx	x,xxx
	$x,xxx	$x,xxx
Net Assets Available for Benefits	$x,xxx	$x,xxx

The weighted average assumed rate of return used in determining the actuarial present value of accumulated plan benefits was (number specified) percent for both 19X2 and 19X1.

CHAPTER 18 FOOTNOTES

1. Statement of Financial Accounting Standards No. 13, **Accounting for Leases** (Stamford, Connecticut: FASB, 1976).

2. **Ibid.**

3. **Ibid.**

4. **Ibid.**

5. **Ibid.**

6. **Ibid.**

7. APB Opinion No. 8, **Accounting for the Cost of Pension Plans** (New York: AICPA, 1966).

8. Statement of Financial Accounting Standards No. 36, **Disclosure of Pension Information** (Stamford, Connecticut: FASB, 1980).

QUESTIONS

1. Define the following terms:
   1. Lease
   2. Lessor
   3. Lessee
   4. Executory costs ~Lease Cost~
   5. Bargain purchase option
2. Why is leasing sometimes more attractive than ownership?
3. From the standpoint of the lessee, there are two types of leases: (1) capital leases and (2) operating leases. State the criteria for the classification of leases by lessees.
4. Briefly describe the accounting procedures followed by a lessee in accounting for an operating lease.
5. Briefly describe the accounting procedures followed by a lessee in accounting for a capital lease.
6. What supplementary footnote disclosures must be made by lessees for operating and capital leases?
7. Under what circumstances would a lessee use the interest rate implicit in a lease (instead of the lessee's own incremental borrowing rate) in computing the present value of the minimum lease payments?
8. A hospital leases equipment having a 12-year estimated useful life. The lease term is 10 years. Assuming the lease is properly classified as a capital lease, should the lessee depreciate the leased equipment over 10 years or 12 years? Explain.
9. What criteria are used by a lessor in classifying leases as either direct-financing leases, sales-type leases, or operating leases?
10. What are **initial direct costs**, and how are they accounted for by hospital lessors?
11. Distinguish between a direct-financing lease and a sales-type lease from the standpoint of a hospital lessor.
12. With respect to leasing arrangements, what is the difference between an ordinary annuity and an annuity due?
13. What is the nature of a "sale-and-leaseback" arrangement?
14. Define the following terms:
    1. Pension plan
    2. Past service cost
    3. Normal cost
    4. Prior service cost
    5. Vested benefits
15. A hospital has a funded pension plan. What is the minimum amount of pension cost that must be charged to expense in any given year? What is the maximum amount?
16. What supplementary footnote disclosures must be made by a hospital having a pension plan?

17.   If past service costs are amortized over 20 years and funded over 15 years, will this result in an asset or a liability to be reported in the hospital's balance sheet? Explain.

EXERCISES

E1.   Corn Hospital leased equipment to Shuck Hospital on 5/1/87. At that time, the collectibility of the minimum lease payments was not reasonably predictable. The lease expires on 5/1/89. Shuck could have bought the equipment from Corn for $900,000 instead of leasing it. Corn's books showed a book value for the equipment on 5/1/87 of $800,000. Corn's depreciation on the equipment in 1987 was $200,000. During 1987, Shuck paid $240,000 in rentals to Corn, and Corn incurred maintenance and other related costs under the terms of the lease of $18,000 in 1987. After the lease with Shuck expires, Corn has an agreement to lease the equipment to Silk Hospital for another two years.

Required. (1) What net amount of income did Corn derive from this lease for 1987? (2) What amount of expense was incurred by Shuck from this lease for 1987?

E2.   On 1/1/87, Flip Hospital signed a ten-year noncancelable lease for certain equipment. The terms of the lease called for Flip to make annual payments (beginning 12/31/87) of $30,000 for ten years with title to pass to Flip at the end of this period. The equipment has an estimated useful life of 15 years with no salvage value. Flip uses the straight-line method of depreciation. Flip appropriately accounted for this lease as a capital lease. The lease payments were determined to have a present value of $184,338 with an effective interest rate of 10%.

Required. (1) What amount should Flip record as interest expense for 1987? (2) What amount should Flip record as 1987 depreciation expense?

E3.   Fox Company, a dealer in advanced technology equipment, leased equipment to Tiger Hospital on 7/1/87. The lease is appropriately accounted for as a sale by Fox and as a purchase by Tiger. The lease is for a 10-year period (the useful life of the asset) expiring 6/30/97. The first of ten annual payments of $500,000 was made on 7/1/87. Fox had purchased the equipment for $2,675,000 on 1/1/87, and established a list selling price of $3,375,000 on the equipment. The present value of the lease payments at 7/1/87 was $3,165,000, assuming a 12% interest rate.

Required. Assuming that Tiger Hospital uses the straight-line depreciation method, what is the total amount of depreciation and interest expense that Tiger Hospital should record for the year ended 12/31/87?

E4.   Following are ten multiple choice items relating to accounting for leases.

_____ 1.   Equal monthly rental payments for a particular lease should be charged to rental expense by the lessee for which of the following:

Capital Lease Operating Lease

	Capital Lease	Operating Lease
a.	Yes	No
b.	Yes	Yes
c.	No	No
d.	No	Yes

_____ 2.   For which of the following transactions would the use of the present value of an annuity due concept be appropriate in calculating the present value of the asset obtained or liability incurred at the date of occurrence?

    a.   A capital lease is entered into with the initial lease payment due one month subsequent to the signing of the lease agreement.
    b.   A capital lease is entered into with the initial lease payment due upon the signing of the lease agreement.
    c.   An operating lease is entered into with the initial lease payment due one month subsequent to the signing of the lease agreement.
    d.   An operating lease is entered into with the initial lease payment due upon the signing of the lease agreement.

  3.   In a lease that is recorded as an operating lease by the lessee, the equal monthly rental payments should be

    a.   Allocated between interest expense and depreciation expense.
    b.   Allocated between a reduction in the liability for leased assets and interest expense.
    c.   Recorded as a reduction in the liability for leased assets.
    d.   Recorded as rental expense.

_____ 4.   In a lease that is record as a capital lease by the lessee, the equal monthly rental payments should be

    a.   Allocated between interest expense and depreciation expense.
    b.   Allocated between a reduction in the liability for leased assets and interest expense.
    c.   Recorded as a reduction in the liability for leased assets.
    d.   Recorded as rental expense.

_____ 5.   Lease Y contains a bargain purchase option and the lease term is equal to 75 percent of the estimated economic life of the leased property. Lease Z contains a bargain purchase option and the lease term is less than 75 percent of the estimated economic life of the issued property. How should the lessee classify these leases?

	Lease Y	Lease Z
a.	Operating lease	Operating lease
b.	Operating lease	Capital lease
c.	Capital lease	Capital lease
d.	Capital lease	Operating lease

6. The appropriate valuation of property obtained under an operating lease on the balance sheet of the lessee is

a. $--0--
b. The absolute sum of the lease payments.
c. The present value of the sum of the lease payments discounted at an appropriate rate.
d. The market value of the leased property at the date of the inception of the lease.

7. What are the three types of period costs that a lessee experiences with capital leases?

a. Lease expense, interest expense, amortization expense.
b. Interest expense, depreciation expense, executory costs.
c. Depreciation expense, executory costs, lease expense.
d. Executory costs, interest expense, lease expense.

8. Under a capital lease, the excess of aggregate rental payments over the present value of such payments should be recognized as expense by the lessee

a. In increasing amounts during the lease term.
b. In constant amounts during the lessee term.
c. In decreasing amounts during the lease term.
d. None of the above.

Required. Select the best answer to each of the above multiple-choice items.

E5. Following the multiple-choice items relating to accounting for hospital pension plans.

1. Which of the following costs is not a part of the defined maximum for pension cost determination?

a. Normal cost.
b. Provision for vested benefits.
c. Interest on overfunding.
d. Ten percent of past service cost.

2. The vested benefits of an employee in a pension plan represent

   a. Benefits to be paid to the retired employee in the current year.
   b. Benefits to be paid to the retired employee in future years.
   c. Benefits accumulated in the hands of a funding agency.
   d. Benefits that are not contingent upon the employee's continuing in the service of the hospital employer.

3. The past service cost in a pension plan

   a. Should be charged to income in the year of the inception of the pension plan.
   b. Should be funded in the year of the inception of the pension plan.
   c. Represent pension cost assigned to years prior to the current balance sheet date.
   d. Represent pension cost assigned to years prior to the inception of the pension plan.

4. APB Opinion No. 8 sets minimum and maximum limits on the annual provision for pension cost. An amount that is always included in the calculation of both the minimum and maximum limit is

   a. Amortization of past service cost.
   b. Normal cost.
   c. Interest on unfunded past and prior service costs.
   d. Retirement benefits paid.

5. Which of the following disclosures concerning pension plans should be made in a hospital's financial statements and accompanying notes?

   a. A statement of the hospital's accounting and funding policies.
   b. The amount of retirement benefits paid during the year.
   c. A description of the actuarial assumptions made.
   d. The amount of unfunded past service costs.

6. The pension expense accrued by a hospital will be increased by interest equivalents when

   a. Amounts funded are less than pension cost accrued.
   b. Amounts funded are greater than pension cost accrued.
   c. The plan is fully funded.
   d. The plan is fully vested.

7. For its defined-benefit pension plans, the hospital should disclose for each complete set of financial statements, as of the most recent benefit information date for which data are available, the actuarial present value of accumulated plan benefits that are

	Vested	Nonvested
a.	Yes	Yes
b.	Yes	No
c.	No	Yes
d.	No	No

8. In the calculation of the maximum limit for the annual provision for pension cost, the past service cost portion of the calculation should not be greater than

   a. Ten percent of the past service cost.
   b. Ten percent of the present value of the vested benefits.
   c. Ten percent of the normal cost.
   d. An amount equivalent to amortization of the past service cost on a forty-year basis.

Required. Select the best answer for each of the above multiple-choice items.

E6. On 1/1/87, Pierce Hospital adopted a noncontributory pension plan for all of its eligible employees. The plan requires Pierce to make annual payments to a funding agency three months after the end of each year. The first payment was due on March 31, 1988. Certain information relating to the plan is as follows:

Normal cost for 1987	$ 200,000
Past service cost at 1/1/87 (unfunded)	1,000,000
Funds held by the funding agency are expected to earn an 8% return.	

Required. Assuming that Pierce elects to maximize its pension expense in accordance with generally accepted accounting principles, what would be the amount of accrued pension expense at 12/31/87?

E7. Johnson Hospital adopted a pension plan in 1987 on a funded, noncontributory basis. Johnson elected to amortize past service costs over 12 years and to fund past service costs over 10 years. Normal costs are to be funded as incurred each year. The following schedule reflects both amortization of the past service costs and funding for the years 1987 and 1988:

	1987	1988
12-year accrual	$100,000	$100,000
Reduction for interest	-0-	835
Past service pension cost	100,000	99,165
10-year funding	113,909	113,909
Balance sheet deferred charge--		
Balance	13,909	28,653
Increase	13,909	14,744
Normal cost	70,000	75,000

Required. How much pension expense should Johnson record in (1) 1987 and (2) 1988?

PROBLEMS

P1. On 1/1/87, Brewer Hospital leased equipment from Carlson Company under a 10-year lease requiring annual rental payments of $12,000, commencing 12/31/87. The equipment has an estimated economic life of 10 years but no expected salvage value. An 8% interest rate is appropriate in the circumstances. Assume that the straight-line depreciation method is employed.

Required. Assuming that this lease is properly classified as an operating lease, make all necessary entries by Brewer Hospital for 1987.

P2. Refer to the data of Problem 1 above.

Required. Assuming that this lease is properly classified as a capital lease, make all necessary entries by Brewer Hospital for 1987 and 1988.

P3. Refer to the data of Problem 1 above, but assume that the annual rental payments are to commence on 1/1/87.

Required. Assuming that this lease is properly classified as a capital lease, make all necessary entries by Brewer Hospital for 1987 and 1988.

P4. On 1/1/87, Briscoe Hospital leased equipment to Cotton Clinic under a 10-year lease requiring annual payments of $12,000, commencing 12/31/87. The equipment, which has a book value and fair value of $80,521, has an estimated useful life of 10 years but no expected salvage value. The straight-line method of depreciation is employed.

Required. Assuming that this lease is properly classified as an operating lease, make all necessary entries by Briscoe Hospital for 1987.

P5. Refer to the data of Problem 4 above.

Required. Assuming that this lease is properly classified as a direct-financing lease, make all necessary entries by Briscoe Hospital for 1987 and 1988.

P6. Refer to the data of Problem 4 above, but assume that the equipment had a book value and fair value of $75,521.

Required. Assuming that this lease is properly classified as a sales-type lease, make all necessary entries by Briscoe Hospital for 1987 and 1988.

P7.   On 1/1/87, Burke Hospital sold equipment which had cost $81,963 to Dean
       Medical Center for $86,963, and immediately leased the equipment back under a
       10-year lease requiring annual rental payments of $12,000, commencing 1/1/87.
       The equipment has an estimated useful life of 10 years but no expected salvage
       value. The straight-line method of depreciation is employed.

       Required. (1) Make all necessary entries on the books of Burke Hospital for 1987.
       (2) Make all necessary entries on the books of Dean Medical Center for 1987.

P8.   Paster Hospital has a contributory pension plan for all of its employees. In 1987,
       a total of $100,000 was withheld from the wages of employees and deposited into
       a pension fund administered by an independent trustee. In addition, Paster
       deposited $200,000 of its own money into the fund in 1987. Based on the report
       of actuaries which was received in December of 1987, the 1987 actuarial cost of
       the pension plan was $320,000. As a result of this report, Paster deposited
       $20,000 of its own money into the fund on 1/12/88.

       Required. How much should the provision for pension cost be in Paster's 1987
       income statement?

P9.   In March of 1987, Rocka Hospital adopted a pension plan for its eligible
       employees. Unfunded past service cost was determined to be $7,000,000 and this
       amount will be paid in 10 annual installments of $1,000,000 to an independent
       funding agency. Past service cost will be amortized over 20 years. The following
       additional data are available:

Normal cost for 1987 (paid in 1987)	$560,000
Amortization of past service cost for 1987	650,000

       Required. What is the amount of the deferred pension cost for 1987?

P10.   Approximately one year ago the Newton Hospital, a 300-bed short-term general
       hospital, initiated an emergency outpatient department staffed by full-time,
       hospital-based physicians. Since then the number of outpatient (private
       ambulatory) and emergency service visits have doubled approximately to 36,000
       and 32,000 respectively. It also has approximately 6,000 outpatient (clinic) visits
       per year.

       The board of trustees and the hospital administrator decide to embark upon a
       $3,000,000 building program to construct facilities which would accumulate the
       required services to meet this obvious trend of patients using the hospital's
       outpatient department as their doctor's office. It is estimated that approximately
       1.5 million dollars in donations could be generated from local industries and
       individuals. Construction would begin in three years and would be completed in
       two years.

As the new controller you are informed that the hospital is in desperate financial condition with over 100 days average daily charges uncollected in accounts receivable, accounts payable of approximately six months and operating deficits averaging $75,000 per year for the past five years. Endowment income is approximately $25,000 per year.

Required. You have been assigned the responsibility to present long-range financial recommendations to meet the following:

1. Recommendation on how to offset the deficit operations and increase cash flow.

2. Considerations for possible construction financing and preparation of a five-year financing schedule for the outpatient department construction. Allow $300,000 for contingencies.

P11.   The board of trustees has decided that Memorial Hospital must have a confusatron if it is to render the best possible service. The only decision facing the Board is whether to purchase or rent. The useful life of the confusatron is estimated to be 10 years. Because of the newness of this type of machine and its complexities, it is essential that a factory maintenance and inspection contract be in effect. Such a contract costs $100 per year. However, this contract is included in the rental fee. The alternatives are:

Rental (includes maintenance and inspection)

Year

1	$2,500
2	2,500
3	2,000
4	2,000
5	1,500
6	1,500
7	1,000
8	1,000
9	500
10	500

The annual rent can be paid in 12 equal monthly installments.

Purchase

Because of the lack of sufficient funds, it will be necessary to purchase the confusatron on an extended payment basis. The best terms that can be arranged for a down payment of $2,800 and $800 annual payments for nine years. Interest at 5 percent on the unpaid balance must be added to these payments.

Required. Prepare a schedule which compares the effect on operating expenses and on cash requirements under the rental plan with the effect under the purchase plan for each of the 10 years of the confusatron's life. The hospital uses a constant percentage (20%) on declining-balance method in computing depreciation. Indicate the comparative cost under rental and purchase methods.

P12.   It has been proposed that your hospital purchase a new unit of equipment to replace the present four-year old unit which is in need of major repairs. The relevant facts concerning the equipment are as follows:

	Existing Unit	Proposed Unit
A. Cost data:		
Cost	$ 80,000	$100,000
Accumulated depreciation	70,000	
Rehabilitation cost	70,000	
Annual cost of five-year		
maintenance service contract	15,000	5,000
Estimated salvage value in		
five years		10,000

B.   **Financing data:**
The hospital does not have funds available to pay for either alternative. It has the following choices:

1.   To rehabilitate the equipment, it can obtain a five-year, $70,000 bank loan with annual payments of $18,000.

2.   To buy the new item, the hospital has two alternatives:

a.   A five-year, $100,000 bank loan with annual payments of $27,000 or

b.   A five-year lease with annual payments of $24,000.

C.   **Additional information:**
1.   Equipment is depreciated on a straight-line basis over a five-year life.

2.   If the existing unit is rehabilitated, it will have no salvage or trade-in value.

3.   Loan repayments are made at the end of each year; payments on rental and service contracts are to be made annually in advance.

4.   If the equipment is leased, $5,000 yearly is paid in addition for a maintenance service contract.

5. All patients are covered under Medicare reimbursement principles.

6. Applying the theory of the value of money, assume an 8 percent discount factor. The necessary tables appear in the Appendix of this text.

Required. Which of the three alternatives will cost the least? (1) Rehabilitation of existing equipment? (2) Five-year loan for new equipment? (3) Five-year lease of new equipment? Show all calculations.

PART 5

Financial Reporting and Analysis

19
Reporting Operating Results

The major function of hospital accounting is the provision of quantitative financial information concerning the economic activities and affairs of a hospital enterprise. This information is required for decision-making purposes by hospital managements and by various external users whose actions directly or indirectly influence the future course of hospital operations. Communication of this essential economic information is accomplished through periodic financial reports depicting operating results and financial position. These reports ordinarily include four basic financial statements.

1. Income statement.
2. Statement of changes in fund balances.
3. Balance sheet.
4. Statement of changes in financial position.

The income statement and statement of changes in fund balances are illustrated and discussed in this chapter; the balance sheet is treated in following chapter. Chapter 21 deals with the statement of changes in financial position. In these three chapters, major attention is given to underlying principles, statement format and content, and required supplementary disclosures. Matters of interpretation and analysis are covered in Chapter 22.

NATURE OF THE INCOME STATEMENT

The **income statement** presents, in conformity with generally accepted principles of accounting, the results of a hospital's operations in terms of revenues earned and expenses incurred during a specified period of time. It also may be referred to as the **statement of revenues and expenses**, the **operating statement** or, less desirably, the **statement of profit and loss**. Current practice, however, tends to favor the use of the term **income statement**, and this title is therefore employed in this book.

Unlike the snapshot photograph of financial position provided by the balance sheet, an income statement is somewhat analogous to a moving picture in which a series of events are summarized. It portrays operating results as reflected by revenues earned and expenses incurred over a given time span such as a month, quarter, or year. Thus, the income statement covers a time **segment** of usually a month or longer, whereas the balance sheet relates only to a particular **point** in time. This distinction is seen in the difference in the way the two statements are dated. A balance sheet, for example, may be dated December 31, 19XX, but the income statement must be dated so as to indicate an appropriate **period** of time, e.g., year ended December 31, 19XX.

Historically, the balance sheet was considered to be the primary financial statement, with income statements being viewed only as connecting links between successive balance sheets. Because the measurement and reporting of enterprise income received steadily increasing emphasis over an extended period of years, the relative importance of the two statements was largely reversed. At present, although balance sheets are still assigned a role of secondary importance, there has been a resurgence of interest in improved balance sheet reporting. The balance sheet has many significant uses of its own. As is demonstrated in the following chapter, the information provided in balance sheets is essential for various types of investment and financing decisions.

It is not surprising that the income statement is generally regarded as the most important of the several financial statements that may be prepared for a hospital enterprise. The statement presents measurements of revenues generated from hospital activities during a given period of time and measurements of the expenses incurred in earning such revenues. In this way, the statement compares financial accomplishment with efforts expended. The result is described as **net income** or **net loss**, depending upon the degree of success achieved by the hospital management in dealing with the many factors influencing the amounts of revenues and expenses. It is a major management responsibility to maintain expenses at a level consistent with available revenues or, alternatively, to obtain revenues in amounts sufficient to avoid operating deficits. The income statement provides much of the information needed to evaluate the performance of management in its discharge of this financial responsibility.

Managerial success, of course, has other important facets that may not be reflected in an immediate and direct way through income statements. The degree to which management has maintained the hospital's short-term financial strength and current debt-paying capacity, for example, is appraised by reference to the hospital's balance sheets. In the long-run analysis, however, the ability to secure a favorable balance between revenues and expenses as reported in income statements is the ultimate test of financial management performance. If this balance is not achieved on a continuing basis, serious impairment of the hospital's service capacity is the inevitable result regardless of the quality of "balance sheet" management.

The income statement also has important uses with respect to decision-making groups external to the hospital. Third-party reimbursement contracts with governmental and private payers, for example, are negotiated largely on the basis of income statement data. While long-term creditors may have a primary concern with the assets that are pledged to the payment of hospital debts, they give considerable emphasis to a history of stable and satisfactory operating results in evaluating the credit-worthiness of a hospital. The information provided in historical and projected income statements is also the basis for many critical decisions made by hospital planning agencies and rate review commissions.

ELEMENTS OF INCOME DETERMINATION

The income of a hospital enterprise for a given period of time might be determined in an indirect manner by the **valuation method**. According to this method, the value of the hospital's net assets at the beginning and at the end of the period are compared. If the net assets, excluding capital additions and withdrawals, have increased, there has been **income** in the amount of such increase; a decrease in net assets would represent a

loss. While this is the method of income determination employed by economists, it has not been adopted by accountants to any great extent. The method has theoretical merit, but serious problems arise when attempts are made to apply the method in actual practice to the measurement of operating results on an interim basis during the economic life of an enterprise. It requires a precise definition of "value," a workable means of obtaining an objective measurement of such value, and a general agreement as to what is to be included in net assets. These serious problems have not yet been resolved in a manner satisfactory for accounting purposes.

Accountants have therefore turned to a more direct method of income determination referred to as the **matching method.** According to this method, the net income of a hospital enterprise for a given period is computed as the difference between the amount of revenue earned by the hospital during the period and the amount of expired costs (expenses) applicable to that revenue. The emphasis of the matching method is upon **revenue realization** and **expense recognition** on an interim reporting basis rather than upon periodic net asset valuations as it is according to the valuation method. It should be recognized, however, that the income statement and the balance sheet are fundamentally interrelated. The measurement of revenues and expenses therefore results in a concurrent determination of net assets, but the latter is a matter of secondary consideration. Preference is given to procedures which produce the most accurate and useful determinations of income; resulting net asset values are assigned less importance.

Revenue Realization

The term **revenues** was defined in Chapter 2 as inflows or other enhancements of the assets of an entity or settlements of its liabilities (or a combination of both) during a period from delivering or producing goods, rendering services, or carrying out other activities that constitute the entity's ongoing major or central operations. To put it another way, revenues are gross increases in assets or gross decreases in liabilities, recognized and measured in conformity with generally accepted accounting principles, that result from those types of profit-directed activities of an enterprise that can change owners' equity. Revenues result when an asset, usually cash or a claim to receive cash, is received or a liability is extinguished in exchange for goods and services provided by the enterprise to another entity. Thus, hospitals derive revenues primarily from the provision of services and the sale of products to patients and others, and these revenues are measured in terms of the exchange prices established between the parties involved in such transactions. In most hospitals, revenues may also arise from the receipt of cash or other assets as unrestricted gifts. If noncash assets are involved, these revenues are measured in terms of the fair market values of the assets at the time received.

It is important to recognize that not all increases in assets or decreases in liabilities are revenues. The acquisition of an asset by purchase or by borrowing, for example, is not revenue, nor does revenue result from the liquidation of a liability by cash payment. It also should be noted that receipts of assets whose use is donor-restricted are not recorded initially as revenue to be reported in the hospital income statement. Certain donor-restricted assets eventually may properly be recognized as revenues when specified conditions are met or restrictions are terminated. Other restricted assets, permanent endowments, for example, are never reported as revenues in the income statement (see Chapter 15).

While this briefly describes the general activities that produce hospital revenues, it does not indicate the time period in which such revenues should be recorded in the accounts and included in the hospital income statement. As a general rule, revenues should be regarded as realized when:

1. The earning process is substantially complete.
2. An exchange has occurred.
3. An objectively measurable asset has been captured.

These conditions generally are met when services have been performed and are billable or when assets have been sold and delivered to the buyer. Revenues such as rentals and interest derived from permitting others to use enterprise assets are recognized as the resources are used or as time passes. Revenues obtained in the form of unrestricted gifts are regarded as realized at the time of receipt. Thus, as discussed in Chapter 7, revenues are recognized at specific points in the revenue-producing process. Prior to these points, all valuations are cost measurements; subsequently, accounting measurements are made in terms of realizable values.

Expense Recognition

The term **expenses** was defined in Chapter 2 as outflows or other using up of assets or incurrences of liabilities (or a combination of both) during a period from delivering or producing goods, rendering services, or carrying out other activities that constitute the entity's ongoing major or central operations. Expenses also may be viewed as gross decreases in assets or gross increases in liabilities, recognized and measured in conformity with generally accepted accounting principles, that result from those types of profit-directed activities of an enterprise that can change owners' equity. It was noted that while many decreases in assets and increases in liabilities are recognized in accounting, not all of them result in expenses. The decrease in cash involved in the repayment of a bank loan, for instance, is not an expense. Neither is the incurrence of a liability for the purchase of an item of equipment to be treated as an expense. Thus, an expense generally may be regarded as a decrease in assets not accompanied by an equal increase in liabilities or by an equal increase in other assets.

A **cost** is an expenditure, an outlay of cash or other assets or services, or the incurrence of a liability, in exchange for goods or services. It generally is measured in terms of the amount of cash disbursed or to be disbursed in the exchange. Assets are "unexpired" costs, and expenses are "expired" costs, i.e., costs that are associated with the revenues of a particular time period, either directly or indirectly through assignment to the same period in which the revenues are recognized. The critical problem in income determination is the decision as to how these costs are to be associated with revenues and therefore when they are to be recognized as expenses.

Three principles govern the recognition of expenses to be deducted form revenues in the determination of the net income or net loss of a period. These principles were described in Chapter 2 as:

1. Association of cause and effect (for example, inventory and payroll costs).
2. Systematic and rational allocation (for example, depreciation and insurance costs).

3. Immediate recognition (other incurred costs which cannot be associated either with future revenues or with future time periods).

Application of these principles results in an appropriate and logical association of expired costs (expenses) with the revenues to which they are applicable. This is known in accounting as the **matching concept.**

ILLUSTRATIVE INCOME STATEMENT

For purposes of discussion, the financial statements of a hypothetical hospital are illustrated in this and the following chapter. The income statement and statement of changes in fund balances are presented and discussed here. Illustrations of the hospital's balance sheet and statement of changes in financial position appear in Chapters 20 and 21, along with the notes accompanying the statements. The data in these statements, although somewhat reclassified and disguised, are drawn from the financial reports of an actual hospital. In the interests of clarity, the dollar amounts are stated in thousands of dollars.

Condensed Summary Income Statement

The income statement of Hartsville Hospital is presented as Exhibit A in Figure 19-1. The statement is highly condensed, providing only summary totals of the major classifications of revenue and expense. Detailed information supporting each total is presented in separate schedules, which are illustrated later in this chapter. In this way, the income statement is freed of cumbersome details, and its readability therefore is greatly enhanced. This practice is recommended for income statements developed for internal management purposes as well as for income statements prepared for public use.

Statement Title. The title of the income statement identifies the hospital entity and indicates the reporting period covered. Unless otherwise specified, it may be assumed that the income statement of a hospital relates only to the operations of its Unrestricted Fund. In this case, the statement presents the results of operations in terms of revenues and expenses pertaining to the Unrestricted Fund of Hartsville Hospital. The receipt and disbursement of restricted resources are disclosed in the hospital's statement of changes in fund balances as illustrated subsequently.

The reporting period is clearly indicated as the **year** ended December 31, 1987. (As stated earlier, the statement should not be dated simply as December 31, 1987, with the period of time then ended not being specified.) Thus, it is assumed that Hartsville Hospital employs a "calendar year" accounting period. In actual practice, however, hospitals often find a "natural business year" ending in a summer or early autumn month more desirable. The calendar year is used here for convenience in referring to the data of different fiscal years.

Hartsville Hospital's summary income statement is presented in comparative form; the 1987 operating results are shown in comparison with the prior year's (1986) results. This is an essential feature of satisfactory financial reporting for both internal and external purposes. The presentation of a single year's operating results alone is of

Figure 19-1.
Hartsville Hospital
Income Statement
Years Ended December 31, 1987 and 1986   Exhibit A

	1987	1986
Patient service revenues (Schedule 1)	$8,830	$7,326
Less deductions from patient service revenues (Schedule 2)	1,430	1,465
Net patient service revenues	$7,400	$5,861
Add other operating revenues (Schedule 3)	505	407
Total operating revenues	$7,905	$6,268
Less Operating Expenses:		
Nursing division	$2,560	$2,197
Other professional services division	2,050	1,615
General services division	1,350	1,033
Fiscal and administrative services division (including interest and depreciation)	1,925	1,614
Total operating expenses (Schedule 4)	$7,885	$6,459
Net operating income (loss)	$ 20	$ (191)
Add nonoperating revenues (Schedule 5)	224	176
Net income (loss) for the year	$ 244	$ (15)

The accompanying notes are an integral part of these financial statements.

questionable utility to the user of the statement, and it may even be misleading. The inclusion of comparative data tends to place the current year's figures in proper perspective and emphasizes the fact that a single year is but a brief installment in a continuing financial history. Consider, for example, the added significance of Hartsville Hospital's operating results for 1987 when viewed in comparison with the 1986 figures. A rather spectacular improvement has been affected by the hospital's management, but this fact might not be so clearly evident to many readers were comparative data omitted from the presentation.

Although comparative figures are essential in actual practice, prior year data are excluded from the income statement schedules illustrated in this chapter. This is done in an effort to facilitate the exposition. Considerably more attention is given to the importance of comparative financial statements in Chapter 22 where comparative analytical techniques are fully discussed.

Statement Format and Content. A satisfactory income statement is something more than a haphazard itemization of revenues and expenses. Careful attention should be given to such matters as the system of classification, the order of presentation, the relationships between the various elements and totals, and the terminology used to describe the items appearing in the statement. The objective should be that of full disclosure of all essential information in the clearest and most useful manner.

Industrial corporations sometimes present their income statements in **single-step** format. In this format, all revenues are grouped in a single category and totaled at the top of the statement, and all expenses are totaled in one classification in the lower portion of the statement. The net income then is computed in a single step by subtraction of total expenses from total revenues. While a presentation of this sort has theoretical merit and may be desirable in certain lines of business, it may not be a satisfactory format for the income statements of hospitals.

Traditionally, the income statements of hospitals have been presented in a **multiple-step** format as illustrated for Hartsville Hospital in Figure 19-1. In this form of presentation, the results of operations are depicted through a series of intermediate subtotals or balances, including net patient service revenues, total operating revenues, net operating income, and net income for the year. This provides a more useful indication of the sources of hospital income than would be the case in a single-step format. The multiple-step arrangement also highlights the amount of revenues "lost" due to charity service, bad debts, and contractual adjustments, and it emphasizes the net operating income or loss from regular activities before consideration of unrestricted gifts and other nonoperating revenues.

The summary income statement, of course, can be designed to reflect totals of revenues and expenses different from those shown in Figure 19-1. Examine the possible alternatives suggested in Figure 19-2 where more detail is given with respect to patient service revenues and operating expenses are presented in a natural classification rather than in functional groupings. This can be done without making any changes in the arrangement of the detailed supporting schedules. The choice of totals to be highlighted in the summary income statement depends largely upon the needs of users and the desirability of emphasizing a particular set of relationships and activity totals rather than another.

Figure 19-2.
Hartsville Hospital
Income Statement
Year Ended December 31, 1987

Patient Service Revenues:	
Inpatients	$7,995
Outpatients	835
Total patient service revenues (Schedule 1)	$8,830
Less deductions from patient service revenues (Schedule 2)	1,430
Net patient service revenues	$7,400
Add other operating revenues (Schedule 3)	505
Total operating revenues	$7,905
Less Operating Expenses:	
Salaries and wages	$4,591
Supplies and other expenses	2,799
Depreciation	360
Interest	135
Total operating expenses (Schedule 4)	$7,885
Net operating income	$ 20
Add nonoperating revenues (Schedule 5)	224
Net income for the year	$ 244

The accompanying notes are an integral part of these financial statements.

At this writing, there is some indication that hospitals may make a significant change in the manner in which they measure and report revenues. The HFMA's Principles and Practices Board recently released an exposure draft of a statement proposing that revenues be reported at the amount which a payer has an obligation to pay (rather than at the hospital's full, established rates). If this proposal is adopted, the "revenue deductions" classification would be eliminated from the hospital income statement. The provision for bad debts and charity service would be reported as expenses in amounts equal to the amounts reported as revenue when the related services were rendered. Contractual adjustments would not be reported at all. In this book, however, the traditional method of reporting revenues and revenue deductions is followed.

Supporting Schedules

As indicated, the income statement usually should be presented in condensed form uncluttered by a mass of detail so that the more important relationships are given emphasis. The details supporting the broad totals shown in the statement must be disclosed in accompanying schedules. Five schedules are used in support of classification totals contained in Hartsville Hospital's summary income statement. While all of these schedules normally would be presented in comparative form, prior year data are omitted here for convenience and clarity.

As in the summary income statement, the dollar figures in the schedules are presented in thousands of dollars. Smaller hospitals might round the figures in their financial reports to the nearest hundred dollars. Nothing of significance is lost, and the readability of the statements and schedules is considerably improved. At the very least, consideration should be given to the deletion of cents in reported data.

Patient Service Revenues. The details of the $8,830 total of patient service revenues are presented as Schedule A/1 in Figure 19-3. This schedule provides a classification of these revenues by department or functional activity and the inpatient and outpatient category totals. Even greater amounts of detail may be included if a useful purpose is served. Daily patient service revenues, for example, may be further analyzed by nursing service (medical and surgical, pediatric, obstetric, and intensive care). If provided for in the accounts, these revenues also could be accumulated and reported by type of accommodation or by patients' financial relationship with the hospital.

It is important to note that patient service revenues in this illustration represent the hospital's gross earnings determined on the accrual basis and measured at full established rates, whether collectible or not. When revenues are recognized and recorded in this manner, the income statement will reflect the monetary value of all services provided during the period. This provides management and other concerned parties with a useful measurement of activity volume and gross potential earnings. It would not otherwise be possible to fully determine the financial impact of revenues "lost" due to charity care and contractual adjustments or to adequately evaluate the hospital's policies and practices with regard to such deductions.

Deductions from Patient Service Revenues. The details of the $1,430 total of revenue deductions are presented as Schedule A/2 in Figure 19-4. The schedule provides a classification of these deductions by major types and also shows inpatient and outpatient totals in each category. If desired, this schedule may include additional details, e.g., a classification of contractual adjustments by major categories of third-party payers.

Figure 19-3.
Hartsville Hospital
Patient Service Revenues
Year Ended December 31, 1987   Schedule A/1

	Inpatients	Outpatients	Total
Nursing Division:			
Daily patient services	$4,274		$4,274
Newborn nursery	169		169
Operating room	550	$ 4	554
Recovery room	62		62
Delivery room	113		113
Central supply	269	3	272
Emergency room	63	205	268
Other	10	8	18
Totals	$5,510	$ 220	$5,730
Other Professional Services Division:			
Laboratory	$ 647	$ 100	$ 747
Blood bank	145	11	156
Radiology	548	274	822
Pharmacy	682	80	762
Anesthesia	194	2	196
Inhalation therapy	78	3	81
Cardio-pulmonary	6	4	10
Physical therapy	85	22	107
EKG/EEG	88	26	114
Clinic fees		89	89
Other	12	4	16
Totals	$2,485	$ 615	$3,100
Total patient service revenues	$7,995	$ 835	$8,830

The accompanying notes are an integral part of these financial statements.

Figure 19-4.
Hartsville Hospital
Deductions from Patients Service Revenues
Year Ended December 31, 1987   Schedule A/2

	Inpatients	Outpatients	Total
Charity care (net of specific purpose gifts of $67)	$ 302	$ 261	$ 563
Contractual adjustments	127	16	143
Courtesy discounts and allowances	8	3	11
Provision for doubtful accounts	656	57	713
Total deductions from patient service revenues	$1,093	$ 337	$1,430

The accompanying notes are an integral part of these financial statements.

As noted in Chapter 7, revenue deductions should be presented **net** of related revenues. Hospitals, for example, may receive gifts or grants from donors who restrict the use of such amounts to the assistance of charity patients generally or to the financing of a free clinic. These amounts often are initially recorded in the Specific Purpose Fund, being subsequently transferred as revenue to the Unrestricted Fund as the donor's requirements are fulfilled. In the case of Hartsville Hospital, it is assumed that $67 of specific purpose gifts were so transferred for charity service during 1987. Figure 19-4 therefore presents $563 of charity care, net of the $67 specific purpose transfer indicated parenthetically. All such restricted amounts received in **general support** of charity care are presented in this manner rather than as "other operating revenue." Amounts that are received in behalf of **specific** indigent patients, however, should be credited directly to patients' accounts receivable.

The $1,430 total of revenue deductions is subtracted from gross patient service revenues of $8,830 as shown in the summary income statement. This provides a $7,400 figure that is labeled as "net patient service revenues." Thus, the volume of patient care services for the period is measured in terms of full rates **and** in terms of net realizable or collectible value. Emphasis thereby is given to the very significant fact that patient services having a value of $1,430 were rendered but the amount is not collectible for reasons set forth in Schedule A/2. This does not mean, however, that the entire $7,400 collectible balance of revenues has been in fact collected at the statement date. A substantial portion undoubtedly remains uncollected and is reflected in accounts receivable within the asset section of the year-end balance sheet.

Figure 19-5.
Hartsville Hospital
Other Operating Revenues
Year Ended December 31, 1987   Schedule A/3

Educational program tuition and fees	$ 102
Specific purpose gifts and grants (other than for charity care)	59
Rentals of space to doctors and employees	4
Nonpatient sales of supplies	13
Cafeteria sales	263
Medical record transcript fees	4
Recovery of telephone charges	5
Revenue from gift shop and newsstand (net)	9
Income from vending machines	7
Revenue from parking lot (net)	15
Purchase discounts earned	21
Miscellaneous	3
Total other operating revenues	$ 505

The accompanying notes are an integral part of these financial statements.

Other Operating Revenues. The details of Hartsville Hospital's other operating revenues of $505 are presented as Schedule A/3 in Figure 19-5. As defined in Chapter 7, these revenues are derived from incidental services to patients, from sales to persons other than hospital patients, and from other activities normal to the day-to-day operation of the hospital but not directly related to the provision of healthcare services to patients. Care should be taken to be certain that only those revenue items embraced by this definition are included in this financial statement classification. Items of nonoperating revenues, as indicated in Chapter 7, should be excluded as they are presented more properly in a later section of the statement. Once the appropriate classifications are established, they should be followed on a consistent basis to maintain the necessary degree of comparability between accounting periods.

In the income statement, the other operating revenues are added to the net patient service revenues, resulting in "total operating revenues" of $7,905. This is the amount of revenues available for coverage of the operating expenses shown in the next section of the statement. The illustrative income statement therefore is arranged in a format that provides for and emphasizes this critical comparison of operating revenues and operating expenses.

Operating Expenses. The details of Hartsville Hospital's operating expenses of $7,885 are presented as Schedule A/4 in Figure 19-6. This schedule is designed to provide both a functional and a natural (object of expenditure) classification of expense. It should be recognized that the expenses listed for each of the departments are **direct expenses** only, i.e., those expenses over which the department heads have effective control and, therefore, primary responsibility. For this reason, and only incidentally as a matter of bookkeeping convenience, items such as employee benefits and depreciation are excluded from the departmental expense totals. The reporting of operating expenses in this manner is most useful from a managerial control point of view. It also is appropriate to the needs of the users of general-purpose financial statements.

While the financial accounting process does not measure and record in the ledger accounts the **full costs** of departmental operations or specific services provided to patients, such information is essential to particular purposes of hospital management, third-party payers, and other groups. The necessary full-cost information is developed either by a cost accounting system or through cost-finding procedures performed at regular intervals. In essence, a cost finding is a supplementary analysis of the direct expenses recorded in the accounts, involving interdepartmental expense allocations designed to reveal the separate total costs of individual (or groups of) hospital activities and services.

Data concerning the cost of processing a pound of laundry, the cost of serving a meal, the cost of a laboratory procedure, and the cost of a patient day of service are but a few examples of the kinds of determinations made in the cost-finding procedure. This information is required for purposes of cost-based reimbursement computations, but it also has important managerial uses in rate setting, budgeting, and other areas. A discussion of the mechanics of cost finding, however, is beyond the scope of this book. Readers who wish to pursue the matter should refer to the AHA's **Cost Finding and Rate Setting for Hospitals** manual.

The operating expenses shown in Hartsville Hospital's income statement are the direct expenses of departmental cost centers as recorded in the routine processes of financial accounting. These expenses, totaling $7,885, are deducted from total operating revenues of $7,905, resulting in a "net operating income" of $20 for 1987. This is a significant improvement over the $191 net operating loss reported for the previous year.

Figure 19-6.
Hartsville Hospital
Operating Expenses
Year Ended December 31, 1987   Schedule A/4

	Salaries and Wages	Supplies and Other Expenses	Total
Nursing Division:			
Nursing service	$1,344	$ 133	$1,477
Nursing education	138	174	312
Operating room	186	121	307
Recovery room	43	2	45
Delivery room	71	14	85
Central supply	58	82	140
Emergency room	115	66	181
Other	12	1	13
Total nursing division expense	$1,967	$ 593	$2,560
Other Professional Services Division:			
Laboratory	$ 353	$ 86	$ 439
Blood bank	21	103	124
Radiology	357	142	499
Pharmacy	72	199	271
Anesthesia	86	53	139
Inhalation therapy	36	16	52
Cardio-pulmonary	10	2	12
Physical therapy	62	4	66
EKG/EEG	32	7	39
Clinic	72	74	146
Medical education	105	25	130
Medical records and library	81	11	92
Social service	25	2	27
Other	11	3	14
Total other professional services division expense	$1,323	$ 727	$2,050
General Services Division:			
Dietary	$ 237	$ 386	$ 623
Housekeeping	173	37	210
Laundry and linen	72	46	118
Plant operation	22	109	131
Plant maintenance	161	87	248
Other	15	5	20
Total general services division expense	$ 680	$ 670	$1,350
Fiscal and Administrative Services Division:			
Fiscal services	$ 322	$ 185	$ 507
Administrative services (including interest of $135)	299	274	573
Employee benefits		452	452
Depreciation		360	360
Other		33	33
Total fiscal and administrative services division expense	$ 621	$1,304	$1,925
Total operating expenses	$4,591	$3,294	$7,885

The accompanying notes are an integral part of these financial statements.

Nonoperating Revenues. The details of Hartsville Hospital's nonoperating revenues of $224 are presented as Schedule A/5 in Figure 19-7. As discussed in Chapter 2, all unrestricted gifts, contributions, and bequests must be included in this classification in the year received. The hospital's governing board may place restrictions on these amounts, but the amounts received still must be reported as nonoperating revenues of the Unrestricted Fund. The donors are the only persons who can place legally binding restrictions on gifts.

Figure 19-7.
Hartsville Hospital
Nonoperating Revenues
Year Ended December 31, 1987   Schedule A/5

General contributions	$ 45
Unrestricted income from Endowment Fund	139
Income and gains from Unrestricted Fund investments	18
Miscellaneous	22
Total nonoperating revenues	$ 224

The accompanying notes are an integral part of these financial statements.

The addition of nonoperating revenues to the net operating income results in a total of $244 that is labeled "net income for the year." This may also be referred to as the "excess of revenues over expenses." It represents the net results of activities during 1987 in Hartsville Hospital's Unrestricted Fund in terms of revenues earned and expenses incurred. It can be said that a "profit" of $244 was made, but considerable attention should be drawn to the fact that the hospital barely broke even on the basis of its regular operations. If the nonoperating revenues had not been substantial, Hartsville Hospital might well have found itself to be in a financially uncomfortable situation.

Since unrestricted contributions, investment income, and other sources of nonoperating revenue ordinarily are somewhat uncertain and cannot always be relied upon to offset operating losses, it generally would be imprudent to take them into account in an important way when planning the hospital's program for regular operations. Management's operating plans in most hospitals must be directed into a program designed to avoid an **operating** loss, disregarding for this purpose the possibility of material amounts of nonoperating revenues. This is not to say, however, that nonoperating revenues should not be budgeted. It is important that all revenues be carefully budgeted, but it is unwise to establish an operating program that is heavily dependent upon anticipated revenues from nonoperating sources. When nonoperating revenues are acquired, however, such realized amounts certainly should be taken into account in making plans for the ensuing year.

For external financial reporting purposes, however, the critical figure in the income statement is the amount of net income for the year. All non-operating revenues, regardless of their materiality, must be included in that determination. No attempt should ever be made to "bury" the net income figure through the use of misleading terminology or confusing arrangements of data. The appropriate figure should be clearly labeled "net income for the year" so that it may easily be located and identified by the reader of the statement. In some cases where extraordinary items and other special income adjustments are involved, the presentation of net income requires careful consideration. A discussion of these special considerations appears in a later section of this chapter.

STATEMENT OF CHANGES IN FUND BALANCES

The fundamental accounting equation is often stated as: assets = equities. In accounting, equities (or rights in assets) are of two types. Equities in assets may be held by entities external to the enterprise, i.e., outsiders. These claims are called **liabilities**. The second type of claim against enterprise assets is the **owners' equity**. It is a residual claim in that legal preference is given to the claims of non-owners, i.e., liabilities. Hence, the equation discussed in Chapter 2 was expressed in the following manner: assets − liabilities = owners' equity. In other words, the total of enterprise assets minus the claims of creditors against such assets equals the residual ownership interest in enterprise assets.

In a profit-seeking business enterprise, the owners' equity is the residual interest of the owners of the enterprise, e.g., the stockholders. The owners' equity at any time is the sum of the owners' investments and enterprise profits minus the amount of investment and profit withdrawn from the business by the stockholders. All profits accrue to stockholders, and much of the profits are withdrawn through distribution of dividends.

The nature of the owners' equity in a not-for-profit hospital is less easily defined. It is the residual ownership interest in hospital assets; it is the excess of hospital assets over hospital liabilities. But who are the owners of the not-for-profit hospital? The residual ownership interest in a not-for-profit hospital theoretically resides with the community it serves and with sponsoring organizations, if any, such as a church, university, or governmental unit. Legally, however, the rights and duties incident to ownership usually are invested in the governing body, i.e., the board of trustees or directors. Yet, no part of the hospital's profits or assets can be directed to the personal benefit of the board members.

The concept of owners' equity in a hospital enterprise is also complicated by the fact that hospitals usually receive a substantial amount of assets whose use and disposition is subject to donors' restrictions and against which the general creditors of the hospital may have no claim. In effect, the hospital owners' equity consists of several different residual interests in several different groups of assets. Hospitals typically deal with this problem through the vehicle of fund accounting in which the owners' equity is fragmented into a number of individual **fund balance** accounts. That is, there is a separate fund balance (owners' equity) account for each fund maintained by the hospital. The fund balance account of any fund is the difference between the assets and liabilities recorded in that fund.

The total owners' equity of a hospital, then, is the total of the individual fund balance accounts. This **total** generally is changed in only two ways: (1) by net income or net losses and (2) by the receipt of pure endowments or resources restricted by donors to the acquisition of plant assets. Certain interfund transfers of resources may be made, however, that properly increase the equity balance of one fund and decrease that of another fund. But the total of fund balances is not affected by such transfers.

Unrestricted Fund Balance

The Unrestricted Fund Balance is the difference between the hospital's unrestricted assets (resources having no donor restrictions) and the liabilities properly payable from such assets. Board designations of otherwise unrestricted resources do not affect the total amount of the Unrestricted Fund Balance nor do they alter the legal status of the hospital's general creditors. The rights of such creditors in the hospital's unrestricted assets are not reduced merely by action of the hospital's governing board.

Nevertheless, perhaps for internal management purposes, hospitals will sometimes subdivide the Unrestricted Fund Balance in the accounts so as to show its composition as a result of designations or appropriations made by the board. In other words, separate accounts might be maintained somewhat as follows:

Unrestricted Fund Balance:	
Board-designated for investment	$ 500,000
Board-designated for specific operating purposes	100,000
Board-designated for replacement of plant assets	400,000
Invested in property, plant, and equipment	7,000,000
Unappropriated	1,000,000
Total Unrestricted Fund Balance	$9,000,000

Although the **Hospital Audit Guide** appears to suggest such a disclosure in the hospital's financial statements, the procedure is cumbersome and likely to be confusing rather than helpful. The presentation of a single $9,000,000 fund balance figure is important. It informs the financial statement reader very clearly as to the total resources available to the board for general operating purposes. That is the important disclosure, and it would seem most unwise to reduce its clarity with today's board designations which easily may be reversed tomorrow.

The Unrestricted Fund Balance is increased by the excess of revenues over expenses, i.e., net income, as reported in the hospital's income statement; it is decreased by reported net losses. Transfers to the Unrestricted Fund from the Plant Replacement and Expansion Fund to finance the acquisition of plant assets also increase the Unrestricted Fund Balance by direct credit. Transfers of this type are not reflected as revenue in the income statement. The fair market value of donated plant assets also is credited directly to the Unrestricted Fund Balance account without revenue recognition. Rarely is it appropriate to record direct changes in the Unrestricted Fund Balance account for any other reason. A possible exception is prior period adjustments for correction of errors, a matter discussed later in this chapter.

Restricted Fund Balances

The fund balance of any restricted fund is the difference between the assets and liabilities of that particular fund. It is essential that the integrity of each fund be maintained absolutely so that the fund balance of each fund is clearly identified. The restricted fund balances must not be compromised by unwarranted and artificial interfund transfers.

Restricted fund balances are increased by the receipt of donor-restricted resources and gains from dispositions of investments made of such resources. Interest and dividend income on the investments of specific purpose funds and plant replacement and expansion funds also are credited to the respective fund balance accounts. As noted in Chapter 15, however, income on the investments of endowment funds ordinarily should not be recorded in the endowment funds at all but should be reported in whatever other fund is appropriate in view of donor restrictions, or the absence thereof. Restricted fund balances may also be increased by transfers, other than interfund loans, received from other funds.

Decreases are recorded in restricted fund balances as a result of losses relating to investment transactions and for transfers, other than interfund loans, of resources to other funds. Investment expenses should be recorded in the restricted fund where the related investment income is reported.

A sufficient number of descriptively titled temporary accounts should be employed in the restricted funds to clearly reflect the investment activity, receipt of restricted resources, transfers, and other transactions which increase or decrease the fund balance accounts when the temporary accounts are closed at the end of each fiscal period. In addition, it may be desirable to subdivide the restricted fund balance accounts so as to reflect the composition of the balance of each restricted fund. Some examples are provided below:

Specific Purpose Fund Balance:
      Research grants
      Charity service
      Educational programs
      Other
Plant Replacement and Expansion Fund Balance:
      New building
      New equipment
Endowment Fund Balance:
      Permanent endowments
         Income restricted
         Income unrestricted
      Term endowments
         Income restricted
         Income unrestricted

Unlike the Unrestricted Fund Balance, the restricted fund balances are governed by the stipulations of donors. The composition of these balances therefore is of considerable importance and significance to the external users of hospital financial statements.

Illustrative Statement of Changes in Fund Balances

The income statement, as illustrated above, presents only the change in the Unrestricted Fund Balance that results from the revenues and the expenses of a given period. A net income increases the Unrestricted Fund Balance; a net loss decreases it. Factors other than net income or net loss, however, may cause the amount of the Unrestricted Fund Balance to change. Since these "other" factors are not reflected in the income statement as revenues or expenses, another financial statement is necessary in order to report fully all changes that have occurred in the fund balance. While such a statement could be prepared for the Unrestricted Funds alone, it is considerably more useful when it is developed in a manner that presents **all** changes in the balances of **all** funds. Where this is the case, it is called the **statement of changes in the fund balances.** An illustrative statement of this kind is presented as Exhibit B in Figure 19-8.

Figure 19-8.

Hartsville Hospital

Statement of Changes in Fund Balances

Years Ended December 31, 1987 and 1986   Exhibit B

Unrestricted Fund

	1975	1974
Fund balance, January 1	$7,511	$7,596
Net income (loss) for the year (Exhibit A)	244	(15)
Donated medical equipment	20	
Transfers from Plant Replacement and Expansion Fund for financing of plant asset acquisitions	95	45
Transfers to Plant Replacement and Expansion Fund of third-party reimbursements restricted to plant asset acquisitions	(140)	(115)
Fund balance, December 31	$7,730	$7,511

Restricted Funds

	1975	1974
Specific Purpose Fund:		
Fund balance, January 1	$ 365	$ 352
Restricted gifts and bequests received	106	93
Restricted income from investments	12	10
Gain on sale of investments	1	
Transfers to Unrestricted Fund for:		
Financing of charity care	(67)	(52)
Other operating revenue	(59)	(38)
Fund balance, December 31	$ 358	$ 365
Plant Replacement and Expansion Fund:		
Fund balance, January 1	$ 791	$ 616
Restricted gifts and bequests received	51	74
Restricted income from investments	33	28
Gain on sale of investments	4	3
Transfer to Unrestricted Fund for financing of plant asset acquisitions	(95)	(45)
Transfer from Unrestricted Fund of third-party reimbursements restricted to plant asset acquisitions	140	115
Fund balance, December 31	$ 924	$ 791
Endowment Fund:		
Fund balance, January 1	$1,789	$1,458
Restricted gifts and bequests received	425	326
Gain on sale of investments	7	5
Fund balance, December 31	$2,221	$1,789

The accompanying notes are an integral part of these financial statements.

   The illustrative statement of changes in fund balances begins with the January 1 balance of each fund maintained in Hartsville Hospital's accounts, shows all changes in those fund balances during the year, and indicates the resultant balances at December 31. These ending balances, of course, appear in the hospital's balance sheet which is illustrated in the next chapter in Figure 20-1. In this way, the statement of changes in fund balances accounts for the increase or decrease in fund balances as indicated by successive balance sheets. A full disclosure of these changes is an essential financial reporting requirement.

   In Figure 19-8, the data are arranged in a vertical "report" format. Some accountants, however, prefer to present the statement of changes in fund balances in a columnar format as illustrated in Figure 19-9. The report format is mechanically superior when comparative data are included, but the columnar arrangement may give the reader a better understanding of interfund transfers.

Figure 19-9.
Hartsville Hospital
Statement of Changes in Fund Balances
Year Ended December 31, 1987

	Unre-stricted Fund	Restricted Funds		
		Specific Purpose	Plant Replacement and Expansion	Endowment
Fund balances, January 1	$7,511	$ 365	$ 791	$1,789
Net income for the year (see Exhibit A)	244			
Donated medical equipment	20			
Restricted gifts and bequests received		106	51	425
Restricted income from investments		12	33	
Gain on sale of investments		1	4	7
Transfers to Unrestricted Fund for financing of charity care	*	(67)		
Transfers to Unrestricted Fund for specific operating purposes	*	(59)		
Transfers of third-party reim-bursements restricted to plant asset acquisitions	(140)		140	
Transfers to Unrestricted Fund to finance plant asset acquisitions	95		(95)	
Fund balances, December 31	$7,730	$ 358	$ 924	$2,221

*Specific Purpose Fund transfers are included in the net income reported in the Unrestricted Fund.

Another possibility is a combined presentation of the income statement and the statement of changes in Unrestricted Fund Balance in a single statement as shown in Figure 19-10. This alternative is suggested in the AICPA's **Hospital Audit Guide.**[1] If this format is employed, the "total" column must be included to present the information fairly and to avoid giving the reader the erroneous impression that the amounts reflected in the "other" and "plant" columns are donor-restricted and legally unavailable for general purposes. It must be made clear that all amounts included in this combined statement are unrestricted funds of the hospital, regardless of designations made by the governing board. Presumably, a separate statement of changes in **restricted** fund balances would be prepared.

Figure 19-10.

Hartsville Hospital

Statement of Income and Changes in Unrestricted Fund Balance

Year Ended December 31, 1987

	Operations	Other	Plant	Total
Patient service revenues	$8,830			$8,830
Less deductions from patient service revenues	1,430			1,430
Net patient service revenues	$7,400			$7,400
Add other operating revenues	505			505
Total operating revenues	$7,905			$7,905
Less Operating Expenses:				
Nursing division	$2,560			$2,560
Other professional services division	2,050			2,050
General services division	1,350			1,350
Fiscal and administrative services division	1,925			1,925
Total operating expenses	$7,885			$7,885
Net operating income	$ 20			$ 20
Nonoperating Revenues:				
Unrestricted contributions		$ 45		$ 45
Unrestricted income from Endowment Fund		139		139
Income and gains from board-designated funds		3	$ 15	18
Miscellaneous		1	21	22
Total nonoperating revenues		$ 188	$ 36	$ 224
Net income for the year	$ 20	$ 188	$ 36	$ 244
Fund balance, January 1	198	618	6,695	7,511
Donated medical equipment			20	20
Transfers from Plant Replacement and Expansion Fund for financing of plant asset acquisitions			95	95
Transfer to plant Replacement and Expansion Fund of third-party reimbursements restricted to plant asset acquisitions	(140)			(140)
Intrafund transfers	127	(87)	(40)	
Fund balance, December 31	$ 205	$ 719	$6,806	$7,730

SOME SPECIAL PROBLEMS

The above discussion was centered on basic considerations of income determination and presentation. Certain special problems may be encountered at times, however, with respect to the appropriate treatment of extraordinary gains and losses, prior period adjustments, error corrections, and the effects of accounting changes. These matters have been the subject of much controversy in the past, but recent FASB and AICPA pronouncements are designed to bring about a greater degree of agreement in these areas of financial reporting practice.

Extraordinary Items

The term **extraordinary items** generally refers to gains and losses of an unusual, nonrecurring nature that arise during an accounting period but which are not clearly identifiable with, and do not result from, the normal operating activities of the period. Assume, for example, that a hospital has a sizable gain on the early retirement of its long-term debt or an uninsured loss arising from a fire or other casualty. The question is whether such items should be reported in the hospital's income statement and be included in the determination of the net income for the period. If not, such items presumably would be treated as direct credits or charges to the Unrestricted Fund Balance in the statement of changes in fund balances. Which treatment is correct?

Historically, many accountants have believed that the income statement should reflect only the net results of ordinary and recurring operations under normal conditions without the distortion that would arise from the inclusion of so-called extraordinary items. It was argued that extraordinary items should be reported in the statement of changes in fund balances rather than in the income statement. This point of view came to be known as the **current operating performance concept** of the income statement. An opposing school of thought supported an **all-inclusive concept** of income reporting by which extraordinary items would be presented on the face of the income statement and used in determining the figure reported as net income. This group of accountants was of the opinion that there should be a general presumption that all items of revenues, expense, gain, and loss that are recognized during a period should enter into the net income determination.

While the controversy continues, the preparation of income statements on an all-inclusive basis is clearly favored in current practice. APB Opinion No. 30 requires the inclusion of extraordinary items in income statements in the following manner: [2]

Income before extraordinary items	$xxx,xxx
Extraordinary items (Note)	xxx,xxx
Net income for the year	$xxx,xxx

Thus, the net results of normally recurring (continuing) operations is identified as "income before extraordinary items." Then, either parenthetically or by an appropriate note to the statement, a full disclosure is made of the nature and amounts of extraordinary items on an individual basis. After addition (or deduction) of the net extraordinary items of the period, the last line of the statement should be designated as "net income for the year."

The distinction between ordinary operating items and extraordinary items may not always be entirely clear. In order for a gain or loss to qualify for treatment as an extraordinary item, it must meet both of the following criteria: [3]

1. The underlying event or transaction should possess a high degree of abnormality and be of a type clearly unrelated to, or only incidentally related to, the ordinary and typical activities of the entity, taking into account the environment in which the entity operates.
2. The underlying event or transaction should be of a type that would not reasonably be expected to recur in the foreseeable future, taking into account the environment in which the entity operates.

In addition, the effect of the event or transaction should be material in relation to income before consideration of extraordinary items, or it should be material by other appropriate criteria.

In view of these criteria, the reporting of extraordinary items will be a most infrequent occurrence. The following items, in fact, were listed by the APB as examples of gains and losses which usually should **not** be reported as extraordinary items: [4]

1. Write-down or write-off of receivables, inventories, equipment leased to others, deferred research and development costs, or other intangible assets.
2. Gains or losses from exchange or translation of foreign currencies.
3. Gains or losses on disposal of a segment of a business.
4. Other gains or losses from sale or abandonment of property, plant, or equipment used in the business.
5. Effects of a strike, including those against competitors and major suppliers.
6. Adjustment of accruals on long-term contracts.

Specific mention is also made of the fact that an event or transaction that occurs frequently **in the environment** in which an entity operates cannot be regarded as extraordinary, regardless of its financial effect. This means that large, unrestricted gifts should be reported in the hospital's income statement as ordinary income, not as extraordinary items.

In rare situations where the APB criteria are met, however, certain of the above items might properly be reported as extraordinary gains or losses. Gains and losses such as those in points 1 and 4 above, for example, may be reported as extraordinary items if they are a direct result of an earthquake or other major casualty, an expropriation, or a prohibition under a newly enacted law or regulation. In addition, it should be noted that the FASB has required certain gains or losses to be treated as extraordinary items, even where the above criteria are not met. FASB Statement No. 4, for instance, requires that gains and losses on the extinguishment of debt be reported as extraordinary items. [5]

Special reporting requirements also are established in APB Opinion No. 30 for the income statement presentation and disclosure of the effects of the disposal of a segment of a business. [6] The Board concluded that the results of continuing operations should be reported separately from discontinued operations and that any gain or loss from disposal of a segment of a business should be reported in conjunction with the related results of discontinued operations and **not** as an extraordinary item. If, for example, a hospital discontinues its long-term care operations and sells the facility, the income statement presentation should be as follows:

Income from continuing operations		$xxx,xxx
Discontinued operations:		
Income (loss) from operations of discontinued long-term care facility (Note)*	$xxx,xxx	$xxx,xxx
Gain (loss) on disposal of long-term care facility (Note)	xxx,xxx	_____
Net income for the year		$xxx,xxx

*From the beginning of the fiscal year to the disposal date.

Full disclosure should be made, in appropriate notes to the income statement, of all significant details relating to the discontinued operations. The reader having a special interest in this matter should refer to APB Opinion No. 30.

Prior Period Adjustments

Before the issuance of FASB Statement No. 16, prior period adjustments were usually treated in the same inconsistent manner as were extraordinary items, i.e., some accountants reported such adjustments in the income statement while others reported them in the statement of changes in fund balances. Statement No. 16, however, limits the reporting of prior period adjustments in the statement of changes in fund balances mainly to corrections of accounting errors made in prior periods.[7] The general presumption is that all items of revenue, expense, gain, and loss should be included in the determination of net income. The position of the FASB is so restrictive that the reporting of prior period adjustments in the statement of changes in fund balances is extremely rare.

It is important to note that treatment as prior period adjustments should not be given to the normal, recurring corrections and adjustments which are the natural result of the use of estimates inherent in the accounting process. The following items, for example, generally should not be reported as prior period adjustments:

1. Changes in the estimated remaining lives of depreciable assets.
2. Relatively immaterial adjustments of provisions for liabilities.
3. Adjustments related to the realization of assets (collectibility of accounts receivable or realizability of inventory) arising from economic events occurring subsequent to the date of the financial statements for the prior period.
4. Retroactive Medicare adjustments (as a general rule, and when they do not arise from errors).

The effects of these items are considered to be elements in the determination of net income for the current period in which the previous uncertainty is eliminated.

Accounting Changes

Accounting changes may involve changes in accounting principles and changes in accounting estimates. Where these changes are made, a question arises as to the most appropriate manner of reporting the effects of such changes. Are the effects to be reported retroactively, currently, or prospectively? The following discussion summarizes the guidelines established in APB Opinion No. 20 for reporting changes of these types and for reporting the correction of errors in previously issued financial statements.[8]

Change in Accounting Principle. The term **accounting principle** includes not only accounting principles and practices but also the methods by which they are applied. On occasion, a hospital may choose to make a change in accounting principle, i.e., it may adopt a generally accepted accounting principle different from the one used previously for financial reporting purposes. Such change, for example, may include a change from the FIFO (first-in, first-out) to the LIFO (last-in, first-out) inventory pricing method or a change from the declining-balance to the straight-line depreciation method for plant assets. In any case, the presumption is that an accounting principle once adopted should not be changed but should be applied consistently from one period to the next **unless** the use of an alternate principle can be supported on the basis that it is preferable. A change should not be made without sufficient justification that can be adequately demonstrated.

If a change in accounting principle can be sufficiently supported, the cumulative effect of the change usually should be included in the determination of the net income of the period in which the change is made. The cumulative effect is measured as the difference between (1) the fund balance at the beginning of the period of change and (2) the amount of the fund balance that would have been reported at that date if the new principle had been applied retroactively to all prior periods affected by the change. This cumulative amount should be reported separately in the income statement for the current period between the captions "extraordinary items" and "net income for the year." (The remainder of the income statement data are reported on the basis of the newly adopted principle.) Additionally, the nature and justification for the change must be explained in an appropriate note to the financial statements.

Thus, in regard to a change in accounting principle, the financial statements of prior years generally are **not** revised.[9] The cumulative effect of the change is reported as a special item in the income statement of the year of change. There is no retroactive adjustment.

Change in Accounting Estimate. Many estimates of the effects of future events are widely employed in the preparation of financial statements. These estimates change, however, as new events occur, as more experience is acquired, and as additional information is obtained. Such changes are necessary consequences of the accounting process. Examples of items for which estimates are utilized are uncollectible receivables, inventory obsolescence, service lives and salvage values of depreciable plant assets, and future periods benefited by deferred costs.

As previously discussed in Chapter 16, a change may be made in the estimated remaining service life of a depreciable asset. The effect of such a change is reflected in revised depreciation charges for the current and subsequent periods. A change in the **method** of depreciation, on the other hand, is treated as a change in accounting principle as previously discussed.

Thus, a change in accounting estimate does not require a restatement of account balances for prior years. Such changes are accounted for (1) in the period of change if the change affects that period only or (2) in the period of change and future periods if the change affects both. A description of the nature of such changes and the effect on net income should be provided in a note to the income statement of the period of change.

Error Corrections

The correction of an error in the financial statements of a prior period that is discovered subsequent to the issuance of the statements should be reported as a prior period adjustment in the statement of changes in fund balances in the year the error is discovered. Such errors may arise from mathematical mistakes, incorrect application of accounting principles, or the omission of certain data. If the error is material, its nature and effect on reported income should be disclosed in the period of discovery and correction. The financial statements of subsequent periods need not repeat these disclosures.

CHAPTER 19 FOOTNOTES

1. Committee on Health Care Matters, **Hospital Audit Guide** (New York: AICPA, 1982), pp. 44-45.

2. "Reporting the Results of Operations," **APB Opinion No. 30** (New York: AICPA, 1973), par. 11.

3. **Ibid.,** par. 20.

4. **Ibid.,** par. 23.

5. "Reporting Gains and Losses from Extinguishment of Debt," **Statement of Financial Accounting Standards No. 4** (Stamford, Connecticut: FASB, 1975), par. 8.

6. "Reporting the Results of Operations," **APB Opinion No. 30** (New York: AICPA, 1973), par. 8.

7. "Prior Period Adjustment," **Statement of Financial Accounting Standards No. 16** (Stamford, Connecticut: FASB, 1977), par. 11.

8. "Accounting Changes," **APB Opinion No. 20** (New York: AICPA, 1971).

9. **Ibid.,** par. 19.

QUESTIONS

1. Define the term **income statement.** Why is the income statement generally regarded as the single most important financial statement prepared by the hospital?
2. Distinguish between the **valuation** and **matching** methods of income determination.
3. Define the term **revenue.** In accounting, when should revenue be regarded as realized?
4. Distinguish between the terms **cost** and **expense** as they usually are employed in accounting.
5. State the three principles that govern the recognition of expenses to be deducted from revenue in the determination of the net income or loss of a period.
6. Give the reasons why financial statements prepared on the accrual basis are considered more informative and reliable than statements prepared on the cash basis.
7. What is the relationship between the Unrestricted Fund balance sheet and the Unrestricted Fund income statement?
8. Distinguish between the **single-step** and **multiple-step** format of income statement. Which is preferable for hospitals?
9. Why is a statement of changes in fund balances necessary to a complete presentation of a hospital's operating results for a given period?
10. Distinguish between the **current operating performance** and the **all-inclusive** concepts of income determination.
11. In order for a gain or loss to quality for treatment of an extraordinary item in the hospital's income statement, it must meet certain criteria established by the Accounting Principles Board. State these criteria.
12. Infrequently, items of gain or loss are recorded in the accounts as prior period adjustments. Provide two examples of a prior period adjustment. How are prior period adjustments reported in the hospital's financial statements?
13. Give an example of a change in accounting principle. How should such a change be reported in the hospital's financial statements?
14. Give an example of a change in accounting estimate. How should such a change be reported in the hospital's financial statements?
15. It is discovered that a material mathematical error was made in a prior fiscal year which resulted in a $140,000 misstatement of operating income. How should this error be reported in the hospital's current financial statements?
16. Accounting Principles Board Opinion No. 20 is concerned with accounting changes.

Required. (1) Define, discuss, and illustrate each of the following in such a way that one can be distinguished from the other: (a) an accounting change and (b) a correction of an error in previously issued financial statements. (2) Discuss the justification for a change in accounting principle. (3) Discuss the reporting of a change from an accelerated method to the straight-line method of depreciation.

EXERCISES

E1. Sunny Hospital's general ledger provides the following information at September 30, the end of its fiscal year:

Interest expense	$ 200
Gross revenues – inpatients	9,940
Salaries and wages	6,480
Other operating revenues	720
Depreciation expense	500
Gain on retirement of bonds payable	160
Gross revenues – outpatients	1,750
Supplies and purchased services	4,320
Unrestricted contributions	600
Deductions from revenues	1,140

Required. Prepare in good form an income statement for the year ended September 30.

E2. Sunshine Hospital's general ledger provides the following information at June 30, the end of its fiscal year:

Nursing service expenses	$ 4,000
Depreciation expense	510
Daily patient service revenues	6,250
General services expenses	1,900
Unrestricted contributions	600
Other professional services expenses	2,700
Deductions from revenues	1,140
Interest expense	190
Other professional services revenues	5,440
Fiscal and administrative services	2,200
Other operating revenues	720

Required. Prepare in good form an income statement for the year ended June 30.

E3. Sunlight Hospital had accounts receivable of $1,146 at January 1, 1987. During 1987, cash collections on account amounted to $8,729 and $437 of patients' accounts were written off as uncollectible. At December 31, 1987, the balance of accounts receivable was $1,290 of which it was estimated that perhaps 10 percent would prove to be uncollectible.

Required. Compute the amount of charges made to patients' accounts during 1987.

E4.   Sunbright Hospital had accounts payable due to suppliers of $976 at January 1, 1987. During 1987, payments on accounts payable amounted to $2,883. At December 31, 1987, accounts payable to suppliers amounted to $875.

Required. Compute the cost of supplies purchased during 1987.

E5.   Suntime Hospital's general ledger provides the following information at August 31, the end of its fiscal year:

Deductions from revenues	$ 1,050
Unrestricted contributions	479
Supplies and purchased services	4,410
Gross revenues – outpatients	1,820
Depreciation expense	590
Other operating revenues	660
Salaries and wages	6,340
Gross revenues – inpatients	9,892
Interest expense	235
Extraordinary loss	850

Required. Prepare in good form an income statement for the year ended August 31.

E6.   Sunshade Hospital reports the following changes in the accounts of its Unrestricted Fund for the year ended May 31:

	Increase	Decrease
Cash	$150	
Receivables	310	
Inventory		$ 90
Property, plant and equipment	550	
Accounts payable	180	
Other current liabilities		120
Long-term debt		600

During the fiscal year, $250 was transferred from the Unrestricted Fund to the Plant Replacement and Expansion Fund for the reimbursement of depreciation restricted by third-party payers.

Required. Calculate the net income for the year.

E7. Sunside Hospital's general ledger provides the following information relating to the year ending September 30, 1987:

1. Fund balances, 10/1/86:

Unrestricted Fund	$3,800
Specific Purpose Fund	320
Plant Replacement and Expansion Fund	840
Endowment Fund	2,400

2. Donated medical equipment, $33.
3. Net income for the year, $315.
4. Restricted gifts and bequests received:

Specific Purpose Fund	$ 202
Plant Replacement and Expansion Fund	114
Endowment Fund	500

5. Transfer to Unrestricted Fund from:

Specific Purpose Fund	$ 150
Plant Replacement and Expansion Fund	185

6. Restricted income from investments:

Specific Purpose Fund	$ 95
Plant Replacement and Expansion Fund	87

7. Transfer from Unrestricted Fund to Plant Replacement and Expansion Fund, $125.

8. Gain on sale of investments:

Specific Purpose Fund	$ 5
Plant Replacement and Expansion Fund	12
Endowment Fund	23

Required. Prepare in good form a statement of changes in fund balances for the year ended September 30, 1987.

E8. The following multiple-choice questions relate to the reporting of operating results.

1. On 1/1/84, Trail Hospital purchased an item of equipment for $150,000. The equipment had a five-year useful life and no salvage value. The equipment has been depreciated by the sum-of-years'-digits method. Effective 1/1/87, however, Trail decided to change to the straight-line depreciation method. Trail can justify the change. Trail's 1987 income before depreciation and

before the cumulative effect of the change in accounting principle is $100,000. What amount should Trail Hospital report as net income for 1987?

a. $130,000
b. $100,000
c. $ 70,000
d. $ 40,000

2. Bond Hospital purchased equipment on 1/1/84 for $3,000,000. At the date of acquisition, the equipment had an estimated useful life of six years with no salvage value. The equipment is being depreciated by the straight-line method. On 1/1/87, Bond determined, as a result of additional information, that the equipment had an estimated useful life of eight years from the date of acquisition with no salvage value expected. An accounting change was made in 1987 to reflect the revised estimate of useful life. What should be reported in Bond's 1987 income statement as the cumulative effect on prior years of changing the estimated useful life of the equipment?

a. $ - 0 -
b. $125,000
c. $375,000
d. $500,000

3. Refer to the data of Item 2 above. What should be reported in Bond's 1987 income statement as depreciation expense?

a. $100,000
b. $300,000
c. $375,000
d. $500,000

4. Shannon Hospital began operations on 1/1/86. The financial statements for 1986 and 1987 contained errors as indicated below:

	1986	1987
Ending inventory	$16,000 understated	$15,000 overstated
Depreciation expense	$ 6,000 understated	
Insurance expense	$10,000 overstated	$10,000 understated
Prepaid insurance	$10,000 understated	

In addition, on 12/31/87, fully depreciated equipment was sold for $10,800 cash, but the sale was not recorded until 1988. There were no other errors during 1986 or 1987 and no corrections have been made for any of the errors. What is the total effect of the errors on the 1987 net income?

    a.   Net income overstated by $30,200.
    b.   Net income overstated by $11,000.
    c.   Net income overstated by $5,800.
    d.   Net income understated by $1,800.

5. Refer to the data of Item 4 above. By how much will Shannon's Unrestricted Fund balance at 12/31/87 be overstated or understated?

    a. $10,200 overstated.
    b. $26,200 overstated.
    c. $4,200 overstated.
    d. $26,200 understated.

6. Refer to the data of Item 4 above. What is the total effect of the errors on Shannon's working capital at 12/31/87?

    a.   Overstated by $4,200.
    b.   Understated by $5,800.
    c.   Understated by $6,000.
    d.   Understated by $9,800.

7. The cumulative effect of a change in depreciation methods is reported

    a.   As a separate line item in income from continuing operations.
    b.   As an extraordinary item.
    c.   Between extraordinary items and net income.
    d.   As a prior period adjustment.

8. Which type of accounting change should always be accounted for in current and future periods only?

    a.   Change in accounting principle.
    b.   Change in reporting entity.
    c.   Change in accounting estimate.
    d.   Correction of an error.

Required. Select the best answer for each of the above multiple-choice items.

PROBLEMS

P1. Sunway Hospital provides you with the following trial balance of revenue and expense accounts prepared at September 30, 1987, the end of its fiscal year:

	Dr.	Cr.
Daily patient services		$4,327
Newborn nursery		155
Operating room		583
Recovery room		54
Delivery room		104
Central supply		224
Emergency room		285
Laboratory		786
Blood bank		145
Radiology		847
Pharmacy		755
Anesthesia		188
Inhalation therapy		79
Physical therapy		121
EKG/EEG		108
Other patient service revenues		114
Charity care	$ 295	
Contractual adjustments	131	
Courtesy discounts and allowances	9	
Provision for doubtful accounts	702	
Education program tuition and fees		124
Rental income		61
Cafeteria sales		274
Telephone		11
Revenue from gift shop		6
Income from vending machines		4
Purchase discounts		23
Miscellaneous other operating revenues		14
Nursing service	1,408	
Nursing education	133	
Operating room	191	
Recovery room	69	
Delivery room	75	
Central supply	55	
Emergency room	121	
Laboratory	366	
Blood bank	22	
Radiology	361	
Pharmacy	70	
Anesthesia	85	
Inhalation therapy	39	

Physical therapy	72
EKG/EEG	31
Medical education	75
Medical records and library	84
Social service	22
Other professional services	52
Dietary	723
Housekeeping	310
Laundry and linen	218
Plant operation	231
Plant maintenance	348
Other general services	30
Fiscal services	607
Administrative services	581
Interest	121
Employee benefits	467
Depreciation	375
General contributions	140
Unrestricted income from Endowment Fund	235
Extraordinary gain	375

Required. Prepare a condensed summary income statement for the year ended September 30, 1987, supported by appropriate schedules in good form. Use the divisional classification illustrated in the text.

P2.   The following account balances were taken from the general ledger of Hartfull Hospital at the end of the 1987 fiscal year:

Unrestricted contributions	$ 28,930
Bad debts	53,790
Cafeteria sales	235,520
General services expenses	763,448
Nursing services revenues	3,565,282
Administrative services expenses (including depreciation and interest)	988,296
Extraordinary loss	12,470
Transfers from restricted funds for research and education	92,000
Other professional services expenses	2,499,194
Charity service (net of specific purpose gifts)	194,920
Fiscal services expenses	355,318
Unrestricted income from endowment fund	41,000
Other professional services revenues	2,738,130
Interest income on unrestricted fund investments	14,850
Contractual adjustments	389,620
Rental income	14,680
Other professional services expenses	972,099
Purchase discounts	23,169

Required. Prepare a 1987 income statement for the Unrestricted Fund of Hartfull Hospital.

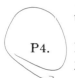

P3. Goodcare Hospital provides you with the following information taken from its Unrestricted Fund accounting records at September 30, 1987, the end of its fiscal year:

Nursing service expense	$134,000
Deductions from revenues	99,000
Income from board-designated investments	7,000
General services expense	108,000
Depreciation expense	12,000
Unrestricted contributions	36,000
Gross patient service revenues	422,000
Fiscal services expense	29,000
Unrestricted income from endowment funds	21,000
Transfers received from specific purpose funds for education and research	23,000
Transfer received from plant replacement and expansion fund for purchase of equipment	52,000
Interest expense	11,000
Unrestricted fund balance, 10/1/86	325,000
Other professional services expense	101,000
Donated equipment	15,000
Other operating revenues	31,000
Prior period adjustment (debit)	14,000
Administrative services expense	22,000

Required. (1) Prepare an income statement for the year ended September 30, 1987. (2) Prepare a statement of changes in the Unrestricted Fund balance for the year ended September 30, 1987.

P4. Baird Hospital provides you with the following information relating to its fiscal year ended December 31, 1987:

Endowment fund balance, 1/1/87	$ 471
Restricted income from investments:	
Specific purpose fund	31
Plant replacement and expansion fund	67
Specific purpose fund balance, 1/1/87	496
Donated equipment	27
Restricted gifts received:	
Specific purpose fund	71
Plant replacement and expansion fund	94
Endowment fund	100
Plant replacement and expansion fund balance, 1/1/87	972

Net income for the year   418
Transfer from plant replacement and
    expansion fund for purchase of plant assets   132
Unrestricted fund balance, 1/1/87   14,703
Loss on sale of investments of plant
    replacement and expansion fund   26
Cumulative effect on prior years of change
    in accounting principle (credit)   34
Transfers from specific purpose fund to
    unrestricted fund for education and research   196
Gain on sale of investments:
    Unrestricted fund   12
    Specific purpose fund   8
    Endowment fund   21
Prior period adjustment for correction of
    accounting error in 1985 (credit)   18
Unrestricted income from investments of endowment fund   37

Required. Prepare an all-funds statement of changes in fund balances for the
year ended 12/31/87.

20
Reporting Financial Position

The financial report of a hypothetical Hartsville Hospital serves as the basis for discussion in this and the immediately preceding chapter. Hartsville Hospital's report consists of the following financial statements:

Exhibit

A	Income Statement
B	Statement of Changes in Fund Balances
C	Balance Sheet
D	Statement of Changes in Financial Position

Exhibits A and B were presented in Chapter 19 where the discussion was directed to the reporting of operating results. In this chapter, Exhibits C and D are presented along with the notes accompanying the hospital's financial statements. The discussion here, however, is concerned mainly with the reporting of financial position. The development of statements of changes in financial position is described and illustrated in Chapter 21. Matters pertaining to the analysis and interpretation of financial statements are dealt with in Chapter 22.

ILLUSTRATIVE BALANCE SHEET

Hartsville Hospital's December 31, 1987, balance sheet is presented as Exhibit C in Figure 20-1. The data are arranged in a vertical or "report" format, with the assets of all funds listed on one page and the liabilities and fund balances listed on a second page. Comparative figures from the prior year (December 31, 1986) are included in the presentation. The notes and supplementary schedules accompanying the hospital's balance sheet are illustrated and discussed at various points throughout this chapter. It should be understood, however, that the notes described here are also relevant to the financial statements illustrated in Chapter 19; the notes are to be considered an integral part of **all** statements included in Hartsville Hospital's financial report. The independent auditor's opinion, as a matter of fact, embraces not only the financial statements but the accompanying notes as well. The two are inseparable.

Figure 20-1.
Hartsville Hospital
Balance Sheet
December 31, 1987 and 1986

	December 31	
	1987	1986

ASSETS

Unrestricted Fund

	1987	1986
Current Assets:		
Cash	$ 268	$ 211
Investments (Note 1)	126	34
Receivables–patients, net of estimated allowances and uncollectibles of $1,007 at December 31,1987, and $987 at December 31,1986 (Note 2)	969	854
Other receivables	42	39
Inventories (Note 3)	296	315
Prepaid expenses	25	29
Total current assets	$ 1,726	$ 1,482
Board-Designated Assets:		
Cash	$ 14	$ 13
Investments (Note 1)	452	429
Total board-designated assets (Note 4)	$ 466	$ 442
Property, Plant and Equipment, net of accumulated depreciation of $4,118 at December 31,1987, and $3,844 at December 31,1986 (Note 5)	$ 8,126	$ 8,185
Other Assets	$ 67	$ 88
Total Unrestricted Fund Assets	$10,385	$10,197

Restricted Funds

	1987	1986
Specific Purpose Fund:		
Cash	$ 2	$ 5
Investments (Note 1)	310	369
Grants receivable	60	
Total Specific Purpose Fund Assets	$ 372	$ 374
Plant Replacement and Expansion Fund:		
Cash	$ 5	$ 8
Investments (Note 1)	763	727
Pledges receivable, net of estimated uncollectibles of $18 at December 31,1987, and $7 at December 31, 1986	127	37
Due from Unrestricted Fund	29	19
Total Plant Replacement and Expansion Fund Assets	$ 924	$ 791
Endowment Fund:		
Cash	$ 34	$ 21
Investments (Note 1)	2,187	1,768
Total Endowment Fund Assets	$ 2,221	$ 1,789

The accompanying notes are an integral part of these financial statements.

Figure 20-1 — *Continued*

	December 31	
	1987	1986
LIABILITIES AND FUND BALANCES		
Unrestricted Fund		
Current Liabilities:		
Current installments of long-term debt (Note 6)	$ 180	$ 180
Notes payable	125	75
Accounts payable	196	202
Accrued expenses payable	238	217
Payroll taxes withheld	81	63
Current advances from third-party payers	75	55
Other current liabilities	42	29
Total current liabilities	$ 937	$ 821
Noncurrent Liabilities:		
Deferred revenues–third-party reimbursement (Note 5)	$ 171	$ 114
Long-term debt–7½% mortgage notes payable, less		
current maturities of $180 (Note 6)	1,320	1,500
Past service pension liability (Note 7)	227	251
Total noncurrent liabilities	$ 1,718	$ 1,865
Total liabilities	$ 2,655	$ 2,686
Unrestricted Fund Balance (Note 8)	7,730	7,511
Total Unrestricted Fund Liabilities and Fund Balance	$10,385	$10,197
Restricted Funds		
Specific Purpose Fund:		
Due to Unrestricted Fund	$ 14	$ 9
Fund balances		
Charity care	$ 108	$ 97
Education and research	213	242
Other	37	26
Total fund balances	$ 358	$ 365
Total Specific Purpose Fund Liabilities and Fund Balances	$ 372	$ 374
Plant Replacement and Expansion Fund:		
Fund balance–restricted by third-party payers	$ 613	$ 568
Fund balance–restricted by others	311	223
Total Plant Replacement and Expansion Fund Liabilities		
and Fund Balances	$ 924	$ 791
Endowment Fund:		
Fund balance—permanent endowments	$ 1,271	$ 939
Fund balance–term endowments	950	850
Total Endowment Fund Liabilities and Fund Balances	$ 2,221	$ 1,789

The accompanying notes are an integral part of these financial statements.

An alternative arrangement of Hartsville Hospital's balance sheet is illustrated in Figure 20-2. This arrangement, regarded by some accountants as preferable to the "report" form, is the horizontal or "account" format. As can be seen in the illustration provided, the assets (debits) are shown on the left side of the statement and are "balanced" against the total of liabilities and fund balances (credits) appearing on the right-hand side. Facing pages may be used where the amount of data involved is excessive for clear presentation on a single page.

Figure 20-2.
Hartsville Hospital
Balance Sheet
December 31, 1987　　　　　　　　　　　　　　　Exhibit C

ASSETS

UNRESTRICTED FUND		
Current Assets:		
Cash		$　268
Investments (Note 1)		126
Receivables–patients (Note 2)	$ 1,976	
Less estimated allowances and uncollectibles	1,007	969
Other receivables		42
Inventories (Note 3)		296
Prepaid expenses		25
Total current assets		$ 1,726
Board-Designated Assets:		
Cash	$　14	
Investments (Note 1)	452	
Total board–designated assets (Note 4)		466
Property, Plant and Equipment (Note 5)	$12,244	
Less accumulated depreciation	4,118	
Net property plant and equipment		8,126
Other Assets		67
Total Unrestricted Fund Assets		$10,385
RESTRICTED FUNDS		
Specific Purpose Fund:		
Cash	$　2	
Investments (Note 1)	310	
Grants receivable	60	
Total Specific Purpose Fund Assets		$　372
Plant Replacement and Expansion Fund:		
Cash	$　5	
Investments (Note 1)	763	
Pledges receivable, net of estimated uncollectibles of $18	127	
Due from Unrestricted Fund	29	
Total Plant Replacement and Expansion Fund Assets		$　924
Endowment Fund:		
Cash	$　34	
Investments (Note 1)	2,187	
Total Endowment Fund Assets		$ 2,221

Figure 20-2—*Continued*

LIABILITIES AND FUND BALANCES

Current Liabilities:

Current installments of long-term debt (Note 6)	$ 180	
Notes payable	125	
Accounts payable	196	
Accrued expenses payable	238	
Payroll taxes withheld	81	
Current advances from third-party payers	75	
Other current liabilities	42	
Total current liabilities		$ 937

Noncurrent Liabilities:

Deferred revenues—third-party reimbursement (Note 5)	$ 171	
Long-term debt—7½% mortgage notes payable, less current maturities of $180 (Note 6)	1,320	
Past service pension liability (Note 7)	227	
Total noncurrent liabilities		1,718
Total liabilities		$ 2,655
Unrestricted Fund Balance (Note 8)		7,730
Total Unrestricted Fund Liabilities and Fund Balance		$10,385

Specific Purpose Fund:

Due to Unrestricted Fund		$ 14
Fund balances		
Charity care	$ 108	
Education and research	213	
Other	37	358
Total Specific Purpose Fund Liabilities and Fund Balances		$ 372

Plant Replacement and Expansion Fund:

Fund balance—restricted by third-party payers	$ 613	
Fund balance—restricted by others	311	
Total Plant Replacement and Expansion Fund Liabilities and Fund Balances		$ 924

Endowment Fund:

Fund balance—permanent endowments	$ 1,271	
Fund balance—term endowments	950	
Total Endowment Fund Liabilities and Fund Balances		$ 2,221

The accompanying notes are an integral part of these financial statements.

Balance sheets, sometimes called statements of financial position or condition, present the financial status of a hospital enterprise in terms of its resources, obligations, and residual ownership equities (fund balances) at given points in time. These statements may be regarded as snapshot photographs of resource-and-obligation situations existing at specified moments in the economic life of the hospital. It is for this reason that

Hartsville Hospital's balance sheet is dated December 31, 1987. The amounts appearing in the statement are applicable only to that particular date. Most of the account balances were different figures on December 30, and a majority of them probably changed to other amounts on January 1 of the following year.

Seventy years ago, the balance sheet was regarded as the primary financial statement. Experience has shown, however, that the long-run viability of economic enterprises and the performance of their managements are best judged on a continuing basis in terms of operating results. While today's balance sheet therefore is considered of secondary importance to the income statement, it is not correct to conclude that the balance sheet is unimportant or without utility. The balance sheet, in providing information concerning assets and liabilities, has many important uses of its own. It reflects short-run solvency for credit purposes, indicates the pattern of resource allocations and choice of financing method by management, reveals commitments that must be met in the future, and otherwise serves as a useful complement to the information provided in income statements. Also, it should be observed that the reduction of the balance sheet to a position of secondary importance is not nearly so pronounced in hospital accounting as it has been in accounting for profit-seeking enterprises. In hospital accounting, considerably more attention is given to accountability and stewardship concerns.

Underlying the financial information presented in the balance sheet are a number of basic assumptions and accounting concepts discussed at length in Chapter 2. The hospital, for example, is considered to be an **accounting entity**, a **going concern**, whose **resources** and **obligations** are measured in terms of **money**, largely on a **historical cost valuation** basis, and reported on the **accrual basis** in conformity with generally accepted accounting principles. **Consistency, conservatism, realization, matching, periodicity**, and **materiality** also have important implications for balance sheet presentations.

The major objective of the balance sheet is to supply the reader with information concerning assets, liabilities, and fund balances that is relevant to the making of rational decisions based upon such data. In view of this objective, the significance of the balance sheet is dependent upon a full disclosure of all **material** information essential to its proper interpretation. Account titles should provide a complete and clearly worded description of each item in the statement. Asset valuation bases should be disclosed. If differing acceptable accounting methods are available, those employed should be indicated. Appropriate details of condensed data within the balance sheet should be provided in supplementary schedules. Accounting changes and their effects should be adequately described. Disclosure of significant events occurring subsequent to the balance sheet date and necessary to a proper evaluation of the hospital's current financial position is also necessary. The requirements of full disclosure can be implemented through clear account descriptions and classifications, informative parenthetical notations in the body of the statement, and in explanatory notes or supplementary schedules.

ELEMENTS OF THE BALANCE SHEET

The basic elements of the balance sheet are assets, liabilities, and equity (fund balances). Definitions of these elements were provided in Chapter 2 as follows:

1.   **Assets:** probable future economic benefits obtained or controlled by a hospital as a result of past transactions.
2.   **Liabilities:** probable future sacrifices of economic benefits arising from present obligations of a hospital to transfer assets or provide services to other entities in the future as a result of past transactions or events.
3.   **Equity:** the residual interest in the assets of a hospital that remains after deducting its liabilities.

The equity of a not-for-profit hospital is represented by accounts called "fund balances." In an investor-owned hospital, the equity is the ownership interest.

The relationship among these three elements of financial position is expressed in the equation: assets = liabilities + fund balances. This equality is the basic formula for the hospital balance sheet.

In addition to assets that may be employed in any manner desired by the governing board, a hospital is also likely to have donated assets whose use is subject to donors' restrictions. The resulting responsibilities of stewardship and the related requirements of accountability give rise to the need for **fund accounting**. As explained in Chapter 4, this involves the segregation of hospital assets, and the related liabilities, into independent subordinate entities, or **funds**, according to legal and other restrictions on their use. The difference between the assets and liabilities of each fund is referred to as the **fund balance**.

As many as four different types of funds may be necessary to provide for a proper accounting and for the reporting of a hospital's financial position. Hartsville Hospital, for example, maintains an Unrestricted Fund and three restricted funds as follows:

1.   **Unrestricted Fund.** This fund includes all of the hospital's resources, and related obligations, not restricted to particular purposes by donors or other external authorities. All of the assets of this fund are available for the financing of general operating activities at the discretion of the governing board.
2.   **Restricted Funds.** These funds include all hospital resources whose use is restricted to particular purposes by donors and other external authorities. The assets of these funds are not currently available for the financing of general operating activities.
     a.   **Specific Purpose Fund.** This fund includes all hospital resources restricted by donors to the financing of charity care, education, research, and other purposes, excluding plant asset acquisitions and endowments.
     b.   **Plant Replacement and Expansion Fund.** This fund includes all hospital resources restricted by donors and third-party payers to the acquisition of plant assets. Investments in plant assets and the liabilities related to such investments, however, are reported as Unrestricted Fund assets and liabilities.
     c.   **Endowment Fund.** This fund includes all donated resources which, by donor restriction, are to be held intact for the production of income.

Each of these funds is self-balancing in terms of the equation mentioned above. This equality of each fund's total assets with the total of its liabilities and balance is the derivation of the term **balance sheet.**

Assets

In accordance with the principles of fund accounting, Hartsville Hospital's assets are segregated by funds in its balance sheet as illustrated in Figures 20-1 and 20-2. Each of the major asset categories are discussed briefly below; detailed treatment was given to these matters in Chapters 10 through 18.

Cash. As indicated in Chapter 10, cash includes petty cash and change funds, cash in banks, and undeposited cash on hand, but these details need not be presented in the balance sheet intended for external users. Amounts of Unrestricted Fund cash set aside by the governing board for noncurrent uses (purchase of plant assets or long-term investments, for example) may be excluded from the "current" classification. Hartsville Hospital, for instance, has $14 of Unrestricted Fund cash so classified at December 31, 1987. Amounts shown as cash in the hospital balance sheet should be the actual cash balances as determined by bank reconciliations and actual counts.

Investments. As is the case with Hartsville Hospital, the assets of each fund maintained by a hospital usually will include investments in securities of one kind or another. The investments of Hartsville Hospital's Unrestricted Fund consist of highly marketable, temporary investments of $126 and $452 of long-term investments. The former appear in the current asset section; the latter are in the board-designated asset classification. Investments of restricted funds may be either short-term or long-term, but the tendency is toward a long-term investments policy in these funds. Short-term investments were described in Chapter 10, and long-term investments were dealt with at length in Chapter 15.

Balance sheet reporting of investments requires disclosure of the basis of valuation. As explained earlier, short-term investments usually are carried at cost, or at the lower of cost or market. The short-term investments included in the current assets section of Hartsville Hospital's Unrestricted Fund, for example, might have been reported as follows:

Investments, valued at the lower of
    cost or market ($128) $ 126

An acceptable alternative in this situation would be:

Investments, at cost (which approximates
    market) $ 126

Short-term investments in marketable equity securities, as indicated in Chapter 10, should be reported at the lower of aggregate cost or market.

As discussed in Chapter 15, long-term investments in marketable equity securities are carried at the lower of aggregate cost or market; long-term investments in debt securities are stated at cost. In the case of investments in bonds, "cost" is adjusted for the amortization of bond discount or premium, if any.

An increasing number of accountants favor the valuation of investments in securities at current market values. This procedure has some merit, but it is not yet a generally accepted practice for hospitals. A widely employed and desirable alternative, however, is the supplementary disclosure of market values. Hartsville Hospital does this in Note 1, which reads as follows:

Note 1. All investments are stated in the balance sheet at cost. For each classi-fication of investments, current market value is higher than cost. The aggregate costs and market values of investments at December 31, 1987, are summarized below:

	Cost	Market Value
Unrestricted Fund:		
Current	$ 126	$ 128
Board-Designated	452	477
Specific Purpose Fund	310	316
Plant Replacement and Expansion Fund	763	805
Endowment Fund	2,187	2,314

If desired, additional information may be provided as to the major types of investment securities held, interest and dividend rates, and current yields. Details of this kind, however, usually are found only in reports prepared for internal management purposes.

Receivables. The receivables reported in Hartsville Hospital's Unrestricted Fund include $969 (net) due from patients and their sponsors. Another $42 of receivables apparently represents amounts due from employees, suppliers, restricted funds, and other miscellaneous sources. If these "other" receivables were significant, material individual sources and amounts would be disclosed. In addition to receivables of the Unrestricted Fund, Hartsville Hospital's balance sheet also includes $60 of grants receivable in the Specific Purpose Fund and $127 of pledges receivable in the Plant Replacement and Expansion Fund. All receivables should be reported at estimated realizable values (see Chapter 11).

Details pertaining to the receivables arising from patient services often are supplied in a footnote or supplementary schedule to the balance sheet. The type and amount of detail varies, but a breakdown of receivables according to source of payment may be very useful. Hartsville Hospital provides such detail in Note 2, as follows:

Note 2. Receivables in all funds are stated in the balance sheet at estimated realizable values. The December 31, 1987, receivables from patient services reported in the Unrestricted Fund are summarized by payer category below:

Governmental Agencies	$ 720
Blue Cross	336
Commercial and Independent Insurers	384
Self-Pay Accounts	396
Charity	140
Total	1,976
Less Allowances for Charity Care, Contractual Adjustments, and Uncollectibles	1,007
Net Receivables	$ 969

Revenues received under reimbursement agreements totaling $4,750 for the current year and $3,920 for the prior year are subject to audit and retroactive adjustment by third-party payers. Provisions for estimated retroactive adjustments under these agreements have been provided.

This note might also include disclosure of the totals of each category of the $1,007 of allowances. A brief statement of the hospital's collection and write-off policies could also be useful to readers. The note should also comment on any "open" prior years subject to audit and retroactive adjustments by third-party payers.

A question may sometimes arise as to the propriety of offsetting advances from third-party payers against receivables from patients. The offsetting of assets and liabilities in the balance sheet, except in rare circumstances, is not permissible in terms of generally accepted accounting principles. As may be seen in Hartsville Hospital's balance sheet, $75 of current advances from third-party payers is reported among the current liabilities of the Unrestricted Fund. In some cases, such advances may properly be reported as noncurrent liabilities, but they generally should not be shown as a reduction of receivables.

Inventories. The presentation of inventories for external reporting purposes must include a disclosure of the inventory valuation method. Additional details, if material, may be provided concerning major categories of inventory, significant changes with respect to sources of supply, and other matters essential to a full disclosure of the hospital's inventory position. Hartsville Hospital presents supplementary inventory information in Note 3, as follows:

Note 3. Inventories are stated in the balance sheet at the lower of cost or market. Cost is determined principally by the first-in, first-out method. The December 31, 1987, inventories are summarized below:

Medical and Surgical Supplies	$ 95
Foodstuffs and Other Dietary Supplies	39
Drugs and Pharmaceuticals	86
Fuel and Other Supplies	76
Total	$296

Considerably more detail would be provided in reports intended for internal management purposes (see Chapters 12 and 14).

Prepaid Expenses. The current assets section of the Unrestricted Fund in Hartsville Hospital's balance sheet reports $25 of prepaid expenses at December 31, 1987. These assets usually arise from prepayments of insurance, interest, rent, and other expense items. If such prepayments are for periods longer than one year, they properly are included in the "other assets" classification in the Unrestricted Fund. Accounting procedures for prepaid expenses were discussed in Chapters 3 and 12.

Board-Designated Assets. As discussed in Chapter 4, hospital governing boards may designate or earmark certain otherwise unrestricted resources for various purposes. These resources, however, should **not** be reported as a part of the hospital's restricted funds but are segregated within the Unrestricted Fund as illustrated in Figure 20-1. The principle of full disclosure requires a supplementary explanation of the purpose of such designations. This information is provided by Hartsville Hospital in Note 4, as follows:

Note 4. The total Unrestricted Fund assets of $10,385 at December 31, 1987, are not subject to any restrictions by donors or other external authorities. Of these unrestricted assets, however, resources of $466 have been designated by the hospital's governing board for renovation and replacement of plant facilities. The board-designated resources are excluded from current assets because they are not expected to be expended during the coming year.

The important point is that board-designated assets carry no legal restrictions as donor-restricted funds do. Board actions can be rescinded whereas donor restrictions can be changed only by approval of the donor or by the court. Board-designated assets therefore should not be commingled with donor-restricted funds.

Property, Plant, and Equipment. The "property, plant, and equipment" asset caption in the Unrestricted Fund reflects the hospital's actual investment in physical resources and facilities used in regular operations. These assets are not reported in a restricted fund classification as this would imply restrictions upon their use or disposition which do not ordinarily exist. If such restrictions should exist, however, those restrictions should be disclosed.

In addition to the required disclosures of the basis of valuation and depreciation method employed for plant assets, an analysis may be provided to show the amounts invested in plant assets by major categories. This information is supplied by Hartsville Hospital in Note 5, as follows:

Note 5. Property, plant, and equipment is stated in the balance sheet at cost. A summary of the accounts and the related accumulated depreciation at December 31, 1987, follows:

	Cost	Accumulated Depreciation	Book Value
Land	$ 421		$ 421
Land Improvements	236	$ 104	132
Buildings and Fixed Equipment	7,952	2,783	5,169
Major Movable Equipment	3,635	1,231	2,404
Totals	$12,244	$ 4,118	$8,126

Depreciation is determined on a straight-line basis for financial reporting purposes. The hospital uses an accelerated depreciation method to determine reimbursable costs under certain third-party reimbursement agreements. Cost reimbursement revenue in the amount of $171, resulting from the difference in depreciation methods, is deferred in the current year and will be taken into income in future years.

Plant asset accounting procedures, depreciation methods, and deferrals of third-party reimbursement revenues related to depreciation methods are discussed fully in Chapter 16.

Liabilities

As with its assets, Hartsville Hospital's liabilities are segregated by funds in its balance sheet illustrated in Figure 20-1. An extended discussion of hospital liabilities appears in Chapters 13, 17, and 18, but certain essential points are repeated below.

Unrestricted Fund. Most of the hospital's liabilities are reported in its Unrestricted Fund in that a substantial majority of such obligations are liquidated by the use of unrestricted resources. These liabilities are presented in two balance sheet classifications: "current liabilities" and "noncurrent liabilities." As explained in Chapter 13, current liabilities are those obligations whose liquidation is reasonably expected to require the use of existing resources properly classifiable as current assets, or the creation of other current liabilities, usually within one year from the balance sheet date. The noncurrent classification, sometimes called **long-term debt**, includes all other liabilities of the Unrestricted Fund.

Hartsville Hospital's balance sheet provides what may be regarded as a typical listing of items in the current liability classification. The noncurrent liabilities consist of the deferred revenues mentioned above in Note 5, mortgage notes payable, and a liability arising from the hospital's pension plan. Disclosures relating to the latter two items are made in Notes 6 and 7 accompanying the financial statements. These notes are reproduced below:

> **Note 6.** The mortgage notes are payable in quarterly installments of $45 with interest at 12.25% through March 31, 1996, and are collateralized by land, buildings, and equipment carried at $2,750. Current maturities of $180, payable in 1988, are included in current liabilities at December 31, 1987.

> **Note 7.** The hospital has a noncontributory pension plan covering substantially all employees. Total pension plan expense for 1987 was $97, which includes amortization of prior service cost over a period of 20 years. The hospital's policy is to fund pension costs accrued. The actuarially computed value of vested benefits at December 31, 1987, exceeds net assets of the pension fund and balance sheet accruals by approximately $320.

Accounting procedures and other matters relating to mortgage notes, pension plan liabilities, leases, and other long-term debts were discussed in Chapters 17 and 18.

Only in unusual cases would liabilities of major significance exist in the restricted funds. Hartsville Hospital, for example, reports a Specific Purpose Fund liability only. This is a nominal amount due to the Unrestricted Fund, and no liabilities of any type appear in the other restricted funds.

Fund Balances

The excess of the assets over the liabilities reported in each fund is referred to as the **fund balance**. Detailed consideration was given to accounting procedures relative to fund balances in Chapters 4 and 19. As indicated there, accounting methods may be employed to permit a disclosure of the **composition** of each fund balance in the financial statements. This information may be desired with respect to the Unrestricted Fund; it is generally essential in connection with the restricted funds.

The composition of the Unrestricted Fund Balance may be determined and represented in a **statement of income and changes in unrestricted fund balance** as was illustrated for Hartsville Hospital in Figure 19-10 in the preceding chapter. Alternatively, this information can be provided in a footnote to the balance sheet. Hartsville Hospital does this in Note 8, as follows:

Note 8. The composition of the Unrestricted Fund Balance at December 31, 1987, is indicated below:

Operations	$ 205
Property, Plant and Equipment	6,806
Other Board-Designations	719
Total Unrestricted Fund Balance	$7,730

While presentation of the details of internal designations may have some external significance, the most important disclosure is a very clear presentation of the $7,730 total of net unrestricted resources.

The composition of the restricted fund balances, on the other hand, is a matter of more importance to users of hospital financial statements. For this reason, the balance of each restricted fund usually should be reported in meaningful subfund groupings. As illustrated in Figure 20-1, Hartsville Hospital provides a breakdown of restricted fund balances as follows:

1. The Specific Purpose Fund balance is classified according to the nature of donors' restrictions, i.e., charity care, education, research, and other.
2. The Plant Replacement and Expansion Fund balance is classified by donor category, i.e., third-party reimbursement agencies and others.
3. The Endowment Fund balance is classified according to the type of endowment, i.e., permanent or term.

In addition to these disclosures, a **statement of changes in fund balances**, as illustrated in Figure 19-8 in the preceding chapter, should be regarded as a basic requirement of external financial reporting by hospitals.

STATEMENT OF CHANGES IN FINANCIAL POSITION

The **income statement** presents the results of hospital operations in terms of revenues earned and expenses incurred during a given time period. A **balance sheet** presents the hospital's financial position in terms of the assets, liabilities, and fund balances existing at a given point in time. The **statement of changes in fund balances** provides a comprehensive summary of the factors causing increases and decreases in the amounts of individual fund balances over a given period of time. For many years, these three financial statements were generally considered to be sufficient for the purposes of external financial reporting by hospitals.

In 1971, however, the Accounting Principles Board recognized the **statement of changes in financial position** as a fourth statement that should be required in fully reporting the financial activities and affairs of an economic enterprise.[1]   This position subsequently was affirmed and specifically made applicable to hospital financial reporting by the AICPA Subcommittee on Health Care Matters.[2]

Illustrative "Funds" Statement

An illustrative statement of changes in financial position for Hartsville Hospital for the year ended December 31, 1987, is presented as Exhibit D in Figure 20-3. This statement has variously been referred to as the "statement of sources and applications of funds," the "statement of resources provided and applied," or simply the "fund statement." To simplify references to this statement in the following discussion, the term **funds statement** will be used. The technically correct name specified by the AICPA, however, is the **statement of changes in financial position**, and that title should be employed in hospital financial reports.

The utility of financial presentations is greatly enhanced by the provision of comparative data. This has been done with respect to the funds statement illustrated in Figure 20-3. It should be pointed out, however, that the derivation of many of the figures cannot be ascertained from the information supplied in this and the immediately preceding chapter.

Nature of the Statement

The three financial statements previously discussed obviously provide much essential information concerning the operating results and financial position of the hospital. Certain important changes in financial position and certain vital aspects of the financing and investing activities of the hospital, however, are not always disclosed by or clearly apparent from an examination of such statements. Consider, for example, the following item appearing in comparative balance sheets.

	December 31	
	1987	1986
Property, plant and equipment (cost)	$4,500	$4,000

It might be concluded from this presentation that new plant assets costing $500 were acquired during 1987. The fact of the matter, however, may be that plant asset additions amounted to $825 while plant assets which had cost $325 were disposed of during the year. These events, and similar offsetting activities in other financial position accounts, ordinarily are not determinable from the information supplied in the three financial statements previously discussed. It is important that such "hidden" information be clearly disclosed.

The purpose of the funds statement therefore is to provide a summary of all operations and all financing and investing activities of the hospital. In this way, it accounts for **all** changes in financial position as reported in successive balance sheets. Although the funds statement is closely related to the other financial statements, it should not be regarded in any sense as a duplication or substitution for them.

Figure 20-3.
Hartsville Hospital
Statement of Changes in Financial Position – Unrestricted Fund
Years Ended December 31, 1987 and 1986   Exhibit D

	1987	1986
Funds Provided by:		
Net operating income (loss)	$ 20	$(191)
Add (deduct) items included in operations not requiring (providing) funds:		
Provision for depreciation	360	342
Increase in deferred revenues–third-party reimbursement	57	29
Revenues restricted to plant asset acquisitions transferred to Plant Replacement and Expansion Fund	(140)	(115)
Funds derived from operations	$297	$ 65
Add nonoperating revenues	224	176
Funds derived from operations and nonoperating revenues	$521	$ 241
Property, plant and equipment expenditures financed by Plant Replacement and Expansion Fund	95	45
Donation of medical equipment	20	..
Decrease in other assets	21	13
Total funds provided	$657	$ 299
Funds Applied to:		
Increase in board-designated assets	$ 24	$ (10)
Purchase of property, plant and equipment	281	59
Addition of medical equipment by donation	20	..
Reduction of long-term debt	180	180
Decrease in past service pension liability	24	24
Increase in working capital (see schedule below)	128	46
Total funds applied	$657	$ 299

Changes in Working Capital

	1987	1986
Increases (decreases) in Current Assets:		
Cash	$ 57	$ (14)
Investments	92	81
Receivables–patients (net)	115	98
Other receivables	3	(6)
Inventories	(19)	35
Prepaid expenses	(4)	(11)
Net increase in current assets	$244	$183
Increases (decreases) in Current Liabilities:		
Current installments of long-term debt	$ ..	$ ..
Notes payable	50	75
Accounts payable	(6)	37
Accrued expenses payable	21	(14)
Payroll taxes withheld	18	9
Advances from third-party payers	20	40
Other current liabilities	13	(10)
Net increase in current liabilities	$116	$137
Increase in working capital	$128	$ 46

The accompanying notes are an integral part of these financial statements.

The funds statement has a long history of use for internal management purposes. It is "new" only in the sense that recently it has become a regularly required external financial report. The statement's utility arises from its presentation of the sources and amounts of resources that were available to the hospital in the past, and the uses that were made of such resources. In summarizing the hospital's investing and financing operations, the information in the statement has important implications for prospective creditors, reimbursement agencies, and other external groups as well as for internal managerial decisions. It can be used in estimating the funds that will be generated in the future and the growth potential of the hospital in terms of its ability to finance expansion and meet added indebtedness. The statement is most useful, of course, when presented in comparative form for two or more years. For managerial purposes, consideration should also be given to the development of a funds statement based upon budgeted data.

It should be carefully noted that the term **funds** has been defined in several ways for purposes of the funds statement. In its narrowest sense, funds may be used simply to denote cash. Others have defined funds as the total of cash and temporary investments, or all monetary assets, or net monetary assets. In the context of the funds statement described here, however, a broadened working capital concept of funds is assumed. In other words, funds means **working capital** (the excess of current assets over current liabilities of the hospital's Unrestricted Fund), **except** that **exchanges** and certain types of **gifts** are reported in the funds statement as both funds provided and funds applied.[3] This view of funds, referred to as the **all financial resources** concept, is preferred according to APB Opinion No. 19 and is widely employed in actual practice.

Preparation of the Statement

The following chapter illustrates the mechanics involved in the preparation of the funds statement under the all financial resources concept. In some cases, the statement can be developed from a relatively simple analysis of the changes in the noncurrent asset, noncurrent liability, and fund balance accounts of the hospital's Unrestricted Fund; complex situations sometimes require the use of special worksheets. Readers who desire to pursue the details of preparing the statement of changes in financial position should refer to Chapter 21.

An analysis of the changes in the noncurrent asset, noncurrent liability, and fund balance accounts provides the information necessary for preparation of the funds statement. First, however, one must be able to identify the changes as being either sources or applications of funds.

The formula for identification of the elements entering into the funds statement may be derived as follows:

1. $A = L + FB$. This is the basic accounting equation upon which the balance sheet rests, i.e., assets = liabilities + fund balance.
2. $CA + NCA = CL + NCL + FB$. This simply is an expansion of the above equation by substitution of CA (current assets) and NCA (noncurrent assets) for A (assets) and, similarly, CL (current liabilities) and NCL (noncurrent liabilities) for L (liabilities).
3. $CA + NCA - CL = NCL + FB$. Here, current liabilities (CL) have been subtracted from each side of equation 2.

4. $CA - CL = NCL + FB - NCA$. Now, noncurrent assets (NCA) have been subtracted from each side of equation 3.

Since $CA - CL$ is working capital or funds, equation 4 is the formula for the funds statement, i.e., funds $= NCL + FB - NCA$.

Given this formula, it follows that an increase in funds occurs when the **value** of the right-hand side of the equation increases. It also may be said that a decrease in funds occurs when the **value** of the right-hand side of the equation decreases. To summarize:

1.   **Sources of funds:**
   a.   **Increases in NCL.** Increases in noncurrent liability accounts are sources of funds, e.g., the issue of mortgage notes or the sale of bonds.
   b.   **Increases in FB.** Increases in the fund balance are sources of funds, e.g., net operating income or transfers of resources from the Plant Replacement and Expansion Fund for financing of plant asset acquisitions.
   c.   **Decreases in NCA.** Decreases in noncurrent asset accounts are sources of funds, e.g., the sale of long-term investments or the sale of plant assets.
2.   **Applications of funds:**
   a.   **Decreases in NCL.** Decreases in noncurrent liability accounts are applications of funds, e.g., the repayment of mortgage notes and other reductions of long-term debt.
   b.   **Decreases in FB.** Decreases in the fund balance are applications of funds, e.g., net operating losses.
   c.   **Increases in NCA.** Increases in noncurrent asset accounts are applications of funds, e.g., purchase of long-term investments or acquisition of new plant assets.

Thus, the "funds equation" may be used as an analytical tool for the identification of changes in noncurrent accounts, including the fund balance, as sources or applications of funds. This also may be done with a special worksheet as illustrated and discussed in the next chapter.

HOSPITAL-RELATED ORGANIZATIONS

Hospitals have long been assisted by auxiliaries, guilds, and similar organizations that are separate entities but often are closely related to the hospitals they serve. In recent years, there has been a trend toward the formation of foundations to raise and hold resources for hospitals. Differing reporting practices have been observed with respect to related organizations of these types. Some practices combine the financial statements of the related organizations with those of the hospital; others do not combine them. The AICPA Subcommittee on Health Care Matters therefore issued a Statement of Position (an amendment to the **Hospital Audit Guide**) in an attempt to resolve the problems of reporting the hospital's relationships with these separate organizations.[4]

Statement of Position No. 81-2 provides that a separate not-for-profit organization is considered to be "related" to a not-for-profit hospital if either of the following conditions exist:

1. The hospital controls the separate organization through contracts and other legal documents that give the hospital authority to direct the separate organization's activities, management, and policies.
2. The hospital is for all practical purposes the sole beneficiary of the separate organization. The hospital should be considered the organization's sole beneficiary if any one of the following three conditions exist:
   a. The separate organization has solicited funds in the name of the hospital, and with the expressed or implied approval of the hospital, and substantially all the funds solicited were intended by the contributor, or were otherwise required, to be transferred to the hospital or used at its discretion or direction.
   b. The hospital has transferred some of its resources to the separate organization, and substantially all the organization's resources are held for the benefit of the hospital.
   c. The hospital has assigned certain of its functions (such as the operation of a dormitory) to the separate organization, which is operating primarily for the benefit of the hospital.

If the hospital controls the separate organization and is its sole beneficiary, the financial statements of the hospital and the related organization may be consolidated or combined in accordance with Accounting Research Bulletin No. 51.[5] Such financial statements sometimes may be necessary for a fair and meaningful presentation of the financial position and operating results of the hospital and the related organization as a single economic unit.

If consolidated financial statements are deemed appropriate, the hospital should follow normal consolidation accounting procedures and should disclose the basis of consolidation in its summary of significant accounting policies as required by APB Opinion No. 22 (see the next section of this chapter). Where combined (rather than consolidated) financial statements are appropriate, the practice generally considered preferable involves presenting the financial statement items of the related organization as a separate restricted fund in the hospital's financial statements. In other words, (1) the balance sheet accounts of the related organization are reported in a separate restricted fund in the hospital's balance sheet, and (2) the income statement accounts of the related organization are reported as a separate restricted fund in the hospital's statement of changes in fund balances.

Under this procedure, the hospital's income statement would be unaffected except to the extent that the related organization makes unrestricted resources available to the hospital during the reporting period. The amounts of such resources should be reported on an accrual basis as nonoperating revenue in the hospital's income statement. Restricted resources made available to the hospital should be accounted for on an accrual basis in accordance with the terms prescribed by the related organization, that is, as resources of the appropriate restricted fund of the hospital.

Statement of Position No. 81-2, however, applies primarily to situations in which the consolidation or combination of financial statements is not appropriate. It states that where the hospital controls the separate organization and is its sole beneficiary, but where the financial statements of the hospital and the related organization are not consolidated or combined, the hospital should do the following: (1) disclose summarized financial information about the related organization in the notes to the hospital's financial statements, and (2) clearly describe the nature of the relationships between the hospital and the related organization.

The following also may occur: (1) the hospital controls the separate organization but is not its sole beneficiary; (2) the hospital does not control the separate organization but is its sole beneficiary; or (3) the hospital does not control the separate organization and is not its sole beneficiary, but the separate organization holds material amounts of resources for the benefit of the hospital or there have been material transactions between the hospital and the separate organization. In such situations, the hospital's financial statements should disclose the existence and nature of the relationship between the hospital and the separate organization. In addition, with respect to material transactions, the hospital's financial statements should disclose the following:

1. A description of the transactions — summarized, if appropriate — for the period reported on, including amounts, if any, and any other information deemed necessary to an understanding of the effects on the hospital's financial statements.
2. The dollar volume of transactions and the effects of any changes in the terms from the preceding period.
3. Amounts due from or to the separate organization, and, if not otherwise apparent, the terms and manner of settlement.

Illustrations of the required disclosures may be found in the AICPA's Statement of Position No. 81-2 and in the author's **External and Internal Reporting by Hospitals.**[6]

DISCLOSURE OF ACCOUNTING POLICIES

In its Opinion No. 22, the Accounting Principles Board concluded that information concerning the major accounting policies of not-for-profit as well as profit-seeking entities is essential for financial statement users.[7] The reporting hospital therefore describes all significant and pertinent accounting policies it has adopted and followed with respect to its presentation of operating results, financial position, and changes in financial position. These disclosures should be considered as an integral part of the financial statements.

The disclosure of accounting policies should identify and describe briefly the accounting principles followed by the hospital as well as the methods of applying them. This is particularly necessary where any of the following are involved:[8]

1. A selection has been made from existing acceptable alternatives;
2. Principles and methods have been used that are peculiar to the industry in which the reporting entity operates, even if such principles and methods are predominantly followed in that industry; and
3. Unusual or innovative applications have been made of generally accepted accounting principles (and, as applicable, of principles and methods peculiar to the industry in which the reporting entity operates).

Usually, the necessary disclosures are given in a separate "Summary of Significant Accounting Policies" preceding the notes to the hospital's financial statements or as the initial note.

To illustrate the requirements of APB Opinion No. 22 and the presentation of notes to accompany financial statements, hypothetical Hartsville Hospital is again used as an example. The notes accompanying Hartsville Hospital's financial statements, which were discussed at various earlier points in this chapter, are now summarized in Figure 20-4, following a statement of accounting policies. It is important to understand that disclosures are preferably made in the body of the financial statement itself; footnotes are employed where disclosures in the body of the statement would be cumbersome or impractical.

Figure 20-4.
Hartsville Hospital
Accounting Policies and Notes Accompanying Financial Statements
Year Ended December 31, 1987

SUMMARY OF SIGNIFICANT ACCOUNTING POLICIES

A summary of significant accounting policies and principles followed by Hartsville Hospital is presented below to assist the reader in evaluating the financial statements and other data in this report. Additional information is included in the notes accompanying the financial statements.

Basis of Financial Reporting

The financial statements for the year ended December 31, 1987, have been prepared on the accrual basis and in accordance with guidelines recommended by the Subcommittee on Health Care Matters of the American Institute of Certified Public Accountants. These guidelines in general provide that assets, liabilities, and related revenues and expenses be segregated into unrestricted and restricted funds. Unrestricted funds include general operating and other hospital-designated funds and gifts, grants, and bequests that are not donor-restricted. Restricted funds include gifts, grants, and bequests, and other resources, that are restricted as to their use by donors and other external entities.

Investments

Investments held by the hospital, and described in Note 1, are stated in the balance sheet at cost. Certain endowment funds held in trust by banks are not included in the balance sheet. The principal balance of those resources held in trust at December 31, 1987, amounted to $140,000 at cost (quoted market value, $182,000). Income from these resources is recorded by the hospital when received and used to cover expenditures of the hospital as specified by the terms of the trust agreement.

Receivables

Receivables, described in Note 2, are stated in the balance sheet at estimated realizable values after provision for uncollectible amounts.

Figure 20-4 — *Continued*

Inventories

Inventories, described in Note 3, are stated in the balance sheet at the lower of cost or market. Cost is determined principally by the first-in, first-out method.

Board-Designated Assets

Board-designated assets, described in Note 4, consist of unrestricted resources that have been designated by the hospital's governing board for the renovation and replacement of certain plant facilities.

Property, Plant, and Equipment

Property, plant, and equipment, described in Note 5, is stated in the balance sheet at cost, except for donated assets which are recorded at fair value when received.

Depreciation

Depreciation of property, plant, and equipment is determined on the basis of the straight-line method for financial reporting purposes. The hospital uses an accelerated depreciation method to determine reimbursable costs under certain third-party reimbursement agreements. Reimbursement revenues arising from the difference in depreciation methods are reported as deferred revenues to be taken into income in future years.

Pension Plan

The hospital pension plan, described in Note 7, covers substantially all employees. The hospital's policy is to fund pension costs as accrued. Prior service costs are being amortized over a period of 20 years.

Cost Reimbursement Agreements

Revenues under certain reimbursement agreements are subject to audit and retroactive adjustments by third-party payers. Provisions for the estimated retroactive adjustments under these agreements have been provided.

NOTES ACCOMPANYING FINANCIAL STATEMENTS

Note 1. All investments are stated in the balance sheet at cost. For each classification of investments, current market value exceeds cost. The aggregate costs and market values of investments at December 31, 1987, are summarized below:

Figure 20-4 —*Continued*

	Cost	Market Value
Unrestricted Fund:		
Current	$ 126	$ 128
Board-Designated	452	477
Specific Purpose Funds	310	316
Plant Replacement and Expansion Funds	763	805
Endowment Funds	2,187	2,314

Note 2. Receivables in all funds are stated in the balance sheet at estimated realizable values. The December 31, 1987, receivables from patient services reported in the Unrestricted Fund are summarized by payer category below:

Governmental Agencies	$ 720
Blue Cross	336
Commercial and Independent Insurers	384
Self-Pay Accounts	396
Charity	140
Total	1,976
Less Allowance for Charity Care, Contractual Adjustments, and Bad Debts	1,007
Net Receivables	$ 969

Revenues received under reimbursement agreements totaling $4,750 for the current year and $3,920 for the prior year are subject to audit and retroactive adjustment by third-party payers. Provisions for estimated retroactive adjustments under these agreements have been provided.

Note 3. Inventories are stated in the balance sheet at the lower of cost or market. Cost is determined principally by the first-in, first-out method. The December 31, 1987, inventories are summarized below:

Medical and Surgical Supplies	$ 95
Foodstuffs and Other Dietary Supplies	39
Drugs and Pharmaceuticals	86
Fuel and Other Supplies	76
Total Inventories	$296

Figure 20-4—*Continued*

Note 4. The total Unrestricted Fund assets of $10,385 at December 31, 1987, are not subject to any restrictions by donors or other external authorities. Of these unrestricted assets, however, resources of $466 have been designated by the hospital's governing board for renovation and replacement of certain plant facilities. The board-designated resources are excluded from current assets because they are not expected to be expended during the coming year.

Note 5. Property, plant, and equipment is stated in the balance sheet at cost. A summary of the accounts and the related accumulated depreciation at December 31, 1987, follows:

	Cost	Accumulated Depreciation	Book Value
Land	$ 421		$ 421
Land Improvements	236	$ 104	132
Buildings and Fixed Equipment	7,952	2,783	5,169
Major Movable Equipment	3,635	1,231	2,404
Totals	$12,244	$4,118	$8,126

Depreciation is determined on a straight-line basis for financial reporting purposes. The hospital uses an accelerated depreciation method to determine reimburseable costs under certain third-party reimbursement agreements. Reimbursement revenues in the amount of $171, resulting from the difference in depreciation methods, is deferred in the current year and will be taken into income in future years.

Note 6. The mortgage notes are payable in quarterly installments of $45 with interest at 12.25% through March 31, 1996, and are collateralized by land, buildings, and equipment carried at $2,750. Current maturities of $180, payable in 1988, are included in current liabilities at December 31, 1987.

Note 7. The hospital has a noncontributory pension plan covering substantially all employees. Total pension plan expense for 1987 was $97, which includes amortization of past service cost over a period of 20 years. The hospital's policy is to fund pension costs as accrued. The actuarially computed value of vested benefits at December 31, 1987, exceeds net assets of the pension fund and balance sheet accruals by approximately $320.

Note 8. The composition of the Unrestricted Fund Balance at December 31, 1987, is indicated below:

Operations	$ 205
Property, Plant, and Equipment	6,806
Other Board-Designations	719
Total Unrestricted Fund Balance	$7,730

CHAPTER 20 FOOTNOTES

1. "Reporting Changes in Financial Position," **APB Opinion No. 20** (New York: AICPA, 1971).

2. Subcommittee on Health Care Matters, **Hospital Audit Guide** – Fourth Edition (New York: AICPA, 1982), p. 38.

3. "Reporting Changes in Financial Position," **APB Opinion No. 20** (New York: AICPA, 1971), par. 8.

4. Subcommittee on Health Care Matters, "Reporting Practices Concerning Hospital-Related Organizations," **Statement of Position No. 81-2** (New York: AICPA, 1981).

5. "Consolidated Financial Statements," **Accounting Research Bulletin No. 51** (New York: AICPA, 1959).

6. Seawell, **External and Internal Reporting by Hospitals** (Chicago: HFMA, 1984), pp. 131-135.

7. "Disclosure of Accounting Policies," **APB Opinion No. 22** (New York: AICPA, 1972), par. 8.

8. **Ibid.,** par. 12.

assets on page (had another) *(handwritten)* *(handwritten: Vary and form)*

QUESTIONS

1. Define the term **balance sheet.** What is the primary objective of the hospital balance sheet?

2. Distinguish between the **report format** and the **account format** for balance sheets. Which is preferable for hospitals?

3. State the **accounting equation** as the basic formula for the balance sheet, and define each of its elements.

4. Identify and briefly describe the four major types of **funds** that would be reported in the balance sheet of a hospital that employs fund accounting. Why are the resources and obligations of each fund reported separately in a hospital's balance sheet?

5. Indicate the basis of valuation in hospital balance sheets for each of the following assets:
    1. Investments in marketable securities:
        a. Corporate stocks.
        b. Corporate bonds.
    2. Accounts receivable
    3. Inventories
    4. Property, plant, and equipment

6. In what three areas is the disclosure of accounting policies in hospital financial statements particularly necessary?

7. What is a **board-designated fund?** How should board-designated assets be reported in a hospital's balance sheet?

8. State the major limitations of the balance sheet as a source of information to external groups interested in a hospital's financial position?

9. The terms **reserve, net worth,** and **surplus** have at times been used in balance sheet account titles. Why is the use of these terms objectionable? What alternative terms are more appropriate?

10. In what sequence should assets be listed in the balance sheet of a hospital?

11. In a hospital balance sheet, plant assets generally are carried at historical cost rather than at market value. Why?

12. What disclosures should be made in a hospital balance sheet with respect to the Unrestricted Fund Balance?

13. What is your understanding of the requirements of **Statement of Position No. 81-2** as set forth in the **Hospital Audit Guide?**

14. Name several matters that should be included in a hospital's "Summary of Significant Accounting Policies."

EXERCISES

E1. The following multiple-choice questions relate to the preparation and presentation of balance sheets:

1. Historical cost is a measurement basis currently used in balance sheets. Which of the following measurement bases also are currently used in balance sheets?

	Current Market Value	Discounted Cash Flow	Replacement Cost
a.	Yes	No	Yes
b.	Yes	Yes	Yes
c.	Yes	No	No
d.	No	Yes	Yes

2. The computation of the current value of an asset using the present value of future cash flows method does not include the

    a.   Cost of alternative uses of funds given up.
    b.   Productive live of the asset.
    c.   Applicable interest rate.
    d.   Future amounts of cash flows.

3. Glenn Hospital purchased certain plant assets under a deferred payment contract on 12/31/87. The agreement was to pay $10,000 at the time of purchase and $10,000 at the end of each year for the next five years. The plant assets acquired should be recorded at

    a.   The present value of an ordinary annuity of $10,000 for five years.
    b. $60,000.
    c. $60,000 plus imputed interest.
    d. $60,000 less imputed interest.

4. Donated plant assets should be reported in the Unrestricted Fund balance sheet at

    a. $--0--
    b.   Some nominal amount established by the governing board.
    c.   Fair market value at date of donation.
    d.   Fair market value at date of donation less accumulated depreciation.

5. The carrying amount of a current marketable equity securities portfolio in the balance sheet of a hospital should be the aggregate

    a.   Cost of the portfolio, whether it is higher than or lower than the aggregate market value.
    b.   Cost of the portfolio, when it is higher than the aggregate market value of the portfolio.
    c.   Market value of the portfolio, whether it is higher than or lower than the aggregate cost of the portfolio.
    d.   Market value of the portfolio, when it is lower than the aggregate cost of the portfolio.

Required. Select the best answer for each of the above multiple-choice items.

E2.   Given the following information for Hartsburg Hospital:

Inventory	$ 550
Long-term debt	5,000
Accumulated depreciation	3,750
Cash and marketable securities	350
Unrestricted fund balance	9,000
Plant and equipment, at cost	16,000
Current liabilities	2,600
Receivables (net)	3,450

Required. Prepare a balance sheet in good form.

E3.   Given the following information for Havencare Hospital:

Long-term investments	$ 419
Accrued expenses payable	668
Cash	107
Current portion of long-term debt	471
Patients' accounts receivable (net)	2,792
Notes payable (current)	100
Mortgage bonds payable	3,900
Unrestricted fund balance	15,102
Short-term investments	235
Inventories	405
Property, plant, and equipment (net)	17,705
Accounts payable	537
Obligations under capital leases	832
Prepaid expenses	72
Other current receivables	187
Other current liabilities	206
Other long-term debt	333
Other noncurrent assets	227

Required. Prepare a balance sheet in good form.

E4.   Barbara Hospital had equipment of $3,400 on 1/1/87. The balance of accumulated depreciation was $1,200 at 1/1/87 and $1,480 at 12/31/87. Depreciation for 1987 was $340. During 1987, equipment having a book value of $110 was sold at a loss of $10. During 1987, new equipment was purchased for $600. What was the amount of equipment, net of accumulated depreciation, at 12/31/87?

PROBLEMS

P1.   Tammy Hospital's general ledger at September 30 provides the following Unrestricted Fund balances:

Board-designated cash	$ 16
Short-term notes payable	80
Deferred revenues (noncurrent)	122
Temporary investments	67
Property, plant, and equipment, at cost	9,140
Accounts payable	195
Cash in bank (undesignated)	239
Accumulated depreciation	2,168
Accrued expenses payable	199
Current advances from third-party payers	75
Receivables – patients	1,172
Miscellaneous noncurrent assets	58
Payroll taxes withheld	62
8.5% mortgage notes payable (of which $160 is payable within one year)	1,360
Inventories	341
Allowance for uncollectible accounts	433
Board-designated investments in securities	526
Past service pension liability (noncurrent)	375
Prepaid expenses (current)	24
Other current liabilities	33

Required. Prepare in good form a September 30 balance sheet for the Unrestricted Fund of Tammy Hospital.

P2.   Downtown Hospital's general ledger at June 30 provides the following balances:

Investments:	
Unrestricted Fund (current)	$ 134
Specific Purpose Fund	379
Plant Replacement and Expansion Fund	802
Endowment Fund	1,463
Receivables – patients	1,874
Accounts payable	247
Cash:	
Unrestricted Fund (current)	242
Specific Purpose Fund	11
Plant Replacement and Expansion Fund	14
Endowment Fund	21
Pledges receivable (construction program)	136
Accrued expenses payable	201
Property, plant, and equipment, at cost	9,475
Allowance for uncollectible accounts	588
Short-term notes payable	150
Inventories	344
7% revenue bonds payable	1,250
Accumulated depreciation	2,749
Deferred revenues (noncurrent)	155

Prepaid expenses (current)	13
Other current liabilities	147
Specific purpose grants receivable	50
Allowance for uncollectible pledges	11
Plant Replacement and Expansion Fund Balance restricted by third-party payers	428
Payroll taxes withheld	66
Specific Purpose Fund Balance:	
Charity Care	119
Research	85
Current advances from third-party payers	25
Endowment Fund Balance – permanent	1,484

Required. Prepare an all-funds balance sheet for Downtown Hospital at June 30. Indicate what additional information is needed to make the necessary supplementary disclosures to this balance sheet.

P3. The following account balances were drawn from the general ledger of Hartfull Hospital at December 31, 1987:

Deferred rental income	$ 1,450
Temporary investments – unrestricted	175,000
Cash – specific purpose fund	10,300
Investments – endowment fund	2,924,029
Specific purpose fund balance	287,460
Notes payable	125,000
Inventories	87,000
Endowment fund balance	2,921,400
Pledges receivable plant fund	184,929
Due to unrestricted fund from specific purpose fund	12,000
Bond payable	2,400,000
Cash – unrestricted fund	192,068
Accrued interest payable	40,163
Accrued interest receivable	8,124
Cash – endowment fund	1,371
Prepaid expenses	9,260
Plant fund balance	1,740,329
Equipment	3,505,345
Accounts payable	72,384
Cash – plant fund	9,267
Accrued payroll	31,270
Land	175,000
Accounts receivable – patients	1,192,563
Due to unrestricted fund from plant fund	25,000
Due to unrestricted fund from endowment fund	4,000
Accumulated depreciation	2,302,679

Unrestricted fund balance	$5,281,116
Investments – specific purpose fund	289,160
Allowance for uncollectible pledges	20,450
Payroll taxes withheld and accrued	9,242
Investments – plant fund	1,591,583
Allowances for uncollectible patients' accounts	122,056
Buildings	5,000,000

Required. Prepare an all-funds balance sheet for Hartfull Hospital at December 31, 1987.

P4.   Mark Hospital provides you with the following information which relates to the year ended June 30, 1988:

Cafeteria sales	$ 240,000
Transfer to unrestricted fund from plant fund for purchase of plant assets	120,000
Cash – unrestricted fund (current)	190,000
Cash – endowment fund	1,000
Accrued salaries and wages payable	32,000
Nursing services expense	2,500,000
Gross revenues – nursing services	3,600,000
Unrestricted contributions	29,000
Donated medical equipment	40,000
Donated resources received – endowment fund	90,000
Land	166,000
Cash plant fund	9,300
Deductions from revenues – bad debts	54,000
General services expense	770,000
Deferred rental income (current)	2,000
Due to unrestricted fund from:	
Specific purpose fund	15,000
Plant fund	34,000
Endowment fund	6,000
Gross revenues – other professional services	2,800,000
Unrestricted income from endowment fund investments	28,000
Investment income – specific purpose fund	17,000
Investment income – plant fund	108,000
Temporary investments – unrestricted fund	180,000
Equipment	3,500,000
Notes payable	80,000
Bonds payable	2,500,000
Cash – specific purpose fund	12,000
Accrued interest receivable	9,000
Accumulated depreciation	2,400,000
Deductions from revenues – charity service	12,000
Other professional services expense	987,000

Prepaid expenses	8,000
Investments — endowment fund	3,000,000
Accounts payable	75,000
Buildings	5,500,000
Inventories	110,000
Rental income	15,000
Fiscal services expense	354,000
Purchase discounts	26,000
Deductions from revenues — contractual adjustments	403,000
Payroll taxes withheld and accrued	7,000
Accrued interest payable	41,000
Donated resources received — specific purpose fund	124,000
Investment gains:	
Specific purpose fund	8,000
Plant fund	3,000
Endowment fund	14,000
Administrative services expense	1,004,000
Donated resources received — plant fund	230,000
Transfers from specific purpose fund	
to unrestricted fund for:	
Charity service	29,000
Research	40,000
Education	52,000
Receivables — patients	1,300,000
Investments — specific purpose fund	290,000
Allowance for uncollectible accounts	140,000
Investments — plant fund	1,600,000
Income on unrestricted fund investments	13,000
Plant fund pledges receivable (net)	206,000

Required. Prepare in good form (1) an income statement for the year ended 6/30/88, (2) a balance sheet at 6/30/88, and (3) a statement of changes in fund balances for the year ended 6/30/88.

21
Reporting Changes in Financial Position

For many years, the primary financial statements generally considered adequate for external financial reporting purposes by hospitals (and other healthcare organizations) were: (1) the *income statement*, which presents the results of hospital operations in terms of revenues earned and expenses incurred during a specified period of time; (2) the *balance sheet*, which reflects the financial position of the hospital in terms of its assets and equities (liabilities and fund balances) at a particular point in time; and (3) the *statement of changes in fund balances*, which provides an analysis of the increase or decrease during a given period in the fund balances (the net assets of each fund maintained by the hospital). These three financial statements contain much of the essential information needed for decision-making by both internal and external users. They do not, however, fully disclose all changes in the hospital's financial position from one period to another. They do not directly provide a complete summary of the amounts of "funds" (financial resources such as cash or working capital, for example) generated and used by the hospital during the reporting period. Even when balance sheets are presented in comparative form, a detailed supplemental analysis usually is required to identify all of the hospital's financing and investing activities.

In 1971, the Accounting Principles Board, recognizing the importance to investors and creditors of information concerning the flow of funds within profit-oriented entities, required that a statement summarizing all changes in financial position be issued as a basic financial statement by business enterprises.[1] The Board concluded that the statement should be based on a broad concept embracing all changes in financial position, and that it should be titled the "statement of changes in financial position" to reflect that broad concept. The *Hospital Audit Guide* makes it clear that these requirements also are applicable to voluntary, not-for-profit hospitals.[2]

Where a fund accounting system is employed to segregate resources into unrestricted and restricted funds, the hospital statement of changes in financial position typically reflects the financing and investing activity only of the Unrestricted Fund. Separate statements of changes in financial position may be prepared for each of the restricted funds if such statements are needed to disclose fully all significant changes in those funds' financial position. The discussion in this chapter, however, is limited to statements of changes in financial position prepared for the Unrestricted Fund.

OBJECTIVES AND USES OF THE STATEMENT

The objectives of the statement of changes in financial position are twofold: (1) to summarize the financing and investing activities of the hospital, including the amount of financial resources generated from operations of the period, and (2) to complete the disclosure of changes in financial position that may not be discernible from examination of the other financial statements. This statement, formerly called the *statement of sources and application of funds,* indicates how the hospital's activities have been financed, and how its financial resources have been used, during the reporting period. The statement provides a summary of the amounts of financial resources generated internally from operations and externally from borrowings, disposals of assets, and other means. It also sets forth the amounts of financial resources applied to certain purposes, such as the acquisition of assets and the retirement of debt.

The statement of changes in financial position assists management and external parties in understanding and evaluating the hospital's financing and investment activities. It accomplishes this objective by providing the answers to such questions as:

(1) What was the amount of financial resources generated during the current period from the hospital's continuing operations, and how were those resources used?

(2) Why did the hospital's cash or working capital position decline during a period when a substantial net income was earned?

(3) How was the acquisition of net plant and equipment financed?

(4) Why was it necessary to borrow money to finance the purchase of new plant and equipment?

(5) How was the hospital able to retire its long-term debt?

(6) What happened to the proceeds from the bond issue?

(7) What happened to the proceeds from the sale of equipment?

(8) Why did the hospital's cash or working capital position improve during a period when a substantial net loss was incurred?

(9) What amount of financial resources will be generated by the hospital during the next year, and how does the hospital plan to use those resources?

(10) How will the hospital be able to accumulate sufficient financial resources during the next ten years to retire its outstanding bonds?

When presented in comparative form covering several years, the statement of changes in financial position may reveal useful information relating to the financial management policies employed in the past, the results of those policies, and policy changes that may be appropriate to meet the hospital's future financial requirements. Many hospitals, for internal management purposes, prepare statements of changes in financial position based on budgets and long-range plans or forecasts. Such statements also may have external uses in connection with negotiations with third-party payors, rate review committees, area planning agencies, and lenders.

Although the statement of changes in financial position is closely related to the other primary financial statements, it is not a substitute for any of them. It is an essential financial statement in its own right in that it provides important information that cannot be easily obtained, if at all, from the other three financial statements.

ALTERNATIVE FORMATS FOR THE STATEMENT

As noted in the previous section, the statement of changes in financial position depicts the flow of "funds" during the reporting period. The term **funds**, in this context, means financial resources; it does not refer to the self-balancing sets of accounts maintained in a fund accounting system. Since confusion, therefore, may result from its use, the term funds should be avoided in connection with the statement of changes in financial position. Expressions such as "sources of funds" and "application of funds" tend to be misunderstood by the less-sophisticated financial statement readers.

Thus, the statement of changes in financial position depicts the flow of *financial resources* during the reporting period. It presents a summary of the amounts of *financial resources provided* and the amounts of *financial resources applied*, each classified in a meaningful manner. It is necessary, however, to define precisely what is meant by "financial resources," since the format in which the statement of changes in financial position is presented is directly dependent upon the definition selected by the hospital.

"Financial resources" may be defined in several different ways. A hospital may choose, for example, to define financial resources to mean either *working capital* or *cash*. While these are the two most widely employed definitions, Opinion No. 19 of the Accounting Principles Board recognizes the need for flexibility and permits other definitions. Whatever definition is selected, however, should result in the most useful portrayal of hospital financing and investing activities.[3]

Working Capital Format

Working capital consists of the excess of current assets over current liabilities as reported in the hospital balance sheet. The adequacy of working capital, the sources from which working capital is derived, and the uses to which working capital is applied are all major concerns to management and to external parties having an interest in a hospital's financial operations and affairs. For this reason, most hospitals define financial resources to mean *working capital*, and present statements of changes in financial position in a *working capital format*. In other words, changes in financial position are expressed in terms of the sources and uses of working capital. Attention is centered, under this format, on the increases and decreases in working capital that arise from changes in noncurrent asset, noncurrent liabilities, and the unrestricted fund balance.

An algebraic equation can be formulated to identify the various sources and uses of working capital. In developing this equation, the following notations are employed:

A	=	assets	L	=	liabilities
CA	=	current assets	CL	=	current liabilities
NCA	=	noncurrent assets	NCL	=	noncurrent liabilities
FB	=	fund balance	WC	=	working capital

The basic accounting equation, $A = L + FB$, then is expanded to read: $CA + NCA = CL + NCL + FB$. Next, NCA and CL are subtracted for each side of the equation to produce: $CA - CL = NCL + FB - NCA$. Because $CA - CL$ is WC, the working capital equation becomes: $WC = NCL + FB - NCA$. Thus, it is evident that there are three possible sources of working capital and three possible uses of working capital:

Sources	*Uses*
1. Increases in NCL,	1. Decreases in NCL,
2. Increases in FB, and	2. Decreases in FB, and
3. Decrease in NCA.	3. Increases in NCA.

Figure 21-1 presents a brief summary of some of the major sources and uses of working capital. The difference between total sources and total uses for a given period represents the increase (or decrease) in the amount of working capital for that period. In this way, the change in working capital during the reporting period is accounted for by the statement of changes in financial position when it is presented in a working capital format.

Figure 21-1.

Sources and Uses of Working Capital

Sources of Working Capital

1. Net income from operations

2. Proceeds from bond issues and other long-term borrowings

3. Proceeds from sales of property, plant, and equipment

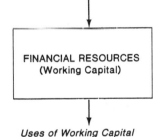

FINANCIAL RESOURCES
(Working Capital)

Uses of Working Capital

1. Net loss from operations

2. Retirement of long-term debt

3. Acquisition of property, plant and equipment

As indicated in Figure 21-1, profitable operations provide working capital. The amount reported as net income in the income statement of the hospital, however, is *not* the amount of working capital generated from operations. In determining net income, certain charges (such as depreciation expense) are made against income but do not require the use of working capital during the reporting period. Certain credits (such as amortization of premium on bonds payable) that also are included in income do not provide working capital. To obtain the amount of working capital generated from operations, these charges must be added back to net income, and the credits must be subtracted from net income. Similar adjustments must be made to a reported net loss to determine the amount of working capital applied to operations of the period. A more complete discussion of this important matter appears in a later section of this chapter.

Cash Format

Some hospitals define financial resources to mean *cash*, and prepare their statements of changes in financial position in a *cash format*. In other words, changes in financial position are expressed in terms of the sources and uses of cash. Emphasis is given, under this format, to the increases and decreases in cash that arise from changes in all of the noncash accounts in the balance sheet. It should be clearly understood, however, that the statement of changes in financial position in a cash format is *not* the same as a statement of cash receipts and disbursements. There are significant differences in both content and presentation.

An algebraic equation also can be formulated to identify the various possible sources and uses of cash. In addition to the notations used for the working capital equation, the following are needed:

$$C \quad = \quad \text{cash}$$
$$OCA = \quad \text{other current assets}$$

The basic accounting equation again is expanded to provide an equation in greater detail: $C + OCA + NCA = CL + NCL + FB$. Then, OCA and NCA are subtracted from each side of this equation to produce the cash equation: $C = CL + NCL + FB - OCA - NCA$. Thus, it may be seen that there are five possible sources of cash and five possible uses of cash:

Sources	*Uses*
1. Increases in CL,	1. Decreases in CL,
2. Increases in NCL,	2. Decreases in NCL,
3. Increases in FB,	3. Decreases in FB,
4. Decreases in OCA, and	4. Increases in OCA, and
5. Decreases in NCA.	5. Increases in NCA.

It should be noted that the sources and uses of cash are much the same as the sources and uses of working capital. The difference arises in the treatment of changes in CL and OCA. Statements of changes in financial position in a cash format present these changes as adjustments of net income (or net loss) to obtain the amount of cash generated from operations. In other words, the amount of cash generated by operations is the amount of working capital generated from operations adjusted for changes in CL and OCA. Thus, the cash format and the working capital format are identical, except that the former presents the amount of cash generated from operations while the latter presents the amount of working capital generated from operations. This matter is examined in greater detail later in this chapter.

THE ALL FINANCIAL RESOURCES CONCEPT

Regardless of the definition of financial resources and the format selected for the statement of changes in financial position, APB Opinion No. 19 requires that the statement be based on an "all financial resources" concept[4] This means that the statement must disclose all significant aspects of the hospital's financing and investing activities even when cash or other elements of working capital are not directly affected by the related transactions.

A hospital may, for example, directly exchange one noncurrent asset for another, or it may directly exchange long-term debt for a noncurrent asset, or it may directly convert an outstanding long-term debt into another long-term debt. A hospital also may receive plant assets by donation in kind. Although these types of transactions occur infrequently, they are important because they may result in significant changes in the hospital's balance sheet accounts.

The above transactions and events do not directly affect either working capital or cash. Under the all financial resources concept, however, such transactions (if significant) must be included in the statement of changes in financial position, regardless of the particular format used. The direct exchange of long-term debt for plant assets, for example, results in an increase in noncurrent liabilities and an increase in noncurrent assets. While the value of the working capital and cash equations is not affected, these changes in noncurrent accounts must be reported in the statement of changes in financial position as financial resources provided and financial resources used. This matter is more fully illustrated and discussed at a later point.

BASIS OF ILLUSTRATIONS

Certain financial statements for a hypothetical Sample Hospital are provided in Figures 21-2, 21-3, and 21-4. These statements, along with other information to be supplied, will serve as a basis for illustrating the preparation of fairly typical statements of changes in financial position of working capital and cash formats, both based on the "all financial resources concept." Some of the more complex presentation problems are dealt with later in this chapter.

Figure 21-2.
Sample Hospital
Condensed Income Statement
Year Ended December 31, 1987
($000's)

Gross patient service revenues	$9,000
Less revenue deduction	980
Net patient service revenues	8,020
Add other operating revenues	830
Total operating revenues	8,850
Less operating expenses	8,520
Operating income	330
Add nonoperating revenues (net)	160
Net income	$ 490

Figure 21-3.
Sample Hospital
Statement of Changes in Unrestricted Fund Balance
Year Ended December 31, 1987
($000's)

Unrestricted fund balance, January 1	$4,100
Add:	
Net income	490
Plant assets donated in kind	40
Unrestricted fund balance, December 31	$4,630

Figure 21-4.
Sample Hospital
Condensed Balance Sheet — Unrestricted Fund
December 31, 1987 and 1986
($000's)

	December 31	
	1987	1986
Cash	$ 300	$ 250
Temporary investments	400	360
Accounts receivable, net of allowances		
for uncollectible accounts	1,440	1,320
Inventories	130	150
Prepaid expenses	30	20
Total current assets	2,300	2,100
Long-term investments	840	600
Property, plant, and equipment, net of		
accumulated depreciation of $3,390 at		
12/31/87 and $3,200 at 12/31/86	5,720	4,800
Total assets	$8,860	$7,500
Accounts payable	$ 640	$ 590
Accrued expenses payable	390	310
Total current liabilities	1,030	900
Long-term debt — bonds payable	3,200	2,500
Total liabilities	4,230	3,400
Fund balance	4,630	4,100
Total liabilities and fund balance	$8,860	$7,500

STATEMENT IN WORKING CAPITAL FORMAT

If Sample Hospital elects to define financial resources as working capital, its statement of changes in financial position should be prepared in a working capital format. Under this format, changes in financial position are expressed in terms of sources and uses of working capital so that the statement accounts for the change in working capital for the year. As indicated in Figure 21-5, the working capital of Sample Hospital increased by $70 during 1987. The total sources of working capital during the year, therefore, must have exceeded the total uses of working capital by $70. To determine what these sources and uses were, an analysis must be made of the changes that occurred during 1987 in the noncurrent asset, noncurrent liability, and fund balance accounts of the hospital.

Figure 21-5.
Sample Hospital
Computations of Increase in Working Capital
Year Ended December 31, 1987
($000's)

	December 31 1987	1986	Increase (Decrease)
Cash	$ 300	$ 250	$ 50
Temporary investments	400	360	40
Receivables (net)	1,440	1,320	120
Inventories	130	150	(20)
Prepaid expenses	30	20	10
Total current assets	2,300	2,100	200
Accounts payable	640	590	50
Accrued expenses payable	390	310	80
Total current liabilities	1,030	900	130
Working capital	$1,270	$1,200	$ 70

Analysis of Account Changes

As indicated earlier, the sources and uses of working capital can be derived from a working capital equation: $WC = NCL + FB - NCA$. The gross changes in each of the accounts positioned on the right-hand side of the equation represent those sources and uses. An analysis of the ledger accounts is necessary to determine the gross changes.

Noncurrent Assets

Sample Hospital's balance sheet presents two categories of noncurrent assets: (1) long-term investments and (2) property, plant, and equipment. Gross increases in these accounts are uses of working capital; gross decreases are sources of working capital.

Figure 21-4 provides the following information concerning the long-term investments of Sample Hospital:

	December 31	
	1987	1986
Long-term investments	$840	$600

Although it might initially appear that new long-term investments of $240 were acquired during the year, an examination of the hospital's ledger accounts indicates that this is not what actually occurred. During 1987, Sample Hospital (1) purchased investments for $440, and (2) sold for $260 investments that had cost $200.

The 1987 statement of change in financial position, therefore, should report the $440 purchase of long-term investment as a *use of working capital*, and the $260 proceeds from the sale of long-term investments as a *source of working capital*, as shown in Figure 21-6. It should be noted that the *sale proceeds*, and not the cost of the investments sold, are reported as the source of working capital. The $60 gain on the sale, of course, is recorded as nonoperating revenue and included in net income. Since the gain itself did not provide working capital, but is included in net income, the $60 gain must be deducted from net income (as shown in Figure 21-6) in determining the amount of working capital generated from operations during 1987. Otherwise, the $60 gain would be counted twice as a source of working capital.

An alternative practice would be to report the $200 cost of investments sold as the amount of working capital provided by the sale. The adjustment of net income for the gain can be avoided in this way, but the procedure described above seems preferable because it discloses the sales price of the investments that were sold. Reporting a $200 source of working capital, when the amount actually was $260, is a misstatement that could be misleading. The alternative practice, therefore, is not followed in the illustrations presented in this chapter.

Sample Hospital's balance sheets also provide the following information concerning property, plant, and equipment:

	December 31	
	1987	1986
Property, plant, and equipment	$9,110	$8,000
Less accumulated depreciation	3,390	3,200
Net property, plant, and equipment	$5,720	$4,800

Again, one might be tempted to draw incorrect conclusions from the net changes in these accounts. It might be assumed, for example, that $1,110 of plant assets were acquired during 1987, and that depreciation expense for the year was $190. The hospital's ledger, however, may reveal that the $1,110 increase in property, plant, and equipment is the net result of several transactions: (1) purchase of new plant assets for $1,770, (2) sale for $450 of plant assets that had cost $700 and on which $210 of depreciation was accumulated, and (3) acquisition by donation in kind of plant assets having a fair value of $40. It also may be discovered that the $190 increase in accumulated depreciation is the net result of (1) depreciation expense of $400 and (2) the elimination of $210 of accumulated depreciation on the plant assets that were sold.

As shown in Figure 21-6, the 1987 statement of changes in financial position reports the $1,770 purchase of plant assets as a use of working capital, and reports the $450 proceeds from the sale of plant assets as a source of working capital. The $40 loss on the sale, because it was charged against income but did not require the use of working capital, is added to net income in determining the amount of working capital provided by operations in 1987. For the same reason, depreciation expense of $400 also is added back to net income.

The addback of depreciation to net income should not be interpreted to mean that depreciation is a source of working capital. An addback is made only because the amount reported as net income is an understatement of the amount of working capital generated from operations. Depreciation, although it was deducted in determining net income, did not require the use of working capital. Revenues provide working capital; expenses do not.

Sample Hospital's entry to record the acquisition by donation in kind of plant assets having a fair value of $40 was:

Property, Plant and Equipment	$ 40	
Unrestricted Fund Balance		$ 40
Receipt of donated equipment.		

The entry results in an increase both in a noncurrent asset and in the fund balance, but the transaction has no direct effect on working capital. Under the all financial resources concept, however, the statement of changes in financial position (shown in Figure 21-6) reports the increase in property, plant, and equipment as a use of working capital, and includes the increase in the fund balance as a source of working capital. A similar treatment would be given to direct exchanges of noncurrent asset items, direct conversions of long-term debt securities, and direct exchanges of long-term debt for noncurrent assets.

Noncurrent Liabilities

Gross increases in noncurrent liability accounts are sources of working capital; gross decreases are uses of working capital. The noncurrent liabilities of Sample Hospital are reported in its balance sheets as follows:

	December 31	
	1987	1986
Long-term debt — bonds payable	$3,200	$2,500

An examination of the hospital's ledger reveals that the increase of $700 in bonds payable is actually the net result of two separate transactions: (1) the retirement of $300 of bonds at face value, and (2) the issuance of $1,000 of additional bonds at face value.

Figure 21-6.
Sample Hospital
Statement of Changes in Financial Position — Unrestricted Fund
Year Ended December 31, 1987
($000's)

Sources of working capital:

Net income	$ 490
Add (deduct) items included in operations not requiring (providing) working capital:	
Depreciation	400
Loss on sale of plant assets	40
Gain on sale of long-term investments	(60)
Working capital provided by operations	870
Proceeds of bond issue	1,000
Proceeds from sale of plant assets	450
Proceeds from sale of long-term investments	260
Receipt of donated plant assets	40
Total sources of working capital	2,620

Uses of working capital:

Purchases of plant assets	1,770
Purchase of long-term investments	440
Retirement of bonds	300
Plant assets acquired by donation in kind	40
Total uses of working capital	2,550
Increase in working capital	$ 70

Increase (decrease) in elements of working capital:

Cash	$ 50
Temporary investments	40
Receivables (net)	120
Inventories	(20)
Prepaid expenses	10
Total current assets	200
Accounts payable	50
Accrued expenses payable	80
Total current liabilities	130
Working capital	$ 70

As illustrated in Figure 21-6, the statement of changes in financial position for 1987, therefore, reports the $300 retirement of bonds as a use of working capital and the $1,000 issue of bonds as a source of working capital. Procedures to be followed in the

Fund Balance

Gross increases in the unrestricted fund balance account represent sources of working capital; gross decreases in the account are uses of working capital. Sample Hospital's statement of changes in unrestricted fund balance, presented in Figure 21-3, provides an analysis of the $530 increase in the fund balance during the year ended December 31, 1987. The increase is composed of the 1987 net income of $490, and a direct credit of $40 arising from the receipt of a plant asset donated in kind. As shown in Figure 21-6, the 1987 statement of changes in financial position reports both the $490 of net income (with appropriate adjustments) and the donation as a source of working capital.

There were no direct charges or other decreases in the fund balance during 1987. When such decreases occur, they generally are reported in the statement of changes in financial position as uses of working capital.

Presentation of the Statement

Based on the foregoing analysis of Sample Hospital's noncurrent asset, noncurrent liability, and fund balance accounts, a statement of changes in financial position can be prepared in a working capital format as shown in Figure 21-6. The statement heading indicates the name of the hospital, the statement title recommended by Opinion No. 19, and the time period covered by the statement. The body of the statement consists of two sections: one for *sources of working capital* (financial resources) and another for *uses of working capital* (financial resources). The "bottom line" of the statement indicates the difference between total sources and total uses of working capital (in this case, the increase in working capital for 1987). As required by Opinion No. 19, this difference is supported by a schedule of the net changes in each element of working capital.[5]

An alternative method of presenting the amount of working capital provided by operations is often used by hospitals having significant nonoperating revenues. This presentation is shown below:

Operating income	$330
Add items included in operations not requiring working capital:	
Depreciation	400
Working capital provided by operations	730
Nonoperating revenues, net (excluding gains and losses on disposals of noncurrent assets)	140
Working capital provided by operations and nonoperating revenues, net	$870

Note that the presentation begins with operating income (rather than net income) as reported in the income statement. The amount of working capital provided by nonoperating revenues is determined as follows:

Nonoperating revenues per income statement	$160
Loss on sale of plant assets	40
Gain on sale of long-term investments	(60)
Working capital provided by nonoperating revenues	$140

An advantage of this method of presentation is that it gives emphasis to the amount of working capital provided by the hospital's continuing and regularly recurring operations.

Workpaper to Develop Statement

The sources and uses of working capital may be derived from ledger account analysis, as was done earlier. In certain cases, however, it may be desirable to prepare a workpaper such as the one illustrated in Figure 21-7. The first two columns list the balances of all balance sheet accounts at the beginning and end of the period. In columns three and four, the net change (debit or credit) in each account is indicated. The final two columns represent adjustments made to eliminate the net changes and determine the sources and uses of working capital for the period. A debit net change in an account, for example, is eliminated by making equal net credit adjustments to the account.

Adjustment (1) eliminates the net changes in all working capital accounts. The debit needed to balance the entry is the increase in working capital, and it is entered in the working capital section under "uses." This is done only to maintain the "balancing" feature of the workpaper. The formal statement of changes in financial position, of course, should not list an increase in working capital as a use of working capital, since this would be tantamount to saying that an increase in working capital is a decrease in working capital.

The second adjustment, in effect, *reverses* the entry made by Sample Hospital to record the purchase of long-term investments. Since the hospital's entry was a debit to long-term investments and a credit to cash, the workpaper adjustment is:

Working Capital Uses	$ 440	
Long-Term Investments		$ 440

This adjustment does not debit cash because the cash "line" previously was eliminated or "closed" by adjustment (1).

Adjustment (3) is a reversal of the hospital's entry to record the sale of long-term investments. The hospital's entry was a debit to cash for $260, a credit to long-term investments for $200, and a credit to nonoperating revenues for the $60 gain. On the workpaper, the reversal entry therefore is:

Long-Term Investments	$ 200	
Fund Balance	60	
Working Capital Sources		$ 260

Cash is not credited in this entry because the cash line on the workpaper previously was closed by adjustment (1). The $60 gain is debited to the fund balance because, when Sample Hospital's books were closed at the end of 1987, the gain (nonoperating revenues) was credited to the fund balance account.

Figure 21-7.
Sample Hospital
Workpaper to Develop Statement of Changes in Financial Position
Unrestricted Fund
Year Ended December 31, 1987
($000's)

	December 31 Balances		Net Changes		Adjustments			
	1987	1986	Dr.	Cr.	Dr.		Cr.	
Cash	300	250	50				(1)	50
Temporary investments	400	360	40				(1)	40
Receivables (net)	1,440	1,320	120				(1)	120
Inventories	130	150		20	(1)	20		
Prepaid expenses	30	20	10				(1)	10
Long-term investments	840	600	240		(3)	200	(2)	440
Property, plant and equipment	9,110	8,000	1,100		(5)	700	(4)	1,770
							(6)	40
Total	12,250	10,700						
Accumulated depreciation	3,390	3,200		190	(8)	400	(5)	210
Accounts payable	640	590		50	(1)	50		
Accrued expenses payable	390	310		80	(1)	80		
Bonds payable	3,200	2,500		700	(10)	1,000	(9)	300
Fund balance	4,630	4,100		530	(3)	60	(5)	40
					(6)	40	(8)	400
					(11)	870		
Total	12,250	10,700	1,570	1,570				

	Working Capital	
	Uses	Sources
Increase in working capital	(1) 70	
Purchase of long-term investments	(2) 440	
Sale of long-term investments		(3) 260
Purchase of plant assets	(4) 1,770	
Sale of plant assets		(5) 450
Plant assets donated in kind	(7) 40	
Receipt of donation of plant assets		(7) 40
Retirement of bonds payable	(9) 300	
Issue of bonds		(10) 1,000
Provided by operations		(11) 870
Total	2,620	2,620

Key to adjustments:
(1) Elimination of net changes in working capital accounts.

(2) Purchase of long-term investments.

   (3) Sale of long-term investments.   (4) Purchase of plant assets.
   (5) Sale of plant assets.   (6) Plant assets donated in fund.
   (7) Recognize donation in kind of   (8) Depreciation for the year.
        plant assets as both source
        and use of working capital.
   (9) Retirement of bonds.   (10) Issue of bonds.
 (11) Funds provided by operations.

Note that the $200 debit adjustment and the $440 credit adjustment to long-term investments eliminates the $240 debit net change in the long-term investments account. At the same time, adjustments (2) and (3) produce the related sources and uses of working capital. The same procedure is followed in adjustments (4) through (10), which eliminate the net change in each of the remaining noncurrent accounts. Adjustment (11) closes the fund balance line of the workpaper by debiting the fund balance for $870, which, of course, is the amount of working capital provided by operations during the year. All the information needed to prepare the statement of changes in financial position in a working capital format appears on the completed workpaper.

Alternate Workpaper to Develop Statement

Another workpaper format is presented in Figure 21-8. This format provides a direct analysis of the gross changes in noncurrent accounts; it avoids the "reversal process" involved in the workpaper illustrated in Figure 21-7. The "working capital" column of Figure 21-8 provides all information needed to prepare the statement of changes in financial position.

STATEMENT IN CASH FORMAT

Assuming that Sample Hospital elects to define financial resources as cash, its statement of changes in financial position will be prepared in a cash format. The statement, under this format, will express changes in financial position in terms of sources and uses of cash, thereby accounting for the change in the cash balance for the year. As shown in Sample Hospital's balance sheets (Figure 21-4), the cash balance increased by $50 during 1987.

The increase in the cash balance of the unrestricted fund can be explained by a statement of cash receipts and disbursements (also known as a "cashflow statement"), as illustrated in Figure 21-9. This statement is simply a classified listing of the debits and credits made to cash during the reporting period. A statement of this kind, however, is not regarded as a substitute for the statement of changes in financial position in a cash format.

Analysis of Account Changes

As indicated earlier, the sources and uses of cash can be derived from a cash equation: $C = CL + NCL + FB - OCA - NCA$. An analysis of the ledger accounts is necessary to determine the *gross* changes in NCL, FB, and NCA. The procedure is identical to that discussed in connection with the working capital format. Under the cash format, however, it is not necessary to determine the gross changes in CL or OCA; only the *net* changes in these accounts need be reported in the statement of changes in financial position. These net changes, as shown before, are presented in the statement as adjustments to net income in determining the amount of cash generated from operations.

In other words, a statement of changes in financial position that is presented in a cash format is substantially the same as a statement presented in a working capital format, with one major exception: the former reports the amount of *cash* provided by operations, while the latter reports the amount of *working capital* provided by operations.

Figure 21-8.
Sample Hospital
Alternate Worksheet for Statement of Changes in Financial Position
Unrestricted Fund Year Ended December 31, 1987
($000's)

		Working Capital	Long-Term Investments	Plant Assets (net)	Bonds Payable	Fund Balance
Balances, 12/31/86		$ 1,200	$600	$4,800	$(2,500)	$(4,100)
Net income		490				(490)
Depreciation expense		400		(400)		
Sale of investments:						
Proceeds	$260	260				
Book value	200		(200)			
Loss	$ 60	(60)				
Purchase of investments		(440)	440			
Sale of plant assets:						
Proceeds	$450	450				
Book value	490			(490)		
Loss	$ 40	40				
Purchase of plant assets		(1,770)		1,770		
Proceeds of bond issue		1,000			(1,000)	
Retirement of bonds		(300)			300	
Donated plant assets:						
Source		40				(40)
Use		(40)		40		
Balances, 12/31/87		$1,270	$840	$5,720	$3,200	$4,630

Presentation of the Statement

Sample Hospital's 1987 statement of changes in financial position, prepared in a cash format, is presented in Figure 21-10. The body of the statement consists of a *sources of cash* section and a *uses of cash* section. The "bottom line" of the statement indicates the difference between total sources and total uses (in this case, the $50 increase in cash for 1987).

Note that the net increases in current asset accounts (other than cash) are deducted from net income; net decreases in these accounts are added to net income. Consider, for example, the deduction from reported net income of the $120 net increase in receivables. Since revenues are credited when receivables are debited, the 1987 income statement will include $120 of revenues that were not collected in cash. Thus, the increase in receivables must be subtracted from net income to obtain the amount of cash generated from operations.

Figure 21-9.
Sample Hospital
Statement of Cash Receipts and Disbursements
Unrestricted Fund
Year Ended December 31, 1987
($000's)

Cash balance, January 1	$ 250
Add cash receipts:	
Collections on receivables	7,900
Proceeds from bond issue	1,000
Other operating revenues	830
Sale of plant assets	450
Sale of temporary investments	370
Sale of long-term investments	260
Nonoperating revenues	130
Total cash receipts	10,940
Total cash available	11,190
Less cash disbursements:	
Payments of operating expenses	6,630
Purchase of plant assets	1,770
Payments of accounts payable	1,350
Purchase of long-term investments	440
Purchase of temporary investments	400
Retirement of bonds	300
Total cash disbursements	10,890
Cash balance, December 31	$ 300

On the other hand, net increases in current liability accounts are added to net income; net decreases in these accounts are deducted from net income. Consider, for example, the $80 increase in accrued expenses payable that is shown as an addition to net income. Since expenses are debited when accrued expenses payable is credited, the 1987 income statement includes expenses that have not yet been paid. Thus, the increase in accrued expenses payable must be added to net income to determine the amount of cash generated from operations of the period.

OTHER FORMATS FOR THE STATEMENT

As indicated earlier, hospital statements of changes in financial position are most often presented in a working capital format although the cash format appears to be gaining in popularity. Other acceptable formats, however, may be used. These include: (1) cash plus temporary investments; (2) quick assets; and (3) total current assets. Because these formats are rarely used in practice, they are not discussed or illustrated in this book.

Figure 21-10.
Sample Hospital
Statement of Changes in Financial Position – Unrestricted Fund
Year Ended December 31, 1987
($000's)

Sources of cash:	
Net income	$ 490
Add (deduct) items included in operations	
not requiring (providing) cash:	
Depreciation	400
Loss on sale of plant assets	40
Gain on sale of long-term investments	(60)
Increase in temporary investments	(40)
Increase in receivables (net)	(120)
Decrease in inventories	20
Increase in prepaid expenses	(10)
Increase in accounts payable	50
Increase in accrued expenses payable	80
Cash provided by operations	850
Proceeds of bond issue	1,000
Proceeds from sale of plant assets	450
Proceeds from sale of long-term investments	260
Receipt of donated plant assets	40
Total sources of cash	2,600
Uses of cash:	
Purchase of plant assets	1,770
Purchase of long-term investments	440
Retirement of bonds	300
Plant assets acquired by donation in kind	40
Total uses of cash	2,550
Increase in cash	$ 50

SPECIAL PROBLEMS OF STATEMENT PRESENTATION

The preceding illustrations were limited in complexity in order to concentrate on the major concepts and elements involved in the development of the statement of changes in financial position. This section deals with some of the special problems that frequently arise in the preparation of the statement.

Adjustments of Net Income

As noted before, income statement changes that do not require the use of working capital are added to reported net income, and income statement credits that do not provide working capital are subtracted from net income, to determine the amount of working capital generated by operations during the reporting period. Examples of items treated as adjustments of net income for this purpose are presented in Figure 21-11.

Previous illustrations included depreciation expense and losses on sales of noncurrent assets as addbacks to net income. It also was shown that gains on sales of noncurrent assets are deducted from reported net income. Like depreciation, amortization of intangible assets (such as goodwill or patents) and deferred charges (such as bond issue costs) also are expenses that are added to net income. Such expenses relate to prior period expenditures being amortized currently, thereby reducing net income but not affecting working capital in the current period. Similarly, the amortization of discount on bonds payable increases interest expense but does not reduce working capital. (Amortization of premium on bonds payable has the opposite effect.) The amortization of a premium on long-term investments in bonds is recorded as a reduction of interest income, reducing net income but not affecting working capital. (Amortization of discount on long-term investments in bonds has the opposite effect).

Because of timing difference in the recognition of certain costs for financial reporting and for reimbursement purposes, a hospital's balance sheet often will include a noncurrent "deferred reimbursement revenue" account. In periods when the timing differences originate, the following entry is made:

Revenue Deductions $xxx,xxx
    Deferred Reimbursement Revenue $xxx,xxx
    Adjustment for timing differences.

Thus, increases in deferred reimbursement revenues reduce the hospital's net income but not its working capital. Such increases are, therefore, added to net income in computing the amount of working capital provided by operations. In periods when timing differences reverse, the above entry is reversed, increasing net income but not the hospital's working capital. Decreases in deferred reimbursement revenues, then, are treated as reductions of net income for the purpose of determining the amount of working capital provided by operations.

Under the equity method of accounting for investments in common stocks, (discussed in Chapter 15) a hospital accrues as income its share of the earnings of the investee. This accrual has the effect of increasing net income without increasing working capital. Income accrued under the equity method of accounting, therefore, must be deducted from net income to arrive at the amount of working capital provided by operations. If the investee has a net loss, the hospital records its share of that loss. Losses accrued under the equity method are added to net income in computing the amount of working capital provided by operations.

Figure 21-11.
Summary of Net Income Adjustments

NET INCOME plus

ADDITIONS	DEDUCTIONS
Depreciation	Gain on sale of noncurrent assets
Loss on sale of noncurrent assets	Amortization of premium on bonds payable
Amortization of intangible assets	Amortization of discount on long-term investments in bonds
Amortization of deferred charges	Decrease in deferred reimbursement revenues
Amortization of discount on bonds payable	Income accrued on investments in common stock (the equity method of accounting)
Amortization of premium on long-term investments in bonds	
Increase in deferred reimbursement revenues	
Loss accrued on investments in common stock (the equity method of accounting)	

less

equals

WORKING CAPITAL PROVIDED BY OPERATIONS

Extraordinary Items

A hospital may, at times, have a gain or loss that is properly classified as an extraordinary item in its income statement. For example, if Sample Hospital had paid $330 to retire certain of its bonds payable with a book value of $300, the 1987 income statement would have been presented as shown in Figure 21-12.

Where extraordinary items exist, APB Opinion No. 19 requires that the statement of changes in financial position report (1) working capital provided by operations exclusive of extraordinary items, (2) the amount of working capital provided or used by the extraordinary items, and (3) working capital provided by operations including extraordinary items.[6] The manner in which these requirements may be met is illustrated in Figure 21-13.

Figure 21-12.
Sample Hospital
Condensed Income Statement
Year Ended December 31, 1987
($000's)

Gross patient service revenues	$9,000
Less revenue deductions	980
Net patient service revenues	8,020
Add other operating revenues	830
Total operating revenues	8,850
Less operating expenses	8,520
Operating income	330
Add nonoperating revenues (net)	160
Income before extraordinary item	490
Extraordinary item:	
Loss on retirement of long-term debt	30
Net income	$ 460

Figure 21-13.
Sample Hospital
Statement of Changes in Financial Position – Unrestricted Fund
(With Extraordinary Items)
Year Ended December 31, 1987
($000's)

Sources of working capital:	
Income before extraordinary items	$ 490
Add (deduct) items included in operations	
not requiring (providing) working capital:	
Depreciation	400

Figure 21-13—*Continued*

Loss on sale of plant assets	40
Gain on sale of long-term investments	(60)
Working capital provided by operations, exclusive of extraordinary items	870
Working capital used by extraordinary item—retirement of bonds payable	330
Working capital provided by operations, including extraordinary item	540
Proceeds of bond issue	1,000
Proceeds from sale of plant assets	450
Proceeds from sale of long-term investments	260
Receipt of donated plant assets	40
Total sources of working capital	2,290

Uses of working capital:

Purchase of plant assets	1,770
Purchase of long-term investments	440
Plant assets acquired by donation in kind	40
Total uses of working capital	2,250
Increase in working capital	$ 40

Increase (decrease) in elements of working capital:

Cash	$ 20
Temporary investments	40
Receivables (net)	120
Inventories	(20)
Prepaid expenses	10
Total current assets	170
Accounts payable	50
Accrued expenses payable	80
Total current liabilities	130
Working capital	$ 40

Because of the extraordinary item, the statement of changes in financial position begins with income before extraordinary items (rather than net income). The amount of working capital used by the extraordinary event was $330, the amount Sample Hospital paid to retire the bonds. Because the working capital, applied to the extinguishment of this debt, is included in the sources of working capital section of the statement, it is excluded from the uses of working capital section. (The reader may find it helpful to compare Figure 21-13 with Figure 21-6.)

If Sample Hospital had paid only $270 to retire bonds payable having a book value of $300, the income statement would have included an extraordinary *gain* of $30. The statement of changes in financial position would report that $270 of working capital was used by the extraordinary event. This is not to say, however, that extraordinary items always result in the *use* of working capital. An unusual and infrequent event (such as an earthquake or flood) may cause the loss of an insured noncurrent asset, the book value of which is less than the insurance recovery. In such a case, the statement of changes in financial position would include working capital provided by an extraordinary event.

Capital Leases

Assume that Sample Hospital entered into a long-term lease of equipment on December 31, 1987. The lease meets the criteria for a capital lease (see Chapter 18), and the first lease payment is due within one year. The entry at the inception of the lease was:

Leased Equipment	$ 500	
Obligation Under Capital Lease – Noncurrent		$ 465
Obligation Under Capital Lease – Current		35
Acquisition of equipment under capital lease.		

The 1987 statement of changes in financial position in a working capital format would report this situation as follows:

> Sources of working capital:
>   Long-term borrowing under capital lease $465
>
> Uses of working capital:
>   Equipment acquired under capital lease   500

If the statement is prepared in a cash format, the same presentation would be made. In addition, the increase in the current portion of the lease obligation would be shown as a net income adjustment (an addback to net income to determine working capital provided by operations).

Nonworking Capital Transactions

The all-financial resources concept requires that all significant financing and investing transactions of the hospital be reported in its statement of changes in financial position, regardless of whether working capital or cash is affected. Occasionally, transactions will occur that change the hospital's long-term financial position but do not affect working capital. These nonworking capital transactions include:

(1)   The direct exchange of long-term debt for noncurrent assets;
(2)   The direct conversion of an outstanding long-term debt for another long-term debt;
(3)   The retirement of long-term debt through a sinking fund classified as noncurrent;
(4)   The acquisition of noncurrent assets by donation in kind; and
(5)   The forgiveness of long-term debt.

In each case, the transaction is reported as both a source and a use of financial resources in the statement of changes in financial position. If Sample Hospital acquires plant assets in exchange for a long-term note, for example, the statement would report the following:

Sources of working capital:
Issuance of mortgage note for plant assets $XXX

Uses of working capital:
Acquisition of plant assets for mortgage note   XXX

Reclassifications

Assets and liabilities may at times be properly reclassified from current to noncurrent, or from noncurrent to current, sections of the hospital's balance sheet. Long-term debt becoming due within one year, for example, should be transferred from the noncurrent to the current liability classification. Since the transfer reduces working capital, the reduction in long-term debt must be reported as a use of working capital in the statement of changes in financial position. A transfer of current liabilities to long-term debt (as in a debt restructuring, or example) is presented as a source of working capital. The same principles would apply if marketable securities were transferred from the noncurrent to the current asset classification in the balance sheet, or if current receivables were reclassified as noncurrent assets.

Net Loss

When the hospital income statement reports a net loss instead of a net income, the net loss (like net income) must be adjusted for charges and credits in the income statement which did not affect working capital during the reporting period. The presentation in the statement of changes in financial position depends upon whether the adjusted net loss indicates a source or use of working capital from operations.

To illustrate, refer again to Figure 21-6 and assume that Sample Hospital's 1987 income statement reports a net loss of $290. The appropriate statement of changes in financial position presentation is:

Sources of working capital:
Net loss $ (290)
Add (deduct) items included in operations
   not requiring (providing) working capital:
Depreciation   400
Loss on sale of plant assets   40
Gain on sale of long-term investments   (60)

Working capital provided by operations $ 90

Assuming that the net loss is $690, the presentation is as follows:

Uses of working capital:
Net loss $ (690)
Add (deduct) items included in operations
   not requiring (providing) working capital:
   Depreciation   400
   Loss on sale of plant assets   40
   Gain on sale of long-term investments   (60)
Working capital applied to operations $ 310

CHAPTER 21 FOOTNOTES

1. "Reporting Changes in Financial Position," **APB Opinion No. 19** (New York: AICPA, 1971), par. 7.

2. Subcommittee on Health Care Matters, **Hospital Audit Guide** (New York: AICPA, 1982), pp. 46-47.

3. "Reporting Changes in Financial Position," **APB Opinion No. 19**, (New York: AICPA, 1971), par. 9.

4. **Ibid.**, par. 8.

5. **Ibid.**, par. 12.

6. **Ibid.**, par. 10.

QUESTIONS

1. What are the objectives of the statement of changes in financial position?
2. If a hospital's annual financial report includes an income statement, balance sheet, and statement of changes in fund balances, why should a statement of changes in financial position also be included?
3. State the formula (equation) for the statement of changes in financial position, assuming a working capital format.
4. List the three possible sources of working capital. Give an example of each.
5. List the three possible uses or applications of working capital. Give an example of each.
6. Is depreciation a source of working capital? Explain.
7. Explain what is meant by the "all financial resources" concept.
8. Odon Hospital reported a net income of $87,400 for 1987. The income statement included the following items, among others:

Loss on sale of long-term investments	$ 13,900
Depreciation expense	141,600
Gain on sale of plant assets	8,300

   In the hospital's 1987 statement of changes in financial position, what amount should be reported as "working capital provided by operations"?
9. Refer to Question 8 above, but assume that Odon Hospital reported a net loss of $87,400 for 1987. In the hospital's 1987 statement of changes in financial position, what amount should be reported as "working capital provided by operations"?
10. Distinguish between a cash-flow statement and a statement of changes in financial position.
11. Delray Hospital's balance sheets provide the following information:

	12/31/87	12/31/86
Long-term investments	$288,300	$262,700

   During 1987, the hospital sold certain long-term investments at a gain or $14,600 and purchased new long-term investments at a cost of $87,500. In the hospital's 1987 statement of changes in financial position, what amount should be reported as a source of working capital from the sale of long-term investments?
12. Explain why the annual provision for bad debts is not added back to net income (as depreciation expense is) to arrive at the amount of working capital provided by operations in a hospital's statement of changes in financial position.

636

Reporting Changes in Financial Position

EXERCISES

E1. Newtown Hospital provides you with the following comparative balance sheets:

	12/31/87	12/31/86
Current assets	$ 600	$ 500
Long-term investments	440	450
Plant and equipment	7,900	7,600
Accumulated depreciation	(1,740)	(1,550)
	$7,200	$7,000
Current liabilities	$ 534	$ 250
7% bonds payable	2,80	3,000
Fund balance	3,866	3,750
	$7,200	$7,000

The following additional information is available:

1. The 1987 income statement reports a net income of $116.
2. Long-term investments which had cost $60 were sold for $75.
3. Plant and equipment was purchased for $500.
4. Depreciation expense for the year was $280.
5. Plant and equipment was sold for $100.

Required. Prepare a statement of changes in financial position for Newtown Hospital for the year ended December 31, 1987.

E2. Oldtown Hospital provides you with the following comparative balance sheets:

	12/31/87	12/31/86
Current assets	$ 200	$ 100
Long-term investments	400	350
Plant and equipment	2,000	1,860
Accumulated depreciation	(900)	(780)
	$1,700	$1,530
Current liabilities	$ 90	$ 40
8% long-term notes payable		500
7% long-term notes payable	600	
Fund balance	1,010	990
	$1,700	$1,530

The 1987 income statement shows a net income of $80. Long-term investments were purchased at a cost of $90; certain other long-term investments were sold for $54. Plant and equipment which had cost $100 (and was 60 percent depreciated) was sold for $32. In 1987, $60 of reimbursed depreciation restricted by third-party payers was transferred to the Plant Replacement and Expansion Fund.

Required. Prepare a statement of changes in financial position for Oldtown Hospital for the year ended December 31, 1987.

E3.   The following are multiple-choice questions relating to the statement of changes in financial position:

1.   The amortization of bond premium on long-term debt should be presented in a statement of changes in financial position as a (an)

a.   Addition to net income.
b.   Deduction from net income.
c.   Use of funds.
d.   Source and use of funds.

2.   How should the amortization of bond discount for a bond issuer be shown on the statement of changes in financial position, defining funds as working capital?

a.   Need not be shown.
b.   Use of funds.
c.   Expense not requiring the use of funds.
d.   Contra-expense item not providing funds.

3.   The working capital format is an acceptable format for presenting a statement of changes in financial position. Which of the following formats is (are) also acceptable?

	Cash	Quick Assets
a.	Acceptable	Not acceptable
b.	Not acceptable	Not acceptable
c.	Not acceptable	Acceptable
d.	Acceptable	Acceptable

4.   If a hospital issues both a balance sheet and an income statement with comparative figures for the prior period, a statement of changes in financial position

a.   Is not necessary, but may be issued at the hospital's option.
b.   Should not be issued.

    c.   Should be issued for each period for which an income statement is presented.

    d.   Should be issued for the current year only.

5. The financial statement which has as its primary function the summarization of the financing and investing aspects of all significant transactions affecting financial position is the

    a.   Balance sheet.

    b.   Income statement.

    c.   Statement of changes in financial position.

    d.   Statement of changes in fund balances.

6. A loss on the sale of equipment should be presented in the statement of changes in financial position as a (an)

    a.   Deduction from net income.

    b.   Addition to net income.

    c.   Source and use of funds.

    d.   Use of funds.

7. A gain on the sale of equipment should be presented in the statement of changes in financial position as a (an)

    a.   Deduction from net income.

    b.   Addition to net income.

    c.   Source and use of funds.

    d.   Source of funds.

8. The receipt of an item of equipment donated in kind to a hospital should be presented in the statement of changes in financial position as a (an)

    a.   Deduction from net income.

    b.   Addition to net income.

    c.   Source and use of funds.

    d.   Source of funds.

Required. Select the best answer for each of the above multiple-choice questions.

E4. Following are comparative balance sheets and other information pertaining to Magnolia Hospital:

Balance Sheets

	12/31/87	12/31/86
Current assets	$ 474,000	$ 320,000
Plant assets	1,230,000	1,200,000
Accumulated depreciation	(436,000)	(420,000)
	$1,268,000	$ 1,100,000
Current liabilities	$ 360,000	$ 160,000
Bond payable	400,000	600,000
Discount on bonds	(12,000)	(20,000)
Fund balance	520,000	360,000
	$1,268,000	$ 1,100,000

The following additional information is available:

1. During 1987, Magnolia sold at no gain or loss equipment with a book value of $76,000 and purchased new equipment costing $150,000.
2. During 1987, bonds with a face and book value of $200,000 were retired, with no gain or loss. They were not current liabilities prior to their retirement.
3. The fund balance was affected only by the 1987 net income or loss.

Required. How much working capital was provided by operations during 1987?

PROBLEMS

P1. Following are comparative balance sheets for Memorial Hospital:

	12/31/87	12/31/86
Cash	$ 170,000	$ 150,000
Accounts receivable (net)	180,000	200,000
Inventories	71,000	60,000
Prepaid expenses	4,000	5,000
Plant and equipment (net)	800,000	750,000
	$1,225,000	$1,165,000
Accounts payable	$ 105,000	$ 120,000
Accrued payroll	65,000	70,000
Other current liabilities	40,000	30,000
Mortgage payable	360,000	400,000
Hospital equity (fund balance)	655,000	545,000
	$1,225,000	$1,165,000

The following additional information is available:

1. Net income for 1987 was $80,000.
2. Depreciation expense for 1987 was $40,000.
3. A payment of $40,000 was made on the mortgage during 1987.
4. During 1987, equipment was purchased for $90,000.
5. During 1987, an unrestricted contribution of $30,000 was received.

Required. (1) Prepare a statement of changes in working capital for 1987. (2) Prepare a statement of changes in financial position for 1987. (3) What other accounting statements are most related to the statement of changes in financial position? (4) List three significant questions regarding past performances which the statement of changes in financial position might answer.

P2.   The following information was obtained from the accounting records of Medicare Hospital:

Balance Sheets

	6/30/87	6/30/86
Current assets:		
Cash	$ 549,600	$ 425,100
Patients' accounts receivable, less allowance for uncollectibles of $81,000 6/30/87 and $108,000 at 6/30/86	337,200	354,100
Inventories	85,000	76,800
Prepaid expenses	46,800	56,200
	1,018,600	912,200
Plant funds:		
Cash (Note #1)	274,600	204,600
Land	100,000	100,000
Buildings	9,200,000	9,200,000
Equipment	1,750,000	1,600,000
Accumulated depreciation	(1,818,000)	(1,518,000)
	$ 10,525,200	$10,498,800
Current liabilities and fund balance:		
Accounts payable	$ 90,000	$ 78,000
Accrued payroll and other expenses	177,100	160,000
Patients' advance payments	5,600	5,000
Fund balance	745,900	669,200
	1,018,600	912,200

Plant funds:	1,910,000	2,110,000
Mortgage payable	7,596,600	7,476,600
Fund balance		
	$10,525,200	$10,498,800

Note #1 – Unexpended plant funds:

Balance, 7/1/86	$204,600
Add (deduct):	
Gifts for plant fund	120,000
Depreciation funded	300,000
Reduction of mortgage	(200,000)
Equipment purchases	(150,000)
Balance, 6/30/87	$274,600

Income Statements
Years Ended June 30

	1987	1986
Gross patient revenues	$5,194,600	$4,700,000
Revenue deductions:		
Charity service	210,000	195,000
Contractual adjustments	651,900	610,000
Bad debts	60,000	48,000
Total deductions	921,900	853,000
Net patient revenues	4,272,700	3,847,000
Operating expenses:		
Administrative and fiscal	330,000	265,000
Dietary	476,000	400,000
Household and property	580,000	460,000
Professional care of patients	2,510,000	2,250,000
Depreciation	300,000	280,000
Total operating expenses	4,196,000	3,655,000
Net income	$ 76,700	$ 192,000

Required. (1) Prepare a statement of changes in working capital for the year ended June 30, 1987. (2) Prepare a statement of changes in financial position for the year ended June 30, 1987.

P3. Following are comparative balance sheets for Memorial Hospital:

	9/30/87	9/30/86
Cash	$ 22,000	$ 20,000
Accounts receivable (net)	680,000	650,000
Other current assets	19,500	16,000
Long-term investments in securities	575,000	550,000
Land	70,000	70,000
Buildings and equipment	1,975,000	975,000
Accumulated depreciation	(565,000)	(550,000)
	$2,776,500	$1,731,000
Accounts payable	$ 65,000	$ 70,000
Accrued payroll	62,000	55,000
Payroll taxes payable	14,500	12,000
Mortgage payable	500,000	500,000
Bonds payable (net of $30,000 discount)	970,000	
Fund balance	1,165,000	1,094,000
	$2,776,500	$1,731,000

The following additional information is available:

1. The hospital does not fund depreciation.
2. Bonds with a face value of $1,000,000 were issued on April 1, 1987, at 97 and are due on April 1, 2007.
3. A check for $25,000 was presented to the hospital as a gift to be used at the discretion of the governing board.
4. No amortization of the bond discount has yet been recorded.

Required. Prepare a statement of changes in financial position for the year ended September 30, 1987.

P4. General Hospital is a not-for-profit voluntary hospital of 148 beds (adults and children). Its Unrestricted Fund is divided into two self-balancing sets of accounts which are called the General Fund and the Plant Fund. Comparative balance sheets and an income statement are provided below:

Balance Sheets

	12/31/87	12/31/86
General fund:		
Cash	$ 149,000	$ 40,000
Accounts receivable	310,000	300,000
Allowance for uncollectible accounts	(21,000)	(20,000)
Inventories	58,000	60,000
Prepaid expenses	7,000	10,000
Total assets	$ 503,000	$ 390,000
Accounts payable	$ 45,000	$ 50,000
Accrued payroll	43,000	40,000
Other current payables	15,000	12,000
Due to plant fund	92,000	
General fund balance	308,000	288,000
Total liabilities and fund balance	$ 503,000	$ 390,000
Plant fund:		
Land	$ 150,000	$ 150,000
Buildings	4,000,000	4,000,000
Accumulated depreciation	(860,000)	(740,000)
Equipment	350,000	300,000
Accumulated depreciation	(160,000)	(140,000)
Cash	28,000	60,000
Investments	100,000	80,000
Due from general fund	92,000	
	$3,700,000	$3,710,000
Mortgage payable	$ 470,000	$ 500,000
Plant fund balance	3,230,000	3,210,000
Total liabilities and fund balance	$3,700,000	$3,710,000

1987 Income Statement

Gross charges to patients	$2,050,000
Less deductions	50,000
Net charges to patients	2,000,000
Other operating revenues	20,000
Total operating revenues	2,020,000

Operating expenses:
Payroll   1,220,000
Supplies   450,000
Other operating expenses   160,000
   Depreciation – buildings   120,000
   Depreciation – equipment   20,000

Total operating expenses   1,970,000

Operating income   50,000
Less interest expense   30,000

Net income for the year $ 20,000

The following additional information is available:

1. Make-up of investment portfolio:

	12/31/87	12/31/86
Corporate stocks	$ 30,000	$ 10,000
U.S. Treasury bills	70,000	70,000

2. Accounts receivable over 90 days old   50,000   40,000
3. Census days for 1987 (adults and children), 47,619
4. Percentage of occupancy, 88%
5. Equipment purchases for 1987:
    From general fund $18,000
    From plant fund   32,000
6. Mortgage principal payment from the general fund in 1987, $30,000.
7. There was a stock donation received in the plant fund of $20,000 in 1987. It will be used for plant expansion.
8. In January, 1988, in accordance with hospital policy of funding depreciation, a transfer of cash will be made from the general fund to the plant fund in an amount equal to the 1987 depreciation less the amounts spent by the general fund in 1987 for equipment purchases and the mortgage principal payment.

Required. (1) Prepare a schedule of changes in working capital for 1987. (2) Prepare a statement of changes in financial position for 1987.

P5. Mark Hospital's preclosing trial balance at 12/31/86 is presented below:

	Dr.	Cr.
Cash	$ 310	
Accrued interest receivable	40	
Accounts receivable	1,460	
Allowance for uncollectible accounts		$ 170
Inventories	180	
Prepaid expenses	35	
Long-term investments	990	
Plant assets	6,100	
Accumulated depreciation		1,300
Accounts payable		390
Accrued expenses payable		210
Deferred revenues		50
Bond payable		2,500
Fund balance		3,225
Patient service revenues		8,900
Deductions from revenues	800	
Other operating revenues		670
Nursing service expense	3,200	
Other professional service expense	2,100	
General services expense	1,600	
Fiscal and administrative expense	1,500	
Depreciation expense	570	
Other operating expenses	320	
Nonoperating revenues		190
	$18,405	$18,405

The following additional information relates to 1987 activities:

1. Patient service revenues total $9,600.
2. Collections were as follows on accounts receivable:

Cash	$8,600
Deductions from revenues	750
Credited to accounts receivable	$9,350

3. The hospital sold long-term investments (cost $50) for $58.
4. The hospital sold plant assets (cost $250, accumulated depreciation $170) for $65.
5. Other cash receipts were as follows:

Other operating revenues	$ 680
Nonoperating revenues	170
Proceeds of new bond issue	3,500

6. Operating expenses vouchered were as follows:

Nursing services	$3,100
Other professional services	2,000
General services	900
Fiscal and administrative services	1,500
Other operating expenses	260

7. Depreciation expense for the year was $550.
8. Vouchers issued for other items were as follows:

Purchases of inventory	$ 900
Purchases of long-term investments	500
Purchase of plant assets	1,500
Retirement of bonds payable	2,500

9. Checks issued in payment of vouchers totaled $12,300.
10. Cost of supplies used during the year was as follows:

Nursing services	$ 210
Other professional services	140
General services	490
Fiscal and administrative services	70

11. Accrued interest receivable at 12/31/87 was $55.
12. The allowance for uncollectible accounts at 12/31/87 should be adjusted to a balance of $195.
13. Prepaid expenses at 12/31/87 total $49.
14. Accrued expenses payable at 12/31/87 total $234 (make the necessary adjustment through nursing service expenses).
15. Deferred revenues at 12/31/87 total $75 (make the necessary adjustment through other operating revenues).

Required. (1) Prepare a statement of changes in financial position worksheet for 1987. (2) Prepare a formal statement of changes in financial position for 1987.

P6.   Bruce Hospital provides you with the following comparative balance sheets:

	12/31/87	12/31/86
Cash	$ 140	$ 290
Accrued interest receivable	50	40
Accounts receivable	1,800	1,600
Allowance for uncollectible accounts	(200)	(180)
Inventories	170	130
Prepaid expenses	60	70
Long-term investments	1,000	750
Plant assets	7,000	6,800
Accumulated depreciation	(1,900)	(1,300)
	$8,120	$8,200

Accounts payable	$ 300	$ 290
Accrued expenses payable	210	240
Deferred revenues	80	90
Bonds payable	3,000	3,000
Fund balance	4,530	4,580
	$8,120	$8,200

The following additional information is available:

1. During 1987 certain long-term investments were sold at a loss of $40, and new long-term investments were purchased for $400.

2. During 1987, certain plant assets (cost $250, accumulated depreciation $240) were sold for $22.

3. During 1987, an old $3,000, 7% bond issue was retired at face value, and a new $3,000, 6% bond issue was sold at face value.

4. The 1987 income statement reported a net loss of $50.

Required. (1) Prepare a statement of changes in financial position worksheet for 1987. (2) Prepare a formal statement of changes in financial position for 1987.

22
Analysis and Interpretation of Financial Statements

The emphasis in this book has been directed primarily to the development and managerial uses of accounting information in the **internal** financial administration of the hospital. It has been shown that hospital managements make many critically important operating and financial decisions based upon data contained in income statements, balance sheets, statements of changes in fund balances and financial position, statistical summaries, and a wide variety of detailed, special-purpose reports generated by the hospital's information system. Accounting, as the essential component of such a system, makes an indispensable contribution to financial management within the hospital. The accounting process, however, is by no means entirely management-oriented.

Many groups outside the hospital enterprise are also vitally interested in its financial affairs, and they make extensive use of information provided by hospital accounting. Included among these external users are:

1. Creditors (suppliers, banks, and other lenders).
2. Third-party payers (governmental agencies, Blue Cross, commercial insurers, and other reimbursement groups).
3. Hospital-related organizations (hospital, medical, and other healthcare associations, churches, schools, fraternal orders, and other sponsoring or associated organizations).
4. Governmental taxing and regulatory authorities.
5. Hospital planning agencies and rate-review commissions.
6. Investors (bond holders and, in investor-owned hospital corporations, stockholders).
7. Securities exchanges, brokers, and investment bankers.
8. Employees and their labor unions.
9. General public (including donors, foundations, researchers, and students).

Some of these groups are interested in the hospital's operating performance; others are interested in its financial strength and debt-paying ability; still others are concerned with the management's stewardship responsibilities and accountability, or with the hospital's compliance with laws, regulations or contractual agreements. Whatever their interests and points of view may be, all of these groups have a common need for financial information about hospitals.

Outsiders generally do not have access to the detailed data that are made available to the hospital management and governing board. In most instances, outsiders must rely upon the information provided in the hospital's published financial reports in making intelligent decisions in the areas with which they are concerned. This chapter considers the analysis of financial statements in such reports by outsiders, but the reader should recognize that internal management is highly concerned with many of the same questions that are raised by external users of hospital financial reports. Many of the analytical techniques that are described here are also useful for internal management purposes. Some, in fact, have already been discussed in earlier chapters of this book.

ROLE OF INDEPENDENT AUDITORS

The financial statements of a hospital are the representations of its management. They are prepared by hospital employees working as accountants and responsible to the hospital administration. In certain circumstances, there may be an understandable bias on the part of these accountants to report the hospital's financial position and operating results in the most favorable light or otherwise according to the desires of the management. This tendency undoubtedly exists; hospital accountants have a certain loyalty to their institutions and to the field of hospital accounting generally. This loyalty, however, would be seriously misplaced if it were used as an excuse for shoddy, misleading, or fraudulent financial reporting. It should be recognized that the best interests of the business of hospitals are not served in this way and that there are legal and moral responsibilities to external groups that must be strictly observed.

Yet, the fact remains that the hospital's financial statements are prepared by hospital employees who are not independent of the management whose performance and stewardship is measured in those statements. What assurance, then, does the user of a hospital financial report have that the figures are reasonably accurate and that all significant information is fully disclosed? While serious errors and intentional falsifications are not likely to exist, the objectivity, competence, and integrity of those who prepare the financial statements may be questioned.

As a result, most hospitals engage certified public accountants to make an independent verification and examination of the accounts and to render an opinion as to the fairness of the representations in the financial statements. An unqualified audit report usually reads somewhat as follows:

> We have examined the balance sheet of Hartsville Hospital at December 31, 1987, and the related statements of income, changes in fund balances and changes in financial position for the year then ended. Our examination was made in accordance with generally accepted auditing standards, and accordingly included such tests of the accounting records and such other auditing procedures as we considered necessary in the circumstances.
>
> In our opinion, the statements referred to in the preceding paragraph present fairly the financial position of Hartsville Hospital at December 31, 1987, and the results of its operations and changes in financial position for the year then ended, in conformity with generally accepted accounting principles applied on a consistent basis.

If the external auditors are not completely satisfied with every material aspect of the hospital's financial statements, they will qualify their opinion. The auditors will indicate what they believe to be improperly reported. In addition, they will disclose any matters that they were unable to verify to their satisfaction. There are instances where the auditors' qualifications are so important or extensive that they are unable to render any opinion at all.

Due to the external auditors' professional status, independence, and competence, the auditors' opinion is accepted as authoritative and reliable by all parties concerned. Should those who rely upon the auditors' opinion suffer any loss as a result of such reliance, the auditors may be sued if the audit was not performed in accordance with generally accepted auditing standards.

Briefly, this is the "attest function" of independent auditors. Attestation, however, is by no means their only function. Certified public accountants also provide management or administrative services, including assistance with problems of cost analysis, rate setting, budgeting, and computer installations. They also render tax services and consult with hospital managements on financial, personnel, and other business matters. The auditors' advice and recommendations in these areas sometimes are as valuable as the audit itself.

It is a widely held notion that the major purpose of an audit is to detect embezzlements and other frauds. The detection of fraud, however, is largely incidental to the main purpose of an audit, which is to provide a basis for forming an opinion as to the fairness of the financial statement presentations. Often an audit will uncover fraud, but it will not always necessarily do so. Although auditors perform certain procedures designed to detect common types of fraud, embezzlements occasionally may go undiscovered over a period of several audits.

There also is a common misconception that the auditors' opinion means that each figure in the financial statements is precisely accurate to the penny and that other auditors would arrive at identical amounts. The auditors make no guarantee of this kind. An unqualified opinion means only that the amounts in the financial statements are, in the auditors' opinion, fairly stated. In other words, the information is reasonably accurate in all significant respects in terms of the ordinary uses of financial statements. The determination of net income and financial position is to some extent a matter of opinion, estimates, and judgment. Other auditors may well arrive at different results, but these results are not likely to be materially different unless alternative generally accepted accounting principles are followed.

BASIC ANALYTICAL PROCEDURES

Consider this statement: "The currents assets of Hartsville Hospital amount to $1,726 at December 31, 1987." Does this information have any particular significance? No. An absolute dollar amount standing alone has little, if any, meaning. The financial statement analyst therefore finds it necessary to employ certain devices to ascertain, measure, and evaluate relationships among financial data and the changes that occur over a period of time. The analyst is interested, for example, not so much in the amount of current assets but in the relationship between, say, current assets and current liabilities and in the changes in this relationship **over time**. Comparative data are essential.

The presentation of a single year's operating results and financial position is of questionable utility to financial statement users. Inherent in such a presentation is a tendency to overemphasize the significance of the figures. The 12-month fiscal period is but a relatively brief time segment in the business history of a hospital. Economic factors having a major influence on the hospital's financial status have a history of sudden and substantial change. Comparative financial statements bring attention to the fact that single-year statements merely are periodic installments in a continuing financial history. They provide reference to past performance and place the current year statements in proper perspective.

It is essential, however, that prior year figures shown for comparative purposes be in fact comparable with those of the current year. All matters and changes in practice which affect comparability should be disclosed. In APB Statement No. 4, the following conditions were established for comparative statements:[1]

1. The presentations are in good form, i.e., the arrangement within the statements is identical.
2. The content of the statements is identical, i.e., the same items from the underlying accounting records are classified under the same captions.
3. Accounting principles are not changed or, if changed, the effects of the changes are disclosed.
4. Changes in circumstances or in the nature of the underlying transactions are disclosed.

The reporting periods, of course, should be of equal and regular lengths, and the factor of consistency in practices and procedures must be present. If the criteria mentioned here are not met, the comparisons could be misleading and erroneous conclusions might be drawn from them.

When accounting changes are made, APB Opinion No. 20 requires special procedures in the presentation of comparative statements.[2] The requirements were discussed earlier in this book, but they are summarized below:

1. A change in accounting principle generally requires no restatement of financial statements of prior periods included for comparative purposes, but the effect of the change on the net income of the current and prior periods must be disclosed.
2. A change in accounting estimate is accounted for in present and subsequent periods, with disclosure of its effect on net income, but the financial statements of prior periods included for comparative purposes are reported without change.
3. A change in the reporting entity requires the restatement of the financial statements of all prior periods included for comparative purposes.

Horizontal Analysis

Horizontal analysis of comparative statements consists of the development of data relating to absolute (dollar amount) and relative (percentage) changes which have occurred over a period of time. The significance of the absolute amounts of change is made more evident by the expression of such changes in percentage terms. Consider, for example, the following:

1. **Balance Sheet Analysis:**

	December 31		Increase (Decrease)	
	1987	1986	Amount	Percent
Current assets	$1,726	$1,482	$244	16.5%

2. **Income Statement Analysis:**

	Year Ended 12/31		Increase (Decrease)	
	1987	1986	Amount	Percent
Deductions from patient service revenues	$1,430	$1,465	$ (35)	(2.4%)

The percentage increase or decrease is determined by dividing the dollar amount of change by the base year (1986 in this example) figure, i.e., $244/$1,482 = 16.5%. Where the base year figure is zero or a negative value, the dollar change cannot be expressed as a percentage.

Figure 22-1 illustrates a horizontal analysis of the Hartsville Hospital balance sheet (Unrestricted Fund only) presented in Chapter 20. A horizontal analysis of Hartsville Hospital's condensed income statement, discussed in Chapter 19, is illustrated in Figure 22-2. In each case, both dollar changes and percentage changes are provided to show the absolute as well as the relative changes that have taken place between 1986 and 1987. Although not illustrated here, a similar analysis could be made of Hartsville Hospital's statements of changes in fund balances and financial position.

Figure 22-1.
Hartsville Hospital
Condensed Comparative Balance Sheets – Unrestricted Fund
Horizontal Analysis
December 31, 1987 and 1986

Assets	December 31		Increase (Decrease)	
	1987	1986	Amount	Percent
Current Assets:				
Cash	$ 268	$ 211	$ 57	27.0%
Temporary investments	126	34	92	270.6
Receivables–patients (net)	969	854	115	13.5
Other receivables	42	39	3	7.7
Inventories	296	315	(19)	(6.0)
Prepaid expenses	25	29	(4)	(13.8)
Total current assets	1,726	1,482	244	16.5
Board-designated assets	466	442	24	5.4
Property, plant and equipment (net)	8,126	8,185	(59)	(.7)
Other assets	67	88	(21)	(23.9)
Total assets	$10,385	$10,197	$ 188	1.8

Figure 22-1—*Continued*

Liabilities and Fund Balance

Current Liabilities:				
Current installments of long-term debt	$ 180	$ 180	$ ..	..
Notes payable	125	75	50	66.7
Accounts payable	196	202	(6)	(3.0)
Accrued expenses payable	238	217	21	9.7
Payroll taxes withheld	81	63	18	28.6
Advances from third-party payers	75	55	20	36.4
Other	42	29	13	44.8
Total current liabilities	937	821	116	14.1
Noncurrent Liabilities:				
Deferred revenues	171	114	57	50.0
Long-term debt	1,320	1,500	(180)	(12.0)
Past service pension liability	227	251	(24)	(9.6)
Total noncurrent liabilities	1,718	1,865	(147)	(7.9)
Total liabilities	2,655	2,686	(31)	(1.2)
Unrestricted Fund Balance	7,730	7,511	219	2.9
Total liabilities and fund balance	$10,385	$10,197	$ 188	1.8

Figure 22-2.
Hartsville Hospital
Condensed Comparative Income Statements
Horizontal Analysis
Years Ended December 31, 1987 and 1986

	1987	1986	Increase (Decrease) Amount	Percent
Patient service revenues	$8,830	$7,326	$1,504	20.5%
Deductions from patient service revenues	1,430	1,465	(35)	(2.4)
Net patient service revenues	7,400	5,861	1,539	26.3
Other operating revenues	505	407	98	24.1
Total operating revenues	7,905	6,268	1,637	26.1
Operating Expenses:				
Nursing services	2,560	2,197	363	16.5
Other professional services	2,050	1,615	435	26.9
General services	1,350	1,033	317	30.7
Fiscal and administrative services	1,925	1,614	311	19.3
Total operating expenses	7,885	6,459	1,426	22.1
Net operating income (loss)	20	(191)	211	..
Nonoperating revenues	224	176	48	27.3
Net income (loss) for the year	$ 244	$ (15)	$ 259	..

Where more than two years are involved in a horizontal analysis, trend percentages often are employed. Each figure in the base year statement (the earliest year) is considered to represent 100 percent, and the figures in succeeding statements are expressed as a percentage of the base figure. Examine, for example, the illustration in Figure 22-3 of a portion of Hartsville Hospital's income statements.

Figure 22-3.
Hartsville Hospital
Trend Analysis of Operating Results
Five Years Ended December 31, 1987

| | Year Ended December 31 | | | | |
Amounts	1987	1986	1985	1984	1983
Patient service revenues	$8,830	$7,326	$7,205	$6,930	$6,487
Deductions from patient service revenues	1,430	1,465	1,132	988	741
Net patient service revenues	$7,400	$5,861	$6,073	$5,942	$5,746
Other operating revenues	505	407	478	527	492
Total operating revenues	$7,905	$6,268	$6,551	$6,469	$6,238
Trend Percentages					
Patient service revenues	136.1%	112.9%	111.1%	106.8%	100.0%
Deductions from patient service revenues	193.0	197.7	152.8	133.3	100.0
Net patient service revenues	128.8%	102.0%	105.7%	103.4%	100.0%
Other operating revenues	102.6	82.7	97.2	107.1	100.0
Total operating revenues	126.7%	100.5%	105.0%	103.7%	100.0%

While comparative data covering two or more years have unquestionable value, hospital managements and external users of financial statements should exercise caution in drawing conclusions from an extended array of comparative data. Changes in the purchasing power of the dollar tend to distort comparisons of data relating to more than a short period of time. Such data may reflect growth and progress when, in fact, the hospital has merely stood still or even moved backward in real terms, i.e., volume of service. Therefore, such data should always be evaluated in conjunction with service volume statistics.

In Figure 22-3, for example, it can be seen that gross patient service revenues in 1987 were 136.1 percent of such revenues in 1983, the base year. Does this mean that the volume of patient services has grown 36.1 percent over this five-year period? Or, has there been a seven percent annual rate of inflation which is reflected in Hartsville Hospital's service rates? What has been the trend for this period in patient days of service, in number of meals served, and in other statistical measurements of the volume of hospital services? The progression pattern of change reflected in Figure 22-3 is also very interesting.

Trend percentages can be extremely useful in bringing out unusual relationships that might not be noticed in an examination of dollar amounts alone. The technique, of course, can be applied equally well to the balance sheet and other financial statements, but no illustration is provided here.

Vertical Analysis

The vertical analysis of comparative statements involves the development of component percentages which express the relationships among related data within each individual statement. This procedure is also referred to as **common-size analysis,** and the percentages sometimes are called **structural ratios.**

In the Hartsville Hospital balance sheet illustrated in Figure 22-4, the base figure for asset analysis is total assets, and all other figures in the statement are expressed as percentages of the base figure. The December 31, 1987, cash balance of $268, for example, is 2.6 percent ($268/$10,385) of the total assets of the Unrestricted Fund. The base figure for the analysis of liabilities and fund balance is their combined total (same as total assets), and each component item is converted to a percentage of that base. It may be said, for example, that total liabilities at December 31, 1987, are 25.6 percent of total assets ($2,655/$10,385). This type of analysis is helpful in evaluating the balance sheet in terms of management's allocation of resources. It also indicates the sources from which the assets have been financed, i.e., the hospital's capital structure.

Figure 22-4.
Hartsville Hospital
Condensed Comparative Balance Sheets – Unrestricted Fund
Vertical Analysis
December 31, 1987 and 1986

Assets	December 31, 1987 Amount	Percent	December 31, 1986 Amount	Percent
Current Assets:				
Cash	$ 268	2.6%	$ 211	2.1%
Temporary investments	126	1.2	34	.3
Receivables–patients (net)	969	9.3	854	8.4
Other receivables	42	.4	39	.4
Inventories	296	2.9	315	3.1
Prepaid expenses	25	.2	29	.2
Total current assets	$ 1,726	16.6%	$ 1,482	14.5%
Board-designated assets	466	4.5	442	4.3
Property, plant and equipment (net)	8,126	78.3	8,185	80.3
Other assets	67	.6	88	.9
Total assets	$10,385	100.0%	$10,197	100.0%

Liabilities and Fund Balance				
Current Liabilities:				
Current installments of long-term debt	$ 180	1.7%	$ 180	1.8%
Notes payable	125	1.2	75	.7
Accounts payable	196	1.9	202	2.0
Accrued expenses payable	238	2.3	217	2.1
Payroll taxes withheld	81	.8	63	.6
Advances from third-party payers	75	.7	55	.5
Other	42	.4	29	.3
Total current liabilities	$ 937	9.0%	$ 821	8.0%
Noncurrent Liabilities:				
Deferred revenues	$ 171	1.7%	$ 114	1.1%
Long-term debt	1,320	12.7	1,500	14.7
Past service pension liability	227	2.2	251	2.5
Total noncurrent liabilities	$ 1,718	16.6%	$ 1,865	18.3%
Total liabilities	$ 2,655	25.6%	$ 2,686	26.3%
Unrestricted Fund Balance	7,730	74.4	7,511	73.7
Total liabilities and fund balance	$10,385	100.0%	$10,197	100.0%

For certain analytical purposes it may be more useful to develop component percentages for current assets, using total current assets as the 100 percent figure. This is illustrated in Figure 22-5, where it can be seen, for example, that cash is 15.5 percent of total current assets at December 31, 1987. A similar analysis, of course, could be made of current liabilities or total liabilities. It may also be helpful to compute the percentage of each current asset to the total of current liabilities. These latter alternatives, however, are not illustrated here.

Figure 22-5.
Hartsville Hospital
Component Percentage Analysis of Current Assets
December 31, 1987 and 1986

	December 31, 1987		December 31, 1986	
	Amount	Percent	Amount	Percent
Cash	$ 268	15.5%	$ 211	14.2%
Temporary investments	126	7.3	34	2.3
Receivables–patients (net)	969	56.1	854	57.6
Other receivables	42	2.4	39	2.6
Inventories	296	17.2	315	21.3
Prepaid expenses	25	1.5	29	2.0
Total current assets	$ 1,726	100.0%	$ 1,482	100.0%

Vertical analysis may also be applied to the hospital's income statement. Such an analysis is illustrated in Figure 22-6, using the Hartsville Hospital statement. In this case, total operating revenues is taken as the base figure for the computation of component percentages. In 1987, for example, the general services division expenses were 17.1 percent ($1,350/$7,905) of total operating revenues. As indicated at the top of the statement, however, the deductions from patient service revenues generally are expressed as a percentage of gross patient service revenues. Otherwise, the component percentage would be distorted to the extent of other operating revenues to which the deductions are not related. In other words, while 1987 deductions are 18.1 percent ($1,430/$7,905) of total operating revenues, it is more meaningful to say that the deductions are 16.2 percent ($1,430/$8,830) of gross patient service revenues, or 16.2 cents of each dollar billed to patients for hospital services.

Figure 22-6.
Hartsville Hospital
Condensed Comparative Income Statements
Vertical Analysis
Years Ended December 31, 1987 and 1986

	1987 Amount	1987 Percent	1986 Amount	1986 Percent
Patient service revenues	$8,830	100.0%	$7,326	100.0%
Deductions from patient service revenues	1,430	16.2	1,465	20.0
Net patient service revenues	$7,400	83.8%	$5,861	80.0%
Net patient service revenues (above)	$7,400	93.6%	$5,861	93.5%
Other operating revenues	505	6.4	407	6.5
Total operating revenues	$7,905	100.0%	$6,268	100.0%
Operating Expenses:				
Nursing services	$2,560	32.4%	$2,197	35.0%
Other professional services	2,050	25.9	1,615	25.8
General services	1,350	17.1	1,033	16.5
Fiscal and administrative services	1,925	24.3	1,614	25.7
Total operating expenses	$7,885	99.7%	$6,459	103.0%
Net operating income (loss)	$ 20	.3%	$ (191)	(3.0)%
Nonoperating income	224	2.8	176	2.8
Net income (loss) for the year	$ 244	3.1%	$ (15)	(.2)%

In their external reports, hospitals often present operating expenses in a natural classification rather than in the functional classification provided in Figure 22-6. In such cases, a vertical analysis of the income statement would develop component percentages as illustrated in Figure 22-7.

The information developed in the analysis shown in Figure 22-7 often is most meaningful to many external users as it provides an insight into Hartsville Hospital's operating activities. Of each dollar of the hospital's revenue from patient services, for example, 90.5 cents is derived from inpatient services and 9.5 cents comes from outpatient services. Only 83.8 cents of each revenue dollar is actually collected, however. In terms of total operating revenues, 93.6 cents of each dollar results from patient services and only 6.4 cents is generated from other operating sources. Of each dollar of total operating revenues, 99.7 percent is taken by operating expenses of which the greater part (63.8 cents) is employee compensation. Hartsville Hospital's operating margin is only three-tenths of a penny. Although an additional 2.8 cents of income is obtained from nonoperating sources, the hospital's continuing ability to provide quality health care services and to maintain its productive capacity generally must be evaluated largely in terms of operating income without substantial reliance being placed on uncertain nonoperating sources.

The statements of changes in fund balances and financial position also may be subjected to vertical analysis in order to bring out significant relationships that might otherwise be overlooked. Whatever statement is so analyzed, the trend of component percentages over a period of years should be considered. In addition, where supporting schedules are provided to show the details of financial statement totals, the individual items in such schedules may be expressed as percentages of the totals they support.

Figure 22-7.
Hartsville Hospital
Alternative Condensed Comparative Income Statement
Vertical Analysis
Year Ended December 31, 1987

	Amount	Percent
Patient Service Revenues:		
Inpatients	$7,995	90.5%
Outpatients	835	9.5
Total patient service revenues	$8,830	100.0%
Deductions from patient service revenues	1,430	16.2
Net patient service revenues	$7,400	83.8%
Net patient service revenues (above)	$7,400	93.6%
Other operating revenues	505	6.4
Total operating revenues	$7,905	100.0%
Operating Expenses:		
Salaries and wages (including employee benefits)	$5,043	63.8%
Supplies and other expenses	2,347	29.7
Depreciation	360	4.5
Interest	135	1.7
Total operating expenses	$7,885	99.7%
Net operating income	$ 20	.3%
Nonoperating revenues	224	2.8
Net income for the year	$ 244	3.1%

Ratios

A ratio is the quotient which results when one number is divided by another. It is one number expressed in terms of another; it is an expression of the quantitative relationship between the two numbers. A ratio may be stated as a common fraction, decimally, or in percentage form. If, for example, the inventory of a hospital is $50 and the current assets are $400, the ratio of inventory to total current assets is 1/8, 0.125, or 12 1/2 percent. It may be said, then that the inventory is 1/8th of total current assets, or that for every $1 of current assets the hospital has $0.125 invested in inventory, or that the inventory is 12 1/2 percent of total current assets, or that the ratio of inventory to current assets is 1 to 8. The ratio is found by dividing one number ($400), called the base, into the other number ($50). Ratios are used in financial analysis to expedite comparisons and make relationships more intelligible. It should be recognized, however, that computing a ratio does not add any information not already inherent in the figures that are being compared.

Many different ratios can be computed from the data in financial statements. The analyst, however, does not compute all possible ratios. Many, such as the ratio of prepaid expenses to nonoperating revenues, would be totally meaningless. The analyst must select those ratios which have significance and relevance for the purposes of the analysis. In the following pages of this chapter, the discussion is directed to the selection, computation, and interpretation of a number of ratios commonly employed in financial analysis.

Internal and External Standards

Assume that a hospital has total current assets of $400 at December 31, 1987. Is this amount of current assets excessive, inadequate, or "about right"? Seeing this $400 total of current assets in the balance sheet, should the hospital management and its creditors be elated, depressed, or indifferent? How can a judgment be made as to the adequacy of the current asset figure?

As stated before, a single figure standing alone is meaningless. To have meaning, a figure must be related to something else. A standard of comparison is necessary. Such standards may be either **internal** or **external** standards.

In the foregoing illustrations, the comparisons involved the financial data of a single hospital over a period of time or within the statements of a single year. To form a judgement concerning the $400 of current assets mentioned above, for example, a horizontal analysis would be helpful:

	December 31		Increase (Decrease)	
	1987	1986	Amount	Percent
Current Assets	$400	$320	$80	25%

In this case, the prior year figure is the standard of comparison. The $400 of current assets at December 31, 1987, represents an increase of $80 or 25 percent over the prior year. The significance of the $400 figure is improved, but it is not possible to say on the basis of this comparison that the amount is adequate.

If another figure (total assets) is added, the significance of the current asset figures may be increased by vertical analysis:

	December 31		Increase (Decrease)	
	1987	1986	Amount	Percent
Current assets	$ 400	35%	$ 320	32%
Total assets	$ 1,142	100%	$ 1,000	100%

Now it is seen that current assets at the end of 1987 represent a greater percentage (35% vs. 32%) of total assets, although total assets have increased. No conclusion can be drawn from these internal comparisons, however, as to the adequacy of $400 current asset figure. Perhaps at December 31, 1987, the current asset total **should be** $571, or 50 percent of total assets! Or perhaps this current asset total **should be** $286, or only 25 percent of total assets.

Still another internal comparison can be made by introducing the current liability figure. Examine the following ratio:

	December 31	
	1987	1986
1. Current assets	$400	$300
2. Current liabilities	$250	$150
Ratio of current assets to current liabilities (1 ÷ 2)	1.60	2.00

In common parlance, the **current ratio** at December 31, 1987, is 1.6 to 1. The ratio is substantially lower than it was a year ago. Since this ratio generally is regarded as an indicator of short-term debt-paying ability, it might be concluded that the current financial strength of the hospital has deteriorated in comparison with the prior year in terms of the current ratio. Yet, it does not follow that the December 31, 1987, current assets are inadequate or that the current ratio is "too low."

Like a single dollar-figure standing alone, a single ratio standing alone is also meaningless. A ratio may have significance, but only when it is compared with some standard. Therefore, in interpreting ratios developed from information in a hospital's financial statements, the analyst (management or external user) cannot conclude that the ratios indicate favorable or unfavorable conditions unless they are judged by valid standards. Even where useful standards are available, however, the intelligent interpretation of ratios is a difficult art.

Standards of comparison itemized by Kennedy and McMullen in their widely used text are summarized below:[3]

1. Mental standards of the analyst, i.e., a general conception of what is adequate or normal which has been gained by personal experience and observation.
2. Ratios based on the records of the past financial and operating performance of the individual business.
3. Ratios developed by using the data included in budgets, i.e., "goal ratios."
4. Ratios of selected competing companies, especially the most progressive and successful ones.
5. Ratios of the industry of which the individual company is a member.

Thus, computed ratios may be compared with standard ratios taken from historical or budgeted data of the same hospital, or the comparison may be made with standard ratios arising from external sources, i.e., other individual hospitals, groups of hospitals by type, size and region or the hospital industry taken as a whole.

Ratio analysis has been an important financial tool among profit-seeking enterprises for many years. The hospital industry until recently, however, has made limited use of this technique due to the lack of appropriate ratio values for use as standards of comparison. As stated by Berman and Weeks:[4]

For the most part, hospitals have just adopted the standard ratios developed by other industries and have attempted to apply them directly to their own operating situation. Unfortunately, this approach has not been successful, for these borrowed standards have not been based upon the unique operating parameters of the hospital industry. The standards which hospitals have traditionally used have thus not only been erroneous and irrelevant but also have acted to confuse rather than clarify balance sheet evaluation.

In recent years, however, considerable work has been done toward the development of hospital ratios by research agencies, public accounting firms, and hospital associations, both local and national. The Hospital Financial Management Association, for example, provides a Financial Analysis Service which generates financial ratio norms and ranges on a trend and peer group comparison basis.[5] This service, available on a subscription basis, has been extremely useful to many hospitals. Particularly valuable is the comparison of the performance of one hospital with that of similar institutions within the same geographic area.

However, it must be recognized that no two hospitals are exactly alike. Each has its own characteristics which may greatly influence its financial relationships. Variations in financial ratios between hospitals or between a hospital and a seemingly similar group of hospitals may arise from many factors that could distort or, in some instances, even invalidate ratio comparisons.

ANALYSIS OF OPERATING RESULTS

The management of a not-for-profit hospital is charged with the task of maintaining a satisfactory relationship between revenues and expenses, i.e., one that permits the hospital to provide the volume and quality of services desired by the community it serves. Opinions may differ as to precisely what this relationship should be. There are those who maintain a belief that the financial operating objective should be to break even. Given the pressures of changes in demand for healthcare services, advancing technology, inflation, fixed-price reimbursement systems, and other socioeconomic forces, however, most authorities are convinced that a "profit" objective is both necessary and justifiable.

Without an excess of revenues over expenses, it is argued, the hospital's financial position will deteriorate rapidly. The development of new or improved healthcare delivery systems, programs, and facilities will be impossible; even funds for replacement of worn-out and inefficient plant assets to maintain existing productive capacity will not be available. It will become more and more difficult to pay annual interest charges on debt and to retire obligations as they mature. As a result, difficulty will be encountered in obtaining bank loans and in selling bonds to investors. Suppliers will be wary of extending credit, and payrolls will be increasingly hard to meet. Pay scales will lag behind other industries, and qualified personnel will be attracted elsewhere. The hospital may limp along for a period of years, but its eventual demise as a viable and effective service-producer will be inevitable.

These results can be predicted with certainty, at least for the proprietary hospital having owners, partners, and stockholders. In profit-seeking enterprises of any kind, the financial objective is quite clear: a satisfactory long-run return on capital investment consistent with social responsibilities and ethical standards. While a maximum financial return on investment objective is hardly applicable to the not-for-profit hospital, a "no-profit-at-all" objective seems totally unrealistic to most observers in view of current and emerging conditions in the hospital industry.

Some of the more widely used ratios generally applied in the analysis of the operating results of both investor-owned and not-for-profit hospitals are described below. These ratios usually are referred to as profitability ratios. Computations are based on the data in Hartsville Hospital's 1987 and 1986 financial statements provided earlier in this chapter.

Net Income Ratio

The net income ratio is a primary measure of profitability in the hospital industry. It reflects the percentage of operating revenues (net of revenue deductions) that the hospital has been able to bring down into net income. The computation is:

$$\frac{\text{Net Income}}{\text{Total Operating Revenues}}$$

In 1987, for example, Hartsville Hospital had a net income ratio of 3.1% ($244/$7,905). The hospital was able to turn 3.1 cents of each dollar of operating revenues into net income.

Where net income includes significant amounts of nonoperating income that is generally nonrecurring and largely unrelated to continuing operations, the operating income ratio usually is more meaningful and useful than the net income ratio. The operating income ratio is computed by dividing the hospital's operating income by total operating revenues. In 1987, Hartsville Hospital had an operating income ratio of .3% ($20/$7,905).

Return on Equity

Another primary indicator of profitability is the rate of return earned on the hospital's equity. The computation is:

$$\frac{\text{Net Income}}{\text{Average Unrestricted Fund Balance*}}$$

*In the case of an investor-owned hospital corporation, the denominator is the average stockholders' equity.

In 1987, Hartsville Hospital had a net income of $244. The Unrestricted Fund Balance was $7,511 at the beginning of the year and $7,730 at the end of the year. The average Unrestricted Fund Balance for the year, therefore, was $7,620 ($15,241/2). The return on equity is 3.2% ($244/$7,620).

Return on Total Assets

The rate of return earned on total assets generally is regarded as the best indicator of profitability. The computation is:

$$\frac{\text{Net Income}}{\text{Average Unrestricted Fund Assets}}$$

The Unrestricted Fund of Hartsville Hospital had total assets of $10,197 at the beginning of 1987 and $10,385 at the end of 1987. Average Unrestricted Fund assets for the year, therefore, were $10,291 ($20,582/2). The 1987 return on total assets was about 2.4% ($244/$10,291).

Some additional ratios commonly computed for investor-owned hospital corporations are indicated below:

1. **Earnings per Share.** Net income divided by the number of shares of capital stock outstanding. Cash dividends paid per share also are computed and reported.
2. **Price-Earnings Ratio.** Market price per share of capital stock divided by earnings per share.
3. **Income Yield.** Earnings per share divided by market price per share of capital stock. The dividend yield is computed by dividing earnings per share by market price per share.
4. **Book Value per Share.** Net assets divided by number of shares of capital stock outstanding.

These ratios are used to evaluate profitability and the investment qualities of capital stock. No further discussion of these ratios as applied to profit-oriented businesses is provided here. The interested reader should refer to general intermediate accounting and finance textbooks.

Because profits are necessary for the survival of most hospitals, a judgment must be made as to what amount that profit figure should be. Some use of the net income, return on equity, and return on total assets ratios may be appropriate for this purpose. A percentage relationship between operating income and operating revenues (or between operating income and total assets) could be established, for example, as a goal or standard against which actual operating results might be measured. A hospital management, however, is more likely to have an absolute dollar amount in mind as a financial operating objective. This amount is determined as the figure required to produce the cash flow needed to meet specific financial requirements such as the retirement of long-term debt, the financing of new plant asset acquisitions, or the generation of additional working capital. The plans of management in this regard sometimes are described in the hospital's financial report.

ANALYSIS OF FINANCIAL POSITION

The evaluation of a hospital's financial position by its management and by groups external to its management closely parallels the analysis made of enterprises in other industries. Many of the same ratios are used. It is important, however, to recognize that hospitals have unique characteristics. Certain rules of thumb and standard ratio values related to commercial businesses often are not applicable to hospitals. Much remains to be done in the development of appropriate ratio values for hospitals. The best comparison a particular hospital employs at present is one in which its ratios are evaluated against those of carefully selected similar institutions, especially the most progressive and successful ones, located in the same geographical area. The external analyst also will find this to be the most rewarding procedure.

While operating performance and financial strength are treated separately here, both are important considerations regardless of the point of view taken by the analyst. One cannot afford to ignore the information in the balance sheet when appraising operating results or to bypass the income statement in evaluating the financial strength of a hospital. Careful attention must also be given to the information provided in statements of changes in fund balances and in financial position.

Evaluation of Current Financial Position

A hospital's current financial strength is a matter of importance not only to its management but also to various external groups including bankers, third-party reimbursement agencies, and suppliers. If the hospital is to be able to repay bank loans and its other short-term obligations promptly and in full, it must maintain a sound current financial position. The hospital must have an adequate amount of working capital; it must sustain a satisfactory degree of liquidity; and it must not overinvest in receivables or inventories. Some of the ratios usually applied to obtain insights into the presence or absence of these desired conditions are summarized below; these and other ratios were discussed at greater length and from a managerial viewpoint in Chapter 14. The figures employed in the computations shown here are drawn from the financial statements illustrated earlier in this chapter.

Current Ratio. One of the most widely used measures of current financial strength is the **current ratio**. It indicates the number of dollars of current assets for each dollar of current liabilities. It shows the number of times the current assets will "pay off" the current debts of the hospital. Following is a computation of Hartsville Hospital's current ratio:

		December 31	
		1987	1986
1.	Current assets	$1,726	$1,482
2.	Current liabilities	937	821
3.	Current ratio (1 ÷ 2)	1.84	1.81

A popular rule of thumb is that the current ratio should be 2 to 1, or higher. This is an erroneous notion. There is no one value for the current ratio that is applicable to all hospitals. For one hospital, a 1.5 to 1 ratio may be more than adequate; for another, a 2.5 to 1 ratio might be dangerously low. It also is worth noting that while a particular current ratio may be satisfactory at the end of one year, it may not be satisfactory for the same hospital at the end of the next year. At any rate, if a hospital is always able to pay its current debts promptly and without undue strain, then the current ratio, whatever it is, must be adequate.

Quick Ratio. One should not rely too heavily on the current ratio as an infallible indicator of the current debt-paying ability of a hospital. It does not, for example, take into account the composition of either current assets or current liabilities. For this reason, the **quick ratio**, sometimes called the **acid test**, is also computed. It is a more severe test of current debt-paying ability in that it takes into account the composition of the hospital's current assets:

		December 31	
		1987	1986
Cash		$ 268	$ 211
Temporary Investments		126	34
Receivables		969	854
1.	Quick Assets	$1,363	$1,099
2.	Current Liabilities	$ 937	$ 821
3.	Quick Ratio (1 ÷ 2)	1.45	1.34

An extreme modification of the quick ratio is the division of cash, or the total of cash and temporary investments, by current liabilities.

Current Asset Turnover. The **current asset turnover** is said to be an indicator of how "hard" the management of a hospital "works" the current assets, i.e., the intensity of current asset utilization. Hartsville Hospital's turnovers are computed below:

		December 31	
		1987	1986
1.	Total operating revenues	$7,905	$6,268
2.	Current assets	1,726	1,482
3.	Current asset turnover (1 ÷ 2)	4.58	4.23

Some analysts make the computation using total operating **expenses** rather than revenues as the numerator; others prefer to use **working capital** rather than current assets as the denominator, i.e., a **working capital turnover**. In any event, a high turnover generally is indicative of efficient and productive employment of current resources.

Analysis of Receivables. The amount of receivables from patient services in a hospital's balance sheet should not exceed a reasonable proportion of the charges made to patients' accounts during a relevant period. This relationship may be clarified by computation of the **accounts receivable turnover**:

	December 31	
	1987	1986
1. Net Patient Service Revenues*	$7,400	$5,861
2. Receivables — Patients**	969	854
3. Receivables Turnover (1 ÷ 2)	7.64	6.86

*This figure should exclude revenues rendered on a cash basis
and not recorded through accounts receivable.
**Average accounts receivable for the year may be used instead
of the year-end figure.

This ratio indicates the number of times during the year the receivables were "turned over," i.e., collected. An increase in this turnover may be regarded as a favorable sign with respect to the effectiveness of the credit and collection function.

Another ratio employed by hospitals in the analysis of receivables is the **number of days' charges uncollected** and in receivables. This ratio is computed for Hartsville Hospital below:

	December 31	
	1987	1986
1. Days in One Year	365	365
2. Receivables Turnover	7.64	6.86
3. Number of Days' Charges Uncollected (1 ÷ 2)	48	53

It may be roughly concluded that, on the average, the quality of receivables management may have improved somewhat. The analyst must recognize, however, that this ratio is an average, i.e., some patients' accounts may be 200 days old and others are only a few days old. It also should be noted that where the information is available, both the receivables turnover and the number of days' charges uncollected should be computed by major categories of patients and third-party payers as emphasized in Chapter 14.

Analysis of Inventories. As is true of receivables, a hospital can have an excessive investment in inventories. There should be a reasonable relationship between inventories and total current assets. In addition, the relationship between inventories and total cost of supplies used may be computed as an **inventory turnover** as shown below:

	December 31	
	1987	1986
1. Total Cost of Supplies Used*	$1,838	$1,671
2. Inventories**	296	315
3. Inventory Turnover (1 ÷ 2)	6.21	5.30

*This information may not be disclosed in financial reports.
**Average inventory for the year may be more appropriate.

The fact that Hartsville Hospital "turned over" its inventories a greater number of times in 1987 than in 1986 generally is a favorable indication as to the quality of inventory management.

In addition to turnover, the **average number of days' supply in inventories** may be calculated:

		December 31	
		1987	1986
1.	Days in One Year	365	365
2.	Inventory Turnover	6.21	5.30
3.	Number of Days' Supply (1 ÷ 2)	59	69

In evaluating inventories, it must be recognized that a hospital can be **understocked** as well as **overstocked**. Either extreme is undesirable. Mention also should be made of the fact that where the information is available, both the inventory turnover and the number of days' supply should be computed by major categories of inventory to properly take into account the differing characteristics of various types of supplies used by hospitals.

Summary. The above discussion of the evaluation of current financial position is summarized in the program below:

1. **Adequacy of current resources?**
   a.   Current ratio.
   b.   Composition of current assets and current liabilities:
       (1)   Ratio of cash balance to debts due immediately.
       (2)   Percentage analysis of current assets.
       (3)   Quick ratio.
   c.   Comparison with other hospitals and industry standards.
2. **Quality of current resources?**
   a.   Average number of days' charges in receivables.
   b.   Average number of days' supply in inventories.
   c.   Comparison with other hospitals and industry standards.
3. **Management of current resources?**
   a.   Current asset (or working capital) turnover.
   b.   Accounts receivable:
       (1)   Turnover.
       (2)   Average number of days' charges uncollected.
       (3)   Component percentage of total current assets.
   c.   Inventories:
       (1)   Turnover.
       (2)   Average number of days' supply.
       (3)   Component percentage of total current assets.
   d.   Comparison with other hospitals and industry standards.

4. **Trend of adequacy, quality, and management of current resources?**
   a. Component percentage trend of current assets and current liabilities over several recent periods.
   b. Horizontal analysis of current assets and current liabilities for several recent periods.
   c. Comparison of current ratios, quick ratios, turnovers, etc., for several recent periods.
   d. Comparison of trends with other hospitals and industry trends.

The application of this program to the financial data of a hospital should enable the internal or external analyst to make an intelligent and useful judgment as to the hospital's current financial position.

Evaluation of Long-Run Financial Position

Many external users of hospital financial statements are interested in the hospital's long-run financial strength as well as in its current financial position. Holders of hospital bonds and mortgages, for instance, require assurance of the ability of the hospital to pay current interest charges. At the same time, they are concerned about the long-run safety of their investments. An intelligent appraisal of a hospital's long-run financial position is also essential to sound long-term financing decisions and long-range planning considerations either on an individual hospital or areawide basis. Such an analysis is also helpful in evaluating the consequences of long-term commitment decisions previously made and implemented.

In studying a hospital's long-run financial position, an analysis may be made of (1) changes in the absolute and relative amounts invested by the hospital in the various categories of assets and (2) changes in the absolute and relative amounts of the sources of its assets. An abbreviated analysis of this kind is illustrated for Hartsville Hospital in Figure 22-8.

Figure 22-8.
Hartsville Hospital
Asset and Capital Structure
December 31, 1987 and 1986

	1987 Amount	1987 Percent	1986 Amount	1986 Percent	Increase Amount	(Decrease) Percent
Current assets	$ 1,726	16.6%	$ 925	10.3%	$ 801	86.6%
Property, plant and equipment	8,126	78.3	7,876	87.7	250	3.2
Other assets	533	5.1	181	2.0	352	194.5
Total	$10,385	100.0%	$8,982	100.0%	$1,403	15.6
Current liabilities	$ 937	9.0%	$ 663	7.4%	$ 274	41.3
Noncurrent liabilities	1,718	16.6	3,011	33.5	(1,293)	(42.9)
Total liabilities	$ 2,655	25.6%	$3,674	40.9%	$(1,019)	(27.7)
Fund balance	7,730	74.4	5,308	59.1	2,422	45.6
Total	$10,385	100.0%	$8,982	100.0%	$1,403	15.6

The above analysis raises many interesting questions concerning the changes that have occurred in the hospital's asset and capital structure over the five-year period. As can be seen, there has been a substantial shift in the allocation of resources from noncurrent to current assets. It would appear, from both the long-run and short-term points of view, that Hartsville Hospital has a more appropriate balance to its asset structure in 1987 than it had in 1983 when 87.7 percent of its assets consisted of property, plant, and equipment. Further analysis of the amount invested in plant assets may be made in terms of **assets per bed**, which naturally vary with the age of the hospital facility, type of construction, depreciation method, and other factors. Some analysts also use the **ratio of operating revenues to plant assets** as a rough indicator of the productivity of hospital investment in property, plant, and equipment. One should be cautious in drawing conclusion from such measurements.

Although not involved in Figure 22-8, the study of a hospital's asset structure should also include an examination of the assets held in the restricted funds. This is particularly true with respect to the Plant Replacement and Expansion Funds where material amounts of resources might be available for long-run financial purposes. In addition, should the hospital have term endowments, their amounts and termination dates should be considered in appraising the hospital's long-term financial strength. Assets of the Specific Purpose Funds, being restricted to specified operating purposes, generally are considered only in evaluations of current financial position.

Also revealed by the analysis in Figure 22-8 is a substantial shift in the capital structure from liabilities to noncreditor sources of asset financing. At the end of 1983, debt was the source of 40.9 percent of the hospital's assets, but the ratio declined to only 25.6 percent at December 31, 1987. Analysts generally refer to this as the **debt ratio**; its complement (fund balance divided by total assets) may be called the **equity ratio**. In some cases, the two ratios are combined into a **debt/equity ratio**, i.e., total liabilities divided by fund balance. These ratios reflect the relationship between debt and nondebt sources of asset financing, thereby serving as indicators of the soundness of the hospital's capital structure.

The decline in Hartsville Hospital's debt ratio from 40.9 percent in 1983 to 25.6 percent in 1987 generally would be regarded as a significant improvement in the hospital's long-run financial position. In other words, only 25.6 cents of each dollar of hospital assets are being supplied by creditors at present. This is a more conservative, less risky ratio than that of five years ago. There is a much greater margin of safety for creditors and considerably less long-term debt pressure from the point of view of hospital management. When operating results are unsatisfactory, a high debt ratio tends to place the hospital in a rather precarious financial situation. In addition, should a hospital need to borrow additional long-term funds, a high debt ratio would not be regarded with favor by prospective bondholders or other lenders.

It should be recognized, however, that a reasonably high debt ratio may be advantageous under certain conditions. A hospital having a high debt ratio, for example, is said to be highly **leveraged**. An alternate term for financial leverage is **trading on the equity**. The principle of leverage is to earn a greater percentage return on borrowed funds than the interest rate paid for the use of that money, e.g., earning, say, 12% on money borrowed at, say, an 8% interest cost. It is a neat trick when it works. When unsuccessful, it can have disastrous results.

A reasonably high debt ratio may also be advantageous during extended periods of inflation. If, for example, $1,000,000 is borrowed today to be repaid ten years hence and there is a 5 percent annual rate of inflation, the loan would be repaid with dollars presumably having a purchasing power value of only $500,000 in today's terms. The purchasing power gain, although not recognized in the accounting process, is very real.

In addition to the hospital's debt ratio, current and prospective bond-holders and other long-term lenders are also interested in the safety of their investments as measured by the **times interest earned** ratio. In 1987, for example, Hartsville Hospital earned its interest charges 2.81 times as computed below:

1. Net Income for the Year* $244
2. Interest Expense   135
3. Total $379
4. Times Interest Earned (3 ÷ 2)   2.81

    *Net operating income may be used instead, resulting in a more
    conservative ratio.

The higher the ratio the more favorable it is for all parties concerned. How high the ratio should be to be regarded as satisfactory is a more difficult question. It can be said, however, that the acceptability of the ratio depends largely upon the stability of the hospital's past and potential net earnings.

The hospital's asset and capital structure as reflected in its balance sheet should always be viewed in conjunction with its statement of changes in financial position. Preferably, this latter statement should be presented in comparative form covering several prior periods so that trends in the sources and applications of funds may be clearly discerned. This permits an appraisal of the effectiveness of management's past investing and financing policies in bringing the hospital to its present financial position. Above all, it must be recognized by all external groups that a successful hospital seldom remains the same; it either changes and grows, or it stagnates. A hospital must be able to finance the development of new programs and services while moving in new directions as demand and technology change. An essential element of long-term financial strength is satisfactory operating results; a healthy hospital must have the ability to generate additional funds when they are needed.

SUMMARY

The information presented in hospital financial statements can be of great value in appraising a hospital's operating results and financial position. All parties concerned with hospital activities can make important uses of this information if it is interpreted intelligently. It must be recognized, however, that financial statements have certain limitations and that, in the last analysis, intangible and unmeasurable nonfinancial factors often may be more important than dollars of earnings, assets, and liabilities. Users of hospital financial reports should be aware of the dangers of attaching excessive significance to income statements and balance sheets so that undesirable price tags are placed on human life, health, and happiness.

CHAPTER 22 FOOTNOTES

1. APB Statement No. 4, **Basic Concepts and Accounting Principles Underlying Financial Statements of Business Enterprises** (New York: American Institute of Certified Public Accountants, 1970), par. 1024.24.

2. APB Opinion No. 20, **Accounting Changes** (New York: American Institute of Certified Public Accountants, 1971).

3. Ralph D. Kennedy and Stewart Y. McMullen, **Financial Statements — Form, Analysis, and Interpretation** (Homewood, Illinois: Richard D. Irwin, Inc., 1973), p. 297.

4. Howard J. Berman and Lewis E. Weeks, **The Financial Management of Hospitals** (Ann Arbor, Michigan: Health Administration Press, School of Public Health, The University of Michigan, 1974), p. 336.

5. For a detailed description of the ratios included in the HFMA's Financial Analysis Service, see the author's **External and Internal Reporting by Hospitals** (Chicago: HFMA, 1984), Chapter 14.

QUESTIONS

1. Name five major external groups having an interest in hospital financial reports. Briefly indicate some of the reasons why each group is concerned with the information contained in such reports.

2. What assurance does an external user of hospital financial reports have that the figures in the report are reasonably accurate and that all significant information is properly disclosed?

3. "An audit by a firm of professional accountants will always detect embezzlements. It also serves as a guarantee that each figure in a set of financial statements is accurate to the penny." Do you agree? Explain.

4. Hospital financial reports often include comparative financial data covering two or more consecutive years. What is the value of comparative data? Why should the reader be cautious about drawing conclusions from such presentations? What major conditions must exist before comparability can be achieved?

5. What are **common-size** financial statements?

6. What is **vertical analysis** and how is it used in the interpretation of financial statements?

7. What is **horizontal analysis** and how is it used in the interpretation of financial statements?

8. State the advantages and disadvantages of using ratios and percentages in the analysis of financial statements.

9. State the formula for the computation of (1) the working capital ratio, (2) inventory turnover, and (3) average number of days' service uncollected.

10. Set up the headings for a form you would recommend for the presentation of a comparative balance sheet.

11. Are statistical data used for the same purpose or purposes as accounting data? Explain the uses of statistical data in connection with accounting data.

12. Community Hospital, a 350-bed institution, maintains its records in the manner prescribed by the AICPA **Hospital Audit Guide.** The accounts of the hospital include an Unrestricted Fund, a Specific Purpose Fund, a Plant Replacement and Explanation Fund, and an Endowment Fund. You have been requested to prepare financial statements to be distributed to:

    1. The various division supervisors (director of nursing, food service manager, etc.)
    2. The hospital administrator
    3. The hospital board
    4. All hospital employees
    5. The general public

    Required. Discuss the type of financial statements that you would prepare for each of the above groups. Include a description of the contents of each statement. Explain any differences between the statements to be used by the various groups.

13. "A hospital with a current ratio of 4 to 1 has greater current financial strength than does a hospital with a current ratio of only 2 to 1." Do you agree? Explain.

14. Assume that you are examining the latest financial report of a hospital from the point of view of one of its bondholders. In what would you be particularly interested? Explain.

15. The performance ratios of one hospital may be compared with that of another hospital. List some of the major factors which might tend to distort or invalidate such comparisons.

16. State how each of the following is computed and explain what might be indicated by the results of the computation:
    1. Quick ratio
    2. Current asset turnover
    3. Operating ratio
    4. Debt/equity ratio
    5. Times interest earned

EXERCISES

E1. Headline Hospital provides you with the following information:

	December 31	
	1987	1986
Cash	$ 200	$ 120
Temporary investments	250	180
Receivables (net)	1,300	1,150
Inventories	400	370
Prepaid expenses	50	80
Total current assets	2,200	1,900
Property, plant and equipment (net)	7,800	7,100
Total assets	$10,000	$ 9,000
Current liabilities	$ 740	$ 475
Long-term debt	3,530	3,205
Fund balance	5,730	5,320
Total liabilities and fund balance	$10,000	$ 9,000

In addition to the above balance sheet data, the following income statement information is available:

| | Year ended 12/31 ||
	1987	1986
Gross patient service revenues	$6,600	$5,900
Deductions from revenues	660	480
Net patient service revenues	5,940	5,420
Other operating revenues	390	325
Total operating revenues	6,330	5,745
Less operating expenses	5,920	5,240
Net income for the year	$ 410	$ 505

Required. Develop a horizontal analysis of the above statements. Comment on what you believe to be the major points revealed in your analysis.

E2.   Refer to the Headline Hospital data provided above in Exercise 1.

Required. Convert the financial statements to common size. Comment on what you believe to be the major points revealed by your analysis.

E3.   Refer to the Headline Hospital data provided above in Exercise 1.

Required. Compute the following ratios and comment briefly on the significance of each ratio:

1. Current ratio

2. Quick ratio

3. Current asset turnover

4. Accounts receivable turnover

5. Days' charges in receivables

6. Inventory turnover

7. Days' supply in inventories

E4.   Refer to the Headline Hospital data provided above in Exercise 1.

Required. Compute the following ratios and comment briefly on the significance of each ratio:

1. Operating revenues to plant assets

2. Debt/equity ratio

3. Times interest earned (assume that interest charges are $280 in 1987 and $250 in 1986)

E5.   Refer to the Headline Hospital data provided above in Exercise 1.

Required. Prepare a ratio analysis of operating results, including the net income ratio, return on total assets and operating ratio. Comment on the results of your analysis.

PROBLEMS

P1.   You are the new controller of Community Hospital, a nonfederal, not-for-profit, general hospital. Your first assignment is that of analyzing the hospital's financial statements and related statistical data for the most recent fiscal years. In addition to the financial and statistical data, you are given the following supplemental information:

1. Blue Cross pays billed charges rather than a per diem rate.

2. County Welfare pays a negotiated per diem rate which at present is total cost less depreciation.

3. There is no outpatient clinic.

4. Supply prices are up approximately 5 percent from 1986.

5. A general salary increase, averaging 4 percent, went into effect January 1, 1987. At the same time, all room and nursery charges were raised $1.50 per day.

6. A new air-conditioning system was completed early in 1987. Among the 1987 equipment purchases was an autoanalyzer for the laboratory. Equipment retirements for the year were nominal.

7. The three-year school of nursing earned its accreditation in March of 1987. One of the accreditation requirements was the reduction of student hours of service by approximately 10 percent and an increase in classroom hours.

8. There are no anesthetists on the hospital payroll.

9. The housekeeping department provides a checkout service upon discharge of patients. This service includes stripping the bed, washing the furniture, making the bed, cleaning the toilet, and wet-mopping the floor.

10. An analysis of the increase in Plant Fund Balance shows miscellaneous donations for equipment totaling $7,500 and interest earned on Plant Fund investments totaling $8,486.

Required. Taking into account the above information, analyze the financial statements and related statistical data provided.

1. List your major findings.

2. Indicate areas of strength and areas of weakness.

3. Indicate where action or further investigation is required.

4. Wherever applicable, delineate methods of measurement or comparison.

5. State clearly any assumptions which you feel are necessary.

Community Hospital
Comparative Balance Sheets   **EXHIBIT A**
December 31, 1987 and 1986

	1987	1986	Increase Amount	(Decrease) Percent
Unrestricted Fund				
Current Assets:				
Cash on hand and in checking	$ 127,699	$ 198,333	$(70,634)	(35.6)%
Cash in savings	30,000	25,000	5,000	20.0
Accounts receivable-patients	1,087,792	959,744	128,048	13.3
Allowance for uncollectibles	(90,322)	(77,739)	12,583	16.2
Accounts receivable-other	10,400	15,128	(4,728)	(31.3)
Inventories − general store	76,752	71,001	5,751	8.1
− drugs	69,106	65,878	3,228	4.9
Prepaid expenses	29,622	35,051	(5,429)	(15.5)
Total current assets	1,341,049	1,292,396	48,653	3.8%
Plant Assets:				
Land and improvements	120,540	120,540	− −	− −%
Accumulated depreciation	(30,057)	(25,236)	4,821	19.1
Buildings	7,602,696	7,587,462	15,234	.2
Accumulated depreciation	(1,859,219)	(1,707,165)	152,054	8.9
Equipment	2,225,400	1,991,043	234,357	11.8
Accumulated depreciation	(987,928)	(875,976)	111,952	12.8
Cash	9,865	16,525	6,660	(40.3)

	1987	1986	Increase (Decrease) Amount	Percent
Investments	$ 162,820	$ 180,938	$ (18,118)	(10.0)
Total plant assets	7,244,117	7,288,131	(44,014)	(.6)%
Total unrestricted fund assets	$8,585,166	$8,580,527	$ 4,639	Neg.

Unrestricted Funds

Current Liabilities:

	1987	1986	Amount	Percent
Accounts payable	$ 118,336	$ 126,265	$ (7,929)	(6.3)%
Salaries and wages payable	113,811	99,240	14,571	14.7
Other current liabilities	2,523	31,122	1,401	4.5
Total current liabilities	264,670	256,627	8,043	3.1%
Mortgage payable	340,000	400,000	(60,000)	(15.0)
Total liabilities	604,670	656,627	(51,957)	(7.9)%
Current fund balance	1,076,379	1,035,769	40,610	3.9
Plant fund balance	6,904,117	6,888,131	15,986	.2
Total unrestricted fund liabilities and fund balances	$8,585,166	$8,580,527	$ 4,639	Neg.

Endowment Fund

	1987	1986	Amount	Percent
Cash	$ 22,107	$ 21,171	$ 846	4.0%
Investments	86,624	86,624		
Total assets	$ 108,641	$ 107,795	$ 846	8%
Endowment fund balance (restricted)	$ 108,641	$ 107,795	$ 846	8%

Community Hospital
Income Statement   **EXHIBIT B**
Years Ended December 31, 1987 and 1986

	1987	1986	Increase Amount	(Decrease) Percent
Routine service-inpatients	$2,905,126	$2,633,744	$271,382	10.2%
Revenue from ancillary services	2,751,087	2,679,361	71,726	2.6
Revenue from emergency room	95,370	94,333	1,037	1.1
Gross operating revenue	5,751,583	5,407,438	344,145	6.4%
Less adjustments and allowances	253,069	234,004	19,065	8.1
Net operating revenue	5,498,514	5,173,434	325,080	6.3%
Operating Expenses:				
Administration and general	570,675	525,196	45,479	8.7%
Dietary	510,618	475,535	35,083	7.4
Household and property	753,951	709,561	44,390	6.3
Nursing service	1,480,633	1,397,447	83,186	6.0
Emergency room	61,605	58,299	3,306	5.7
Other professional care	1,841,900	1,708,339	133,561	7.8
Depreciation	270,827	256,122	14,705	5.7
Total operating expenses	5,490,209	5,130,499	359,710	7.0%
Gain from operations	8,305	42,935	(34,630)	(80.7)%
Other revenue	50,805	47,234	3,571	7.6
Total	59,110	90,169	(31,059)	(34.4)%
Less interest expense	18,500	21,500	(3,000)	(14.0)
Net income	$ 40,610	$ 68,669	$(28,059)	(40.9)%

Community Hospital
Miscellaneous Statistics
Years Ended December 31, 1987 and 1986

EXHIBIT C

	1987	1986	Increase (Decrease) Amount	Percent
Number of beds	420	420		
Number of bassinets	40	40		
Patient days-adults and children	136,437	133,371	3,066	2.3%
-newborn	10,658	10,952	(294)	(2.7)
Discharges-adults and children	17,952	18,023	(71)	(.4)
-newborn	2,175	2,191	(16)	(.7)
Outpatient visits or procedures:				
Emergency room (visits)	21,096	20,885	211	1.0
Radiology (procedures)	28,071	26,372	1,699	6.4
Laboratory (procedures)	32,447	31,594	853	2.7
Other (visits)	4,561	4,433	128	2.9
Average daily census:				
Adults and children	374	365	9	2.5
Newborn	29	30	(1)	(3.3)
Total personnel	747	723	24	3.3
Total payroll	$3,128,692	$2,950,210	$178,482	6.0

Community Hospital
Department Reports
Years Ended December 31, 1987 and 1986

EXHIBIT D

	1987	1986	Increase (Decrease) Amount	Percent
Administration:				
Salaries	$ 252,850	$ 240,815	$ 12,035	5.0%
Supplies, printing, postage	26,438	25,422	1,016	4.0
Telephone and telegraph	32,829	32,119	710	2.2
Dues and memberships	4,333	3,820	513	13.4
Institute and education	3,925	4,014	(89)	(2.2)
General insurance	15,235	12,625	2,610	20.7
Other	21,810	20,444	1,366	6.7
Total	357,420	339,259	18,161	5.4%

	1987	1986	Increase (Decrease) Amount	Percent
Employee Benefits:				
Health insurance	$ 33,741	$ 32,727	$ 1,014	3.1%
Life insurance	5,424	5,272	152	2.9
Retirement plan	25,664	25,285	379	1.5
FICA	128,405	103,575	24,830	24.0
Workmen's compensation	9,586	8,860	726	8.2
Other	10,435	10,218	217	2.1
Total	213,255	185,937	27,318	14.7
Personnel	56	56		
Dietary:				
Salaries	209,223	192,882	16,341	8.5
Raw food	266,321	248,666	17,655	7.1
Other	35,074	33,987	1,087	3.2
Total	510,618	475,535	35,083	7.4
Personnel	72	69	3	4.3
Meals served	395,667	373,438	22,229	6.0
Housekeeping:				
Salaries	230,665	221,142	9,523	4.3
Supplies and other	43,964	41,831	2,133	5.1
Personnel	75	74	1	1.4
Laundry:				
Salaries	101,901	89,548	12,353	13.8
Supplies and other	18,574	15,941	2,633	16.5
Personnel	36	33	3	9.1
Pounds of laundry processed	2,387,650	2,147,730	239,920	11.2
Linen Service:				
Salaries	7,339	7,071	268	3.8
Supplies and other	45,192	40,935	4,257	10.4
Personnel	3	3		

	1987	1986	Increase (Decrease)	
			Amount	Percent
Plant Operation and Maintenance:				
Salaries	$ 97,675	$ 93,559	$ 4,116	4.4%
Supplies	34,619	33,034	1,585	4.8
Fuel	39,280	40,122	(842)	(2.1)
Water and sewage	18,338	18,103	235	1.3
Electricity	63,018	57,186	5,832	10.2
Purchased services	43,537	41,307	2,230	5.4
Total	296,467	283,311	13,156	4.6
Personnel	23	23		
Nursing Service:				
Daily patient service revenue	2,905,126	2,633,744	271,382	10.2
Salaries	1,305,277	1,236,058	69,219	5.6
Supplies and other expense	51,174	48,278	2,896	6.0
Personnel	281	270	11	4.1
Emergency Room:				
Revenue	95,370	94,333	1,037	1.1
Salaries	46,588	44,118	2,470	5.6
Supplies and other expense	15,017	14,181	836	5.9
Personnel	10	10		
Visits	21,096	20,885	211	1.0
Operating Rooms:				
Revenue	322,850	320,285	2,565	.8
Salaries	212,870	202,734	10,136	5.0
Supplies and other expense	83,228	77,206	6,022	7.8
Personnel	53	49	4	8.2
Operations	9,928	9,820	108	1.0
Delivery Room:				
Revenue	75,831	76,182	(351)	(.5)
Salaries	63,403	60,098	3,305	5.5
Supplies and other expense	9,521	9,094	427	4.7
Personnel	13	13		
Deliveries	2,198	2,213	(15)	(.7)
Anesthesia:				
Revenue	97,167	96,301	866	.9
Supplies and other expense	42,916	40,602	2,314	5.7

	1987	1986	Increase (Decrease) Amount	Increase (Decrease) Percent
Radiology:				
Revenue-Diagnostic	$ 539,188	$ 517,952	$ 21,236	4.1%
-Therapy	130,797	125,405	5,392	4.3
Salaries	110,382	100,898	9,484	9.4
Professional fees	266,654	229,412	37,242	16.2
Supplies and other expense	129,631	118,602	11,029	9.3
Personnel	20	19	1	5.2
Diagnostic exams	42,398	40,690	1,708	4.2
Therapy treatments	15,197	14,543	654	4.5
Laboratories:				
Revenue	558,082	538,855	19,227	3.6
Salaries	132,914	130,319	2,595	2.0
Professional fees	98,222	95,449	2,773	2.9
Supplies and expense	49,185	45,608	3,577	7.8
Personnel	27	28	(1)	(3.6)
Exams	243,704	237,760	5,944	2.5
Pharmacy:				
Revenue	571,791	558,390	13,401	2.4
Salaries	46,768	44,121	2,647	6.0
Drugs	203,530	189,294	14,236	7.5
Other expense	1,088	1,056	32	3.0
Personnel 9 9				
Inhalation Therapy:				
Revenue	116,735	112,788	3,947	3.5
Salaries	31,640	30,134	1,506	5.0
Supplies and expense	20,454	18,939	1,515	8.0
Personnel	7	7		
Physical Therapy:				
Revenue	84,430	82,658	1,772	2.1
Salaries	43,678	41,401	2,277	5.5
Supplies and expense	2,355	2,252	103	4.6
Personnel	8	8		
Treatments	22,819	22,155	664	3.0
Central Service:				
Salaries	85,738	78,746	6,992	8.9
Supplies and expense	3,932	3,672	260	7.1
Personnel	24	23	1	4.3

	1987	1986	Increase (Decrease) Amount	Percent
Medical-Surgical:				
Revenue-supplies	$141,012	$140,247	$ 765	.5%
Revenue-IV solutions	113,204	110,298	2,906	2.6
Cost of supplies	90,953	82,460	8,493	10.3
Cost of IV solutions and supplies	60,225	55,972	4,253	7.6
Medical Records:				
Salaries	48,388	46,172	2,216	4.8
Supplies and expense	4,225	4,098	127	3.1
Personnel	12	12		
School of Nursing:				
Salaries	94,622	83,902	10,720	12.8
Supplies and expense	29,560	29,209	351	1.2
Personnel	16	15	1	6.7
Students	157	163	(6)	(3.7)
Nurses' Residence:				
Salaries	6,771	6,492	279	4.3
Supplies and expense	3,078	3,290	(212)	(6.4)
Personnel	2	2		

P2.   Following are the condensed balance sheets and income statements of Rayshow Hospital:

Rayshow Hospital
Balance Sheets
December 31, 1987 and 1986
($ in 000's)

	1987	1986
Cash and marketable securities	$ 1,498	$ 1,375
Receivables, net of allowance for uncollectible accounts of $711 at 12/31/87 and $605 at 12/31/86	5,211	4,893
Inventories	545	512
Prepaid expenses	852	704

Total current assets	8,106	7,484
Long-term investments	3,167	2,899
Fixed assets, net of accumulated depreciation of $9,461 at 12/31/87 and $8,147 at 12/31/86	20,365	19,972
Other assets	2,420	2,128
Total assets	$34,058	$32,483
Current liabilities	$ 4,278	$ 3,541
Long-term debt	11,900	12,500
Total liabilities	16,178	16,041
Fund balance	17,880	16,442
Total liabilities and fund balance	$34,058	$32,483

Rayshow Hospital
Income Statements
Years Ended December 31, 1987 and 1986
($ in 000's)

	1987	1986
Gross patient service revenues	$35,492	$31,754
Less revenue deductions	5,821	5,017
Net patient service revenues	29,671	26,737
Add other operating revenues	1,455	1,080
Total operating revenues	31,126	27,817
Less operating expenses:		
Depreciation	1,314	1,175
Interest	710	756
Other operating expenses	28,357	25,158
Total operating expenses	30,381	27,089
Operating income	745	728
Add nonoperating revenues (net)	693	445
Net income	$ 1,438	$ 1,173

Required. Compute the following ratios for 1987 and 1986, and indicate whether the change in the ratio is favorable or unfavorable.

1. Current ratio.
2. Quick ratio.
3. Number of days' revenue in net receivables.
4. Average payment period for current liabilities.
5. Days' cash on hand.
6. Fund balance to total assets (equity financing ratio).
7. Cash flow to total debt.
8. Long-term debt to fund balance.
9. Times interest earned.
10. Debt service coverage (assuming annual $600 principal payments on long-term debt).
11. Total asset turnover.
12. Current asset turnover.
13. Inventory turnover.
14. Return on total assets.
15. Return on equity (fund balance).
16. Operating income ratio.

Appendix A

This Glossary includes selected general accounting terms and certain special terms encountered in hospital financial management. Many of these definitions have been adapted from a variety of sources, including:

APB Accounting Principles (New York: AICPA, 1973).

Berman, Howard J., and Weeks, Lewis E., **The Financial Management of Hospitals** (Ann Arbor, Michigan: Health Administration Press, School of Public Health, The University of Michigan, 1974).

Chart of Accounts for Hospitals (Chicago: AHA, 1976).

Eric L. Kohler, **A Dictionary for Accountants** (Englewood Cliffs, New Jersey: Prentice-Hall, Inc., 1970).

Hospital Audit Guide (New York: AICPA, 1982).

Statement of Financial Accounting Concepts No. 2 (Stamford Connecticut: FASB, 1980).

Statement of Financial Accounting Concepts No. 3 (Stamford Connecticut: FASB, 1980).

Uniform Hospital Definitions (Chicago: AHA, 1968).

A

Accelerated Depreciation. Depreciation by a method, such as sum-of-years'-digits or double-declining-balance, which results in the write-off of the cost of a depreciable asset at a more rapid rate than would occur by the straight-line method.

Accounting. The accumulation and communication of historical and projected economic data relating to the financial position of an enterprise and the results of its operations, and the interpretation of the results thereof for purposes of managerial planning and control and for use by decision-making groups external to the enterprise.

Accounting Cycle. The procedures involved in maintaining a set of accounting records throughout an accounting period.

Accounting Equation. An equation which is both the basic formula for the balance sheet and the foundation of double-entry accounting. Usually written: Assets = Liabilities + Fund Balances.

Accounting Period. The period of time covered by an income statement. This period generally is not less than one month nor longer than one year.

Accounting Principles. A body of rules, standards, and conventions which determines the manner in which transactions are recorded and in which data are presented in financial statements.

Accounts Payable. Liabilities arising from the purchase of goods and services from suppliers on credit.

Accounts Receivable. Assets arising from the provision of services or the sale of goods to patients on credit.

Accounts Receivable Aging Schedule. An analysis of accounts receivable according to the length of time the accounts have been outstanding.

Accounts Receivable Turnover. Charges to patients' accounts during a given period divided by the amount of accounts receivable.

Accrual Basis of Accounting. A method of accounting by which revenues are recognized when earned and expenses are recognized when incurred, regardless of the flow of cash.

Accrued Expenses. Expenses which have been incurred but not yet paid.

Accrued Income. Income which has been earned but not yet received in cash.

Accumulated Depreciation. The accumulation to date of depreciation expense, that is, the total portion of the original cost of depreciable assets which already has been allocated to expense in prior and current periods.

Adjusting Entry. An entry which is necessary to adjust account balances to conform with the accrual basis at the end of the accounting period.

Admission. (1) An inpatient admission is the formal acceptance by a hospital of a patient who is to receive physician, dentist, or allied services while lodged in the hospital. (2) An outpatient admission is the formal acceptance by the hospital of a patient who is not to be lodged in the hospital while receiving physician, dentist, or allied services at the hospital.

Allowance. The difference between gross revenue from services rendered and amounts received, or to be received, from patients or third-party payers. Allowances are to be distinguished from uncollectible accounts resulting from credit losses.

Allowance for Uncollectible Accounts. A balance sheet valuation account reflecting the estimated amount of accounts and notes receivable which will prove to be uncollectible by reason of charity care, contractual adjustments, courtesy discounts, and bad debt losses.

Amortization. (1) The systematic allocation of an item to revenue or expense over a number of accounting periods. (2) The repayment of a loan on an installment basis.

Annuity. A series of rents (receipts or payment) to be paid or received periodically in the future.

Annuity Funds. Funds given to an institution as consideration for an agreement to pay periodically to the donor, or specified designation persons, stipulated amounts for the period set forth in the agreement.

Assets. The economic resources of a hospital enterprise that are recognized and measured in conformity with generally accepted accounting principles. Assets are probable future economic benefits obtained or controlled by a particular entity as a result of past transactions or events (SFAC No. 3).

Average Daily Census. The average number of inpatients maintained in the hospital each day for a given period of time.

Average Length of Stay. The average number of days of service rendered to each inpatient discharged during a given period.

B

Bad Debt. An account receivable which, although the patient has the ability to pay, is regarded as uncollectible and is charged as a credit loss.

Balance Sheet. A statement of financial position showing the hospital's assets, liabilities, and fund balances at a given date.

Board-Designated Funds. Unrestricted funds set aside by action of the hospital's governing board for specific purposes or projects.

Board-Designated Investment Funds. Unrestricted funds which, at the discretion of the governing board, have been designated for investment to produce income as if they were endowment funds.

Bond. A written promise under seal to pay a sum of money at some definite future time.

Bond Discount or Premium. The difference between the par or face value of a bond and the amount received (by the issuer) or paid (by the investor) when a bond is issued or purchased.

Bond Indenture. The contract between the bondholders and the hospital issuing the bonds.

Bond Sinking Fund. A fund in which assets are accumulated in order to liquidate bonds at their maturity date, or earlier.

Book Value. The amount at which an asset or liability item is carried in the accounting records of the hospital.

Break-Even Point. The volume of revenue where revenues and expenses are exactly equal, i.e., the level of activity where there is neither a gain nor a loss from operations.

Budget. A financial plan for future operations.

C

Capital Expenditure. An expenditure chargeable to an asset account where the asset acquired has an estimated life in excess of one year and is not intended for sale in the ordinary course of operations. The opposite of revenue expenditure.

Capital Expenditure Budgeting. The process of planning and controlling expenditures for property, plant, and equipment items.

Capital Lease. A lease under which the lessee records an asset and a liability, accounting for the lease as an installment purchase of the leased property.

Cash Basis of Accounting. A method of accounting by which revenues are recognized only when cash is received and expenses are recorded only when cash is disbursed.

Cash Budget. A projection of cash receipts, disbursements, and balances for a given future period of time.

Cash-Flow Statement. A statement of actual or projected cash receipts and disbursements for a given period of time.

Chart of Accounts. A listing of account titles, with account numbers, indicating the manner in which transaction data are to be classified in the accounting records.

Chattel Mortgage. A mortgage on personal property, excluding real estate.

Closing the Books. The process of transferring the balances in the revenue and expense accounts, including revenue deductions, to the fund balance account at the end of the fiscal year.

Coinsurance Clause. In fire insurance, for example, a policy clause which limits the liability of the insurance company to a determinable percentage of the loss suffered by the insured.

Collateral. Assets that are pledged to secure a loan.

Comparability. The qualitative characteristic of accounting information that enables users to identify similarities in differences between two sets of economic phenomena (SFAC No. 2).

Compensating Balances. Cash deposits required by a bank as partial compensation for lending and other services which it provides to a hospital.

Completeness. The inclusion in reported information of everything material that is necessary for faithful representation of the relevant phenomena (SFAC No. 2).

Composite Depreciation. Depreciation of a number of similar assets as a group rather than on a unit-by-unit basis.

Compound Interest. Interest that is computed on the principal amount invested or borrowed **and** on any interest earned (on such principal) that has not been paid.

Conditional Sales Contract. A method of financing the acquisition of new equipment by installment payments over a period of months. The seller retains title until all payments have been completed.

Conservatism. A prudent reaction to uncertainty to try to ensure that uncertainty and risks inherent in business situations are adequately considered (SFAC No. 2).

Consistency. Conformity from period to period with unchanging policies and procedures (SFAC No. 2).

Contingent Liabilities. Possible future liabilities which may arise upon the happening of some future event.

Contractual Patient. One of a group of patients for whom the hospital has agreed to provide specific inpatient or outpatient facilities and services, payment for which is made to the hospital on the basis of a contract between an outside agency and the hospital.

Contractual Replacement Funds. Funds set aside by agreement with third-party payers for renewal and replacement of property, plant, and equipment.

Contribution Clause. In fire insurance, for example, a policy clause which limits the liability of the insurance company to a pro rata portion of a loss of property insured by more than one company.

Contribution Margin. The excess of revenues over variables costs.

Control. The process of assuring, insofar as possible, that the objectives of an organization are realized. Its principal elements are (1) the communication of plans, (2) performance appraisal, (3) corrective action, and (4) follow-up.

Control Account. A general ledger account, the detail of which is contained in a subsidiary ledger, e.g., accounts receivable.

Controllable Cost. In the short-run, a cost whose amount is controllable by someone in the organization. It is usually a variable cost.

Controller. The title usually given to the executive responsible for the accounting function in an organization.

Cost. The present value surrendered, or promised to be surrendered, in the future, in exchange for goods and services received. Expired costs are expenses; unexpired costs are assets.

Cost Basis of Accounting. The use of historical, objectively determined cost as the basis of accounting for most assets.

Cost Center. An organizational unit whose costs are separately accumulated in the accounts.

Cost Control. The attempt to maintain actual costs at, or below, budgeted levels.

Cost Finding. The segregation of direct costs by cost centers and the allocation of overhead costs to revenue-producing and other centers by inpatient, outpatient, and other classifications.

Cost or Market, Lower of. A valuation basis for inventories and temporary investments.

Credit. As a noun, an entry or balance on the right-hand side of an account. As a transitive verb, to make an entry on the right-hand side of an account.

Current Assets. Those assets which are cash and will be converted into cash or consumed in the normal operations of the hospital within one year from the balance sheet date.

Current Liabilities. Those liabilities which will be discharged by the use of current assets in the normal course of business within one year from the balance sheet date.

Current Ratio. The ratio of current assets to current liabilities.

D

Days' Revenue in Receivables. The average number of days of billings in accounts receivable and uncollected at a given point in time.

Debenture Bond. A bond not secured by specific assets but only by the general credit standing of the issuer.

Debit. As a noun, an entry or balance on the left-hand side of an account. As a transitive verb, to make an entry on the left-hand side of an account.

Deductions from Revenues. Revenues uncollectible by reason of charity care, contractual adjustments, courtesy discounts, and bad debts.

Default. Failure to fulfill a contract, e.g., failure to pay interest or principal on a debt.

Deferred Revenue. Future revenue which has been collected or billed but not yet earned; hence, a liability.

Depreciation Expense. That portion of the original cost of a tangible plant asset allocated to a particular accounting period.

Discounting of Receivables. A method of short term financing where patient receivables are used to secure a loan from a financial institution.

Dishonor. To refuse to honor (pay) a promissory note at maturity.

Donated Services. The estimated monetary value of service of personnel who receive no monetary compensation or partial compensation for their services. The term is usually applied to services rendered by members of religious orders, societies, or similar groups to hospitals operated by or affiliated with such organizations.

E

ECF. Extended care facility, e.g., a nursing home.

Effective Yield Method. A method of amortizing discount or premium on bonds payable, utilizing compound interest and present value concepts.

Endowment Funds. Funds with stipulations by the donors that the principal of the funds be maintained intact and that only the income from investments of the resources may be expended. See **Term Endowment Funds.**

EOQ. Economic order quantity, i.e., the optimum (least cost) quantity of goods which should be purchased in a single order.

Equities. Rights in assets, e.g., fund balances. Equity is the residual interest in the assets of an entity that remains after deducting its liabilities (SFAC No. 3).

Executory Costs. Insurance, property taxes, and maintenance costs associated with leased assets.

Expenses. Costs that have been used up or consumed in carrying on some activity and from which no measurable benefit will extend beyond the present. Expenses are expired costs and ordinarily are accompanied by the surrendering of an asset or by the incurring of a liability. Expenses are outflows or other using up of assets or incurrences of liabilities (or a combination of both) during a period from delivering or producing goods, rendering services, or carrying out other activities that constitute the entity's ongoing major or central operations (SFAC No. 3).

Extraordinary Gains and Losses. Gains or losses unusual in amount and nonrecurring in nature.

F

Factoring. The process of selling or assigning receivables to a factor as a means of obtaining short-term financing.

Feedback Value. The qualitative characteristic of accounting information that enables users to confirm or correct prior expectations (SFAC No. 2).

FICA. Federal Insurance Contributions Act, commonly known as Social Security.

FIFO. First-in, first-out. A method of inventory costing.

Fixed Costs. Costs which remain substantially the same in total amount within a given range of output during a given period of time.

Flexible Budget. A budget prepared in such a manner that it can be adjusted by interpolation to reflect what expenses should be at any level of activity within a relevant range.

Functional Classification. The grouping of expenses according to the operating purposes (patient care, education, research, etc.) for which costs are incurred. Revenues also may be classified functionally.

Fund. A self-contained accounting entity set up to account for a specific activity or project.

Fund Accounting. A system of accounting in which the hospital's resources, obligations, and fund balances are segregated into logical groups of accounts according to legal restrictions and administrative requirements. Each account group, or fund, constitutes a subordinate accounting entity.

Fund Balance. The excess of assets over liabilities (owners' equity). An excess of liabilities over assets is known as a **deficit** in fund balance.

Funded Debt. Long-term debt.

Funds Functioning as Endowment. See Board-Designated Funds.

Funds Held in Trust by Others. Funds held and administered, at the direction of the donor, by an outside trustee for the benefit of an institution or institutions.

G

General Fund. The name sometimes given to the Unrestricted Fund.

Governing Board. The policy-making body of the hospital. Some of the responsibilities usually attributed to the governing board may be assumed by appropriate committees.

Gross Margin Method. A method of estimating the amount of inventory at a given point in time.

Gross Revenues. The value, at the hospital's full established rates, of service rendered and goods sold to patients during a given time period.

H

HCFA. Health Care Financing Administration.

HMO. Health Maintenance Organization.

I

Imprest Cash Fund. See Petty Cash Fund.

Income Statement. A financial statement indicating the results of operations of an enterprise in terms of revenues earned and expenses incurred for a given period of time. Also referred to as an **operating statement,** a **statement of income and expense,** or a **profit and loss statement.**

Insolvency. The inability to meet matured obligations.

Interest. A charge for the use of money.

Interim Financial Statements. Financial statements prepared at a date other than the end of the fiscal year, e.g., monthly balance sheets and income statements.

Internal Auditing. The work performed by a hospital's internal auditors.

Internal Control. The plan of organization and all the coordinate methods and measures adopted within a hospital to safeguard its assets, check the accuracy and reliability of its accounting data, promote operational efficiency, and encourage adherence to prescribed managerial policies.

Inventory. The aggregate of those items of tangible personal property which (1) are held for sale in the ordinary course of business, (2) are in process of production for sale, or (3) are to be consumed currently in the production of goods or services to be available for sale.

Inventory Control. The process of regulating the amount and types of supplies in inventory.

Inventory Turnover. Cost of supplies used divided by the average inventory for the period.

J

Journal. A book of original entry wherein transactions are recorded in chronological sequence.

L

Land Improvements. Improvements made to land, including sidewalks, parking lots, driveways, fencing, and shrubbery. Land improvements are depreciable.

Ledger. The group of accounts used in recording the transactions of the hospital. A book of secondary entry.

Liabilities. The economic obligations of the hospital as recognized and measured in conformity with generally accepted accounting principles. The probable future sacrifices of economic benefits arising from present obligations of a particular entity to transfer assets or provide services to other entities in the future as a result of past transactions or events (SFAC No. 3).

LIFO. Last-in, First-out. An inventory costing method.

Line of Credit. An arrangement whereby a financial institution commits itself to lend up to a specified maximum amount during a specified period.

Liquidity. A hospital's financial position and its ability to meet currently maturing obligations.

Living Trust Funds. Funds acquired by a hospital subject to agreement whereby resources are made available to the hospital on condition that the hospital pay periodically to a designated person, or persons, the income earned on the resources acquired for the lifetime of the designated person, or persons, or for a specified period.

Lock-Box Plan. A procedure used to speed up collections and to reduce float with regard to such collections.

Long-Term Investments. Investments, generally in securities, which the hospital intends to hold for longer than one year from the balance sheet date.

Long-Term Liabilities. Liabilities that are not payable within one year from the balance sheet i.e., all liabilities except current liabilities.

M

Management. The direction of resources to the attainment of desired objectives through planning and control.

Marginal Cost. The addition to total cost resulting from the production of an additional unit of service or product.

Marginal Revenue. The addition to total revenue resulting from the sale of an additional unit of service or product.

Marketable Security. Short-term investments in securities which can be readily sold without significant loss of principal.

Matching. An accounting principle which requires the recognition of related revenues and expenses in the same period.

Materiality. The magnitude of an omission or misstatement of accounting information that, in the light of surrounding circumstances, makes it probable that the judgment of a reasonable person relying on the information would have been changed or influenced by the omission or misstatement (SFAC No. 2).

Mortgage. A pledge of designated property as security for a loan, e.g., mortgage bonds.

N

Net Assets. The excess of assets over liabilities, i.e., fund balance.

Net Income. The excess of revenues over expenses for a given period of time as presented in the income statement.

Net Loss. The excess of expenses over revenues for a given period of time as presented in the income statement.

Net Revenues. The excess of gross revenues from patient services over revenue deductions. Also called **net earnings from patient services**.

Neutrality. Absence in reported accounting information of bias intended to attain a predetermined result or to induce a particular mode of behavior (SFAC No. 2).

Nonexpendable Funds. See Endowment Funds.

Normal Cost. In accounting for pension plans, the annual cost of future retirement benefits earned by employees during a given year.

Notes Receivable Discounted. Notes receivable which have been discounted with recourse at a financial institution.

O

Objective Evidence. A requirement in accounting that all transaction entries be supported, insofar as possible, by properly executed documents.

Object of Expenditure Classification. A method of classifying expenditures according to their natural classification such as salaries and wages, employee benefits, supplies, and purchased services.

Operating Lease. A lease that does not qualify for treatment as a capital lease under the criteria provided in SFAS No. 13.

Operating Ratio. Total operating expenses divided by total operating revenues.

Opportunity Cost. The measurable advantage foregone in the past or that may be sacrificed as a result of a decision involving alternatives.

Organization Chart. A diagrammatic illustration of the manner in which a hospital is organized internally.

Outliers. Under the Medicare prospective payment system (PPS), cases that are assigned to a particular DRG that have either unusually long lengths of stay or unusually high costs compared to other cases in that DRG.

Overstocked. Excessive inventories.

P

Past Service Cost. In accounting for a pension plan, the cost that is associated with employee services prior to inception of the plan. This cost usually is expensed over a period not less than 10 years.

Patient Day. The unit of measure denoting lodging facilities provided and services rendered to one inpatient between the census-taking hour on two successive days.

Payback Period. The period of time it will take a new item of equipment to produce revenues or result in savings equal to its cost.

Percentage of Occupancy. The ratio of actual patient days to maximum patient days as determined by bed capacity during any given period of time.

Periodic Inventory System. A system of accounting for purchased goods and supplies by which items purchased are charged to expense accounts rather than to inventory.

Permanent Funds. See Endowment Funds.

Perpetual Inventory System. A system of accounting for inventories under which a continuous, day-to-day record is kept of inventory levels.

Petty Cash Fund. A small fund of cash maintained for the purpose of making minor disbursements for which the issuance of a check would be inconvenient or impractical.

Physical Inventory. The actual inventory as determined by physical count, usually at the end of a reporting period.

Planning. The process of establishing programs for the achievement of objectives.

Plant Assets. Physical properties used for hospital purposes, i.e., land, land improvements, buildings, and equipment. The term does not include real estate or properties of restricted or unrestricted funds not used for hospital operations.

Plant Replacement and Expansion Funds. Funds donated for renewal or replacement of hospital plant.

Pooled Investments. Assets of two or more funds consolidated for investment purposes.

Position Control Plan. A management tool for controlling the number of employees on the hospital payroll and for assuring the utilization of each employee to the point of maximum effectiveness.

Posting. The process of transferring the information in the journals to the ledger.

PPS. Prospective payment system, under which hospitals are paid a fixed price-per-case based on diagnosis-related groups (DRGs) of patients.

Predictive Value. The qualitative characteristic of accounting information that helps users to increase the likelihood of correctly forecasting the outcome of past or present events (SFAS No. 2).

Preemptive Right. The right of existing stockholders to purchase a new issue of capital stock before it is offered to the general public.

Preferred Stock. A type of stock which has preference over common stock with respect to dividends or to assets in case of liquidation, or both.

Prepaid Expense. An expense-type outlay which benefits (is applicable to) subsequent accounting periods and therefore is an asset.

Prepaid Income. See Deferred Revenue.

Present Value. The value today of a future receipt or payment, or successive receipts or payments, discounted at the appropriate discount rate.

Profit and Loss Statement. A less satisfactory term for **income statement**.

Prior Service Cost. In accounting for a pension plan, the cost that is assigned to all periods prior to the date of an actuarial valuation or amendment of the plan.

PSRO. Professional Standards Review Organization.

Purchase Order. A business document used in purchasing.

Q

Qualified Audit Report. An audit report including one or more qualifications or exceptions.

Quantity Discount. A reduction in unit purchase cost received by those who purchase supplies in a quantity in excess of a certain amount.

Quick Assets. Cash, temporary investments, and receivables.

Quick Ratio. The ratio of quick assets to current liabilities.

R

Ratio. The quotient which results when one number is divided by another.

Receiving Report. A business document in which a record is made of incoming quantities of supplies.

Record Date. The date on which a list of stockholders is prepared to determine those who are entitled to receive a declared dividend.

Referred Outpatient. One who is admitted exclusively to a special diagnostic or therapeutic facility or service of the hospital for diagnosis or treatment on an ambulatory basis.

Refunding. The process of replacing one debt with another, usually having a lower interest cost.

Registered Bond. A type of bond that has the principal and usually the interest payable only to the owner as recorded by the issuer.

Relative Value Units. Index numbers assigned to various procedures based on the relative amounts of labor, supplies, and capital required to perform the procedure.

Relevance. The capacity of accounting information to make a difference in a decision by helping users to form predictions about the outcomes of past, present, or future events, or to confirm or correct prior expectations (SFAC No. 2).

Reliability. The qualitative characteristic of accounting information that assures that the information is relatively free from error and bias, and faithfully represents which it purports to represent (SFAC No. 2).

Reserve. A generally undesirable term in accounting usage but sometimes employed, e.g., **reserve for bad debts** and **reserve for depreciation.**

Responsibility Accounting. A system of accounting which accumulates and communicates historical and projected monetary and statistical data relating to revenues and controllable expenses classified according to the organizational units producing the revenues and responsible for incurring the expenses.

Restricted Funds. Funds restricted by donors for specific purposes. The term refers to specific purpose, plant replacement and expansion, and endowment funds.

Retirement of Indebtedness Funds. Funds required by external sources to be used to meet debt service charges and the retirement of indebtedness on plant assets. The term **sinking funds** is sometimes used to describe these funds.

Revenue. Revenue results from the sale of goods and the rendering of services and is measured by the charge made to patients and others for goods and services furnished to them. It also includes gains from the sale or exchange of assets, interest, and dividends earned on investments and unrestricted donations of resources to the hospital. Revenues are inflows or other enhancements of assets of an entity or settlements of its liabilities (or a combination of both) during a period from delivering or producing goods, rendering services, or other activities that constitute the entity's ongoing major or central operations (SFAC No. 3).

Revenue Expenditure. An expenditure charged against operations.

ROP. Reorder Point. In inventory management, the point in time at which a new order should be placed for supplies.

S

Salvage Value. The estimated amount for which a plant asset can be sold at the end of its useful life. Also called residual or scrap value.

Self-Responsible Patient. A patient who pays either all or part of his hospital bill from his own resources as opposed to third-party payment.

Semivariable Costs. Costs which are partly variable and partly fixed in behavior in response to changes in volume.

Share of Pooled Investments. The proportion of pooled investments including accumulated gains or losses owned by a particular fund, usually expressed by a number (units) indicating the fractional ownership of total shares in the pool or by a percentage expressing the portion of the total pool owned by the particular fund.

Sinking Fund. See Retirement of Indebtedness Funds.

Specific Identification Method. A system of inventory costing. Also applied in the determination of the costs of securities sold.

Specific Purpose Fund. Funds restricted by donors for a specific purpose or project. Board-designated funds are not restricted funds.

Statement of Changes in Financial Position. A financial statement summarizing the movement of funds (working capital or cash) within a hospital for a given period of time.

Statement of Changes in Fund Balances. A financial statement setting forth the changes that have occurred in the amount of the fund balances during a given period of time.

Stock Dividend. A dividend paid in the form of additional shares of stock.

Stockout. A condition wherein demand exists for inventory items which are currently not on hand.

Stock Right. A transferable warrant issued by a corporation in connection with the sale of a new issue of stock.

Stock Split. An action taken by a corporation to increase the number of shares outstanding, other than by sale, in order to reduce the market price of the stock to a level more attractive to investors.

Straight-Line Method. A method of depreciation. Also a method of amortizing bond premium and discount.

Subordinate Debentures. Bonds having a claim on assets only after the senior debts have been paid off in the event of liquidation.

Subsidiary Ledger. A group of accounts which is contained in a separate ledger and which supports a single account (a control account) in the general ledger.

SYD. Sum-of-years'-digits. An accelerated method of depreciation.

T

Tangible Asset. An asset having physical existence, e.g., equipment.

Temporary Fund. Name formerly given to Specific Purpose Fund.

Temporary Investments. Investments, generally in marketable securities, which a hospital does not intend to hold for more than one year from the balance sheet date.

Term Endowment Funds. Donated funds which by the terms of the agreement become available either for any legitimate purpose designated by the governing board or for a specific purpose designated by the donor upon the happening of an event or upon the passage of a stated period of time.

Term Loan. A loan generally obtained from a bank or insurance company with a maturity greater than one year. Term loans are generally amortized.

Timeliness. Having accounting information available to a decision-maker before it loses its capacity to influence decisions (SFAC No. 2).

Trade Credit. Debt arising from transactions in which supplies and services are purchased on credit from suppliers.

Trial Balance. A list of the accounts in a ledger, with their balances, at a given date.

U

Unamortized Bond Discount (or Premium). That portion of bond discount (or premium) which has not yet been amortized by charges (credits) to bond interest expense.

Understandability. The qualitative characteristic of accounting information that enables users to perceive its significance (SFAC No. 2).

Unemployment Taxes. Taxes levied by federal and state governments to finance payments to the unemployed.

Unexpended Plant Funds. See Plant Replacement and Expansion Funds.

Unexpired Cost. An asset. See **Cost.**

Unrestricted Funds. Funds which bear no external restrictions as to use or purpose, i.e., funds which can be used for any legitimate purpose designated by the governing board as distinguished from funds restricted externally for specific operating purposes, for plant replacement and expansion, and for endowment.

Useful Life. An estimate made of the number of years an item of plant and equipment will be used by a hospital.

V

Variable Cost. A cost which varies directly in total with changes in the level of activity.

Verifiability. The ability through consensus among measurers to ensure that information represents which it purports to represent or that the chosen method of measurement has been used without error or bias (SFAC No. 2).

Voucher System. A system for the processing and control of cash disbursements.

W

Weighted Average Costing. A method of determining the cost of supplies used and the valuation of inventory.

Working Capital. Generally, the excess of current assets over current liabilities. Sometimes called **net working capital.**

Worksheet. A device used in accounting to facilitate the preparation of financial statements.

Y

Yield. The actual rate of return on an investment as opposed to the nominal rate of return.

Appendix B

PRESENT AND FUTURE VALUE OF MONEY

Hospital managers are continually involved with investing and borrowing decisions. Funds are invested today in the expectation of realizing periodic cash returns in the future; funds are borrowed today in return for a promise to repay a certain sum or sums of money in the future. These decisions are complicated by the fact that a dollar paid or received today has a different value than one dollar paid or received in some future period, i.e., money has a time value. The **timing** of cash inflows has an important effect on the value of an investment (asset), and the **timing** of cash outflows has an important effect on the value of a commitment (liability). Measurement of these values is essential to sound decision-making in many areas and requires an understanding of compound interest, annuities, and present value concepts.

Reference has been made to these concepts at various points in the text in connection with notes receivable and payable, leases, amortization of bond premium and discount, bond sinking funds, pension plans, evaluation of capital expenditure proposals, and other matters. This Appendix provides an introduction to the computation of present and future values by the use of compound interest tables (see Tables 1-4 of this Appendix). A more extensive treatment of these matters can be found in most intermediate accounting textbooks.

INTEREST

Interest is the fee charged for the use of money for a given time period. **Simple interest** is the fee charged for **one** period of time (assuming that the interest itself does not earn interest). If, for example, a hospital invests a sum of $1,000 at 8 percent simple interest per annum for one year, the interest on the investment will be $80 ($1,000 X .08). Simple interest, however, normally is applicable only to short-term (one year or less) investment and borrowing situations.

Many critical investment and borrowing decisions involve more than one time period, and the term **compound interest** refers to interest that is computed on the principal amount invested or borrowed **and** on any interest earned (on such principal) that has not been paid. If, for example, a hospital invests a sum of $1,000 at 8 percent interest per annum compounded annually, the interest earned for two one-year periods will be $166.40, as follows:

Year

1	$1,000 x .08 =	$ 80.00
2	$1,080 x .08 =	86.40
		$166.40

Thus, compound interest is the growth of principal for **two** or **more** time periods, assuming that the growth (interest) in each time period is added to the principal at the end of the period and earns a return in all subsequent periods. Except for short-term lending and borrowing involving one year or less, compound interest is the typical interest computation applied in business decision-making by the hospital manager.

The mathematics of compound interest can become quite complex and, for this reason, tables have been constructed to facilitate computations. Four of these tables are provided at the end of this Appendix, and the following discussion relates to the use of these tables.

AMOUNT OF A SINGLE SUM

Table 1 indicates the amount to which $1 invested today will accumulate at **i** compound interest for **n** periods (a n\i). Assume, for example, that a hospital invests $1 today at 8 percent interest, compounded annually. To what amount would this $1 accumulate in five years? The answer ($1.4693) may be found in Table 1 in the 8 percent column on the n = 5 line. To determine the amount to which, say, $50,000 invested today would accumulate in five years at 8 percent annual interest, compounded annually, $50,000 is multiplied by the 1.4693 factor. This provides an answer of $72,465. The amount to which $50,000 invested today at 8 percent interest, compounded semiannually, would accumulate in five years is $74,010, i.e., 4 percent interest each six months for 10 six-month periods ($50,000 X 1.4802).

PRESENT VALUE OF A SINGLE SUM

Table 2 indicates the present value of $1 due in **n** periods at **i** rate of compound interest per period (p n\i). Assume, for example, that a hospital agrees to pay $1 to another party at a date five years in the future. What is the value of that promise today, assuming that money is worth 8 percent per year, compounded annually? The answer ($0.6806) may be found in Table 2 in the 8 percent column on the n = 5 line. To determine the value of a promise to pay $50,000 at a date five years from now with money worth 8 percent compounded annually, $50,000 is multiplied by the .6806 factor to obtain the answer ($34,030). The present value of $50,000 due in five years at 8 percent annual interest compounded semiannually is $33,780 ($50,000 multiplied by .6756).

AMOUNT OF AN ANNUITY

The above discussion considers only the accumulation of a single sum, but many investment and borrowing situations are encountered in which a **series** of dollar amounts ("rents") are to be paid or received periodically in the future. When a series of **equal** periodic rents occurs at the **end** of each period, the situation is referred to as an **ordinary annuity**. The amount of an ordinary annuity may be expressed by the formula Ao n\i, and the factors are provided in Table 3.

Suppose, for example, that a hospital deposits $10,000 at the end of each year for five years in a savings account that will earn 6 percent annual interest compounded annually. What amount will have accumulated in the account at the end of the fifth year? The answer is $56,371 ($10,000 X 5.6371). Or, given annual interest of 6 percent compounded annually, what amount must be deposited in a savings account at the end of each year for five years if $56,271 is to be accumulated at the end of the fifth year? The answer is $10,000 ($56,371 divided by 5.6371).

In an annuity due, **equal** periodic rents occur at the **beginning** of each period and interest continues to accumulate for one period after the last rent. The amount of an annuity due is the amount of an ordinary annuity for n + 1 periods minus one rent. For example, to what amount will an annuity due of $1 accumulate at i compound interest for **n** periods? The formula may be stated as $(Ao \overline{n + 1}\backslash i) - 1$. If i is 6 percent and **n** is 5, the answer is $5.9753 ($6.9753 − $1.00). Or, if $2,000 is deposited in a savings account on January 1 of each year for five years, what amount will have accumulated at December 31 of the fifth year if the account earns 6 percent annual interest compounded annually? The answer is $11,951 ($2,000 X 6.9753, minus $2,000). And, of course, if the amount to be accumulated is known, the required equal annual deposits (rents) can be calculated, i.e., $11,951 = (R X 6.9753) − R, and R equals $2,000.

PRESENT VALUE OF AN ANNUITY

The present value of an ordinary annuity, shown in Table 4, is the amount which if invested today at i interest would be just sufficient to permit the withdrawal of equal rents (R) at the end of each of **n** periods. The present value of an ordinary annuity may be expressed by the following formula: $Po \overline{n}\backslash i$.

What present cash payment, for example, would be equivalent to an annuity of $5,000 paid at the END of each year for the next five years if money is worth 6 percent annually? The answer is $21,062 ($5,000 X 4.2124). Or, if $50,000 is invested today in a savings account that earns 6 percent annually, what equal amounts can be withdrawn at the end of each of the next five years so as to exactly exhaust the fund at the end of the fifth year? The answer is $11,870 ($50,000 divided by 4.2124).

The present value of an **annuity due** is the present value of an ordinary annuity of n − 1 periods **plus** one additional rent. The formula may be stated as $(Po \overline{n - 1}\backslash i) + 1$. What present cash payment, for example, would be equivalent to an annuity of $5,000 paid at the beginning of each year for the next five years if money is worth 6 percent annually? The answer is $22,326 ($5,000 X 3.4651, plus $5,000). Or, given a debt of $40,000 with interest at 6 percent annually, what five equal annual payments (the first to be paid at once) must the hospital make to extinguish the debt? The answer is $8,958, i.e., $40,000 = (R x 3.4651) + R, and solve for R.

Table 1

Table 1

Amount of $1 = a \overline{n}| i$

n	Rate of interest, %										
	.5	1.0	1.5	2.0	2.5	3.0	4.0	5.0	6.0	8.0	10.0
1	1.0050	1.0100	1.0150	1.0200	1.0250	1.0300	1.0400	1.0500	1.0600	1.0800	1.1000
2	1.0100	1.0201	1.0302	1.0404	1.0506	1.0609	1.0816	1.1025	1.1236	1.1664	1.2100
3	1.0151	1.0303	1.0457	1.0612	1.0769	1.0927	1.1249	1.1576	1.1910	1.2597	1.3310
4	1.0202	1.0406	1.0614	1.0824	1.1038	1.1255	1.1699	1.2155	1.2625	1.3605	1.4641
5	1.0253	1.0510	1.0773	1.041	1.1314	1.1593	1.2167	1.2763	1.3382	1.4693	1.6105
6	1.0304	1.0615	1.0934	1.1262	1.1597	1.1941	1.2653	1.3401	1.4185	1.5869	1.7716
7	1.0355	1.0721	1.1098	1.1487	1.1887	1.2299	1.3159	1.4071	1.5036	1.7138	1.9487
8	1.0407	1.0829	1.1265	1.1717	1.2184	1.2668	1.3686	1.4775	1.5938	1.8509	2.1436
9	1.0459	1.0937	1.1434	1.1951	1.2489	1.3048	1.4233	1.5513	1.6895	1.9990	2.3579
10	1.0511	1.1046	1.1605	1.2190	1.2801	1.3439	1.4802	1.6289	1.7908	2.1589	2.5937
11	1.0564	1.1157	1.1779	1.2434	1.3121	1.3842	1.5395	1.7103	1.8983	2.3316	2.8531
12	1.0617	1.1268	1.1956	1.2682	1.3449	1.4258	1.6010	1.7959	2.0122	2.5182	3.1384
13	1.0670	1.1381	1.2136	1.2936	1.3785	1.4685	1.6651	1.8856	2.1329	2.7196	3.4523
14	1.0723	1.1495	1.2318	1.3195	1.4130	1.5126	1.7317	1.9799	2.2609	2.9372	3.7975
15	1.0777	1.1610	1.2502	1.3459	1.4483	1.5580	1.8009	2.0789	2.3966	3.1722	4.1772
16	1.0831	1.1726	1.2690	1.3728	1.4845	1.6047	1.8730	2.1829	2.5404	3.4259	4.5950
17	1.0885	1.1843	1.2880	1.4002	1.5216	1.6528	1.9479	2.2920	2.6928	3.7000	5.0545
18	1.0939	1.1961	1.3073	1.4282	1.5597	1.7024	2.0258	2.4066	2.8543	3.9960	5.5599
19	1.0994	1.2081	1.3270	1.4568	1.5987	1.7535	2.1068	2.5270	3.0256	4.3157	6.1159
20	1.1049	1.2202	1.3469	1.4859	1.6386	1.8061	2.1911	2.6533	3.2071	4.6610	6.7275
21	1.1104	1.2324	1.3671	1.5157	1.6796	1.8603	2.2788	2.7860	3.3996	5.0338	7.4002
22	1.1160	1.2447	1.3876	1.5460	1.7216	1.9161	2.3699	2.9253	3.6035	5.4365	8.1403
23	1.1216	1.2572	1.4084	1.5769	1.7646	1.9736	2.4647	3.0715	3.8197	5.8715	8.9543
24	1.1272	1.2697	1.4295	1.6084	1.8087	2.0328	2.5633	3.2251	4.0489	6.3412	9.8497
25	1.1328	1.2824	1.4509	1.6406	1.8539	2.0938	2.6658	3.3864	4.2919	6.8485	10.8347
26	1.1385	1.2953	1.4727	1.6734	1.9003	2.1566	2.7725	3.5557	4.5494	7.3964	11.9182
27	1.1442	1.3082	1.4948	1.7069	1.9478	2.2213	2.8834	3.7335	4.8223	7.9881	13.1100
28	1.1499	1.3213	1.5172	1.7410	1.9965	2.2879	2.9987	3.9201	5.1117	8.6271	14.4210
29	1.1556	1.3345	1.5400	1.7758	2.0464	2.3566	3.1187	4.1161	5.4184	9.3173	15.8631
30	1.1614	1.3478	1.5631	1.8114	2.0976	2.4273	3.2434	4.3219	5.7435	10.0627	17.4494
35	1.1907	1.4166	1.6839	1.9999	2.3732	2.8139	3.9461	5.5160	7.6861	14.7853	28.1024
40	1.2208	1.4889	1.8140	2.2080	2.6851	3.2620	4.8010	7.0400	10.2857	21.7245	45.2593
45	1.2516	1.5648	1.9542	2.4379	3.0379	3.7816	5.8412	8.9850	13.7646	31.9204	72.8905
50	1.2832	1.6446	2.1052	2.6916	3.4371	4.3839	7.1067	11.4674	18.4202	46.9016	117.3909

Table 2

Present Value of $1 = p\,\overline{n}\,i$

n	Rate of interest, % .5	1.0	1.5	2.0	2.5	3.0	4.0	5.0	6.0	8.0	10.0	15.0	20.0	25.0
1	.9950	.9901	.9852	.9804	.9756	.9709	.9615	.9524	.9434	.9259	.9091	.8696	.8333	.8000
2	.9901	.9803	.9707	.9612	.9518	.9426	.9246	.9070	.8900	.8573	.8264	.7561	.6944	.6400
3	.9851	.9706	.9563	.9423	.9286	.9151	.8890	.8638	.8396	.7938	.7513	.6575	.5787	.5120
4	.9802	.9610	.9422	.9238	.9060	.8885	.8548	.8227	.7921	.7350	.6830	.5718	.4823	.4096
5	.9754	.9515	.9283	.9057	.8839	.8626	.8219	.7835	.7473	.6806	.6209	.4972	.4019	.3277
6	.9705	.9420	.9145	.8880	.8623	.8375	.7903	.7462	.7050	.6302	.5645	.4323	.3349	.2621
7	.9657	.9327	.9010	.8706	.8413	.8131	.7599	.7107	.6651	.5835	.5132	.3759	.2791	.2097
8	.9609	.9235	.8877	.8535	.8207	.7894	.7307	.6768	.6274	.5403	.4665	.3269	.2326	.1678
9	.9561	.9143	.8746	.8368	.8007	.7664	.7026	.6446	.5919	.5002	.4241	.2843	.1938	.1342
10	.9513	.9053	.8617	.8203	.7812	.7441	.6756	.6139	.5584	.4632	.3855	.2472	.1615	.1074
11	.9466	.8963	.8489	.8043	.7621	.7224	.6496	.5847	.5268	.4289	.3505	.2149	.1346	.0859
12	.9419	.8874	.8364	.7885	.7436	.7014	.6246	.5568	.4970	.3971	.3186	.1869	.1122	.0687
13	.9372	.8787	.8240	.7730	.7254	.6810	.6006	.5303	.4688	.3677	.2897	.1625	.0935	.0550
14	.9326	.8700	.8118	.7579	.7077	.6611	.5775	.5051	.4423	.3405	.2633	.1413	.0779	.0440
15	.9279	.8613	.7999	.7430	.6905	.6419	.5553	.4810	.4173	.3152	.2394	.1229	.0649	.0352
16	.9233	.8528	.7880	.7284	.6736	.6232	.5339	.4581	.3936	.2919	.2176	.1069	.0541	.0281
17	.9187	.8444	.7764	.7142	.6572	.6050	.5134	.4363	.3714	.2703	.1978	.0929	.0451	.0225
18	.9141	.8360	.7649	.7002	.6412	.5874	.4936	.4155	.3503	.2502	.1799	.0808	.0376	.0180
19	.9096	.8277	.7536	.6864	.6255	.5703	.4746	.3957	.3305	.2317	.1635	.0703	.0313	.0144
20	.9051	.8195	.7425	.6730	.6103	.5537	.4564	.3769	.3118	.2145	.1486	.0611	.0261	.0115
21	.9006	.8114	.7315	.6598	.5954	.5375	.4388	.3589	.2942	.1987	.1351	.0531	.0217	.0092
22	.8961	.8034	.7207	.6468	.5809	.5219	.4220	.3418	.2775	.1839	.1228	.0462	.0181	.0074
23	.8916	.7954	.7100	.6342	.5667	.5067	.4057	.3256	.2618	.1703	.1117	.0402	.0151	.0059
24	.8872	.7876	.6995	.6217	.5529	.4919	.3901	.3101	.2470	.1577	.1015	.0349	.0126	.0047
25	.8828	.7798	.6892	.6095	.5394	.4776	.3751	.2953	.2330	.1460	.0923	.0304	.0105	.0038
26	.8784	.7720	.6790	.5976	.5262	.4637	.3607	.2812	.2198	.1352	.0839	.0264	.0087	.0030
27	.8740	.7644	.6690	.5859	.5134	.4502	.3468	.2678	.2074	.1252	.0763	.0230	.0073	.0024
28	.8697	.7568	.6591	.5744	.5009	.4371	.3335	.2551	.1956	.1159	.0693	.0200	.0061	.0019
29	.8653	.7493	.6494	.5631	.4887	.4243	.3207	.2429	.1846	.1073	.0630	.0174	.0051	.0015
30	.8610	.7419	.6398	.5521	.4767	.4120	.3083	.2314	.1741	.0994	.0573	.0151	.0042	.0012
35	.8398	.7059	.5939	.5000	.4214	.3554	.2534	.1813	.1301	.0676	.0356	.0075	.0017	.0004
40	.8191	.6717	.5513	.4529	.3724	.3066	.2083	.1420	.0972	.0460	.0221	.0037	.0007	.0001
45	.7990	.6391	.5117	.4102	.3292	.2644	.1712	.1113	.0727	.0313	.0137	.0019	.0003	.0000
50	.7793	.6080	.4750	.3715	.2509	.2281	.1407	.0872	.0543	.0213	.0085	.0009	.0001	.0000

Table 3

Amount of an Ordinary Annuity of $1 = Ao $\overline{n}|\,i$

n	Rate of interest, % .5	1.0	1.5	2.0	2.5	3.0	4.0	Rate of interest, % 5.0	6.0	8.0	10.0
1	1.0000	1.0000	1.0000	1.0000	1.0000	1.0000	1.0000	1.0000	1.0000	1.0000	1.0000
2	2.0050	2.0100	2.0150	2.0200	2.0250	2.0300	2.0400	2.0500	2.0600	2.0800	2.1000
3	3.0150	3.0301	3.0452	3.0604	3.0756	3.0909	3.1216	3.1525	3.1836	3.2464	3.3100
4	4.0301	4.0604	4.0909	4.1216	4.1525	4.1836	4.2465	4.3101	4.3746	4.5061	4.6410
5	5.0503	5.1010	5.1523	5.2040	5.2563	5.3091	5.4163	5.5256	5.6371	5.8666	6.1051
6	6.0755	6.1520	6.2296	6.3081	6.3877	6.4684	6.6330	6.8019	6.9753	7.3359	7.7156
7	7.1059	7.2135	7.3230	7.4343	7.5474	7.6625	7.8983	8.1420	8.3938	8.9228	9.4872
8	8.1414	8.2857	8.4328	8.5830	8.7361	8.8923	9.2142	9.5491	9.8975	10.6366	11.4359
9	9.1821	9.3685	9.5593	9.7546	9.9545	10.1591	10.5828	11.0266	11.4913	12.4876	13.5795
10	10.2280	10.4622	10.7027	10.9497	11.2034	11.4639	12.0061	12.5779	13.1808	14.4866	15.9374
11	11.2792	11.5668	11.8633	12.1687	12.4835	12.8078	13.4864	14.2068	14.9716	16.6455	18.5312
12	12.3356	12.6825	13.0412	13.4121	13.7956	14.1920	15.0258	15.9171	16.8699	18.9771	21.3843
13	13.3972	13.8093	14.2368	14.6803	15.1404	15.6178	16.6268	17.7130	18.8821	21.4953	24.5227
14	14.4642	14.9474	15.4504	15.9739	16.5190	17.0863	18.2919	19.5986	21.0151	24.2149	27.9750
15	15.5365	16.0969	16.6821	17.2934	17.9319	18.5989	20.0236	21.5786	23.2760	27.1521	31.7725
16	16.6142	17.2579	17.9324	18.6393	19.3802	20.1569	21.8245	23.6575	25.6725	30.3243	35.9497
17	17.6973	18.4304	19.2014	20.0121	20.8647	21.7616	23.6975	25.8404	28.2129	33.7502	40.5447
18	18.7858	19.6147	20.4894	21.4123	22.3863	23.4144	25.6454	28.1324	30.9057	37.4502	45.5992
19	19.8797	20.8109	21.7967	22.8406	23.9460	25.1169	27.6712	30.5390	33.7600	41.4463	51.1591
20	20.9791	22.0190	23.1237	24.2974	25.5447	26.8704	29.7781	33.0660	36.7856	45.7620	57.2750
21	22.0840	23.2392	24.4705	25.7833	27.1833	28.6765	31.9692	35.7193	39.9927	50.4229	64.0025
22	23.1944	24.4716	25.8376	27.2990	28.8629	30.5368	34.2480	38.5052	43.3923	55.4568	71.4027
23	24.3104	25.7163	27.2251	28.8450	30.5844	32.4529	36.6179	41.4305	46.9958	60.8933	79.5430
24	25.4320	26.9735	28.6335	30.4219	32.3490	34.4265	39.0826	44.5020	50.8156	66.7648	88.4973
25	26.5591	28.2432	30.0630	32.0303	34.1578	36.4593	41.6459	47.7271	54.8645	73.1059	98.3471
26	27.6919	29.5256	31.5140	33.6709	36.0117	38.5530	44.3117	51.1135	59.1564	79.9544	109.1818
27	28.8304	30.8209	32.9867	35.3443	37.9120	40.7096	47.0842	54.6691	63.7058	87.3508	121.0999
28	29.9745	32.1291	34.4815	37.0512	39.8598	42.9309	49.9676	58.4026	68.5281	95.3388	134.2099
29	31.1244	33.4504	35.9987	38.7922	41.8563	45.2189	52.9663	62.3227	73.6398	103.9659	148.6309
30	32.2800	34.7849	37.5387	40.5681	43.9027	47.5754	56.0849	66.4388	79.0582	113.2832	164.4940
35	38.1454	41.6603	45.5921	49.9945	54.9282	60.4621	73.6522	90.3203	111.4348	172.3168	271.0244
40	44.1588	48.8864	54.2679	60.4020	67.4026	75.4013	95.0255	120.7998	154.7620	259.0565	442.5926
45	50.3242	56.4811	63.6142	71.8927	81.5161	92.7199	121.0294	159.7002	212.7435	386.5056	718.9048
50	56.6452	64.4632	73.6828	84.5794	97.4843	112.7969	152.6671	209.3480	290.3359	573.7702	1163.9085

Table 4

Table 4

Present Value of an Ordinary Annuity of $1 = Po $\overline{n}$| i

n	Rate of interest, %													
	.5	1.0	1.5	2.0	2.5	3.0	4.0	5.0	6.0	8.0	10.0	15.0	20.0	25.0
1	.9950	.9901	.9852	.9804	.9756	.9709	.9615	.9524	.9434	.9259	.9091	.8696	.8333	.8000
2	1.9851	1.9704	1.9559	1.9416	1.9274	1.9135	1.8861	1.8594	1.8334	1.7833	1.7355	1.6257	1.5278	1.4400
3	2.9702	2.9410	2.9122	2.8839	2.8560	2.8286	2.7751	2.7232	2.6730	2.5771	2.4869	2.2832	2.1065	1.9520
4	3.9505	3.9020	3.8544	3.8077	3.7620	3.7171	3.6299	3.5460	3.4651	3.3121	3.1699	2.8550	2.5887	2.3616
5	4.9259	4.8534	4.7826	4.7135	4.6458	4.5797	4.4518	4.3295	4.2124	3.9927	3.7908	3.3522	2.9906	2.6893
6	5.8964	5.7955	5.6972	5.6014	5.5081	5.4172	5.2421	5.0757	4.9173	4.6229	4.3553	3.7845	3.3255	2.9514
7	6.8621	6.7282	6.5982	6.4720	6.3494	6.2303	6.0021	5.7864	5.5824	5.2064	4.8684	4.1604	3.6046	3.1611
8	7.8230	7.6517	7.4859	7.3255	7.1701	7.0197	6.7327	6.4632	6.2098	5.7466	5.3349	4.4873	3.8372	3.3289
9	8.7791	8.5660	8.3605	8.1622	7.9709	7.7861	7.4353	7.1078	6.8017	6.2469	5.7590	4.7716	4.0310	3.4631
10	9.7304	9.4713	9.2222	8.9826	8.7521	8.5302	8.1109	7.7217	7.3601	6.7101	6.1446	5.0188	4.1925	3.5705
11	10.6770	10.3676	10.0711	9.7868	9.5142	9.2526	8.7605	8.3064	7.8869	7.1390	6.4951	5.2337	4.3271	3.6564
12	11.6189	11.2551	10.9075	10.5753	10.2578	9.9540	9.3851	8.8633	8.3838	7.5361	6.8137	5.4206	4.4392	3.7251
13	12.5562	12.1337	11.7315	11.3484	10.9832	10.6350	9.9856	9.3936	8.8527	7.9038	7.1034	5.5831	4.5327	3.7801
14	13.4887	13.0037	12.5434	12.1062	11.6909	11.2961	10.5631	9.8986	9.2950	8.2442	7.3667	5.7245	4.6106	3.8241
15	14.4166	13.8651	13.3432	12.8493	12.3814	11.9379	11.1184	10.3797	9.7122	8.5595	7.6061	5.8474	4.6755	3.8593
16	15.3399	14.7179	14.1313	13.5777	13.0550	12.5611	11.6523	10.8378	10.1059	8.8514	7.8237	5.9542	4.7296	3.8874
17	16.2586	15.5623	14.9076	14.2919	13.7122	13.1661	12.1657	11.2741	10.4773	9.1216	8.0216	6.0472	4.7746	3.9099
18	17.1728	16.3983	15.6726	14.9920	14.3534	13.7535	12.6593	11.6896	10.8276	9.3719	8.2014	6.1280	4.8122	3.9279
19	18.0824	17.2260	16.4262	15.6785	14.9789	14.3238	13.1339	12.0853	11.1581	9.6036	8.3649	6.1982	4.8435	3.9424
20	18.9874	18.0456	17.1686	16.3514	15.5892	14.8775	13.5903	12.4622	11.4699	9.8181	8.5136	6.2593	4.8696	3.9539
21	19.8880	18.8570	17.9001	17.0112	16.1845	15.4150	14.0292	12.8212	11.7641	10.0168	8.6487	6.3125	4.8913	3.9631
22	20.7841	19.6604	18.6208	17.6580	16.7654	15.9369	14.4511	13.1630	12.0416	10.2007	8.7715	6.3587	4.9094	3.9705
23	21.6757	20.4558	19.3309	18.2922	17.3321	16.4436	14.8568	13.4886	12.3034	10.3711	8.8832	6.3988	4.9245	3.9764
24	22.5629	21.2434	20.0304	18.9139	17.8850	16.9355	15.2470	13.7986	12.5504	10.5288	8.9847	6.4338	4.9371	3.9811
25	23.4456	22.0232	20.7196	19.5235	18.4244	17.4131	15.6221	14.0939	12.7834	10.6748	9.0770	6.4641	4.9476	3.9849
26	24.3240	22.7952	21.3986	20.1210	18.9506	17.8768	15.9828	14.3752	13.0032	10.8100	9.1609	6.4906	4.9563	3.9879
27	25.1980	23.5596	22.0676	20.7069	19.4640	18.3270	16.3296	14.6430	13.2105	10.9352	9.2372	6.5135	4.9636	3.9903
28	26.0677	24.3164	22.7267	21.2813	19.9649	18.7641	16.6631	14.8981	13.4062	11.0511	9.3066	6.5335	4.9697	3.9923
29	26.9330	25.0658	23.3761	21.8444	20.4535	19.1885	16.9837	15.1411	13.5907	11.1584	9.3696	6.5509	4.9747	3.9938
30	27.7941	25.8077	24.0158	22.3965	20.9303	19.6004	17.2920	15.3725	13.7648	11.2578	9.4269	6.5660	4.9789	3.9950
35	32.0354	29.4086	27.0756	24.9986	23.1452	21.4872	18.6646	16.3742	14.4982	11.6546	9.6442	6.6166	4.9915	3.9984
40	36.1722	32.8347	29.9158	27.3555	25.1028	23.1148	19.7928	17.1591	15.0463	11.9246	9.7791	6.6418	4.9966	3.9995
45	40.2072	36.0945	32.5523	29.4902	26.8330	24.5187	20.7200	17.7741	15.4558	12.1084	9.8628	6.6543	4.9986	3.9998
50	44.1428	39.1961	34.9997	31.4236	28.3623	25.7298	21.4822	18.2559	15.7619	12.2335	9.9148	6.6605	4.9995	3.9999

Index

ratio, 228, 662, 695
revenues, 172
Organization chart
budgeting prerequisite, 149
fiscal services division, 11
illustrated, 7, 101, 219
reports conform to, 219
Outpatient revenues
accounting for, 179-180
internal controls, 183
Owners' equity, 22-23, 558

Past service cost of pension plan, 527, 695
Patient days of service rendered, 104, 695
Patient service revenues
accounting for, 177
budgeting procedures, 210
internal controls, 183
schedule of, 553
Pattillo, J., 236
Payback period, 476, 695
Payroll
accounting procedures, 193-201
accrued, 196, 352
budgeting procedures, 214-215
checking account, 253
computation of, 194-195
deductions, 195
employees' earnings records, 195
employment practices, 193
importance of, 193
internal controls, 201-202
overtime premium pay, 197
pension and retirement plans, 200
personnel manuals, 214
position control plan, 201, 214
taxes, 195
vacation pay, 198, 353
withholdings, 195
workmen's compensation, 198
Pension and retirement plans
accounting for, 526
advantages of, 200
contributory vs. noncontributory, 200, 526
disclosures, 529

funded vs. unfunded, 526
liability for, 528
normal cost, 527
past service cost, 527
Percentage of occupancy, 104, 695
Periodic inventory system, 325, 695
Periodicity principle, 29
Perpetual inventory system, 325, 695
Personnel manual, 214
Petty cash, 259, 695
Physicians' orders, 178
Plant assets
accounting for, 444-478
acquisition of, 444
balance sheet presentation, 589
budgeting procedures, 475-478
buildings, 445-446
classification of, 445
component of unrestricted fund, 37
construction in progress, 447
cost of, 447
defined, 444, 696
depreciation of, 455-465
disposal of, 471
donated, 454
equipment, 446-447
exchanges of, 450-452
internal controls, 454-455
involuntary conversion of, 472
land, 445
land improvements, 445
leasing of, 515
purchase contracts for, 452
records, 454-455
repairs, 454
salvage value, 457
service lives, 457
Plant replacement and expansion fund
balance account, 86, 591
balance sheet presentation, 84
chart of accounts, 95-96
defined, 87-88, 696
statement of changes in fund balances, 86
Pledges receivable, 39
Pooled investments, 425-431, 696
Position control plan, 201, 214, 696
Posting, 51, 696